NURSING RESEARCH
IN CANADA

Methods, Critical Appraisal, and Utilization

GERI LoBIONDO-WOOD, RN, PhD, FAAN

Director of Nursing Research and Evidence-Based
    Practice, Planning and Development
The University of Texas
MD Anderson Cancer Center
Houston, Texas

Adjunct Associate Professor
University of Texas Health Sciences Center
School of Nursing
Nursing Systems and Technology
Houston, Texas

JUDITH HABER, PhD, APRN, BC, FAAN

The Ursula Springer Leadership Professor in Nursing
Associate Dean for Graduate Programs
New York University
College of Nursing
New York, New York

Canadian Editors

CHERYLYN CAMERON, RN, PhD

Associate Vice President
University Partnership Centre, Research and Scholarship
Georgian College
Barrie, Ontario

MINA D. SINGH, RN, PhD

Coordinator, Program Evaluation Unit
York Institute for Health Research
Toronto, Ontario

Associate Professor
School of Nursing
York University
Toronto, Ontario

Third Canadian Edition

ELSEVIER

Library and Archives Canada Cataloguing in Publication

LoBiondo-Wood, Geri
 Nursing research in Canada: methods, critical appraisal, and utilization/
Geri LoBiondo-Wood, Judith Haber.—3rd Canadian ed./
Canadian editors, Cherylyn Cameron, Mina D. Singh
Includes biographical references.
ISBN 978-1-926648-54-5
 1. Nursing–Research–Canada–Textbooks. I. Haber, Judith II. Cameron, Cherylyn, 1958– III. Singh, Mina D. IV. Title.
RT81.5.N8724 2012 610.73072'071 C2011-907013-8

Vice President, Publishing: Ann Millar
Managing Editor: Roberta A. Spinosa-Millman
Developmental Editor: Jerri Hurlbutt
Publishing Services Manager: Jeffrey Patterson
Project Manager: Mary G. Stueck
Copy Editor: Anne Ostroff
Proofreader: Claudia Forgas
Cover, Interior Design: Teresa McBryan
Typesetting and Assembly: Toppan Best-set Premedia Limited

Elsevier Canada
905 King Street West, 4th Floor, Toronto, ON, Canada M6K 3G9
Phone: 1-866-896-3331
Fax: 1-866-359-9534

3 4 5 6 7 8 9 16 15 14

NURSING RESEARCH
IN CANADA

Methods, Critical Appraisal,
and Utilization

Contents

Author Biographies

Geri LoBiondo-Wood, RN, PhD, FAAN, is the Director of Nursing Research and Evidence-Based Practice, Planning and Development at the MD Anderson Cancer Center, Houston, Texas, and an Adjunct Associate Professor at the University of Texas Health Sciences Center at Houston (UTHSC-Houston), School of Nursing. She received her Diploma in nursing at St. Mary's Hospital School of Nursing in Rochester, New York; her Bachelor's and Master's degrees from the University of Rochester; and her PhD in Nursing Theory and Research from New York University. At MD Anderson Cancer Center, Dr. LoBiondo-Wood developed and implemented the Evidence-Based Resource Unit Nurse (EB-RUN) Program, which is a hospital-wide program that involves all levels of nurses in the application of research evidence to practice. She also has implemented a mentorship program for nurses wishing to conduct research. Dr. LoBiondo-Wood also teaches research and evidence-based practice principles to undergraduate, graduate, doctoral, and doctor of nursing practice students at UTHSC-Houston, School of Nursing. She has extensive experience guiding nurses and other health care professionals in the development and utilization of research in clinical practice. Dr. LoBiondo-Wood is currently a member of the Editorial Board of *Progress in Transplantation* and a reviewer for *Nursing Research* and *Nephrology Nursing Journal.* Her research and publications focus on chronic illness and the impact of solid organ transplantation on pediatric or adult recipients and their families throughout the transplant process. At MD Anderson Cancer Center, her research focuses on symptom clusters in adult patients with cancer.

Dr. LoBiondo-Wood has been active locally and nationally in many professional organizations, including the Southern Nursing Research Society, the Midwest Nursing Research Society, and the North American Transplant Coordinators Organization.

She has received local and national awards for teaching and contributions to nursing. In 1997, she received the Distinguished Alumnus Award from New York University, Division of Nursing Alumni Association. In 2001 she was inducted as a Fellow of the American Academy of Nursing, and in 2007 to The University of Texas Academy of Health Science Education.

Judith Haber, PhD, APRN, BC, FAAN, is the Ursula Springer Leadership Professor in Nursing and Associate Dean for Graduate Programs in the College of Nursing at New York University. She received her undergraduate nursing education at Adelphi University in New York, and she holds a Master's degree in Adult Psychiatric–Mental Health Nursing and a PhD in Nursing Theory and Research from New York University. Dr. Haber is internationally recognized as a clinician and educator in psychiatric–mental health nursing. She has extensive clinical experience in psychiatric nursing, having been an advanced practice psychiatric nurse in private practice over 30 years, specializing in treatment of families coping with the psychosocial sequelae of acute and chronic catastrophic illness. Dr. Haber is currently on the Editorial Board of the *Journal of the American Psychiatric Nurses Association (JAPNA).* Her areas of research involvement include tool development, particularly in the area of family functioning. She is internationally known for developing the Haber Level of Differentiation of Self Scale. Another program of research addresses physical and psychosocial adjustment to illness, focusing specifically on women with breast cancer and their partners. On the basis of this research, she and Dr. Carol Hoskins have written and produced an award-winning series of evidence-based psycho-educational videotapes, *Journey to Recovery: For Women with Breast Cancer and Their Partners,* which has been tested in a randomized clinical trial funded by the National Cancer Institute.

Dr. Haber has been active locally and nationally in many professional organizations, including the American Nurses Association, the American Psychiatric Nurses Association (APNA), and the American Academy of Nursing. She has received numerous local, state, and national awards for public policy, clinical practice, and research, including the APNA Psychiatric Nurse of the Year Award in 1998 and 2005, the APNA Outstanding Research Award in 2005, and the 2007 New York University College of Nursing Distinguished Alumnus Award. In 1993, she was inducted as a Fellow of the American Academy of Nursing.

CANADIAN EDITORS

Cherylyn Cameron, RN, PhD, is the Associate Vice President of the University Partnership Centre, Georgian College. She received her Bachelor of Science in Nursing degree from the University of Alberta and a Master of Arts degree in education from Central Michigan University. She received her doctorate in theory and policy studies in education from the Ontario Institute for Studies in Education (OISE)/University of Toronto. Her dissertation, "The Lived Experience of Transfer Students from a Baccalaureate Nursing Program," won the Best Dissertation award from the Council for Study of Community Colleges in the United States. Dr. Cameron currently teaches courses as an adjunct professor for Central Michigan University in the Master of Arts degree in education program with a community college specialization. At Georgian College, she works with university partners to provide degree-level studies for college students and is responsible for research and scholarship at the college. Her research interests include college-university relations, student experiences, transfer from college to university, and the implementation of best practice guidelines.

Mina D. Singh, RN, PhD, is an Associate Professor at York University School of Nursing and Coordinator of the Program Evaluation Unit at the York Institute for Health Research. She received her Bachelor of Science in Nursing degree from the University of Toronto and started her clinical nursing neurosurgery program but spent most of her career in mental health and public health nursing. Her interests in program evaluation encouraged her to pursue her education in quantitative research. She earned her doctorate in measurement and evaluation from the University of Toronto. Her current interests, in her role as a specialist in quantitative methods, relate to program evaluation in health care and nursing education. She also conducts research in chronic disease prevention and cultural diversity in health care.

Contributors

Susan Adams, RN, PhD
Associate Director
Research Translation and Dissemination Core
Gerontological Nursing Interventions Research Center
College of Nursing
University of Iowa;
Director
National Nursing Practice Network
Iowa City, Iowa

Julie Barroso, PhD, ANP, APRN, BC, FAAN
Associate Professor and Specialty Director
Adult Nurse Practitioner Program;
Research Development Coordinator
Office of Research Affairs
Duke University School of Nursing
Durham, North Carolina

Carol Bova, PhD, RN, ANP
Associate Professor of Nursing and Medicine
Graduate School of Nursing
University of Massachusetts, Worcester
Worcester, Massachusetts

Barbara Davies, RN, PhD
Professor
School of Nursing
Faculty of Health Sciences
University of Ottawa;
Co-Director, Nursing Best Practice Research Unit
University of Ottawa and RNAO
Ottawa, Ontario

Nancy C. Edwards, RN, BScN, MSc, PhD
Full Professor
Department of Epidemiology and Community Medicine
School of Nursing
University of Ottawa
Ottawa, Ontario

Stephanie Fulton, MSIS
Assistant Library Director
Research Medical Library
The University of Texas
MD Anderson Cancer Center
Houston, Texas

Julie Gaudet, RN, MN (Admin.)
Professor
School of Nursing
Centre for Health Sciences
George Brown College
Toronto, Ontario

Nancy E. Kline, PhD, RN, CPNP, FAAN
Director, Center for Evidence-Based Practice and Research
Department of Nursing
Memorial Sloan-Kettering Cancer Center
New York, New York

Barbara Krainovich-Miller, EdD, APRN, BC,
    ANEF, FAAN
Clinical Professor
College of Nursing
New York University
New York, New York

Barbara Paterson, RN, MEd, PhD
Professor and Dean
Thompson Rivers University
School of Nursing
Kamloops, British Columbia

Joan Samuels-Dennis, RN, PhD
Assistant Professor, Faculty of Health
School of Nursing
York University
Toronto, Ontario

Helen J. Streubert, EdD, RN, CNE, ANEF
Vice President of Academic Affairs
Our Lady of the Lake University
San Antonio, Texas

Susan Sullivan-Bolyai, DNSc, CNS, RN
Associate Professor
Graduate School of Nursing and Department of Pediatrics
University of Massachusetts, Worcester
Worcester, Massachusetts

Sally Thorne, RN, PhD, FCAHS
Professor
School of Nursing
University of British Columbia
Vancouver, British Columbia

Marita Titler, RN, PhD, FAAN
Professor of Nursing, Rhetaugh Dumas Endowed Chair
Associate Dean of Practice and Clinical Scholarship
    Development
University of Michigan School of Nursing
Ann Arbor, Michigan

Judith Wuest, RN, BScN, MN, PhD
Professor Emerita, Faculty of Nursing
University of New Brunswick
Fredericton, New Brunswick

Reviewers

Davina Banner, RN, PhD
Assistant Professor
School of Nursing
University of Northern British Columbia
Prince George, British Columbia

Barbara Brady-Fryer, BSc, MN, PhD, RN
Instructor
Baccalaureate in Nursing Program
Grant MacEwan University
Edmonton, Alberta

Shelley Cobbett, MN, RN, Gnt, EdD
Adjunct Assistant Professor
School of Nursing—Yarmouth Campus
Dalhousie University
Halifax, Nova Scotia

Cheryl Forchuk, RN, MScN, PhD
Associate Director, Nursing Research
Arthur Labatt Family School of Nursing
The University of Western Ontario
London, Ontario

Angela Gillis, RN, PhD
Professor
School of Nursing
St. Francis Xavier University
Antigonish, Nova Scotia

Patricia Grainger, RN, BN, MN
Nurse Educator
Centre for Nursing Studies
St. John's, Newfoundland

Cindy Murray, RN, MN, PhD
Assistant Professor
School of Nursing
Memorial University of Newfoundland
St. John's, Newfoundland

Kathy Quee, RN, MSN
Clinical Placement Advisor
Chair, Research Ethics Board
British Columbia Institute of Technology
Burnaby, British Columbia

Louise Racine, RN, MScN, PhD
Associate Professor
College of Nursing
University of Saskatchewan
Saskatoon, Saskatchewan

Jasna K. Schwind, RN, PhD
Associate Professor
Daphne Cockwell School of Nursing
Ryerson University
Toronto, Ontario

Kathy F. Spurr, BSc, RRT, MHI, FCSRT
Assistant Professor
School of Health Sciences
Dalhousie University
Halifax, Nova Scotia

Dr. Darlene Steven, RN, PhD
Full Professor
School of Nursing
Lakehead University
Thunder Bay, Ontario

Lela V. Zimmer, BScN, PhD
Assistant Professor
School of Nursing
University of Northern British Columbia
Prince George, British Columbia

Acknowledgements

This major undertaking was accomplished with the help of many people, some of whom made direct contributions to the new edition and some of whom contributed indirectly. We acknowledge with deep appreciation and our warmest thanks the following people who made this third Canadian edition possible:

- Nursing educators across Canada who provided valuable and insightful comments that helped to direct the revisions featured in this edition and contributed to improving the content
- Our students, particularly the nursing students of the Georgian College, Seneca College, and York University Second-Entry programs, who inspired us with their feedback and willingness to use the information in this text by becoming research assistants
- Ann Millar, Publisher, Elsevier Canada, who had faith in us and provided much-needed guidance and discussion
- Roberta A. Spinosa-Millman, Managing Editor, who got us started with encouragement, a sense of humour, and great insight
- Jerri Hurlbutt, Developmental Editor, who encouraged us with positive feedback, made sense of the process, and extended deadlines graciously

- Anne Ostroff, Copy Editor, and Mary Stueck, Senior Project Manager, whose attention to detail ensured that we had a very readable text for our students
- Teresa McBryan, Design Manager, who redesigned this edition so that it is a pleasure to look at and read
- Our vignette contributors, whose willingness to share their wisdom and evidence of their innovative research made a unique contribution to this edition
- All of the reviewers, who provided thoughtful feedback not only on the first and second editions but also on the third Canadian edition manuscript
- Our families, who supported us and picked up the "loose ends" while we wrote and revised:

To my husband John Cameron, who has always been there loving, supporting, and encouraging me. Thanks for keeping our family and household together so that I could stay focused on this third edition.

Cherylyn Cameron

To my husband Neranjan, my daughter Sandhya, and my parents Ram and Betty Laljie, for their support and encouragement.

Mina D. Singh

Preface

The foundation of the third Canadian edition of *Nursing Research in Canada: Methods, Critical Appraisal, and Utilization* continues to be the belief that nursing research is integral to all levels of nursing education and practice. Since the first edition of this textbook, we have seen the depth and breadth of nursing research grow: More nurses are conducting research and using research evidence to shape clinical practice, education, administration, and health policy.

The Canadian Nurses Association promotes the notion that nurses must provide care that is based on the best available scientific evidence. This is an exciting challenge to meet. Nurses are using the best available evidence, combined with their clinical judgement and patient preferences, to influence the nature and direction of health care delivery and to document outcomes related to the quality and cost effectiveness of patient care. As nurses continue to develop a unique body of nursing knowledge through research, decisions about clinical nursing practice will be increasingly evidence informed.

As editors, we believe that all nurses not only need to understand the research process but also need to know how to critically read, evaluate, and apply research findings in practice. We realize that understanding research, as a component of evidence-informed practice, is a challenge for every student, but we believe that the challenge can be accomplished in a stimulating, lively, and learner-friendly manner.

Consistent with this perspective is a commitment to advancing implementation of the evidence-informed practice paradigm. Understanding and applying nursing research must be an integral dimension of baccalaureate education, evident not only in the undergraduate nursing research course but also throughout the curriculum. The research role of baccalaureate graduates calls for evidence-informed practice competencies; central to this are critical appraisal skills: that is, nurses should be competent research consumers.

Preparing students for this role involves developing their critical thinking and reading skills, thereby enhancing their understanding of the research process, their appreciation of the role of the critiquer, and their ability to actually appraise research critically. An undergraduate course in nursing research should develop this basic level of competence, which is an essential requirement if students are to engage in evidence-informed clinical decision making and practice. This is in contrast to a graduate-level research course, in which the emphasis is on carrying out research, as well as understanding and appraising it.

The primary audience for this textbook remains undergraduate students who are learning the steps of the research process, as well as how to develop clinical questions, critically appraise published research literature, and use research findings to inform evidence-informed clinical practice. This book is also a valuable resource for students at the master's and doctoral levels who want a concise review of the basic steps of the research process, the critical appraisal process, and the principles and tools for evidence-informed practice.

This text is also a key resource for doctoral students who are preparing to be experts at leading evidence-informed initiatives in clinical settings. Furthermore, it is an important resource for practising nurses who strive to use research evidence as the basis for clinical decision making and development of evidence-informed policies, protocols, and standards, rather than rely on tradition, authority, or trial and error. It is an important resource for nurses who collaborate with nurse-scientists in the conduct of clinical research and evidence-informed practice.

Building on the success of the second edition, we maintain our commitment to introduce evidence-informed practice and research principles to baccalaureate students, thereby providing a cutting-edge research consumer foundation for their clinical practice.

Nursing Research in Canada: Methods, Critical Appraisal, and Utilization prepares nursing students and practising nurses to become knowledgeable nursing research consumers in the following ways:

- By addressing the evidence-informed practice role of the nurse, thereby embedding evidence-informed competence in the clinical practice of every baccalaureate graduate.
- By demystifying research, which is sometimes viewed as a complex process.
- By using an evidence-informed approach to teaching the fundamentals of the research process.
- By teaching the critical appraisal process in a user-friendly but logical and systematic progression.
- By promoting a lively spirit of inquiry that develops critical thinking and critical reading skills, facilitating mastery of the critical appraisal process.
- By developing information literacy, searching, and evidence-informed practice competencies that prepare students and nurses to effectively locate and evaluate the best available research evidence.
- By elevating the critical appraisal process and research appreciation to a position of importance comparable to that of producing research. Before students become research producers, they must become knowledgeable research consumers.

- By emphasizing the role of evidence-informed practice as the basis for informing clinical decision making and nursing interventions that support nursing practice, demonstrating quality and cost-effective outcomes of nursing care delivery.
- By presenting numerous examples of recently published research studies that illustrate and highlight each research concept in a manner that brings abstract ideas to life for students new to the research and critical appraisal process. These examples are a critical link for reinforcement of evidence-informed concepts and the related research and critiquing process.
- By showcasing, in **Research Vignettes,** the work of renowned nurse researchers whose careers exemplify the links among research, education, and practice.
- By providing numerous pedagogical chapter features, including **Learning Outcomes, Key Terms, Key Points,** new **Critical Thinking Challenges, Helpful Hints, Evidence-Informed Practice Tips,** new **Practical Applications**, and revised **Critical Thinking Decision Paths,** as well as numerous tables, boxes, and figures. At the end of each chapter that presents a step of the research process, we feature a revised section titled **Appraising the Evidence,** which reviews how each step of the research process should be evaluated from a consumer's perspective. This section is accompanied by an updated **Critiquing Criteria** box.
- By providing a **Study Guide** that promotes active learning and assimilation of nursing research content.
- By offering an Evolve site presenting free **Evolve Resources for Instructors** that includes a Test Bank, an Instructor's Manual, PowerPoint slides, critiquing exercises, an Image Collection, and new critical appraisal activities. There are also Evolve

resources for both the student and faculty that include a research article library, an audio glossary, and instructions on how to write proposals for funding.

The third edition of *Nursing Research in Canada: Methods, Critical Appraisal, and Utilization* is organized into six parts. Each part is preceded by an introductory section and opens with an exciting "Research Vignette" by a renowned nurse researcher.

Part One, Research Overview, contains six chapters. Chapter 1, "The Role of Research in Nursing," provides an excellent overview of research and evidence-informed practice processes that shape clinical practice. This chapter introduces the role research plays in practice and education, the roles of nurses in research activities, a historical perspective, and future directions in nursing research. The style and content of this chapter are designed to make subsequent chapters more user-friendly. Chapter 2, "Theoretical Framework," focuses specifically on how theoretical frameworks guide and inform knowledge generation through the research process. Chapter 3, "Critical Reading Strategies: Overview of the Research Process," addresses students directly and highlights critical thinking and critical reading concepts and strategies, thereby facilitating students' understanding of the research process and its relationship to the critical appraisal process. This chapter introduces a model evidence hierarchy that is used throughout the text.

The next two chapters address foundational components of the research process. Chapter 4, "Developing Research Questions, Hypotheses, and Clinical Questions," focuses on how research questions, hypotheses, and evidence-informed practice questions are derived, operationalized, and critically appraised. Numerous clinical examples illustrating different types of research questions and hypotheses maximize student understanding. Students are also taught how to develop clinical questions that are used to guide evidence-informed inquiry. Chapter 5, "Finding and Appraising the Literature," showcases cutting-edge information literacy content, providing students and nurses with the tools necessary to effectively search, retrieve, manage, and evaluate research studies and their findings. This chapter also develops research consumer competencies that prepare students and nurses to critically read, understand, and appraise a study's literature review and framework. The final chapter in this section, Chapter 6, "Legal and Ethical Issues," provides an overview of the increased emphasis on the legal and ethical issues facing researchers in Canada.

Part Two, Qualitative Research, contains two interrelated qualitative research chapters. Chapter 7, "Introduction to Qualitative Research," provides a framework for understanding qualitative research designs and literature, as well as the significant contribution of qualitative research to evidence-informed practice. Chapter 8, "Qualitative Approaches to Research," presents, illustrates, and, in examples from the literature, showcases major qualitative methods. This chapter highlights the questions most appropriately answered through the use of qualitative methods.

Part Three, Quantitative Research, contains Chapters 9 ("Introduction to Quantitative Research"), 10 ("Experimental and Quasiexperimental Designs"), and 11 ("Nonexperimental Designs"). These chapters delineate the essential steps of the quantitative research process, with published, current clinical research studies used to illustrate each step. Links between the steps and their relationship to the total research process are examined.

Part Four, Processes Related to Research, describes the specific steps of the research process for qualitative and quantitative studies. The chapters make the case for linking an evidence-informed approach with essential steps of the research process by teaching students how to critically appraise the strengths and weaknesses of each step of the research process. Students learn how to select participants (Chapter 12, "Sampling"), gather data (Chapter 13, "Data-Collection Methods"), analyze the results (Chapter 15, "Qualitative Data Analysis," and Chapter 16, "Quantitative Data Analysis"), and present their results (Chapter 17, "Presenting the Findings"). Chapter 14, "Rigour in Research," gives students the tools for assessing the quality and trustworthiness of a study.

Part Five, Critiquing Research, makes the case for linking an evidence-informed approach with essential steps of the research process by teaching students how to critically appraise the strengths and weaknesses of each step of the research process. Each chapter critiques two examples of actual published research. Chapter 18, "Critiquing Qualitative Research," focuses on qualitative research, whereas Chapter 19, "Critiquing Quantitative Research," is based on the quantitative research process.

Part Six, Application of Research: Evidence-Informed Practice, contains the final chapter in the book. Chapter 20, "Developing an Evidence-Informed Practice," provides a dynamic review of evidence-informed models. These models can be applied—step by step, at the organizational or individual patient level—as frameworks for implementing and evaluating the outcomes of evidence-informed health care.

Stimulating critical thinking is a core value of this text. Innovative chapter features such as Critical Thinking Decision Paths, Evidence-Informed Practice Tips, Helpful Hints, Practical Applications, and Critical Thinking Challenges enhance critical thinking and promote the development of evidence-informed decision-making skills. To be consistent with previous editions, we now promote critical thinking by including sections called "Appraising the Evidence," which describe the critical appraisal process related to the focus of the chapter. In addition, Critiquing Criteria are included in this section to stimulate a systematic and evaluative approach

to reading and understanding qualitative and quantitative research literature and evaluating its strengths and weaknesses. Extensive Internet resources are provided on the accompanying Evolve site that can be used to develop evidence-informed knowledge and skills.

The Evolve Web site that accompanies the third Canadian edition provides interactive learning activities that promote the development of critical thinking, critical reading, and information literacy skills designed to develop the competencies necessary to produce informed consumers of nursing research. Instructor resources are available at a passcode-protected Web site that gives faculty access to all instructor materials online, including the Instructor's Manual, Image Collection, PowerPoint Slides, a Test Bank that allows faculty to create examinations through the use of the ExamView test generator program, and more.

The development and refinement of an evidence-informed foundation for clinical nursing practice is an essential priority for the future of professional nursing practice. The third Canadian edition of *Nursing Research in Canada: Methods, Critical Appraisal, and Utilization* will help students develop a basic level of competence in understanding the steps of the research process that will enable them to critically analyze research studies, evaluate their merit, and judiciously apply evidence in clinical practice. To the extent that this goal is accomplished, the next generation of nursing professionals will include a cadre of clinicians who inform their practice by using theory and research evidence, combined with their clinical judgement, and specific to the health care needs of patients and their families in health and illness.

Cherylyn Cameron
ccameron@georgianc.on.ca

Mina Singh
minsingh@yorku.ca

To the Student

We invite you to join us on an exciting nursing research adventure that begins as you turn the first page of the third Canadian edition of *Nursing Research in Canada: Methods, Critical Appraisal, and Utilization.* The adventure is one of discovery! You will discover that the nursing research literature sparkles with pride, dedication, and excitement about the research dimension of professional nursing practice. Whether you are a student or a practising nurse whose goal is to use research evidence as the foundation of your practice, you will discover that nursing research and a commitment to evidence-informed practice positions our profession at the forefront of change. You will discover that evidence-informed practice is integral to meeting the challenge of providing quality health care in partnership with patients and their families and significant others, as well as with the communities in which they live. Finally, you will discover the richness in the "who," "what," "where," "when," "why," and "how" of nursing research and evidence-informed practice, and you will develop a foundation of knowledge and skills that will equip you for clinical practice today and into the future.

We think you will enjoy reading this text. Your nursing research course will be short but filled with new and challenging learning experiences that will develop your evidence-informed practice skills. The third Canadian edition of *Nursing Research in Canada: Methods, Critical Appraisal, and Utilization* reflects cutting-edge trends for developing evidence-informed nursing practice. The six-part organization and special features in this text are designed to help you develop your skills in critical thinking, critical reading, information literacy, and evidence-informed clinical decision making, while providing a user-friendly approach to learning that expands your competence to deal with these new and challenging experiences. The companion *Study Guide,* with its chapter-by-chapter activities, will serve as a self-paced learning tool to reinforce the content of the text. The accompanying Evolve Web site offers "summative" review material to help you reinforce the concepts discussed throughout the book.

Remember that evidence-informed practice skills are used in every clinical setting and can be applied to every patient population or clinical practice issue. Whether your clinical practice involves primary care or specialty care and provides inpatient or outpatient treatment in a hospital, clinic, or home, you will be challenged to apply your evidence-informed practice skills and use nursing research as the foundation for your evidence-informed practice. The third Canadian edition of *Nursing Research in Canada: Methods Critical Appraisal, and Utilization* will guide you through this exciting adventure, where you will discover your ability to play a vital role in contributing to the building of an evidence-informed professional nursing practice.

Cherylyn Cameron
ccameron@georgianc.on.ca

Mina D. Singh
minsingh@yorku.ca

Research Overview

RESEARCH **VIGNETTE**

How Nurses Use and Respond to Research

Barbara Paterson, RN, MEd, PhD
Professor and Dean
Thompson Rivers University
School of Nursing
Kamloops, British Columbia

A few years ago, I was fortunate to work as a nurse scholar on an acute care medical unit in a large urban hospital. This experience gave me an opportunity to observe first-hand how nurses use and respond to research. During that time, one of the staff nurses on the unit made a comment that I believe captures many Canadian nurses' attitudes toward research. She said, "I used to think that nursing research was bunk. Just something we had to learn in school that I could put away with my textbooks when I graduated. I thought that we learned research in school because the professors were hoping to convince some of us to go on to graduate school. I really didn't see it as having anything to do with the real world of bedside nursing." She added that because of our regular research discussions on the unit and our continual efforts to use research findings in the care of patients, her attitude about research had changed. She said, "When I saw research as relevant to what I did and not just some pie-in-the-sky idea from school, I began to use research as a tool—something that helped me do my job better."

Practising nurses' positive attitudes toward research are not unique. During the 3 years I worked on the unit, I observed as nurses searching for research evidence to answer their practice questions, chatting with each other about research articles, and quoting research findings to patients and other health care professionals. Put simply, these nurses used research to "do the job" of nursing more effectively. For example, they consulted research articles to find solutions to several practice issues on the unit, such as how to help an anxious patient cope with invasive procedures; how to help nurses deal with their feelings about patients who use illegal injection drugs and leave the hospital in compromised medical conditions, against medical advice; and how best to structure nursing assignments so that patients receive the care they need.

Sometimes, when nurses discovered that little research existed about the issues that arose, they were forced to imagine how other research might apply. For example, when the nurses became concerned that some patients were not eating enough and not eating nutritionally sound foods, they consulted the research about the nutritional status of hospitalized patients. As it turned out, the existing research had been conducted largely in long-term care facilities and, to a lesser extent, in surgical units. Therefore, the existing research did not address the nurses' particular concerns pertaining to the nutritional status of patients who use injection drugs, late-night admissions of homeless patients who might not have eaten before admission, and patients with neurological deficits who experienced difficulty handling cutlery and cups.

Nevertheless, the nurses were able to apply some findings of the research conducted in long-term care facilities to their unit. For example, the nurses learned that if patients are fed by nursing staff who are in a hurry, those patients' nutritional status was often poor. Many of the unit's patients required assistance in feeding, and the findings of research conducted in long-term care facilities caused the nurses to reflect on the staff who fed the patients and how long the feeding took. This consideration, in turn, caused the nurses to change the feeding directions they gave to support staff (e.g., unit assistants) and to reinforce the fact that it is the nurse's responsibility to make sure that the patient has eaten enough.

The nurses also initiated research on the unit. For example, they were continually frustrated by the behaviour of many patients who use injection drugs. The nurses reported that these patients were often hostile, manipulative, and noncompliant. Hospital statistics demonstrated that this particular patient population accounted for most of the nurses' security calls. Several nurses said they dreaded working with this type of patient.

Initially, they suggested strategies that were inadequate or unrealistic (e.g., building a seclusion room in the unit for patients who use injection drugs). Ultimately, the nurses decided to seek advice from the hospital's chemical dependency experts. After consulting with the nurses, the chemical dependency team developed a program of workshops and conducted weekly rounds over the course of a year to help nurses better understand and care for patients who use injection drugs.

Because other units had similar issues with the same patient population, the nurses decided to report the results of the program to others in a tangible way, as research findings. The nurses formally evaluated the program that had been created by the chemical dependency experts. For example, the nurses administered questionnaires and participated in group interviews. The research revealed that most nurses no longer dreaded caring for patients who used illegal injection drugs. The nurses better understood the behaviour of these patients and what could be done to help them. After a presentation of the research findings, the nurses celebrated their accomplishments of the program with a cake and coffee party on the unit.

Another example of nurses' initiating research involved investigating whether nurses' medication errors could be decreased by using personal digital assistants (PDAs), such as Palm Pilot devices. The idea for the research project arose when the nurses discovered that many of the medication errors occurred because nurses did not recognize that a new order had been provided, misread the order, or forgot that a medication had not been administered. The nurses submitted a proposal for the research project and received funding for it from the University of British Columbia. The first component of this research consisted of observing the nurses' administering medication and writing documentation. On the basis of the observations, the nurses then developed a program for PDAs that told nurses which medications should be given and which had not yet been administered. This program included the ability to link to other information about patients and their medications. In the end, the research confirmed that the use of PDAs did reduce medication errors. Subsequently, the research findings were submitted to a publishing company that may incorporate them into new PDA software for nurses.

Commitment to research does not occur overnight, and some nurses are more excited by research than are others. In 3 years, however, the nurses I worked with began to see research in a new light: as something they *needed* to care for patients effectively. When I told the nurses mentioned in this vignette that I was writing this piece, one nurse said, "They will read it and think that our stories do not represent the real world. They will think it can't happen in most hospitals or for most nurses. They will think that research took place in our case only because you were here with us and you understood research." If that nurse is correct and that is what you are thinking, I invite you to consider the following: To inspire nurses to use research as a method of helping them do their jobs more effectively, what if all we need is someone who believes that research can do just that? What if that someone is you? Are you prepared to be the nurse who says to colleagues, "Let's see what research has been done about that. I bet someone has studied it and that the results will be helpful to us."

After reading this section and this book, I hope that you will use research as the foundation of your nursing practices. I have seen how much research influences practising nurses, and I'm here to tell you that it works. ■

CHAPTER 1

The Role of Research in Nursing

Cherylyn Cameron

LEARNING OUTCOMES

After reading this chapter, you will be able to do the following:

- State the significance of research to the practice of nursing.
- Identify the role of the consumer of nursing research.
- Discuss the differences in trends within nursing research in Canada.
- Describe how research, education, and practice are related to each other.
- Evaluate the nurse's role in the research process as it relates to the nurse's level of education.
- Identify future trends in nursing research.
- Formulate the priorities for nursing research in the twenty-first century.

KEY TERMS

consumer	evidence-informed practice	phenomena
data	generalizability	research
evidence-based practice		

STUDY RESOURCES

Go to Evolve at http://evolve.elsevier.com/Canada/LoBiondo/Research for Audio Glossary, how-to instructions for Writing Proposals for Funding, and additional research articles for practice in reviewing and critiquing.

WE INVITE YOU TO JOIN US on an exciting nursing research adventure that begins as you read the first page of this chapter. The adventure is one of discovery! You will discover that the nursing research literature sparkles with pride in, dedication to, and excitement about this dimension of professional nursing practice. As you progress through your educational program, you are taught how to ensure quality and safety in practice through acquiring knowledge of the various sciences and health care principles. Another component critical for clinical knowledge is research knowledge as it applies to practising from an evidence-informed approach.

Whether you are a student or a practising nurse whose goal is to use research as the foundation of your professional practice, you will discover that nursing research and evidence-informed practice position the nursing profession at the cutting edge of change and improvement in patients' outcomes. You will also discover that nursing research is integral to achieving the goal of providing quality outcomes in partnership with patients, their families and significant others, and the communities in which they live. Finally, you will discover the "who, what, where, when, why, and how" of nursing research and develop a foundation of knowledge, evidence-informed practice, and competencies that will equip you for twenty-first century nursing practice.

Your nursing research adventure will be filled with new and challenging learning experiences that develop your evidence-informed practice skills. Your critical thinking, critical reading, and clinical decision-making skills will expand as you develop clinical questions, search the research literature, evaluate the research evidence found in the literature, and make clinical decisions about applying the best available evidence to your practice. For example, you will be encouraged to ask important clinical questions, such as the following:

- What makes an intervention effective with one group of patients who have a diagnosis of congestive heart failure but not with another?
- What is the effect of using computers to educate children about self-management of asthma?
- What is the experience of men who undergo prostate surgery and therapy?
- What is the quality of studies on therapeutic touch?
- What nursing-delivered smoking cessation interventions are most effective?

This book will help you begin your adventure into evidence-informed nursing practice by giving you the tools to use research as a foundation for evidence-informed practice.

SIGNIFICANCE OF RESEARCH AND EVIDENCE-INFORMED PRACTICE IN THE FIELD OF NURSING

The health care environment is changing at an increasingly rapid pace. Hinshaw (2000), in portraying twenty-first–century nursing, stated that "an unprecedented explosion of nursing knowledge guided practice and advanced the health and well-being of individual clients, families, and communities" (p. 117). Carper (1978) described four fundamental patterns of knowing in nursing: (1) empirical knowledge ("empirics"), the science of nursing; (2) aesthetics, the art of nursing; (3) the component of personal knowing; and (4) ethics, the component of moral knowledge of nursing. Empirical knowledge, which is based on research findings, represents "one source of knowledge within a larger body of knowledge" (Tarlier, 2005, p. 131). The challenges associated with nursing's rapid pace of growth can best be met by integrating evidence-informed knowledge into nursing practice. Nursing research provides specialized scientific knowledge that empowers nurses to anticipate and meet these constantly shifting challenges and maintain the profession's societal relevance.

In learning about nursing research, it is important to differentiate among the terms *research, evidence-based practice,* and *evidence-informed practice.* **Research** is the systematic, rigourous, logical investigation that aims to answer questions about nursing phenomena. **Phenomena** can be defined as occurrences, circumstances, or facts that are perceptible by the senses. Phenomena, such as the expression of pain or loss, are the circumstances of interest to nurses.

There are two types of research: quantitative and qualitative. You will be introduced to these two types of research in more depth in Chapter 2. The methods used by nurse researchers are the same methods used in other disciplines; the difference is that nurses study questions relevant to nursing practice. Nurse researchers also conduct research collaboratively with researchers from other disciplines. Through the conducting of research, they produce knowledge that is reliable and useful for clinical practice. The methods and findings of studies provide evidence that is evaluated, and their applicability to practice is used to inform clinical decisions.

In the past 20 years, many health care disciplines have adopted the tenets of evidence-informed practice to provide the best health care possible for their patients. The roots of evidence-informed practice stem from Dr. Archie Cochrane's investigation of the efficacy of health care, particularly in the work of the medical profession. His work resulted in the establishment of the Cochrane Collaboration, which provides systemic reviews of health care interventions. In 1996, Sackett and colleagues defined "evidence-based medicines" as the "conscientious, explicit, and judicious use of current best evidence in making decisions about the care of individual patients" (p. 71). Since then, most health professions have adopted the tenets of **evidence-based practice.**

Much of the evidence used as a basis for practice is from research that has been completed, written about in papers, and then published. Published research studies are assessed so that decisions about application to clinical practice can be made, which results in practice that is evidence based. According to the Canadian Nurses Association (CNA), "Evidence-based nursing refers to the incorporation of evidence from research, clinical expertise, client preferences and other available resources to make decisions about clients" (CNA, 2002). Through research utilization efforts, knowledge obtained from research is transformed into clinical practice, which results in nursing practice that is evidence based.

Evidence-informed practice extends beyond the early definitions of evidence-based practice described previously. Building upon the foundation of evidence-based practice, evidence-informed practice also involves acknowledging and considering the myriad factors beyond such evidence as local indigenous knowledge, cultural and religious norms, and clinical judgement. With evidence-informed practice, the methods for gathering evidence (use of published research studies) are the same as the processes used for evidence-based practice; however, the evidence also incorporates expert opinion, clinical expertise, patient preference, and other resources (CNA, 2010b). It is important to remember that evidence-informed practice focuses on a more inclusive and interactive process:

> Evidence-informed decision-making is a continuous interactive process involving the explicit, conscientious and judicious consideration of the best available evidence to provide care. It is essential to optimize outcomes for individual clients, promote healthy communities and populations, improve clinical practice, achieve cost-effective nursing care and ensure accountability and transparency in decision-making within the health-care system.
>
> *(CNA, 2010b, p. 1)*

For example, to understand the importance of evidence-informed practice, consider the work of Dr. Judith Ritchie, who won the Canadian Health Services Research Foundation's 2010 Excellence through Evidence Award for her work on the successful implementation of best practice guidelines to reduce falls, manage pain, and protect skin integrity among patients. It has been estimated that as a result of the implementation of best practices, the incidence of pressure ulcers was reduced from 21% to 10.6% in 5 years. Not only does this result in better outcomes for patients, but the potential cost savings are estimated at $2.9 million for every 1,000 people (CNA, 2009).

When you first read about the research and the evidence-informed practice processes, you will notice that both processes may seem similar. Each begins with a question. The difference is that in a research study, the question is tested with a design appropriate for the question and with specific methods (sample, instruments, procedures, and data analysis). In the evidence-informed practice process, a question is used to search the literature for studies already completed that you will critically appraise in order to answer your clinical question.

It is proposed that all nurses share a commitment to the advancement of nursing science by conducting research and using research evidence in practice. Scientific investigation promotes accountability, which is one of the hallmarks of the nursing profession and a fundamental competency for all registered nurses (CNA, 2010a). What does this mean for you as a nurse? There is a consensus that the research role of the baccalaureate and master's graduate calls for the skills of critical appraisal; that is, you must be a knowledgeable consumer of research, whereby you can appraise research evidence and use existing standards to determine the merit and readiness of research for use in clinical practice: "Nurses support, use and engage in research and other activities that promote safe, competent, compassionate and ethical care, and they use guidelines for ethical research that are in keeping with nursing values" (CNA, 2008, p. 9). Therefore, to use research (evidence-informed practice), you may not necessarily be able to conduct research, but you can understand and appraise the steps of the research process in order to read the research

literature critically and use it to inform your clinical decisions.

Throughout this text, the steps of the research and evidence-informed practice processes are described. The steps are systematic and orderly and relate to the development of evidence-informed practice. Understanding the step-by-step process that researchers use will help you develop the assessment skills necessary to judge the soundness of research studies. Chapter 20 will describe how you can implement evidence into practice to improve patient outcomes.

Throughout the chapters, research terms pertinent to each step are identified and illustrated with many examples from the research literature. Four published research studies are found in the appendixes and used as examples to illustrate significant points in each chapter. Judging not only the study's strength and quality but also a study's applicability to practice is key. Before you can judge a study, it is important to understand the differences between and among studies. Many different study designs exist, which you will see as you read through this text and the appendixes. There are standards not only for critiquing the soundness of each step of a study but also for judging the strength and quality of evidence provided by a study and determining its applicability to practice.

This chapter provides an overview of the role that research plays in practice and education, the roles of nurses in research activities, a historical perspective, and future directions in nursing research.

RESEARCH: THE ELEMENT THAT LINKS THEORY, EDUCATION, AND PRACTICE

Research links theory, education, and practice. Theoretical formulations supported by research findings may become the foundations of theory-informed practice in nursing. Your educational setting, whether a nursing program or the health care organization where you are employed, provides an environment in which you, as a student or an employee, can learn about the research process. In the setting of a nursing program or a health care organization, you can also explore different theories and begin to evaluate them in light of research findings. See the Practical Application box for an example of applying theory to nursing practice.

Practical Application

Consider the research program that focused on building knowledge about improving the health and health care of women who experience intimate partner abuse. This program extended for more than a decade and focused on the experiences of women who left abusive partners, the health of the women after leaving the relationships, and the degree of health care improvement for women after they left their abusive partners (Ford-Gilboe, Wuest, Varcoe, & Merrit-Gray, 2006). The knowledge gained from this body of interrelated research led to the development of comprehensive interventions to support the health and quality of life of women who leave abusive partners.

The findings of that 2006 study have had enormous implications both for nurses and for other health care professionals, who make up the interdisciplinary health care team that works with women who experience intimate partner violence. Meaningful intervention is crucial for these women because health problems persist after they leave their partners. Many of these women report continued abuse and harassment from their ex-partners and experience financial hardships. Although health care workers have an interest in improving health care for these women, most health care workers do not have the knowledge required to address their patients' needs in a meaningful and effective way. As the researchers noted, "the vast majority of health practitioners [are] unprepared to recognize and respond to [intimate partner violence] in ways that are sensitive to the complexity of women's experiences and respectful of women's safety and choices" (Ford-Gilboe et al., 2006, p. 148).

The example in the Practical Application box is an attempt to answer a question that you may have asked before taking this course: "How will the theory and research content of this course relate to my nursing practice?" The **data**

from each study discussed thus far have clearly demonstrated implications for society and practice. In an era of continuing concern about health care costs, empirically supported programs that are cost effective without compromising quality are essential. Many researchers directly evaluate the cost effectiveness of treatment models; for example, Forchuk and colleagues (2005) found that a transition discharge model of care for patients experiencing chronic mental illness helped the patients achieve discharge from a psychiatric hospital early, by an average of 116 days, which resulted in considerable cost savings. Several studies have demonstrated that the use of research-based interventions is more likely to result in better outcomes than traditional or ritual-based nursing care (McGinty & Anderson, 2008; Williams, 2004).

At this point in your study of nursing research, you may be wondering how education in nursing research links theory and practice. The answer is twofold. First, learning about nursing research will provide you with an appreciation and understanding of the research process so that you can more easily become a participant in research activities. Second, learning the value of nursing research helps you to become an intelligent *consumer* of research. A **consumer** of research actively uses and applies research. To be a knowledgeable consumer, you must have knowledge about the relevant subject matter, the ability to discriminate and to evaluate information logically, and the ability to apply the knowledge gained. You need not actually conduct research to be able to appreciate and use research findings in practice. Rather, to be an intelligent consumer, you must understand the research process and develop the critical evaluation skills needed to judge the merit and relevance of evidence before applying it to practice. The success of evidence-informed practice depends on your ability, as a consumer of research, to understand the research process and to evaluate the evidence.

ROLES OF THE NURSE IN THE RESEARCH PROCESS

Every nurse practising in the twenty-first century has a role to play in the research process. The Canadian Association of Schools of Nurses (CASN) (n.d.) states that it "strongly supports nursing research and the training of nurse researchers across Canada [and] works to encourage and improve the quality of nursing research, as well as to promote research findings and support Canada's current and upcoming nursing research leaders." More specifically, CASN's objectives include the education of nurse scholars/researchers; securing of sufficient funding for nursing scholarship/research; enhancement of scholarship/research cooperation; dissemination of scholarship/research; and cooperation with other nursing and non-nursing organizations, provincial, national, and international.

The Canadian Registered Nurse Examination (CRNE) outlines competencies related to research on which examination questions for licensing to practise are based. The following sections from the Registered Nurse examination competencies explicitly highlight the importance of research for practice (CNA, 2010a):

Professional Practice
. . . Registered nurses are expected to use knowledge and research to build an evidence-informed practice . . . . The registered nurse . . . uses evidence and critical inquiry to challenge, change, enhance or support nursing practice (e.g., questioning accepted practice, participating in research). [Competency PP-15]

Nurse–Client Partnership
. . . The registered nurse . . . supports the informed choice of the client in making decisions about care (e.g., right to refuse, right to request care, right to choose, right to participate in research). [Competency NCP-9]

Nursing Practice: Health and Wellness
. . . Nursing practice is influenced by continuing competency, determinants of health, life phases, demographics, health trends, economic and political factors, evidence-informed knowledge and research . . . . The registered nurse . . . incorporates research about health risks and risk/harm reduction to support evidence-informed practice (e.g., second-hand smoke, Pap smears). [Competency HW-20]

On a provincial level, each province in Canada has its own standards for entry into nursing practice, and many of these standards have specific related research competencies. For example, the College of Nurses of Ontario (2009) outlined the following competencies that incorporate research:

Engages in nursing or health research by reading and critiquing research reports and identifying research opportunities. [Competency 35]
    Supports involvement in nursing or health research through collaboration with others in conducting research, participating in research, and implementing research findings into practice. [Competency 36]

Nurses must also be intelligent consumers of research; that is, they must understand all steps of the research process and their interrelationships. The registered nurse interprets, evaluates, and determines the credibility of research findings. The nurse discriminates between interesting findings for which further investigation is required and those that are sufficiently supported by evidence before applying findings to practice. The nurse should then use these competencies to advance the nursing or interdisciplinary evidence-informed practice projects (e.g., developing clinical standards, tracking quality improvement data, or coordinating implementation of a pilot project to test the efficacy of a new wound care protocol) of the workplace committees to which he or she belongs.

Registered nurses are also responsible for generating clinical questions to identify nursing issues that necessitate investigation and for participating in the implementation of scientific studies. Clinicians often generate research ideas or questions from hunches, gut-level feelings, intuition, or observations of patients or nursing care. These ideas often become the seeds of research investigations.

For example, Paterson (2002) related the story of Vini and Suzanne, two nurses working in an intensive care unit. They observed that the blood pressure of a certain patient dropped each time he received acetaminophen for a fever. He then needed to receive additional treatment for the corresponding low blood pressure. This situation raised several questions for Vini and Suzanne, and they wondered whether treating the fever was truly beneficial and what the effects of leaving the fever untreated would be. They spoke to other health care professionals, conducted a literature review, and concluded that treatment with antipyretics, such as acetylsalicylic acid, should not be applied immediately and that, in some patients, leaving the fever untreated had clear benefits. Vini and Suzanne subsequently disseminated their research findings to their colleagues and other health care professionals at a critical care conference. The example of these two nurses exemplifies the circularity between practice that generates research and research that improves practice. Systematic collection of data about a clinical problem, such as the one identified by Vini and Suzanne, contributes to the refinement and extension of nursing practice.

Registered nurses may participate in research projects as members of interdisciplinary or intradisciplinary research teams in one or more phases of a project. For example, a staff nurse may work on a clinical research unit in which a particular type of nursing care is part of an established research protocol (e.g., for pain management, prevention of falls, or treatment of urinary incontinence). In situations such as these, the nurse administers care according to the format described in the protocol. The nurse may also be involved in collecting and recording data relevant to the administration of, and the patient's response to, nursing care.

As important as the generation of research is the sharing of research findings with colleagues. Examples of such sharing include developing an article or presentation for a research or clinical conference on the findings of a study and sharing

the findings of a research report that was critiqued, found to have merit, and believed to have the potential for application to practice. In a more formal way, it may involve joining a health care agency's research committee or its quality assurance or quality improvement committee, in which research articles, integrative reviews of the literature, and clinical practice guidelines are evaluated for evidence-informed clinical decision making.

Nurses who have graduate degrees must also be sophisticated consumers of research and are specially prepared to conduct research as co-investigators or primary investigators. At the master's level, nurses are prepared to be active members of research teams. Nurses with master's-level training can assume the role of clinical expert, collaborating with an experienced researcher in proposal development, data collection, data analysis, and interpretation. Nurses with master's degrees enhance the quality and relevance of nursing research by providing not only clinical expertise but also evidence-informed knowledge about the way clinical services are delivered. Nurses with master's-level training also facilitate the investigation of clinical problems by enabling a climate that is open to nursing research and by engaging in evidence-informed practice projects. At the master's level, nurses conduct research investigations to monitor the quality of nursing in clinical settings and to help others apply scientific knowledge to nursing practice.

To achieve the greatest expertise in appraising, designing, and conducting research, nurses must complete PhDs. Nurses with doctoral degrees develop theoretical explanations for phenomena relevant to nursing, develop methods of scientific inquiry, and use a variety of methods to modify or extend existing knowledge so that it is relevant to nursing (or to other areas of health care). In addition to their role as researchers, nurses with doctoral-level training act as role models and mentors to guide, stimulate, and encourage other nurses who are developing their research skills. Nurses with doctoral degrees also collaborate and consult with social, educational, and health care institutions or governmental agencies in their respective research endeavours. These nurses then disseminate their research findings to the scientific community, clinicians, and—as appropriate—the general public through scientific journal articles and presentations for nursing research conferences.

Another essential responsibility of nurses, regardless of the level of education they achieve, is to pay special regard to the ethical principles of research, especially the protection of human participants. For example, nurses caring for patients who are participating in research on antinausea chemotherapy must ensure that the patients have signed the informed consent form and that all their questions are answered by the research team before they begin participation. Furthermore, if patients have an adverse reaction to the medication, nurses must not administer more doses until they have notified an appropriate member of the research team (see Chapter 6). Not all nurses must or should conduct research, but all nurses must play some part in the research process. Nurses at all educational levels—whether they are consumers, researchers, or both—need to view the research process as integral to the growing professionalism in nursing.

As a professional, you must take time to read research studies and evaluate them, using the standards congruent with scientific research. Also, you will need to use the critiquing process in order to identify the strengths and weaknesses of each study. Bearing in mind that each study has its limitations, you should consider whether sound and relevant evidence from one particular study can be used in other settings as well. Chapter 20 will expand on how to bring research into your nursing practice.

HISTORICAL PERSPECTIVE*

Nursing research has undergone many changes and developments since the 1970s. In addition, the groundwork for the research that exists today was laid in the late nineteenth century and throughout the twentieth century. Box 1-1 shows the major milestones in the development of nursing research.

Nineteenth Century

In the mid-nineteenth century, nursing as a formal discipline began to take root with the ideas and practices of Florence Nightingale. Her concepts have contributed to, and are congruent with, the current priorities of nursing research. Promotion of health, prevention of disease, and care of the sick were central ideas of her practice and publications. Nightingale believed that systematic collection and exploration of data were necessary for nursing. Her collection and analysis of data on the health status of British soldiers during the Crimean War led to a variety of reforms in health care. Nightingale (1863) also noted the need for measuring the outcomes of nursing and medical care and had expertise in statistics and epidemiology. Other than Nightingale's work, little research was conducted during the early years of development of the field of nursing. Schools of nursing had just begun to be established and were unequal in their ability to educate, whereas nursing leadership had just started to develop.

Twentieth Century

In the twentieth century, research focused mainly on nursing education, but some patient- and technique-oriented research was also evident (see Box 1-1). In 1923, in the United States, the

---

*This section (i.e., from pp. 11 to 15) is adapted with permission from Potter, P., Perry, A. G., Ross-Kerr, J., & Wood, M. (Eds.), (2010). *Canadian fundamentals of nursing* (4th ed., pp. 80–82). Toronto: Elsevier Canada.

BOX 1-1

HISTORICAL MILESTONES IN THE DEVELOPMENT OF NURSING RESEARCH

1858 and 1863	Florence Nightingale publishes *Notes on Matters Affecting the Health, Efficiency and Hospital Administration of the British Army* and *Notes on Hospitals*
1920	Public health courses are offered at the universities of British Columbia, Alberta, Toronto, McGill, Dalhousie, and Western Ontario
1932	The Weir report, sponsored by the Canadian Nurses Association and the Canadian Medical Association, calls for better nursing education and service
1952	The American Nurses Association first publishes *Nursing Research*
1959	The first Canadian nursing master's degree program is launched at the University of Western Ontario
1964–1965	The first nursing research project is funded by a Canadian federal granting agency *International Journal of Nursing Studies* and *International Nursing Index* are launched
1969–1970	*Nursing Papers*, the forerunner of the *Canadian Journal of Nursing Research*, is published at McGill University
1971	McGill University launches the Centre for Nursing Research, and the first national Canadian conference on nursing research is held; both are financed by the Department of National Health and Welfare
1978	Heads of university nursing schools and deans of graduate studies attend the Kellogg National Seminar on Doctoral Education in Nursing
1982	The Alberta Foundation for Nursing Research, the first funding agency for nursing research, is established The Working Group on Nursing Research is established by the Medical Research Council of Canada (MRC)
1985	The report of the Working Group on Nursing Research is released by the MRC
1988	The MRC and the National Health Research and Development Program establish a joint initiative to structure nursing research grants
1991	The first fully funded Canadian nursing PhD programs are launched first at the University of Alberta, followed by the University of British Columbia, McGill University, and the University of Toronto
1994	McMaster University launches its nursing PhD; MRC's mandate includes health research
1999	The Nursing Research Fund is launched with a $25 million grant over 10 years; the Canadian Health Services Research Foundation (CHSRF) administers the funds The PhD nursing program is launched at the University of Calgary
2000	Five CHSRF/Canadian Institutes of Health Research (CIHR) Chairs Awards are granted to nursing
2002	The Office of Nursing Policy organizes a think tank called, "Pathfinding for Nursing Science in the 21st Century," which advocates for a coordinated voice for nursing science
2004	A forum on doctoral education is held in Toronto under the auspices of the Canadian Association of Schools of Nursing to develop a national position paper on the PhD in nursing for Canada The Canadian Consortium for Nursing Research and Innovation is established to develop a strategic plan, build partnerships, and advocate for funding to support research programs and infrastructure
2003–2010	PhD programs in nursing were initiated at Dalhousie University, Queen's University, Université Laval, Université de Montréal, Université de Sherbrooke, University of Victoria, University of Western Ontario, University of Ontario, and University of Saskatchewan

Adapted from Potter, P., Perry, A. G., Ross-Kerr, J., & Wood, M. (Eds.), (2010). *Canadian fundamentals of nursing* (4th ed., p. 81). Toronto. Elsevier Canada.

Committee for the Study of Nursing Education studied the preparation of educators, administrators, and public health nurses and the clinical experiences of nursing students, publishing the results in the Goldmark report (Committee for the Study of Nursing Education, 1923). This report identified gaps in the educational background of nurses. As a result of the Goldmark report, the method for educating nurses changed, and more university-based nursing curricula were developed. A decade later in Canada, a similar comprehensive study of nursing and nursing education was carried out by Dr. George Weir, sponsored jointly by the CNA and the Canadian Medical Association. The so-called Weir report (Weir, 1932) documented serious problems in nursing education and drew attention to the need for changes to improve standards in education and practice. The Weir report's recommendation that authority and responsibility for schools of nursing be vested within provincial systems of education was revolutionary at the time, and more than half a century passed before it was fully implemented across the country.

Changes in the educational system for nurses were crucial for the development of nursing research. In Canada, the establishment of university nursing courses in 1918, followed by master's degree programs in the 1950s and 1960s and by doctoral programs in the 1990s and 2000s, was key to the development of nursing research.

The first nursing research journal, *Nursing Research,* was established in the United States in 1952. The first nursing research journal published in Canada, *Nursing Papers* (later called the *Canadian Journal of Nursing Research*), was established at McGill University in 1969. Other journals were later established; today, nurses publish their research, both within nursing and in interdisciplinary fields, in dozens of journals.

In 1971, McGill University established the Centre for Nursing Research. In the same year, the first National Conference on Nursing Research in Canada was held in Ottawa. These conferences were held annually or biennially for several years. Papers of the early conferences were published as monographs. The number of nursing research conferences increased and began to be sponsored by professional, research, and academic organizations. In addition, nurses began to participate in the research conferences of interdisciplinary groups, such as the Canadian Association on Gerontology.

The two major factors in the development of nursing research have been the establishment of research training through doctoral programs and the establishment of funding to support nursing research. Throughout the 1970s and 1980s, university faculties and schools of nursing built their research resources so that they could mount doctoral programs. The first provincially approved doctoral nursing program was established at the University of Alberta Faculty of Nursing in 1991. The University of British Columbia School of Nursing was established later that year, and programs at McGill University and the University of Toronto followed in 1993. In the late 1990s and early 2000s, other programs were launched, bringing the total to 15.

Growing awareness of the importance of nursing research gradually led to the availability of research funds. In 1999, in response to intensive lobbying by the CNA, the federal government established the Nursing Research Fund, budgeting $25 million for nursing research (i.e., $2.5 million over each of the following 10 years), with the Canadian Health Services Research Foundation (CHSRF) to administer the funds. The research areas targeted for support included nursing policies, management, human resources, and nursing care. Each year, $500,000 is designated for the Open Grants Competition, $500,000 for the Canadian Nurses Foundation for research on nursing care, $500,000 for nursing chairs, $750,000 for training (postdoctoral fellowships and student grants), and $250,000 for knowledge networks and dissemination activities. Five chairs in nursing research were funded by this initiative, representing excellence in nursing research across Canada (CHSRF, n.d.). The incumbents were charged with developing research capacity in one particular area of nursing. Currently, more than 20 nurse researchers hold research chairs funded by the Canada Research Chairs and private funds (Jeans, 2005). Box 1-2 lists many of the national organizations and programs that provide funding or coordination for nursing research in Canada. Unfortunately, the Nursing Research Fund expired in 2009. Several nursing organizations are currently lobbying intensively for a new government fund of $55 million over another 10 years.

Nursing research has focused progressively on evidence-informed practice in response to demands to justify care practices and systems by improving patient outcomes and controlling costs. The scope of nursing research has also broadened to include historical and philosophical inquiry. The establishment of the Centre for Philosophical Nursing Research at the University of Alberta exemplifies this new direction. Training centres have also been funded by the CHSRF to increase training for graduate nursing students and to increase research capacity in nursing and related disciplines. For example, the Ontario Training Centre in Health Services and Policy Research comprises six Ontario universities for the purpose of enhancing health services and policy research. The centre's headquarters are located at McMaster University and involve collaboration with the University of Toronto, York University, University of Ottawa, Laurentian University, and Lakehead University (Web site: http://www.otc-hsr.ca).

Since the 1990s, some of the original nursing research pathfinders and many new ones have conducted research on a wide range of clinical topics, describing phenomena and testing interventions. The existence of the many nursing journals shows the growth in the variety, quality, and depth of research available for potential use in practice. In a report funded by the CHSRF, an analysis of the CIHR database revealed a wide diversity of nursing research topics in Canada. Of

---

BOX 1-2

NURSING RESEARCH NATIONAL ORGANIZATIONS*

- The Canadian Health Services Research Foundation (CHSRF) provides evidence-informed decision making and change in Canada's health care system. Until 2009, the funding was distributed through the Nursing Research Fund to develop nursing researchers and support research in areas such as nursing recruitment, retention, management, and emergent issues from health service restructuring. CHSRF also supports the Research, Exchange, and Impact for System Support (REISS) program to maximize the effect of nursing research on decision making within the Canadian health care system.
- The Canadian Institutes of Health Research (CIHR) provide funding for several institutes, including the Institute of Health Services and Policy Research, that are dedicated to supporting innovative research, capacity building, and knowledge transfer to improve the delivery of health care services.
- Partnership programs funded by CHSRF and CIHR include the Capacity for Applied and Developmental Research and Evaluation (CADRE) program and the Partnerships for Health System Improvement. These programs provide awards to individuals and teams of researchers.
- The Canadian Nursing Foundation (CNF) depends on the contributions of the public and private sectors to provide funding to support research addressing policy and to support clinical nursing research. The CNF also provides scholarships for undergraduate and graduate education.
- The Canadian Association for Nursing Research (CANR) is a national organization whose mission is to support research-based nursing practice and provides awards to recognize the outstanding research contribution of nurses.
- The Office of Nursing Policy at Health Canada has a mandate to improve the health of Canadians. One of the priorities is to focus on strengthening nursing sciences by describing issues and opportunities, increasing the number of researchers and identifying actions, and identifying directions to move the nursing science agenda forward (Office of Nursing Policy, 2009).
- The Canadian Consortium for Nursing Research and Innovation (CNRI) was formed under the leadership of the Office of Nursing Policy to gather stakeholders from a variety of nursing organizations to provide leadership and direction to advance nursing science in Canada.

*List of organizations from the Office of Nursing Policy (2006).

TABLE 1-1

RESEARCH THEMES IN CANADA

HEALTH ISSUES	HEALTH SERVICE ORGANIZATIONS	HEALTH PROMOTION
Chronic illness	Delivery and structure of health care	Tobacco use
Reproductive health	Reducing disparities and improving access	AIDS/HIV
Pain	Hospital restructuring	Abuse
End-of-life/palliative care	Models of health care delivery	Obesity

AIDS, acquired immune deficiency syndrome; *HIV*, human immunodeficiency virus.

the studies, 67% were conducted in the areas of health issues, health service organizations, and health promotion. Not surprisingly, the research on health issues was dominant; the majority of studies focused on (1) chronic illness; (2) reproductive health; (3) pain; and (4) end-of-life/palliative care (Table 1-1; Jeans & Associates, 2008). Nurses have made significant research contributions to health care. Naturally, nurses are far from finished with their quest for knowledge and research, but the nursing leaders of the twentieth century have—by example—paved the way for those who will emerge in the new millennium.

Nursing research capacity has expanded greatly in Canada, as evidenced by increased numbers of doctoral programs and graduates, increased funding, and the development of research teams and centres. However, the profession still faces many challenges. Despite the increased number of doctoral programs and graduate students, research-prepared faculty to supervise the research of the graduate students are in short supply. In addition, the databases that researchers depend on for funding information are not coordinated, and many do not include classifications specifically for nursing (Jeans & Associates, 2008). Moreover, the uptake of research in practice has resulted in the proliferation of best practice guidelines; however, there is a dearth of documentation assessing the "impact of nursing research on health care services and health policy" (Jeans & Associates, 2008, p. 21).

FUTURE DIRECTIONS

In the twenty-first century, the continuing expansion of nursing research provides numerous opportunities for nurses to study important research questions, promote health care, and ameliorate the side effects of illness and the consequences of treatment while also optimizing the health outcomes of patients and their families (Jennings & McClure, 2004). Villeneuve and MacDonald (2006), in *Toward 2020: Visions for Nursing* (p. 99), included the following prediction:

> . . . nurse researchers in 2020 [will] conduct studies that place less emphasis on nurses and nursing processes than was the case 20 years [earlier], focusing instead on health, the needs of clients and communities, and providing sound evidence to guide policy and practice. Research conducted by nurses [will be] interdisciplinary. Research to determine more cost-effective ways to provide safe, high-quality health and illness services [will be] led by nurse researchers.

Major shifts in the delivery of health care include the following:
- An emphasis on community-based care
- An emphasis on reducing disparities in health care
- A focus on health promotion and risk reduction
- An increase in severity of illness in inpatient settings
- An increased incidence of chronic illness
- An expanding population of older people

• An emphasis on provider accountability through a focus on quality and cost outcomes

• The use of technology to serve human needs

In accordance with these trends, nurse researchers are beginning to focus on the development of quantitative and qualitative research programs and clinically based outcome studies. Strategies that enhance nurses' focus on outcomes management through evidence-informed quality improvement activities and the use of research findings for effective clinical decision making also are being refined and identified as priorities (see Chapter 20). Evidence-informed practice guidelines, standards, protocols, and critical pathways are becoming benchmarks for cost-effective, high-quality clinical practice. Also, nurse researchers and nurse leaders will become increasingly visible at the national level, functioning in policymaking roles, representing the field of nursing on expert panels, and lobbying for more funding dollars. The extent of growth in nursing research is evidenced by the establishment of the Nursing Research Fund, which will provide financial support for research opportunities identified by the community of nurse researchers.

Promoting Depth in Nursing Research

Depth in nursing science becomes evident when research is replicated. Research programs that include a series of studies in a similar area, each of which builds on a prior investigation, promote *depth* in nursing science (Whittemore & Grey, 2002). Moreover, to maximize use of resources and to prevent duplication, researchers must develop intradisciplinary and interdisciplinary networks in similar areas of study (Larson, 2003). Researchers from a variety of professions can come together to delineate common and unique aspects of patient care (i.e., medicine, nursing, and respiratory therapy). Cluster studies, multiple-site investigations, and programs of research facilitate the accumulation of evidence that supports or negates a theory. Furthermore, the

increasing emphasis on health services research promotes scientific inquiry, which in turn leads to a better understanding of health care delivery and issues that cross disciplines, such as resource utilization and policymaking (Aiken, Clarke, Cheung, Sloane, & Silber, 2003; Buerhaus, Staiger, & Auerbach, 2000).

The work of Dr. Nancy Edwards, the director of the Community Health Research Unit, provides an excellent example of depth in nursing research. Working in partnership with Public Health and Long-Term Care–City of Ottawa, the University of Ottawa, and a large team of co-researchers, Dr. Edwards is enhancing the scientific and evidence-informed practice in public health. One of her areas of study is the incidence, causes, and prevention of falls among older adults. For example, in one study, investigators collected qualitative data on older adults' beliefs about falls and prevention behaviour; the key findings guided further study on the use of fall-prevention devices, such as grab bars in bathrooms (Community Health Research Unit, 2005). In a more recent research study, Dr. Edwards and colleagues (2006) focused on the development and testing of tools to assess use of physical restraint.

Dr. Edwards's work illustrates the value of building replication studies into research programs. Stone and colleagues (2002) proposed that the adoption of research findings in practice, with their potential risks and benefits (including the cost of implementation), should be based on a series of replicated studies that provide a body of evidence, thereby increasing the degree to which the findings can be applied and generalized. When appropriate, a greater focus on **generalizability** is important if the evolving science is to be considered reliable and usable in health care settings and in health care policies. As such, future replication studies will yield more credible results and will play a crucial role in developing depth in nursing science (Fahs, Stewart, & Kalman, 2003).

Dr. Edwards's work also highlights why research training is likely to become an increasingly essential component of a research career plan. A larger cadre of nurse researchers who begin their research careers at a young age is important for the development of research programs like Dr. Edwards's. The goal is to increase the longevity of research careers, enhance the discipline's science development, promote mentoring opportunities, prepare the next generation of researchers, and provide leadership in health care for interdisciplinary health care debates.

Nurse researchers should also be committed to developing publicly and privately funded research programs and to subscribing to a life of periodic education and retraining supported by awards, grants, and fellowships. Research programs facilitate growth in the depth and breadth of research expertise and recognize that some researchers must be retrained as they develop or shift the emphasis of their research, seek to broaden their scientific background, and acquire new research capabilities.

An International Perspective

The continuing development of a national and international research environment is essential to the nursing profession's mission to establish a global research community (Chang, 2000; Hegyvary, 2004). The opportunities for cross-cultural and cross-national studies on subjects of common interest are consistent with the priority for global research (Hegyvary, 2004; Hinshaw, 2000).

Because of nursing's emphasis on the cultural aspects of care and the influence of such factors on practice, international research is likely to increase. Access to multiple populations as a function of globalization allows the testing of nursing science from various perspectives. Interaction with colleagues from other countries provides a rich context for the generation and dissemination of research (Dickenson-Hazard, 2004; Ward, 2003).

International research projects are often focused on comparative research in which a phenomenon is studied in more than one country,

usually by a single researcher conducting research in his or her home country and then travelling to the other international sites. Because of the financial and logistical limitations to this method, however, the number of international collaborative research projects has increased. Nurse researchers participating in collaborative international research projects are well positioned to play a large role in improving health care globally (Chiang-Hanisko, Ratchneewan, Ludwick, & Martsolf, 2006).

International organizations committed to the goal of health care for all help create natural research partnerships. For example, the World Health Organization (WHO, n.d.) has established a series of collaboration centres in order to advance health care for the global community. One such centre works toward maximizing the contribution of nursing and midwifery and provides relevant research and clinical training to nurses worldwide.

Research Priorities

As the number of nurses with doctoral degrees increased, and as nursing chairs were created and funding was expanded, a distinct set of Canadian nursing research priorities emerged (Box 1-3). Funding agencies often determine research priorities on the basis of their particular needs and interests. In 2007, the CHSRF's priority research themes included (1) managing the delivery of high-quality services in the health care workplace; (2) managing the safe delivery of high-quality services in the health care workplace; (3) providing primary health care; and (4) providing nursing leadership, organization, and policy. These themes were established after consultation with health sector administrators, policymakers, and researchers across Canada. For example, under the rubric of primary health care, policymakers were particularly interested in research dedicated to exploring which models of primary health care work best in specific contexts (CHSRF, 2007).

CANADIAN NURSING RESEARCH PRIORITIES

PRIORITY 1: NURSING PRACTICE

- Context (including determinants of health, health reform, and ethical issues)
- Populations (vulnerable groups and specific clinical populations, particularly First Nations, Métis, and Inuit)
- Interventions (wide range, from health promotion to comfort measures)

PRIORITY 2: OUTCOMES

- Development of valid measures for multiple dimensions
- Links with clinical judgement

PRIORITY 3: ENHANCED LINKS BETWEEN RESEARCH AND PRACTICE

- Development of a body of nursing knowledge

Adapted from Potter, P., Perry, A. G., Ross-Kerr, J., & Wood, M. (Eds.), (2010). *Canadian fundamentals of nursing* (4th ed., p. 80). Toronto: Elsevier Canada.

The CIHR's nursing grants funded $11.6 million for 105 research projects in 2005. Although the availability of funding contributes to interest in nursing research, only 15% of nurses' applications to the CIHR were successful in procuring funding.

In 2006, 50 Canadian nursing leaders identified additional priorities for nurses during a Nursing Leadership, Organization, and Policy Network Day sponsored by the CHSRF. Several research themes were identified as requiring further research, including "human resources planning and management, nursing roles and scopes of practice, education, worklife, staffing, leadership, and use of research through knowledge transfer and exchange" (CHSRF, 2006, p. 7).

Reducing health disparities in underserviced communities and vulnerable populations is another major topic that will shape the focus of future nursing- and interdisciplinary-related research agendas. For example, the health concerns of mothers and infants will continue to spur research that deals effectively with the maternal–neonatal mortality rate. Individuals of all ages who have sustained life-threatening illnesses will live with the help of new life-sustaining technology that will in turn create new demands for self-care and family support. Cancer, heart disease, arthritis, asthma, chronic pulmonary disease, diabetes, and Alzheimer's disease, prevalent during middle age and later life, will be responsible for expenditures of large proportions of the available health care resources. Human immunodeficiency virus/acquired immune deficiency syndrome (HIV/AIDS), a chronic illness that affects men, women, and children, will continue to have a significant effect on health care delivery.

Another vulnerable population, those with mental health illness, will be served by a better understanding of mental disorders, which will emerge as a result of advancements in psychobiological knowledge and research initiatives. Mental health illnesses will continue to be a major public health issue; depression has been cited as the number one mental illness worldwide (WHO, 2001). Alcohol and drug abuse will continue to be responsible for significant health care expenses. Finally, as national initiatives are launched to improve end-of-life care, the shortage of nurses—as clinicians and investigators—will become a major problem worldwide (WHO, 2001). Investigations that address quality-of-care outcomes related to nursing are a top priority for psychiatric nurses in the twenty-first century (President's New Freedom Commission on Mental Health, 2003), as are nursing contributions to end-of-life research (Matzo & Sherman, 2001).

Undoubtedly, one of the most exciting research opportunities for nurses in the future relates to genetics and the human genome, where study prospects range from basic biological topics to clinical decision making and behavioural interventions (J. K. Williams, Tripp-Reimer, Schutte, & Barnette, 2004).

In terms of the priority given to clinical research issues, the funding of investigations has increasingly emphasized populations of interest. For example, the historical exclusion of women as participants in clinical research is well documented; minority women in particular were even more likely to be excluded from research studies. As a result, research data on the health of minority women traditionally were extremely scarce. Nurse researchers such as Josephine Etowa in Canada are addressing this gap in research.

Along with national nursing research initiatives, specific nursing interest groups frequently establish their own research priorities specific to their specialty. Some associations provide funds to support research initiatives. The Canadian Association of Critical Care Nurses, for example, established a small research grant to support specific research activities. The grant will be awarded to a researcher whose work is related directly to the clinical practice of critical care nurses (Canadian Association of Critical Care Nurses, 2007).

International research priorities are influenced by social, political, and economic factors. Typically, international organizations such as the United Nations and the WHO prioritize health research that will affect the most marginalized of the world's population. As such, the eight goals identified by the United Nations (2000) focus on poverty, vulnerable populations (i.e., women and children), and the specific health issues. The goals are as follows:

- Eradicate extreme poverty and hunger
- Achieve universal primary education
- Promote gender equality and empower women
- Reduce child mortality
- Improve maternal health
- Combat HIV/AIDS, malaria, and other diseases
- Ensure environmental sustainability
- Develop a global partnership for development

The global research priorities established by the United Nations and the WHO influence the development of research priorities for international nursing organizations such the International Council of Nurses. The nursing research priorities listed by this council include "health, illness and care delivery services that emphasise quality and cost-effective care, community-based care, nursing workforce and health care reform" (International Council of Nurses, 2007, p. 2).

Other types of research investigations (e.g., those involving historical, feminist, or case study methods) embody the rich diversity of nursing research methods. The nursing profession must continue to value and promote creativity and diversity in research endeavours at all educational levels as a way of empowering nurses for the future. As opportunities are recognized and gaps in science are observed, nurses will conduct, critique, and use nursing research in ways that publicly demonstrate how nursing care makes a difference in patients' lives.

Nurse researchers will have an increasingly strong voice in shaping public policy relating to health care. Shaver (2004) stated that disciplines such as nursing—because of its focus on treatment of chronic illness, health promotion, independence in health, and care of the acutely ill, all of which are heavily emphasized values for the future—will be central to the shaping of health care policy in the future. Research evidence that supports or refutes the merit of health care needs and programs focusing on these issues will be timely and relevant. Thus, nursing and its science base are strategically placed to shape health policy decisions (Fitzpatrick, 2004).

Communication of nursing research has also become increasingly important. Research findings continue to be disseminated in professional arenas (e.g., international, national, regional, and local electronic and print publications and conferences), as well as in consultations and staff development programs implemented on site through Webinars and Web sites. Dissemination of research findings in the public sector has also gained importance.

Increasingly, nurse researchers are asked to testify at governmental hearings and to serve on commissions and task forces related to health care. Nurses are quoted in the media when health care topics are addressed, and their visibility has expanded significantly. For example, Sue Johanson, RN, host of the *Sunday Night Sex Show,* brought more than 35 years of experience in sex education to the public discourse on sex. In addition to addressing all aspects of sex in a non-judgemental manner on her show, Ms. Johanson has written several books and wrote a weekly column on health for the *Toronto Star.* Although retired in 2008, Ms. Johanson still lectures to a wide range of audiences. Dissemination of research through the public media provides excellent exposure of health-related information to thousands of potential viewers, listeners, and readers.

Nurses have a research heritage to be proud of. They also have a challenging and exciting future ahead of them. Both researchers and consumers of research need to engage in a united effort to gather and assess research findings that make a difference in the care that is provided and in the lives that are touched by their commitment to evidence-informed nursing practice.

CRITICAL THINKING CHALLENGES

- How can you access evidence-informed practice information when practising in the field?
- What assumption underlies the recommendation that the role of the nursing graduate in the research process be primarily that of a knowledgeable consumer?
- What effects will evidence-informed patient outcome studies have on the practice of nursing?
- Discuss how research will contribute to the development of intradisciplinary and interdisciplinary networks.
- How are research priorities established by organizations and professional bodies?

KEY POINTS

- Nursing research expands the unique body of scientific knowledge that forms the foundation of evidence-informed nursing practice. Research is the component that links education, theory, and practice.
- Nurses become knowledgeable consumers of research through educational processes and practical experience. As consumers of research, nurses must have a basic understanding of the research process and must demonstrate critical appraisal skills to evaluate the strengths and weaknesses of research before applying the research to clinical practice.
- Nursing research blossomed in the second half of the twentieth century: Graduate programs in nursing expanded, research journals began to be published, and funding for graduate education and nursing research increased dramatically.
- All nurses, whether they possess baccalaureate, master's, or doctoral degrees, have a responsibility to participate in the research process.
- The role of the baccalaureate graduate is to be a knowledgeable consumer of research. Nurses with master's and doctoral degrees are obliged to be researchers and sophisticated consumers of research studies.
- A collaborative research relationship within the nursing profession will extend and refine the scientific body of knowledge that provides the grounding for theory-informed practice.
- The future of nursing research will focus on the extension of scientific knowledge. Collaborative research relationships between education and practice will multiply. Programs of research studies and replication of studies will become increasingly valuable.
- Research studies will emphasize clinical issues, problems, and outcomes. Priority will be given to research studies that focus on health promotion, care for the health needs of vulnerable groups, and the development of cost-effective health care systems.
- Both consumers of research and nurse researchers will engage in a collaborative effort to further the growth of nursing research and accomplish the profession's research objectives.

REFERENCES

Aiken, L., Clarke, S. P., Cheung, R. B., Sloane, D. M., & Silber, J. H. (2003). Education levels of hospital nurses and patient mortality. *Journal of American Medical Association, 290,* 1617-1623.

Buerhaus, P., Staiger, D., & Auerbach, D. (2000). Implications of a rapidly aging nursing workforce. *Journal of the American Medical Association, 283*(22), 2948-2954.

Canadian Association of Critical Care Nurses. (2007). *CACCN research grant*. Retrieved from http://findarticles.com/p/articles/mi_m5PTW/is_3_18/ai_n31153665/?tag=content;col1

Canadian Health Services Research Foundation. (2006). *Looking forward, working together: Priorities for nursing leadership in Canada*. Retrieved from http://www.chsrf.ca/Migrated/PDF/NLOP_e.pdf

Canadian Health Services Research Foundation. (2007). *Primary research themes*. Retrieved from http://www.chsrf.ca/research_themes/ph_e.php

Canadian Health Services Foundation (2008). *2008 Annual report on the nursing research fund*. Retrieved from http://www.chsrf.ca/Programs/PastPrograms/NursingResearchFund.aspx

Canadian Nurses Association. (2002). Position statement: *Evidence-based decision-making and nursing practice*. Retrieved from http://www.cna-aicc.ca

Canadian Nurses Association. (2008). *Code of ethics for registered nurses*. Retrieved from http://www.cna-nurses.ca/CNA/documents/pdf/publications/Code_of_Ethics_2008_e.pdf

Canadian Nurses Association. (2009). *Strengthening Canada's health system by advancing health through nursing science*. Retrieved from www.cna-nurses.ca/CNA/documents/pdf/MP_leave_behind_e.pdf

Canadian Nurses Association. (2010a). *Canadian Registered Nurse Examination: Competencies*. Retrieved from http://www.cna-aiic.ca/CNA/nursing/rnexam/competencies/default_e.aspx

Canadian Nurses Association. (2010b). *Evidence-informed decision-making and nursing practice*. Retrieved from http://www.cna-aiic.ca/CNA/documents/pdf/publications/PS113_Evidence_informed_2010_e.pdf

Carper, B. A. (1978). Fundamental patterns of nursing. *Advanced Nursing Science, 1*(1), 13-24.

Chang, W. Y. (2000). Priority setting for nursing research. *Western Journal of Nursing Research, 22,* 119-121.

Chiang-Hanisko, L., Ratchneewan R., Ludwick, R., & Martsolf, D. (2006). International collaborations in nursing research: Priorities, challenges and rewards. *Journal of Research in Nursing, 11*(4), 307-322.

College of Nurses of Ontario. (2009). *National competencies in the context of entry level registered nurse practice*. Toronto: Author.

Committee for the Study of Nursing Education. (1923). *Nursing and nursing education in the United States. Report of the committee and report of a survey by Josephine Goldmark*. New York: Macmillan.

Community Health Research Unit. (2005). *Research projects funded in 2005*. Retrieved from http://aix1.uottawa.ca/~nedwards/chru/english/research2005.html

Dickenson-Hazard, N. (2004). Global health issues and challenges. *Journal of Nursing Scholarship, 36*(1), 6-10.

Edwards, N., Danseco, E., Heslin, K., Ploeg, J., Santos, J., Stansfield, M., & Davies, B. (2006). Development and testing of tools to assess physical restraint use. *Worldviews Evidence Based Nursing, 3*(2), 73-85.

Fahs, P. S., Stewart, L. L., & Kalman, M. (2003). A call for replication. *Journal of Nursing Scholarship, 35*(1), 67-72.

Fitzpatrick, J. J. (2004). Translating clinical research into research policy. *Applied Nursing Research, 17*(2), 71.

Forchuk, C., Martin, M. L., Chan, Y. L., & Jensen, E. (2005). Therapeutic relationships: From psychiatric hospital to community. *Journal of Psychiatric and Mental Health Nursing, 12,* 556-564.

Ford-Gilboe, M., Wuest, J., Varcoe, C., & Merrit-Gray, M. (2006). Developing an evidence-based health advocacy intervention for women who have left an abusive partner. *Canadian Journal of Nursing Research, 38,* 147-167.

Hegyvary, S. T. (2004). Working paper on grand challenges in improving global health. *Journal of Nursing Scholarship, 36,* 96-101.

Hinshaw, A. S. (2000). Nursing knowledge for the 21st century: Opportunities and challenges. *Journal of Nursing Scholarship, 32,* 117-123.

International Council of Nurses. (2007). *Nursing research*. Retrieved from http://www.icn.ch/images/stories/documents/publications/position_statements/B05_Nsg_Research.pdf

Jeans, M. E. (2005). Shared leadership for nursing research. *Nursing Leadership (Toronto, Ontario), 15*(1), 20-23.

Jeans, M. E., & Associates. (2008). *Nursing research in Canada: A status report*. Retrieved from http://www.canr.ca/documents/NursingResCapFinalReport_ENG_Final.pdf

Jennings, B. M., & McClure, M. L. (2004). Strategies to advance health quality. *Nursing Outlook, 52,* 17-22.

Larson, E. (2003). Minimizing disincentives for collaborative research. *Nursing Outlook, 51,* 267-271.

Matzo, M., & Sherman, D.W. (Eds.), (2001). *Palliative care nursing: Quality care to the end of life*. New York: Springer.

McGinty, J., & Anderson, G. (2008). Predictors of physician compliance with American Heart Association Guidelines for acute myocardial infarction. *Critical Care Nurse Quarterly*, *31*(2), 161-172.

Nightingale, F. (1863). *Notes on hospitals*. London: Longman Group.

Office of Nursing Policy. (2006). *Nursing issues: Research*. Retrieved from http://www.hc-sc.gc.ca/hcs-sss/pubs/nurs-infirm/onp-bpsi-fs-if/2006-res-eng.php

Office of Nursing Policy. (2009). *Office of Nursing Policy overview*. Retrieved from http://www.hc-sc.gc.ca/ahc-asc/branch-dirgen/spb-dgps/onp-bpsi/overview-apercu-eng.php

Paterson, B. (2002). An answer for Sandra. *Canadian Nurse*, *98*(4), 14.

Potter, P., Perry, A. G., Ross-Kerr, J., & Wood, M. (Eds.), (2010). *Canadian fundamentals of nursing* (4th ed.). Toronto: Elsevier Canada.

President's New Freedom Commission on Mental Health. (2003). *Achieving the promise: Transforming mental health care in America: Final report* [DHHS Pub. No. SMA-03-3832]. Rockville, MD: U.S. Department of Health and Human Services.

Sackett, D. L., Rosenberg, W., Gray, J. A., Haynes, R., & Richardson, W. (1996). Editorial: Evidence based medicine: What it is and what it isn't. *British Medical Journal*, *312*(7023), 71.

Shaver, J. (2004). Improving the health of communities: The position. *Nursing Outlook*, *52*, 116-117.

Stone, P. W., Curran, C. R., & Bakken, S. (2002). Economic evidence for evidence-based practice. *Journal of Nursing Scholarship*, *34*(3), 277-282.

Tarlier, D. (2005). Mediating the meaning of evidence through epistemological diversity. *Nursing Inquiry*, *12*, 126-134.

United Nations. (2000). *Millennium development goals*. Retrieved from http://www.un.org/millenniumgoals/bkgd.shtml

Villeneuve, M., & MacDonald, J. (2006). *Toward 2020: Visions for nursing*. Ottawa: Canadian Nurses Association.

Ward, L. S. (2003). Race as a cross-variable in research. *Nursing Outlook*, *51*(3), 120-125.

Weir, G. M. (1932). *Survey of nursing education in Canada*. Toronto: Macmillan. [Note that this publication is often referred to as the Weir report or the Weir survey.]

Whittemore, R., & Grey, M. (2002). The systematic development of nursing interventions. *Journal of Nursing Scholarships*, *34*(2), 115-120.

Williams, D. O. (2004). Treatment delayed is treatment denied. *Circulation*, *109*, 1806-1808.

Williams, J. K., Tripp-Reimer, T., Schutte, D., & Barnette, J. (2004). Advancing genetic nursing knowledge. *Nursing Outlook*, *52*(3), 73-79.

World Health Organization. (2001). *The world health report 2001—mental health: New understanding, new hope*. Geneva, Switzerland: Author.

World Health Organization. (n.d.). *Networks of WHO collaborating centres*. Retrieved from http://www.who.int/collaboratingcentres/networks/networksdetails/en/index1.html

FOR FURTHER STUDY

ⓔvolve   Go to Evolve at http://evolve.elsevier.com/Canada/LoBiondo/Research for Audio Glossary, how-to instructions for Writing Proposals for Funding, and additional research articles for practice in reviewing and critiquing.

CHAPTER 2

Theoretical Framework

Joan Samuels-Dennis | Cherylyn Cameron

LEARNING OUTCOMES

After reading this chapter, you will be able to do the following:

- Define key concepts in the philosophy of science.
- Identify and differentiate between theoretical/empirical, aesthetic, personal, sociopolitical, and ethical ways of knowing.
- Identify assumptions underlying the post-positivist, critical, and interpretive/constructivist views of research.
- Compare inductive and deductive reasoning.
- Differentiate between conceptual and theoretical frameworks.
- Describe how a framework guides research.
- Differentiate between conceptual and operational definitions.
- Describe the relationships among theory, research, and practice.
- Discuss levels of abstraction related to frameworks guiding research.
- Describe the points of critical appraisal used to evaluate the appropriateness, cohesiveness, and consistency of a framework guiding research.

KEY TERMS

aim of inquiry
concept
conceptual definition
conceptual framework
constructivism
constructivist paradigm
context
critical social theory
critical social thought
deductive reasoning

epistemology
hermeneutics
hypothesis
inductive reasoning
methodology
model
ontology
operational definition
paradigm
philosophical beliefs

post-positivism
post-positivist paradigm
qualitative research
quantitative research
text
theoretical framework
theory
values
variables
worldview

STUDY RESOURCES

Go to Evolve at http://evolve.elsevier.com/Canada/LoBiondo/Research for Audio Glossary, how-to instructions for Writing Proposals for Funding, and additional research articles for practice in reviewing and critiquing.

THE NATURE OF KNOWLEDGE

ON A DAILY BASIS, NURSES DEVISE clinical questions that, if answered, improve upon the care they provide to individuals, families, and communities. A medical/surgical nurse may ask, "How do pediatric and adult patients experience surgical pain, and how, in turn, can we enhance pain management for both groups?" A mental health nurse may ask, "What is the relationship between the use of specific psychotropic medication and heart disease among schizophrenic patients?" A public health nurse might ask, "What factors contribute most significantly to the health of homeless youths living in a specific neighbourhood in Ontario, Canada?"

Each question requires that clinicians/nurse researchers engage in a knowledge development process (Figure 2-1). The process begins with the identification of *knowledge gaps:* the absence of theoretical or scientific knowledge relevant to the phenomenon of interest. *Knowledge generation* next occurs, with the conduct of research that provides answers to well-thought-out research questions. This *knowledge* is then *distributed* through journal articles, textbooks, and public presentations to nurses. Next, the *knowledge* is *adopted,* as nurses alter their practice on the basis of published information or as health care organizations develop policies and protocols that are informed by newly generated knowledge. Finally, *knowledge is reviewed and revised* as new health issues arise, advances in clinical practice occur, or knowledge becomes outdated. In this chapter, we focus specifically on theoretical frameworks and how they guide and inform *knowledge generation.*

Figure 2-2 outlines the various ways by which nurses inform their practice. These include theoretical/empirical, personal, experiential, ethical, aesthetic, and sociopolitical ways of knowing (Chinn & Kramer, 2010; Zander, 2007).

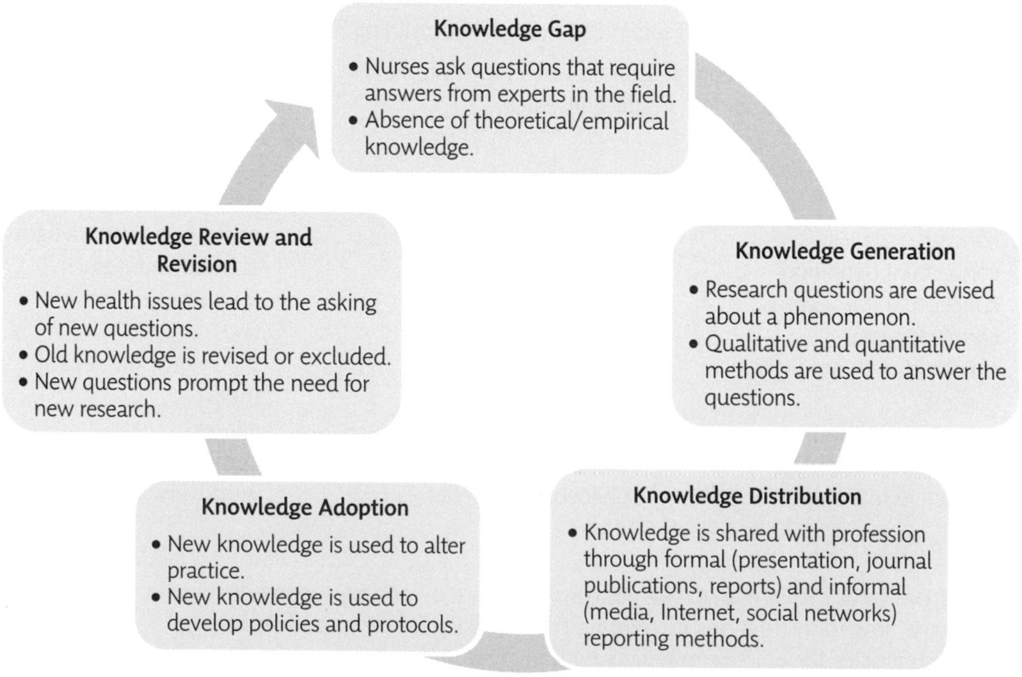

Knowledge Gap
- Nurses ask questions that require answers from experts in the field.
- Absence of theoretical/empirical knowledge.

Knowledge Review and Revision
- New health issues lead to the asking of new questions.
- Old knowledge is revised or excluded.
- New questions prompt the need for new research.

Knowledge Generation
- Research questions are devised about a phenomenon.
- Qualitative and quantitative methods are used to answer the questions.

Knowledge Adoption
- New knowledge is used to alter practice.
- New knowledge is used to develop policies and protocols.

Knowledge Distribution
- Knowledge is shared with profession through formal (presentation, journal publications, reports) and informal (media, Internet, social networks) reporting methods.

FIGURE 2-1 Knowledge development process.

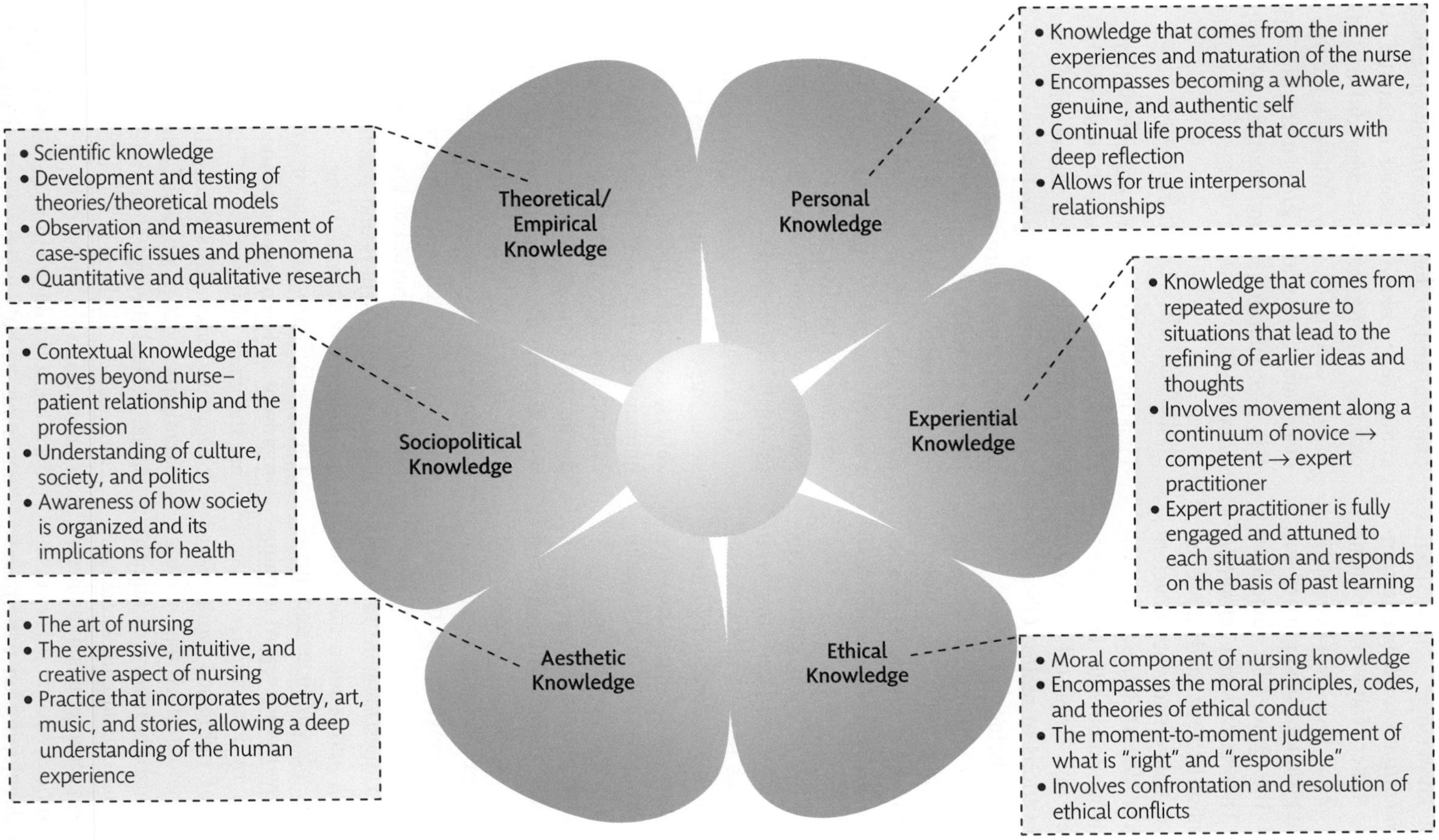
• Scientific knowledge
• Development and testing of theories/theoretical models
• Observation and measurement of case-specific issues and phenomena
• Quantitative and qualitative research
Theoretical/ Empirical Knowledge
Personal Knowledge
• Knowledge that comes from the inner experiences and maturation of the nurse
• Encompasses becoming a whole, aware, genuine, and authentic self
• Continual life process that occurs with deep reflection
• Allows for true interpersonal relationships
• Contextual knowledge that moves beyond nurse–patient relationship and the profession
• Understanding of culture, society, and politics
• Awareness of how society is organized and its implications for health
Sociopolitical Knowledge
Experiential Knowledge
• Knowledge that comes from repeated exposure to situations that lead to the refining of earlier ideas and thoughts
• Involves movement along a continuum of novice → competent → expert practitioner
• Expert practitioner is fully engaged and attuned to each situation and responds on the basis of past learning
• The art of nursing
• The expressive, intuitive, and creative aspect of nursing
• Practice that incorporates poetry, art, music, and stories, allowing a deep understanding of the human experience
Aesthetic Knowledge
Ethical Knowledge
• Moral component of nursing knowledge
• Encompasses the moral principles, codes, and theories of ethical conduct
• The moment-to-moment judgement of what is "right" and "responsible"
• Involves confrontation and resolution of ethical conflicts

FIGURE 2-2 Nursing knowledge.
Based on information from Benner, P. (2004). Using the Dreyfus model of skill acquisition to describe and interpret skill acquisition and clinical judgment in nursing practice and education. *Bulletin of Science, Technology & Society, 24*(3), 188; Benner, P., Tanner, X., & Chesla, C. (1992). From beginner to expert: Gaining a differentiated clinical world in critical care nursing. *Advances in Nursing Science, 14*(3), 13; Chinn, P. L., & Kramer, M. K. (2010). Nursing's fundamental paterns of knowing. In P. Chinn & M. Kramer (Eds.), *Integrated knowledge development in nursing* (8th ed., pp. 1–17). St. Louis: Mosby; and Zander, P. E. (2007). Ways of knowing in nursing: The historical evolution of a concept. *Journal of Theory Construction and Testing, 11*(1), 7–11.

Theoretical/empirical knowledge is most commonly referred to as *scientific knowledge.* In comparison with all the other ways of knowing outlined in Figure 2-2, theoretical/empirical knowledge has gained prominence in nursing and currently serves as the guide for evidence-informed practice. Theoretical and empirical knowledge really cannot be separated; however, theoretical knowing is concerned with developing or testing theories or ideas that nurse researchers have about how the world operate. Theoretical knowing is informed by empirical knowing, which involves observations of reality. Observations may include the following:

1. Speaking with people about their life experiences (e.g., living with Alzheimer's disease) and using their responses to specific and general questions to understand the phenomenon

2. Observing social or cultural interactions (e.g., homeless individuals interacting with service providers) as they naturally occur, interpreting what the interactions might mean for both parties, and using those interpretations to develop theories about health service delivery for that population

3. Delivering an intervention (e.g., a school health program for obese children) and assessing changes in health care–related behaviours (e.g., type of foods consumed, amount of daily exercise) after the delivery of the intervention

4. Using surveys or a questionnaire to ask a large group of men and women questions about experiences of violence and their current symptom levels with regard to pain, digestive problems, or depression.

Taking an example of published work, Erci and colleagues (2003) hypothesized that nursing care guided by Jean Watson's theory of human caring would improve patient outcomes such as quality of life and blood pressure; this hypothesis is an example of *theoretical knowing.* However, it was only through developing an experiment that Erci and colleagues could observe these outcomes (e.g., blood pressure measured every 3 months) among patients who did and did not receive care guided by Watson's theory. These observations provided support for this hypothesis; this support is an example of *empirical knowing.*

PHILOSOPHIES OF RESEARCH

Thus far, we have used a number of terms *(theoretical, empirical, hypothesis)* that may be new to you. Every specialty has characteristic terminology for communicating important features of the work of that specialty. Learning new terminology is part of what nursing students do when they learn research methods and skills. Each research method and all philosophies of science have specialized language that nursing students will encounter in the literature. Thus, to help you comprehend the research you will read, it is important to clarify a few terms.

All research is based on **philosophical beliefs** about the world; these beliefs are the motivating values, concepts, principles, and the nature of human knowledge of an individual, group, or culture, and they are the basis of a **worldview,** or **paradigm.** *Paradigm* is from the Greek word *paradeigma,* meaning "pattern." Paradigms represent a "sets of beliefs and practices, shared by communities of researchers" that guide the knowledge development process (Weaver & Olson, 2006). Therefore, knowing and comprehending these beliefs and practices is important in understanding and using research findings. These beliefs are not right or wrong; rather, they represent different views of the world, and their use the goals of the research.

Nursing research is guided by three research paradigms: post-positivism, constructivism, and social critical theory. These three paradigms are compared in Table 2-1; however, first you need to understand the philosophical language used in the table. **Ontology** (from the Greek word *onto,* meaning "to be") is the science or study of being

TABLE 2-1

BASIC BELIEFS OF RESEARCH PARADIGMS

ITEM/QUESTIONS	POST-POSITIVISM	CRITICAL THEORY	CONSTRUCTIVISM
ONTOLOGY What can be said to exist? Into what categories can we sort existing things?	A material world exists Not all things can be *understood, sensed,* or placed into a cause-and-effect relationship The *senses* provide us with an imperfect understanding of the external/material world	Reality is constructed by those with the most power at particular points in history Reality is plastic and at all time imperfectly understood Over time, reality is shaped by numerous social, political, economical, cultural forces Imperfectly shaped stories become accepted reality	Reality is constructed by individual perception There exists no absolute truth or validity Truth is relative and subjective and based on perception or some particular frame of reference
EPISTEMOLOGY What is knowledge? How is knowledge acquired? How do we know what we know?	Researchers are naturally biased Objectivity (controlled bias) is the ultimate goal Objectivity encourages triangulation and replication of findings across multiple perspectives Objectivity encourages intense scrutiny of research findings from a larger community of scientists and the rejection of poorly conducted research	Research is a transaction that occurs between the researcher and research participant The perceptions (standpoint) of the researcher and the research participants naturally influence knowledge generation/creation Perceptions (standpoints) are determined by context, and so contextual awareness and its relationship to the participants understanding of reality is the focus of the research Objectivity as outlined by the post-positivist is not a desired goal	Research is a transaction that occurs between the researcher and research participant The perceptions (standpoint) of the researcher and the research participants naturally influence knowledge generation/creation Research emphasizes the meaning ascribed to human experiences Context is not emphasized Objectivity as outlined by the post-positivist is not a desired goal
RESEARCHER'S VALUES How do the researcher's values influence the knowledge development process?	All attempts are made to exclude researcher bias Influence denied	Researcher bias is recognized as potentially influential Influence is limited with reflection and bracketing	Researcher bias is recognized as potentially influential Influence is limited with reflection and bracketing

TABLE 2-1			
BASIC BELIEFS OF RESEARCH PARADIGMS—*cont'd*			
ITEM/QUESTIONS	**POST-POSITIVISM**	**CRITICAL THEORY**	**CONSTRUCTIVISM**
METHODOLOGY Within a particular discipline, what principles, rules, and procedures guide the process through which knowledge is acquired?	Inquiry includes experimental, nonexperimental, and qualitative methods and is viewed as a series of logically related steps Research questions/hypotheses are proposed and subjected to empirical testing for the purpose of being proved incorrect rather than correct Research is characterized by careful accounting and control of factors that may influence research findings Research entails the use of qualitative methods to develop hypotheses about people's social world and the meaning/purpose people assign to their actions	Inquiry requires dialogue between the investigator and research participant Dialogue is *transformative* or *consciousness raising* Dialogue brings to the forefront the historical context behind experiences of suffering, conflict, and collective struggles Dialogue increases participants' awareness of actions required to insight change	Inquiry requires dialogue between the investigator and research participant Focus is on interpretation of written texts, art, pictures, and videos Interpretation brings to the forefront the varying ways in which people construct their understanding of their social world and how their interpretation shifts as they interact with others
AIM OF INQUIRY What is the goal of research?	Explanation, prediction, and control	Critique, change and reconstructed reality, and emancipation	Understanding and reconstructed reality
CONTEXT What biographical, life, social, and political factors may influence the research findings?	Focus is on biographical context and its potential to influence research findings Biographical context includes individual characteristics such as race, age, geographic location; it also accounts for past experiences in terms of both timing and content	Focus is on historical, social, and political context Context refers to the social and political climate in which an event or process occurred Social context highlights how structural, economic, representational, and institutional factors of the past influence how people understand an issue today Political context highlights how political dialogue and opinions, legal directives, and government policies of the past influence how people understand an issue.	Focus is on life context, including significant conditions and demands that provide greater understanding of the phenomena being studied; focus also emphasizes time and place

or existence and its relationship to nonexistence. Ontology addresses two primary questions: (1) "What can be said to exist?" and (2) "Into what categories can existing things be sorted?" **Epistemology** (from the Greek word *epistēmē,* meaning "knowledge") is the branch of philosophy that deals with what is known to be "truth." Epistemology addresses three central questions: (1) "What is knowledge?"; (2) "How do we know what we know?"; and (3) "What is the scope/limitation of knowledge?" **Methodology** refers to discipline-specific principles, rules, and procedures that guide the process through which knowledge is acquired. The **aim of inquiry** refers to the goals or specific objectives of the research. **Context** refers to the personal, social, and political environment in which a phenomenon of interest (that "thing of interest") occurs. The context of research studies can include physical settings, such as the hospital or home, or less concrete "environments," such as the context that cultural understandings and beliefs bring to an experience. **Values** are the personal beliefs of the researcher.

Post-positivism is a philosophical orientation that suggests that a material world exists; that is, things can be *sensed* (i.e., seen, touched, heard, tasted). Furthermore, it is governed by the expressed belief that although not all things can be understood or explained, many things can be. In fact, our world can be observed, events and phenomena can be categorized, and we can create theories to explain why some things like *illness* and *health* occur or do not occur. Post-positivism emphasizes the proving/disproving of theories for the purpose of explaining, predicting, and controlling specific outcomes. Post-positivism values objectivity (e.g., observations from a neutral rather than a subjective position) and encourages the intense scrutiny of research findings for the purpose of excluding knowledge that was not developed through a rigorous process.

Constructivism is a philosophical orientation that suggests reality and the way in which we understand our world are largely dependent on our perception. Truth, as viewed by post-positivists, is flawed because truth is never absolute. Truth and our understanding of the world are determined by our life experiences, which in turn inform how we view the world. Knowledge development, from the perspective of the constructivists, is not valuable if it is used simply to prove or disprove theories. Rather, the value of knowledge development lies in the ability to understand how people perceive their world. Knowledge development occurs through observation or dialogue with people, or both, and as a result of paying attention to the language people use to describe life experiences. Constructivists value subjectivity (personal knowing) versus objectivity (quantified knowing), inasmuch as the aim of this form of research is to create an understanding of people and their life experiences from their point of view.

Critical social thought is a philosophical orientation that suggests that reality and our understanding of reality is constructed by people with the most power at a particular point in history. Reality, and our understanding of the world, is always changing, and at all times we have an imperfect understanding of our world. Critical social thought places a strong emphasis on understanding health and illness within the context of history. This perspective supports the understanding that health and other aspects of reality are shaped by numerous social, political, economical, and cultural factors. Such factors include gender, social and economic status, minority versus majority status, and even a country's status as a developed versus developing nation. A strong emphasis is placed on understanding how power imbalances associated with these factors influence health and well-being.

As in constructivism, objectivity is not a goal. Rather, understanding people's experiences from their perspective is highly valued. In addition, the goal of knowledge development is to provide evidence that will support change or the transformation of reality. Critical social thought incorporates feminist theory and what has come to be known as action research. These approaches to research examine how an individual's or a group's position in society shapes that individual's or group's experiences and causes differential or unequal access to resources, power, autonomy, and privilege.

Helpful Hint

All research is based on a paradigm; however, the paradigm is rarely identified in a research report.

Table 2-1 provides an introduction to post-positivism, critical theory, and constructivism and how each might influence nursing research today. The **post-positivist paradigm** is the basis of most quantitative research and, to a smaller extent, qualitative research. Grounded theory, as originally developed by Barney Glaser and Anselm Strauss (1967), is very much based on the cause-and-effect philosophy of the post-positivist paradigm. The **constructivist paradigm** is the basis of most qualitative research that grants importance to **hermeneutics**, which is the interpretation of written, oral, and visual communication. In **critical social theory,** both qualitative and quantitative research are used to highlight historical and current experiences of suffering, conflict, and collective struggles. It is important to note that paradigms guide the development of the research question and the methods used to answer the questions. Some types of research are most congruent with the post-positivist paradigm; others are most congruent with the constructivist or social critical paradigm.

Consider the example of chemotherapy for cancer. A researcher who has a post-positivist orientation may be most interested in answering the question "How effective is tamoxifen in reducing breast cancer among at risk women?" This nurse researcher may use an experiment to address this question. An experiment would involve putting together two groups of at-risk women and then giving one group tamoxifen and the other group a placebo (sugar pills) for a period of time (e.g., 2 years). After 2 years, the nurse researcher would measure how many people in each group developed breast cancer. This approach is guided by the belief that reality can be imperfectly understood through observation and measurement. The aim of the research is to understand exactly how the drug works and under what circumstances. In addition, the goal is to predict who (which type of patient) will benefit most from taking a specific drug such as tamoxifen. The post-positivist researcher recognizes that responses to tamoxifen will be influenced by the biographical or personal context (e.g., age, gender, genetic background, and smoking history), and the researcher will attempt to account for the potential effect these influences might have on the research findings. Knowledge from this type of research will be used to promote evidence-informed practice, health public policy, and the actions of cancer care advocates.

A researcher with a constructivist orientation may be most interested in answering the question "What is the lived experience of women who are being treated for breast cancer?" Qualitative studies based on the constructivist paradigm are guided by the ontological view that multiple realities exist. As Olson (2006) stated, "Phenomena are studied through the eyes of people in their lived situations" (p. 461). For example, the meaning of cancer for a young mother is probably different from that for a grandmother. The meaning of cancer also may be different in Canada than in Japan.

Epistemology includes the view that truth varies and is subjective. Context is important, and description of the experience is vital. When seeking to understand patients' experiences of a treatment, nurse researchers would expect that what is important and "true" for one person may not be so for another. Some of the differences may result from context. The experience may well vary according to where the patient is treated and the patient's characteristics, such as age, gender, and ethnicity. The experience of having cancer may be different for a patient whose mother or father died a painful death from cancer than for a patient who knew people in whom cancer was cured. The values of everyone involved are acknowledged in qualitative research. Again, the finding from this research can be used to support evidence-informed practice and patient-centred care.

A researcher who shares a critical social orientation may be most interested in answering the questions "Does access to cancer treatment vary by racial/ethnic groups?" and "What steps must be taken to ensure equal access to cancer treatment such as tamoxifen?" Such a researcher may use a quantitative approach (e.g., mailing questionnaires to all people who received diagnoses of cancer in the previous 5 years and assessing whether race influenced access to early treatment) to address the first question and a qualitative approach such as focus groups (e.g., speaking with groups of five individuals from various racial/ethnic groups about equal access) to address the second question. This approach is guided by the ontological belief that "reality" is documented by individuals with the most power at particular points in history.

In addition, social critical researchers believe that reality and people's experiences are shaped by numerous social, political, economical, cultural forces. The goal of critical research is to critique, change, and reconstruct reality (tell a different story) and to alleviate the experience of social injustices/inequalities. The research process creates change in study participants, the researcher, and society. This type of research, for example, would attempt to highlight from a historical perspective how the positions of various group (First Nations, Asians, Blacks) and the prestige granted to those groups influence their access to the appropriate treatments for breast cancer.

Findings from these studies would support the researcher and the research participants in becoming "change agents" who advocate for transformations in service delivery practices/policies that intentionally or unintentionally support the unequal access to cancer treatment therapies.

Helpful Hint_____

Values are involved in all research. For the post-positivist, it is vital that values not influence the results of the research. However, for the critical social and constructivist researcher, values and their potential influences on the research results are accepted as a natural part of the research process.

Another way of thinking about paradigms and linking them to research is illustrated in the Critical Thinking Decision Path on p. 32. This algorithm demonstrates that beliefs lead to different questions, which in turn lead to the selection of different research approaches. Qualitative and quantitative research methods are associated with different assumptions that are consistent with each method and are more specific than these global worldviews (positivism, critical theory, and constructivism). These beliefs and approaches lead to different research activities, as illustrated in the decision path.

RESEARCH METHODS: QUALITATIVE AND QUANTITATIVE

Research methods are the techniques, procedures, and processes used by researchers to organize a study in order for it to provide answers to the research question. Research methods can be classified into two major categories: qualitative and quantitative. A researcher chooses between these categories primarily on the basis of the question the researcher is asking. If a researcher wishes to test a cause-and-effect relationship, such as how social support (cause) leads to high blood pressure (effect), quantitative methods are most appropriate. If, however, a researcher wishes to discover and understand the meaning of an experience or process such as death and dying, a

CRITICAL THINKING DECISION PATH

Selecting a Research Process

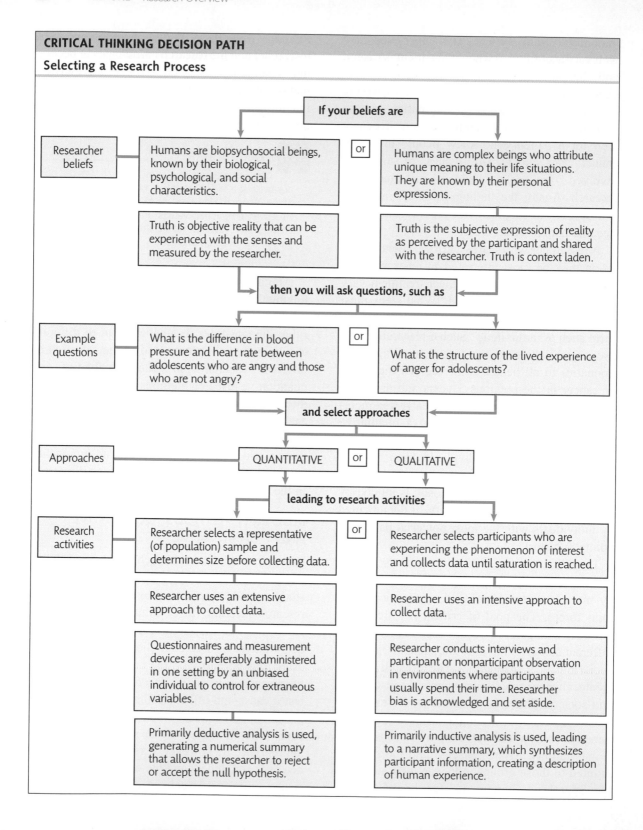

If your beliefs are

Researcher beliefs

Humans are biopsychosocial beings, known by their biological, psychological, and social characteristics.

or

Humans are complex beings who attribute unique meaning to their life situations. They are known by their personal expressions.

Truth is objective reality that can be experienced with the senses and measured by the researcher.

Truth is the subjective expression of reality as perceived by the participant and shared with the researcher. Truth is context laden.

then you will ask questions, such as

Example questions

What is the difference in blood pressure and heart rate between adolescents who are angry and those who are not angry?

or

What is the structure of the lived experience of anger for adolescents?

and select approaches

Approaches

QUANTITATIVE or QUALITATIVE

leading to research activities

Research activities

Researcher selects a representative (of population) sample and determines size before collecting data.

or

Researcher selects participants who are experiencing the phenomenon of interest and collects data until saturation is reached.

Researcher uses an extensive approach to collect data.

Researcher uses an intensive approach to collect data.

Questionnaires and measurement devices are preferably administered in one setting by an unbiased individual to control for extraneous variables.

Researcher conducts interviews and participant or nonparticipant observation in environments where participants usually spend their time. Researcher bias is acknowledged and set aside.

Primarily deductive analysis is used, generating a numerical summary that allows the researcher to reject or accept the null hypothesis.

Primarily inductive analysis is used, leading to a narrative summary, which synthesizes participant information, creating a description of human experience.

qualitative approach would be appropriate. A researcher can also design a study that combines both categories; this approach is discussed later in this chapter.

Qualitative research is a systematic, interactive, and subjective research method used to describe and give meaning to life experiences. Figure 2-3 outlines the qualitative research process. A researcher would choose to conduct a qualitative research study if the question to be answered concerns understanding the meaning of a human experience, such as grief, hope, or loss.

A study completed by de Witt and colleagues (2010) demonstrates the qualitative research process. They conducted a study to understand the "meaning of living alone" from the perspective of older people with Alzheimer's disease or some other form of dementia. Having identified their purpose (Step 1), the authors then selected a small group of people who met the following criteria: (1) they had received a diagnosis of a mild or moderate form of Alzheimer's disease or a related dementia, (2) they had talked about their diagnosis with their physician, (3) they lived alone in the community, (4) they spent the night alone, (5) they were able to speak English, and (6) they were 55 years of age or older. These criteria ensured that the participants of the study were actually experiencing the phenomenon of interest (living alone while suffering with Alzheimer's or dementia) and would be able to provide a rich description about their individual experiences (Step 2). de Witt and colleagues then conducted in-person interviews with eight participants (Step 3).

During the interviews, they asked the participants to share their thoughts on the following: what it is like to live alone with memory loss;

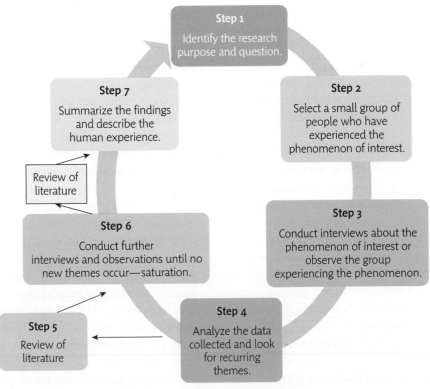

FIGURE 2-3   Qualitative research process.

safety and living alone with memory loss; what it is like to need help and ask for help; and the future. The interviews were recorded and typed out verbatim. Then all eight interviews were reviewed together, and common themes were identified (Step 4). Once the first sets of themes were identified, a second interview was completed with six of the eight participant to ensure that the themes identified were correct and to further clarify the findings (Steps 5 and 6). Existing literature was also reviewed for four primary reasons: (1) to assess what was already known about the topic; (2) to determine how consistent these findings were with previously published research; (3) to further contextualize the findings; and (4) to highlight any knowledge gaps that the study filled (Step 5).

de Witt and colleagues (2010) studied the phenomenon of living alone with dementia in a way totally different from that in any previous studies. Their findings revealed that the human experience related to living alone with dementia was strongly linked to time: *stored time, dreaded time, holding on to time*, and *limited time* (Step 7).

As this example demonstrates, qualitative methods emphasize understanding the meaning of an experience. The context of the experience also plays a role in qualitative research. In this study, past experiences with other people with dementia was a context for *holding back time* or *holding on to now* when facing the risks of living alone with memory loss. As illustrated by this study, qualitative research is generally conducted in natural settings (in this case, the homes of older adults with dementia), and data that are words **(text),** rather than numerical data, are used to describe the experiences being studied. Qualitative data are also collected from a small number of participants, which allows an in-depth study of a particular phenomenon.

Although the methods of qualitative research are systematic, a subjective approach is used; that is, the emphasis is on capturing the personal perceptions of the study participants. Thus, data

from qualitative studies help nurses understand experiences or phenomena that affect patients, and this information in turn leads to improved care and stimulates further research. Chapters 7 and 8 provide an in-depth overview of the underpinnings, designs, and methods of qualitative research.

Whereas the purpose of qualitative research is to create meaning about a phenomenon, that of **quantitative research** is to systematically describe a phenomenon. A researcher would choose to conduct a quantitative research study if the question to be answered concerned testing for the presence of specific relationships, assessing for group differences, clarifying cause-and-effect interactions, or explaining how effective a nursing intervention was. Quantitative methods entail the use of objective, precise, and highly controlled measurement techniques to gather information that can be analyzed and summarized statistically. Figure 2-4 outlines the quantitative research process. Like the qualitative research process, the quantitative research process begins with the development of a research question and a purpose statement that highlight a relationship between two things.

A study completed by Stewart, Reutter, Letourneau, & Makwarimba, (2009) demonstrates the quantitative research process. They addressed the following research question: "What are the effects of a support intervention on homeless youths with respect to the quality, composition, and size of social network; satisfaction with the support received; loneliness and isolation; support-seeking coping; self-efficacy; mental health; and health care–related behaviours?" (Step 1). Unlike the qualitative research process, in which researchers conduct their review of the literature after they have collected their data, the quantitative research process begins with a review of literature such as journal articles, books, government documents, and even Internet sources to determine what is known about the phenomenon of interest and theories that explain the

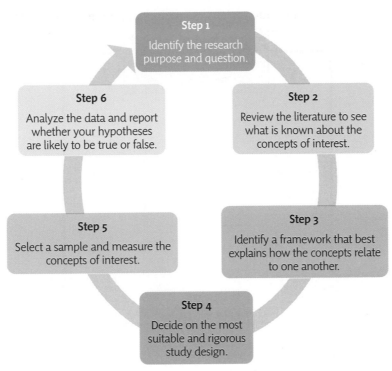

FIGURE 2-4   Quantitative research process.

phenomenon (Step 2). In their introduction and review of the literature, Stewart and colleagues outlined what is already known about the benefits of support for homeless youths. They identified how support is related to each of the six variables identified previously in this chapter. They also provided a diagram or framework that outlines for readers exactly how support influences stress, coping, and health care–related behaviours among homeless youths (Step 3) (Figure 2-5).

An important part of the quantitative research process is to decide which design is most appropriate for answering the research question. The numerous choices include descriptive, correlational, longitudinal, quasiexperimental, and experimental designs. Stewart and colleagues (2009) chose a quasiexperimental design (explained in Chapter 10) to test the effectiveness of the intervention with 70 homeless youths (Step 4). To show how effective the intervention was, all 70 homeless youths participated in the

intervention and completed a questionnaire at three times: before the intervention, midway through the intervention, and at the end of the intervention. The questionnaire assessed the size and characteristics of their social network, their satisfaction with the level of support received, coping behaviours, and depressive symptoms (Step 5). These data were analyzed statistically, and Stewart and colleagues showed that, overall, the authors suggest that the intervention improved the health and well-being of the youths who participated in it (Step 6).

As demonstrated in the article by Stewart and colleagues (2009), quantitative research techniques are systematic, and the methodology emphasizes control of the research process, the environment in which the study is conducted, and how each variable is measured. In contrast to qualitative approaches—in which a question is asked and the participant is responsible for providing an in-depth response—quantitative

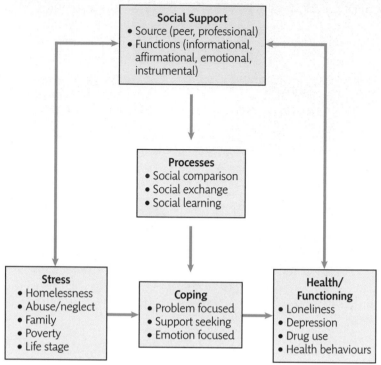

FIGURE 2-5   Model of conceptual foundation.
From Stewart, M., Reutter, L., Letourneau, N., & Makwarimba, E. (2009). A support intervention to promote health and coping among homeless youths. *Canadian Journal of Nursing Research, 41*(2), 54–77.

responses are restricted to a preselected set of responses. Stewart and colleagues, for example, did not ask each homeless youth how the intervention changed his or her coping behaviours; rather, participants responded to a tool that measures two types of coping, which was selected for this study and used to assess how participants' coping behaviour scores changed over three times.

When you read research articles, remember that researchers may vary the steps slightly, depending on the nature of the research problem, but all of the steps should be addressed systematically.

INTRODUCTION TO FRAMEWORKS FOR RESEARCH

When research projects are conducted, particularly within the nursing discipline, great emphasis is placed on including a theoretical framework. For quantitative research projects, a theoretical framework offers researchers and consumers a way to understand how a phenomenon (that thing of interest) comes to exist. Frameworks can be abstract or concrete, but they provide a discipline-specific cause-and-effect explanation of the phenomenon. Furthermore, a framework guides the researcher in determining the questions to be asked/answered by the research project and in the development of the study hypotheses.

The social determinant of health perspective is one example of a theoretical framework that is often used in nursing (Chomik, 2001). This framework, developed by a panel of interdisciplinary experts (policy developers and analysts, community representatives, and health researchers), suggests that people's health and well-being are determined by nine factors; Health Canada recognizes that the last two have a "cross-cutting, influential effect on all other health determinants" (Chomik, p. 13):

1. Socio-economic environment including income, income distribution, and social status; social support networks; education; employment and working conditions; and social environments
2. Physical environment
3. Healthy child development
4. Personal health practices
5. Individual capacity and coping skills
6. Biology and genetic endowment
7. Health and social services
8. Gender
9. Culture/ethnicity

The determinant of health framework guides the researcher in addressing the relationship between health and any of the nine factors just mentioned. The researcher can determine how many factors to focus on and in what way the factors are related to each other and, in turn, to health. In some cases, the researcher may develop a diagram or a pictorial representation of these relationships.

Methodological frameworks serve as a guide for conducting qualitative research studies. Rather than explain how the phenomenon of interest comes to exist, the methodological framework identifies the principles, rules, and procedures that guide the process through which knowledge is acquired. The *human becoming basic research method* (Cody, 1995; Parse, 2005) has been used extensively to guide nursing research. In this method, hermeneutics are used to discover the meaning people assign to their lived experiences as expressed in text and art. The method consists of a dialogue between the researcher and text or art form to answer research questions such as "What does it mean to be human?" (Parse, 2001, p. 172). The analysis is completed in view of the principles of the theory of human becoming (Parse, 1987). Whereas the quantitative project

begins with a theoretical framework, the findings of a qualitative study often lead to the creation of a theoretical framework that conveys an understanding of people's lived experiences.

As a follow-up exercise to this introduction to frameworks for research, read the following story and consider its message for the practising nurse who wishes to critique, understand, and conduct research.

Kate has worked in a coronary care unit (CCU) for nearly 3 years since graduating from nursing school. She has grown more comfortable with her job over time and now believes that she can readily manage the complexities of patient care in the CCU. Recently, she has observed the pattern of blood pressure change when health care professionals enter a patient's room. This observation began when Kate noticed that one of her patients, a 62-year-old woman who had continuous arterial monitoring, showed dramatic increases in blood pressure, as much as 100%, each time the health care team made rounds in the CCU. Furthermore, this elevation in blood pressure persisted after the team left the patient's room, and then her blood pressure slowly decreased to preround levels within the following hour. Conversely, when the nurse manager visited the same patient on her usual daily rounds, the patient engaged calmly in conversation and was often left with lower blood pressure when the nurse manager moved on to the next patient. Kate thought about what was happening and adjusted her work so that she could closely observe the details of this phenomenon over several days.

Team rounds were led by the attending cardiologist and included nurses, pharmacists, social workers, medical students, and nursing students. The team discussed the patient, and, occasionally, she was asked to respond to a question about her history of heart disease or her current experience of chest discomfort. Participants took turns listening to her heart, and the students responded to questions related to her case. In contrast, the nurse manager's visit was a one-on-one meeting in which the patient was given the nurse's full attention. Kate noticed that the nurse manager was especially attentive to the patient's experience. In fact, the nurse manager usually sat and spent time talking to the patient about how her day was going, what she was thinking about while lying in bed, and what feelings were surfacing as she began to consider how life would be when she returned home.

Kate decided to talk to the nurse manager about her observations. The nurse manager, Alison, was pleased that Kate had noticed these blood pressure changes in association with interaction with health care professionals. She told Kate that she, too, noticed these changes during her 8-year experience of working in the CCU. Her observation led her to the theory of *attentively embracing story* (Liehr & Smith, 2000; Smith & Liehr, 2003), which seemed applicable to the observation. Alison had learned the theory as a first-year master's-degree student and now was applying it in practice and beginning plans to use the theory to guide her thesis research. The theory of attentively embracing story proposes that intentional nurse-patient dialogue (communication for a specific purpose), which engages the human story (encourages the patient to discuss her experience), enables connecting with self-in-relation (self-reflection) to create ease (Figure 2-6). As depicted by the theory model, the central concept of the theory is intentional dialogue (purposeful communication), which is what Kate first observed when she noticed Alison interacting with the patient.

Alison was fully attentive to the patient, following her lead in the conversation and pursuing what mattered most to the patient. Alison seemed to obtain a lot of information in a short time, and the patient seemed willing to share information that she was not sharing with other people. According to the theory of attentively embracing story, three concepts—intentional dialogue, connecting with self-in-relation, and creating ease—are intricately connected. Thus, when Kate observed intentional dialogue, she also observed

connecting with self-in-relation as the patient reflected on her experience in the moment and creating ease when she saw the patient's blood pressure decrease after the nurse manager's visit. Alison and Kate shared an understanding that a relationship existed between the patient–health care professional interaction and the patient's blood pressure. They discussed several possible issues that might be affecting this relationship and made a list of research questions related to each issue (Table 2-2). Their list serves only as a reflection of the complexity of the relationship; other issues could generate a research question contributing to understanding of the relationship between the patient–health care professional interaction and the patient's blood pressure. The list developed by Kate and Alison highlights the fact that the relationship cannot be understood with one study; rather, a series of studies may enhance understanding and offer suggestions for

TABLE **2-2**

ISSUES AFFECTING BLOOD PRESSURE CHANGE AND RELATED RESEARCH QUESTIONS

ISSUES	RESEARCH QUESTIONS
Number of people in the patient's room	Is there a difference in BP for patients in the CCU when interacting with one person in comparison with interacting with two or more people?
Involvement of the patient	For the patient in the CCU, what is the relationship between BP and the amount of time spent listening to the health care team's discussion of personal qualities during routine rounds? What is the effect of the nurse-patient intentional dialogue on BP within the hour after the dialogue?
Continuing effect of experience on BP over the next hour	What is the BP pattern of patients in the CCU from the beginning of routine health care rounds until 1 hour after the completion of rounds?
Content of dialogue	What is the relationship between issues discussed during intentional dialogue and BP?
Meaning of experience for the patient	What is the patient's experience of being observed during routine health care rounds? What is the patient's experience of sharing personal matters with a nurse while in the CCU?

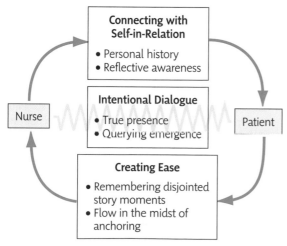

FIGURE 2-6   Attentively embracing story.

BP, blood pressure; *CCU*, coronary care unit.

change. For instance, a thorough understanding may lead to testing different approaches for conducting team rounds.

LINKS CONNECTING PRACTICE, THEORY, AND RESEARCH

Several important aspects of frameworks for research are embedded in the story of Kate and Alison. First, it is important for you to notice the links among practice, theory, and research. Each is intricately connected with the other to create knowledge for the discipline of nursing (Figure 2-7). A **theory** is a set of interrelated concepts that provides a systematic view of a phenomenon. Theory guides practice and research; practice enables testing of theory and generates questions for research; and research contributes to theory building and establishing practice guidelines. Thus, what is learned through practice, theory, and research constitutes the knowledge of the discipline of nursing. From this perspective, each reader is in the process of contributing to the knowledge of the discipline. For example, if you are a practising nurse, you can use focused observation (Liehr, 1992), just as Kate did, to consider the nuances of situations that matter to patient health. Kate noticed the changes in blood pressure occurring with interactions and systematically began to pay close attention to the effect

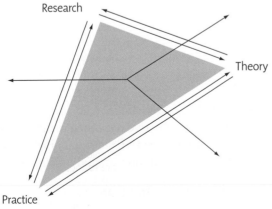

FIGURE 2-7 Discipline knowledge: the theory-practice-research connection.

of different interactions. This logical process often generates the questions that make the most sense for enhancing a patient's well-being.

Another major theme in the story of Kate and Alison can be found in each nurse's approach to the phenomenon of the relationship between the patient–health care professional interaction and blood pressure. Each nurse was using a different approach to look at the situation, but both were systematically evaluating what was observed. This approach is the essence of science: systematic collection, analysis, and interpretation of data. Kate was using **inductive reasoning,** a process of starting with the details of experience and moving to a general picture. Inductive reasoning involves the observation of a particular set of instances that belong to and can be identified as part of a larger set. Alison told Kate that she, too, had begun with inductive reasoning but now was using **deductive reasoning,** a process of starting with the general picture—in this case, the theory of attentively embracing story—and moving to a specific direction for practice and research. In deductive reasoning, the researcher uses two or more related concepts that, when combined, enable the researcher to suggest relationships between the concepts.

Inductive and deductive reasoning are basic in frameworks for research. Inductive reasoning is the pattern of "figuring out what is there" from the details of the nursing practice experience and is the foundation for most qualitative inquiry. Research questions related to the issue of the meaning of experience for the patient (see Table 2-2) can be addressed with the inductive reasoning of qualitative inquiry. Deductive reasoning begins with a structure that guides searching for "what is there." All but the last two research questions listed in Table 2-2 would be addressed with the deductive reasoning of quantitative inquiry.

In view of Alison's use of deductive reasoning guided by the theory of attentively embracing story, we can assume that she has read and critiqued the literature on theoretical frameworks and has chosen *attentively embracing story* to guide her master's thesis research. For Kate to move on in her thinking about research to study the way changes in blood pressure are related to the patient–health care professional interaction, she needs to become well-versed in the importance of theoretical frameworks. As she reads the literature and reviews research studies, she will critique the theoretical frameworks guiding those studies. By critiquing existing frameworks, she will develop the knowledge and understanding needed to choose an appropriate framework for research. As a beginning, Kate is reading this chapter, recognizing that she is critiquing nursing research.

Helpful Hint

Investigators may not always provide a detailed, explicit statement of the one or more observations that led them to their conclusions when using inductive reasoning. Likewise, you will not always find a clear explanation of the structure guiding a study in which deductive reasoning is used.

FRAMEWORKS AS STRUCTURES FOR RESEARCH

Whether you are evaluating a qualitative or a quantitative study, look for the framework that guided the study. In general, in an article in which the researcher is using qualitative inquiry and inductive reasoning methods, the framework is described at the end of the publication, in the discussion section. From the study's findings, the researcher builds a structure for moving forward. For example, in their study on women and violence in improving pregnancy and parenting care for Aboriginal families, D. Smith and colleagues (2006) investigated experiences from community members. These stories were analyzed, and the findings were synthesized at the theoretical level. The researchers moved from the particulars of the experiences of pregnancy and parenting care to a general structure of concepts that included

pregnancy as an opportunity for change, safe health care places and relationships, responsive care, and making interventions safe and responsive. These concepts were described in the context of the participants' stories and relevant literature; thus, a conceptual structure that could be modelled was created.

A **model** is a symbolic representation of a set of concepts that is created to depict relationships. Figure 2-5 shows Stewart and colleagues' (2009) model of *social support*. It highlights the process through which support from peers and professionals influences the stressful life situations, coping behaviours, and health care–related behaviours of homeless youths. In this model, arrows are used to depict a process that explains how social support is related to the social network, stress, and health functioning. For example, the arrow from "social support" to "processes" suggests that social support has an effect on social network comparison, exchange, and learning. Whether this is positive or negative is unknown; however, the social network then influences coping behaviours (problem focused, support seeking, and emotion focused), which in turn influence health care–related functioning (loneliness, depression, drug use, and health behaviours). This model could be the basis for deductive reasoning. An example of a deductive question that could be derived from the model is as follows:

What is the difference in social comparison [an indicator of the quality of the social network] for homeless youths who participate in a supportive intervention, and how does this influence their problem-focused coping skills [one indicator of coping]?

In an article by a researcher who uses quantitative inquiry and deductive reasoning methods, the framework is described at the beginning of the article, before a discussion of study methods.

The Ladder of Abstraction

The ladder of abstraction is a way for you to gain a perspective when reading and thinking about frameworks for research. When you critique the framework of a study, imagine a ladder (Figure 2-8). The highest level on the ladder, the worldview, includes beliefs and assumption or the paradigm to which the research belongs. The middle portion of the ladder includes the framework, theories, and concepts that the researcher uses to articulate the problem, purpose, and structure for the research.

For example, as stated by Stewart and associates (2009), the purpose of their study was to pilot test a comprehensive support intervention for homeless youths that was intended to optimize peer influence, reduce loneliness and isolation, and enhance coping skills. From their review of the literature, which involved reading published research articles about stress and coping among this population and book chapters that theorized about stress and coping, they developed a social

support framework (see Figure 2-5). The framework is used to identify specific concepts of interest, form several hypotheses about how the concepts are related, and logically structure the study's general orientation.

At the lowest level on the ladder of abstraction are variables. **Variables** are the elements that can be observed through the senses. The key empirical aspects of a study—its concepts and variables—are generally articulated through conceptual and operational definitions. A **conceptual definition** is much like a dictionary definition, conveying the general meaning of the concept. However, the conceptual definition goes beyond the general meaning found in the dictionary; the concept is defined as it is rooted in the theoretical literature. The **operational definition** specifies how the concept will be measured: that is, what instruments will be used to capture the essence of the variable.

Helpful Hint

Some research reports embed conceptual definitions in the literature review. The reader should find the conceptual definitions so that the logical fit between the conceptual and the operational definitions can be determined.

Frameworks, Theories, and Concepts

Frameworks, theories, and concepts can be compared with each other from the perspective of abstraction, with concepts being the lowest on the middle portion of the ladder and frameworks the highest. Frameworks, such as the social determinants of health perspective, provide a general orientation to understanding a phenomenon of interest and identify what factors are most significant as we examine various aspects of health, for example. However, a framework does not necessarily reveal how every possible factor relates to one another. The theories specify the relationship between the components of a framework.

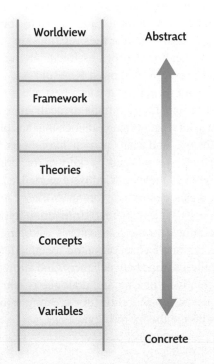

FIGURE 2-8 Ladder of abstraction for evaluating research frameworks.

Theories

As stated earlier, a *theory* is a set of interrelated concepts that serves the purpose of explaining or predicting phenomena. A theory is like a blueprint, a guide for modelling a structure. A blueprint depicts the elements of a structure and the relationship of each element to the other, just as a theory depicts both the concepts that compose it and how they are related. Chinn and Kramer (1999, p. 63) defined a theory as an "expression of knowledge . . . a creative and rigorous structuring of ideas that project a tentative, purposeful, and systematic view of phenomena" (p. 268). For example, consider the relationship between healthy child development, individual capacity and coping, and mental well-being. Several theories that account for the relationship between these variables have been developed by nurse researchers (i.e., Neuman's [1995] systems model). Such models address the ways in which stressful events deplete people's coping resources and, in turn, how both influence the mental health of people (children or adults).

Concepts

At the lower end of the ladder of abstraction, a **concept** is an image or symbolic representation of an abstract idea. Chinn and Kramer (1999, p. 51) defined a concept as a "complex mental formulation of experience." Concepts are the major components of theory and convey the abstract ideas within a theory. In this chapter, the concepts of the theory of attentively embracing story — intentional dialogue, connecting with self-in-relation, and creating ease—have been defined, and their relationships have been modelled. Each concept creates a mental image that is explained further through the conceptual definition. For example, the concept of pain creates a mental image that is based on experience. Its experiential meaning is different for a child who has just fallen off a bike, for an older adult with rheumatoid arthritis, and for a nurse with a doctoral degree who is studying pain mechanisms by using an animal model. These definitions and associated images of the concept of pain incorporate different experiential and knowledge components, all with the same label: *pain.* Therefore, it is important to know the meaning of the concept to the person. For a reader, it is important to know the meaning that the researcher gives to the concepts in a research study.

HYPOTHESIS AND VARIABLES. Chinn and Kramer (1999) defined a **hypothesis** as a "tentative statement of relationship between two or more variables that can be empirically tested (p. 254)." A hypothesis is a best guess or prediction about what one expects to find about the variable outlined in the study. The variables represent the most concrete components of the ladder of abstraction and are derived from the identified concepts of a theory. They represent the measurable properties (what can be observed, measured, or both) of a quantitative study.

As you read this text, you will learn how to articulate a hypothesis, just as Kate formulated a hypothesis about the relationship between patient–health care professional interaction and blood pressure. Although Kate did not label her idea as a *hypothesis,* it was a best guess based on observation. Take a minute to recall an experience from your own nursing practice that has provoked confusion, and state it as a hypothesis. A mismatch between what is known or commonly accepted as fact and what we experience creates a hypothesis-generating moment. Every nurse experiences such moments. Cultivating hypothesis-generating moments requires noticing them, focusing one's observation on specific details and the relationships between them, and allowing time for creative thinking and dialogue (Liehr, 1992); this leads to possibilities for creating a low-level microrange theory or hypothesis.

Frameworks

The Critical Thinking Decision Path on p. 43 takes you through the thinking of a researcher who is about to begin conducting research. You can expect to find some, but not all, of the phases of decision making addressed in a research publication. Beginning with the worldview, the highest rung on the ladder of abstraction, the researcher is inclined to approach a research problem from the perspective of inductive or deductive reasoning. Researchers who pursue an inductive reasoning approach generally do not present a framework before beginning the discussion of methods. This is not to say that the literature will not be reviewed before the methods are introduced. For example, Bottorff and colleagues (2004) were interested in understanding how adolescents view cigarette addiction because an understanding of how adolescents view smoking and addiction can lead to more effective smoking

prevention and cessation programs. Therefore, the point of the literature review is to build a case for doing the research. Researchers do not provide a framework for the study because they are planning an inductive approach to study the problem.

Conversely, researchers who use deductive reasoning must choose between a conceptual and a theoretical framework. In the theory literature, these terms are used interchangeably (Chinn & Kramer, 1999); however, in the case presented in the Critical Thinking Decision Path, each term is distinguished from the other on the basis of whether the researcher is creating the structure or whether the structure has already been created by someone else. In general, each of these terms refers to a structure that provides guidance for research. A **conceptual framework** is a structure

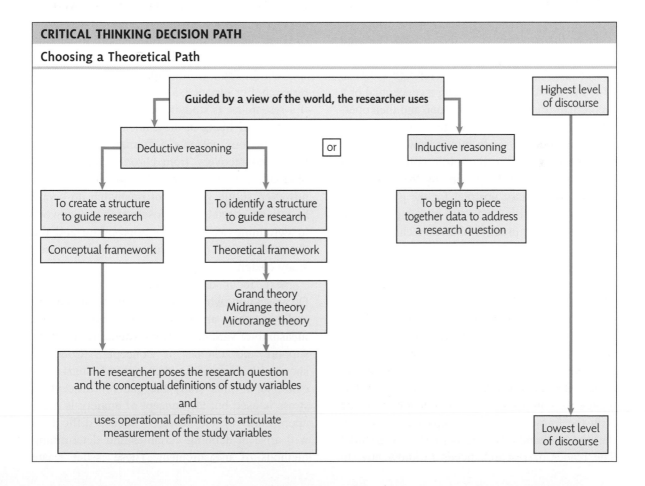

CRITICAL THINKING DECISION PATH

Choosing a Theoretical Path

Guided by a view of the world, the researcher uses

Deductive reasoning   or   Inductive reasoning

Highest level of discourse

To create a structure to guide research

To identify a structure to guide research

To begin to piece together data to address a research question

Conceptual framework

Theoretical framework

Grand theory
Midrange theory
Microrange theory

The researcher poses the research question and the conceptual definitions of study variables

and

uses operational definitions to articulate measurement of the study variables

Lowest level of discourse

of concepts, theories, or both that is used to construct a map for the study. It presents a theory, which explains why the phenomenon being studied exists. Generally, a conceptual framework is constructed from a review of the literature or is developed as part of a qualitative research project. A **theoretical framework** may also be defined as a structure of concepts, theories, or both that is used to construct a map for the study. However, it is based on a philosophical or theorized belief or understanding of why the phenomenon under study exists.

Helpful Hint

When researchers have used conceptual frameworks to guide their studies, you can expect to find a system of ideas, synthesized for the purpose of organizing thinking and providing study direction.

From the perspective of the Critical Thinking Decision Path, theoretical frameworks can incorporate grand, midrange, or microrange theories. Whether the researcher is using a conceptual or a theoretical framework, conceptual and then operational definitions will emerge from the framework. The decision path moves down the ladder of abstraction from the philosophical to the empirical level, tracking thinking from the most abstract to the least abstract for the purposes of planning a research study and accruing evidence to guide nursing practice and research.

APPRAISING THE EVIDENCE

The Framework

The framework for research provides guidance for the researcher as study questions are fine-tuned, methods for measuring variables are selected, and analyses are planned. Once data are collected and analyzed, the framework is used as a basis for comparison. Did the findings coincide with the framework? If discrepancies exist, can they be explained by means of the framework? The reader of research needs to know how to critically appraise a framework for research (see Critiquing Criteria box on the facing page).

The first question posed is whether a framework is presented. Sometimes, a structure may guide the research, but a diagrammed model is not included in the report. You must then look for the study structure in the description of the study concepts. When the framework is identified, consider its relevance for nursing. A nurse does not have to create the framework, but the importance of the study's content for nursing should be clear. The question of how the framework depicts a structure congruent with nursing should be addressed. Sometimes frameworks from very different disciplines, such as physics or art, may be relevant to nursing. The author must clearly articulate the meaning of the framework for the study and link the framework to nursing.

Once the meaning and relationship to nursing are articulated, you will be able to determine whether the framework is appropriate to guide the research. For instance, a blatant mismatch occurs if a researcher is studying students' responses to the stress of being in the clinical setting for the first time but presents a framework of stress related to recovery from chronic illness. Such obvious mismatches do not generally arise; however, subtle versions of mismatch do occur. So you will need to look closely at the framework to determine whether it is appropriate and the "best fit" for the research question and proposed study design.

Next, focus on the concepts being studied. Do you know which concepts are being studied and how they are defined and translated into measurable variables? Does literature exist to support the choice of concepts? Concepts should clearly reflect the area of study; for example, if in a study the general concept of stress is used but the concept of anxiety is more appropriate to the research focus, difficulties will arise in defining variables and determining methods of measurement. These issues relate to the logical consistency within the framework, the concepts being studied, and the methods of measurement.

Throughout the entire critiquing process, from worldview to operational definitions, you are evaluating whether the theoretical framework is appropriate. At the end of a research article, you can expect to find a discussion of the findings as they relate to the model. This final point enables readers to evaluate the framework for use in further research. The discussion may suggest necessary changes to enhance the relevance of the framework for continuing study and thus focus the direction of future research.

Evaluating frameworks for research requires skill that can be acquired only through repeated critique and discussion with other nurses who have critiqued the same publication. The novice reader of research must be patient while these skills are developed. With continuing education and a broader knowledge of potential frameworks, you will build a repertoire of knowledge to enable you to judge the foundation of a research study, the framework for research.

CRITIQUING CRITERIA

1. Is the framework for research clearly identified?
2. Is the framework consistent with a nursing perspective?
3. Is the framework appropriate to guide research on the subject of interest?
4. Are the concepts and variables clearly and appropriately defined?
5. Did the study present sufficient literature to support the selected concepts?
6. Is there a logical, consistent link between the framework, the concepts being studied, and the methods of measurement?
7. Are the study findings examined in relation to the framework?

CRITICAL THINKING CHALLENGES

- Explain the difference between research that is based on a constructivist paradigm and research that is based on a positivist paradigm.
- Discuss how a researcher's values can influence the results of a study. Include an example in your answer.
- You are taking an elective course in advanced pathophysiology. The professor compares the knowledge of various disciplines and states that nursing is an example of a nonscientific discipline, declaring in support of this position that nursing's knowledge has been generated with unstructured methods, such as intuition, trial and error, tradition, and authority. What assumptions has this professor made? Would you counter or support this position?
- Nurse researchers contend that a theoretical framework is essential for systematically identifying the relationship among the chosen variables. If this is true, why do nonnursing research studies not identify theoretical frameworks?
- As a consumer of research, how would you use computer databases to verify tools for measuring operational definitions?
- How would you argue against the following statement: "As a beginning consumer of research, it is ridiculous to expect me to determine whether a researcher's study has an appropriate theoretical framework; I've only had Nursing Theory 101."
- Is it possible for a research study's theoretical framework and variables to be the same?

KEY POINTS

- The scientific approaches used to generate nursing knowledge reflect both inductive and deductive reasoning.
- The interaction among theory, practice, and research is central to knowledge development in the discipline of nursing.
- Conceptual frameworks are created by the researcher, whereas theoretical frameworks are identified in the literature.
- The use of a framework for research is important as a guide to systematically identify concepts and to link appropriate study variables with each concept.
- Conceptual and operational definitions are critical in the evolution of a study, regardless of whether they are explicitly stated.
- In developing or selecting a framework for research, knowledge may be acquired from other disciplines or directly from nursing. In either case, that knowledge is used to answer specific nursing questions.
- Theory is distinguished by its scope. Grand theories are the broadest in scope and at the highest level of abstraction, whereas microrange theories are the most narrow in scope and at the lowest level of abstraction. Midrange theories are in the middle.
- Midrange theories are at a level of abstraction that enhances their usefulness for guiding practice and research.
- When you critique a framework for research, examine the logical, consistent link between the framework, the concepts for study, and the methods of data collection.

REFERENCES

Benner, P. (2004). Using the Dreyfus model of skill acquisition to describe and interpret skill acquisition and clinical judgment in nursing practice and education. *Bulletin of Science, Technology & Society, 24*(3), 188.

Benner, P., Tanner, C., & Chesla, C. (1992). From beginner to expert: Gaining a differentiated clinical world in critical care nursing. *Advances in Nursing Science, 14*(3), 13.

Bottorff, J. L., Johnson, J. L., Moffat, B., Grewal, J., Ratner, P., & Kalaw, C. (2004). Adolescent constructions of nicotine addiction. *Canadian Journal of Nursing Research, 38*, 22-39.

Chinn, P. L., & Kramer, M. K. (1999). *Theory and nursing: Integrated knowledge development.* St. Louis: Mosby.

Chinn, P. L., & Kramer, M. K. (2010). Nursing's fundamental patterns of knowing. In P. Chinn & M. Kramer (Eds.), *Integrated knowledge development in nursing* (8th ed., pp. 1-17). St. Louis: Mosby.

Chomik, T. A. (2001). *The population health template: Key elements and actions that define a population health approach* (Discussion paper). Ottawa: Population and Public Health Branch.

Cody, W. K. (1995). Of life immense in passion, pulse, and power: Dialoguing with Whitman and Parse—A hermeneutic study. In R. R. Parse (Ed.), *Illuminations: The human becoming theory in practice and research* (pp. 269-307). New York: National League for Nursing Press.

de Witt, L., Ploeg, J., & Black, M. (2010). Living alone with dementia: An interpretive phenomenological study with older women. *Journal of Advanced Nursing, 66*(8), 1698-1707.

Erci I. B., Sayan, A., Tortumuoglu, G., Kilic, D., Sahub, O., & Güngörmus, Z. (2003). The effectiveness of Watson's caring model on the quality of life and blood pressure of patients with hypertension. *Journal of Advanced Nursing, 41*(2), 130-139.

Glaser, B. G., & Strauss, A. L. (1967). *The discovery of grounded theory: Strategies for qualitative research.* New York: Aldine.

Hamric, A. B., Spross, J. A., & Hanson, C. M. (2005). *Advanced nursing practice* (3rd ed.). Philadelphia: W. B. Saunders.

Liehr, P. (1992). Prelude to research. *Nursing Science Quarterly, 5*, 102-103.

Liehr, P., & Smith, M. J. (2000). Using story to guide nursing practice. *International Journal of Human Caring, 4*(2), 13-18.

Lincoln, Y., & Guba, E. (2000). Paradigmatic controversies, contradictions, and emerging confluences. In N. K. Denzin & Y. S. Lincoln (Eds.), *Handbook of qualitative research* (2nd ed., pp. 163-188). Thousand Oaks, CA: Sage.

Neuman, B. (Ed.). (1995). *The Neuman systems model* (3rd ed.). San Mateo, CA: Appleton & Lange.

Olson, J. (2006). Understanding paradigms used for nursing research. *Journal of Advanced Nursing, 53*, 459-469.

Parse, R. R. (1987). *Nursing science: Major paradigms, theories, and critiques.* Philadelphia: W. B. Saunders.

Parse, R. R. (2001). *Qualitative inquiry: The path of sciencing.* Sudbury, MA: Jones & Bartlett.

Parse, R. R. (2005). The human becoming modes of inquiry: Emerging sciencing. *Nursing Science Quarterly*, *18*, 297-300.

Smith, D., Edwards, N., Varcoe, C., Martens, P. J., & Davies, B. (2006). Bringing safety and responsiveness into the forefront of care for pregnant and parenting aboriginal people. *Advances in Nursing Science*, *29*(2), E27-E44.

Smith, M. J., & Liehr, P. (2003). *Middle range theory for nursing*. New York: Springer.

Stewart, M., Reutter, L., Letourneau, N., & Makwarimba, E. (2009). A support intervention to promote health and coping among homeless youths. *Canadian Journal of Nursing Research*, *41*(2), 54-77.

Weaver, K., & Olson, J. K. (2006). Understanding paradigms used for nursing research. *Journal of Advanced Nursing*, *53*(4), 459-469.

Zander, P. E. (2007). Ways of knowing in nursing: The historical evolution of a concept. *Journal of Theory Construction and Testing*, *11*(1), 7-11.

FOR FURTHER STUDY

⊖volve Go to Evolve at http://evolve.elsevier.com/Canada/LoBiondo/Research for Audio Glossary, how-to instructions for Writing Proposals for Funding, and additional research articles for practice in reviewing and critiquing.

CHAPTER 3

Critical Reading Strategies: Overview of the Research Process

Geri LoBiondo-Wood | Judith Haber | Cherylyn Cameron

LEARNING OUTCOMES

After reading this chapter, you will be able to do the following:

- Identify the steps that researchers use to conduct quantitative and qualitative research.
- Identify the importance of critical thinking and critical reading for the reading of research articles.
- Identify the steps associated with critical reading.
- Use the steps of critical reading to review research articles.
- Use identified strategies to critically read research articles.
- Use identified critical thinking and critical reading strategies to synthesize critiqued articles.
- Identify the format and style of research articles.

KEY TERMS

abstract	critical reading	critique
assumptions	critical thinking	critiquing criteria

STUDY RESOURCES

Go to Evolve at http://evolve.elsevier.com/Canada/LoBiondo/Research for Audio Glossary, how-to instructions for Writing Proposals for Funding, and additional research articles for practice in reviewing and critiquing.

AS YOU READ THIS TEXT, YOU will learn how the steps of the research process unfold. The steps are systematic and orderly, and they relate to the development of nursing knowledge. Understanding the step-by-step process that researchers use will help you develop the critiquing skills necessary to judge the soundness of research studies you will encounter in the literature. Throughout the chapters in this book, research terms pertinent to each step are identified, defined, and illustrated with many examples from the research literature. Four published research studies are featured in the appendixes, and they used as examples to illustrate significant points in each chapter. Judging not only a study's soundness but also evaluating a study's applicability to practice is a key skill.

Before you can judge a study, you need to understand the differences between and among studies. As you read the chapters and the appendixes, you will encounter many different study designs, as well as standards for critiquing the soundness of each step of a study and for judging both the strength of evidence provided by a study and its application to practice. The steps of the qualitative research process generally proceed in the order outlined in Table 3-1. Table 3-2 outlines the highlights of the general steps associated with quantitative research. Remember that a researcher may vary the steps slightly, depending on the nature of the research problem, but all of the steps should be addressed systematically.

This chapter provides an overview of critical thinking, critical reading, and critiquing skills. The chapter also introduces the overall format of a research article and provides an overview of subsequent chapters in the book. These components of the chapter are designed to help you read research articles more effectively and with greater understanding. You will learn about the research process so that you will be able to practise from a base of evidence to improve patient outcomes.

TABLE 3-1	
STEPS OF THE RESEARCH PROCESS AND JOURNAL FORMAT: QUALITATIVE RESEARCH	
RESEARCH PROCESS STEPS OR FORMAT ISSUES	**USUAL LOCATION IN JOURNAL HEADING OR SUBHEADING**
Identification of the phenomenon	In abstract, introduction, or both
Purpose of research study question	In abstract, at beginning or end of introduction, or in more than one of these locations
Literature review	In introduction, discussion, or both
Design	In abstract, "Introduction" section, "Methods" subsection titled "Design," "Methods" section in general, or more than one of these locations
Sample	In "Methods" subsection titled "Sample," "Subjects," or "Participants"
Legal-ethical issues	In section on data collection, in "Procedures" section, or in description of sample
Data-collection procedure	In "Data Collection" or "Procedures" section
Data analysis	In "Methods" subsection titled "Data Analysis" or "Data Analysis and Interpretation"
Results	In abstract (briefly), In separate section titled "Results" or "Findings"
Discussion and recommendation	In separate "Discussion" or "Discussion and Implications" section
References	At end of article

CRITICAL THINKING AND CRITICAL READING SKILLS

To develop an expertise in evidence-informed practice, you need to be able to critically read all types of research literature. As you read articles, you may notice the difference in style or format between research articles and theoretical or clinical articles. The terms in a research article may be new to you, and the focus of its content is different. Reading research articles can be difficult and frustrating at first, but the best way to become a knowledgeable consumer of research is to use

TABLE **3-2**

STEPS OF THE RESEARCH PROCESS AND JOURNAL FORMAT: QUANTITATIVE RESEARCH

RESEARCH PROCESS STEPS OR FORMAT ISSUES	USUAL LOCATION IN JOURNAL HEADING OR SUBHEADING
Research problem	In abstract, introduction (not labelled as a research problem), or separate subsection titled "Problem"
Purpose	In abstract or introduction, or both; at end of literature review or discussion of theoretical framework; or in separate section titled "Purpose"
Literature review	At end of introduction but not labelled as a literature review; in separate section titled "Literature Review," "Review of the Literature," or "Related Literature"
	Variables reviewed may appear as titles of sections or subsections
Theoretical framework, conceptual framework, or both	In "Literature Review" section (combined) or in separate sections titled "Theoretic Framework" and "Conceptual Framework"; or each concept or definition used in theoretical or conceptual framework may appear as title of separate section or subsection
Hypothesis/research questions	Stated or implied near end of "Introduction" section, which may be labelled; in separate sections or subsection titled "Hypothesis" or "Research Questions"; or, for first time, in "Results" section
Research design	In abstract or introduction (stated or implied) or in section titled "Methods" or "Methodology"
Sample: type and size	"Size": may be stated in abstract, in "Methods" section, or in separate "Methods" subsection as "Sample," "Sample/Subjects," or "Participants"
	"Type": may be implied or stated in any of previous headings described under size
Legal-ethical issues	In section titled "Methods," "Procedures," "Sample," "Subjects," or "Participants" (in all cases, stated or implied)
Instruments (measurement tools)	In section titled "Methods," "Instruments," or "Measures"
Validity and reliability	In section titled "Methods," "Instruments," "Measures," or "Procedures" (specifically stated or implied)
Data-collection procedure	In "Methods" subsection titled "Procedure" or "Data Collection" or in separate section titled "Procedure"
Data analysis	In "Methods" subsection under subheading "Procedure" or "Data Analysis"
Results	In separate section titled "Results"
Discussion of findings and new findings	Combined with results or in separate section titled "Discussion"
Implications, limitations, and recommendations	Combined with discussion or presented in separate or combined major sections
References	At end of article
Communicating research results	In research articles, poster, and paper presentations

critical thinking and critical reading skills when you read research articles. As a student, you are not expected to completely understand a research article. It is also understood that you will find it challenging to critique research articles until you obtain repeated experience doing so. Nor are you expected to develop critiquing skills on your own. An essential objective of this book is to help you acquire critical thinking and critical reading skills. No perfect critique exists; your interpretation will be based on your current knowledge, experience, and understanding. Remember that becoming a competent critical thinker and consumer of research, like learning the steps of the research process, takes time, patience, and experience.

Critical thinking is the rational examination of ideas, inferences, assumptions, principles, arguments, conclusions, issues, statements, beliefs, and actions (Paul & Elder, 2008). As applied to critically reading research, this means that you are engaged in the following:

- Systematic understanding of the research process
- Thinking that displays a mastery of the criteria for critiquing research and evidence-informed practice
- The art of being able to make your thinking better (i.e., clearer, more accurate, or more defensible) by clarifying what you understand and what you do not know

In other words, being a critical thinker means that you are consciously thinking about your own thoughts and what you say, write, read, or do, as well as what other people say, write, or do. While thinking about all of this, you are also questioning the appropriateness of the content, applying standards or criteria, and seeing how the information measures up.

Developing the ability to critically evaluate research articles requires both critical thinking skills and critical reading skills. **Critical reading** is "an active, intellectually engaging process in which the reader participates in an inner dialogue with the writer" (Paul & Elder, p. 461). A critical reader actively looks for **assumptions** (accepted truths), key concepts and ideas, reasons and justifications, supporting examples, parallel experiences, implications and consequences, and any other structured features of the text so as to interpret and assess the text accurately and fairly (Paul & Elder, 2008).

Critical reading is a process that involves the following levels of understanding and allows you to critically assess a study's validity:

Preliminary: familiarizing yourself with the content (skimming the article)

Comprehensive: understanding the researcher's purpose or intent

Analysis: understanding the parts of the study

Synthesis: understanding the whole article and each step of the research process in a study

Box 3-1 provides more in-depth strategies for attaining these levels of understanding.

BOX 3-1

HIGHLIGHTS OF CRITICAL READING PROCESS STRATEGIES

Photocopy the article to be critiqued, and make notations directly on the copy.

STRATEGIES FOR PRELIMINARY UNDERSTANDING

- Keep a research textbook and a dictionary by your side.
- Review the chapters in the textbook on the various steps of the research process.
- Highlight or underline on the photocopy any new terms, unfamiliar terms, and significant sentences.
- Look up the definitions of new terms, and write them on the photocopy.
- Highlight or underline identified steps of the research process.

STRATEGIES FOR COMPREHENSIVE UNDERSTANDING

- Identify the main idea or theme of the article; state it in your own words in one or two sentences.
- Continue to clarify terms that may be unclear on subsequent readings.
- Before critiquing the article, make sure you understand the main points of each reported step of the research process that you identified.

STRATEGIES FOR ANALYSIS UNDERSTANDING

- Using the critiquing criteria, determine how well the study meets the criteria for each step of the process.
- Determine which level of evidence fits the study.
- Write cues, relationships of concepts, and questions on the photocopy.
- Ask fellow students to analyze the same study, using the same criteria, and then compare their results with yours.
- Consult faculty members about your evaluation of the study.

STRATEGIES FOR SYNTHESIS UNDERSTANDING

- Review your notes on the article, and determine how each step discussed in the article compares with the critiquing criteria.
- In your own words, type a one-page summary of the reviewed study.
- Cite article references at the top according to the American Psychological Association (2010) style manual or another reference style.
- In your own words, and using the critiquing criteria, briefly summarize each reported research step.
- In your own words, briefly describe the study's strengths and weaknesses.

Critical thinking and critical reading skills can be further developed by learning the research process. You will find that critical thinking and critical reading skills used in the nursing process can be transferred to understanding the research process and reading research articles. You will gradually be able to read an entire research article and reflect on it by identifying and challenging assumptions, identifying key concepts, questioning methods, and determining whether the conclusions are based on the study's findings. Once you have obtained this competency in critiquing research, you will be ready to synthesize the findings of multiple research studies to use in developing evidence-informed practice.

Critiquing a research study requires several readings. At minimum, you should read it three or four times. The first strategy is to keep your research textbook at your side as you read. Using this book while you read a study may help you do the following:

- Identify the steps of the research process and how the study was conducted
- Clarify unfamiliar concepts or terms
- Question assumptions and rationale
- Assess the study for validity

As you analyze and synthesize an article, you are ready to begin the appraisal process that will help determine a study's worth. An illustration of how to use critical reading strategies is provided by the example in the Practical Application box, which contains excerpts from the abstract, introduction, literature review, theoretical framework literature, and "Methods" and "Procedure" sections of the quantitative study by Wong and associates (2010; see Appendix B). Note that this particular article contains both a literature review and a discussion of the theoretical framework that clearly supports the objectives and purpose of the study. Also note that in the Practical Application box, parts of the text of these sections from the article were deleted so that the examples could be as concise as possible.

Helpful Hint_____

If you still have difficulty understanding a research study after using the strategies related to skimming and comprehensive reading, make another copy of your marked-up research article, include your specific questions or area of difficulty, and ask your professor to read it. Comprehensive understanding and synthesis are necessary for analyzing a research article. Understanding the author's purpose and methods for the study reflects critical thinking and facilitates the evaluation of the study.

STRATEGIES FOR CRITIQUING RESEARCH STUDIES

The evaluation of a research article requires an appraisal or critique of the published study. The **critique** is the process of critical appraisal in which a person objectively and critically evaluates a research report's content for scientific validity or merit and application to practice. It requires some knowledge of the subject matter, as well as knowledge of how to read critically and use critiquing criteria. **Critiquing criteria** are the standards, appraisal guides, or questions used to judge (assess) an article. Guidelines for conducting a critique are presented in the following chapters of this book:

- General principles of qualitative and quantitative research in Chapters 1 through 6
- Criteria for critiques of qualitative research in Chapters 7 and 8
- In-depth exploration of criteria needed for evaluation of quantitative research in Chapters 9 through 11
- Exploration of critiquing criteria for the process related to research such as sampling, data collection, rigour, data analysis and presenting the findings in Chapters 12 through 17
- Summarized examples of critiquing criteria for qualitative studies and an example of a qualitative critique in Chapter 18
- Summarized critiquing criteria and examples of a quantitative critique in Chapter 19

Practical Application
EXAMPLE OF CRITICAL APPRAISAL READING STRATEGIES*

Introductory paragraphs, study's purpose and aims	Health care restructuring in the 1990s in Canada and the Unites States contributed to significant changes in 122 senior nurse leader (SNL) roles, including expansion of their decision-making responsibilities (Murray et al., 1998; Mass et al., 2006; Smith et al., 2006). In some organizations, nurse executives were added to senior executive teams, and in others, their scope of participation in organizational decisions related to budget, strategic planning, quality of care, and a host of challenging organizational issues greatly increased. However, surprisingly little is actually known about the patterns of SNL participation in decision-making (PDM) at the senior executive level of health care organizations and, in particular, the consequences of organizational changes on nurse executive decision-making. Our aim was to describe SNL decision-making processes in terms of the scope and degree of their involvement in strategic and tactical decisions at the executive management level in organizations across Canada.
Literature review: Concepts SNL role changes with restructuring SNL role in organizational decision-making	Substantial changes in the health care system have contributed to new role expectations, higher knowledge requirements, and increased responsibility and accountability for nurse leaders, including: quality and effective coordination of patient services; managing many clinical areas with a broadened span of control; operating merged facilities and decentralized structures; and decision-making in finance, human resources and quality and safety of patient services across the continuum of care (Anthony et al., 2005; Arnold et al., 2006; Duffield et al., 2001; Kleinman, 2003; Upenieks, 2003). Of the published literature on nurse leader decision-making, there is little coherence in topics such as risk propensity (Smith & Friedland, 1998), ethical decision-making (Berggren & Severinsson, 2003; Fonville, 2002), manager role in facilitating staff participation in decision-making (Krairiksh, 2000), middle manager involvement in organizational strategic decision-making (Ashmos et al., 1998) and personality type and decision-making styles (Freund, 1988). Only a small body of research focused on SNLs' organizational decision-making influence (Dwore et al., 2000; Havens, 1998; Banaszak-Holl et al., 1999; Wangsness, 1991).
Theoretical framework	In our framework, PDM...by SNLs in executive management teams is viewed as creating new organizational connections and mechanisms for exchanging information and enriching interpretation of issues that ultimately influence the quality of management decisions. The scope of decision-making is enhanced by involving SNLs at the beginning of decision-making stages (timing), and the breadth of content expertise is expanded by their clinical and professional knowledge. The intensity of PDM is a function of the number and range of decision-making activities involving SNLs. Any decision-making process entails several different fundamental information processing actions from raising issues, clarifying problems, generating and evaluating solutions to making a final choice (Anderson & McDaniel, 1999). The greater the scope and intensity of SNL PDM, the greater the likelihood that they and others perceive them as having an influence on decisions. Last, we propose that decision-making influence is related to the quality of final management decisions reached.
Hypothesis	1) The scope (timing and breadth) and intensity (number of decision activities) of SNL participation in executive decision-making processes positively predicts the degree of SNL decision influence. 2) SNL decision influence positively predicts perceived quality of operational management decisions.
Design	Data were collected by mailed survey from 63 SNLs and 49 chief executive officers (CEOs) in 66 health care organizations in 10 Canadian provinces.
Instrument	We used the Participation in Strategic Decision-Making Scale (Banaszak-Holl et al., 1999) to measure SNL decision-making processes.

*For references cited in this box, please see Appendix B.
Adapted from Wong, C. A., Laschinger, H., Cummings, G. G., Vincent, L., & O'Connor, P. (2010). Decisional involvement of senior nurse leaders in Canadian acute care hospitals. *Journal of Nursing Management, 18,* 122-133.

In analyzing a research report, you must evaluate each step of the research process and ask whether each step of the process meets the criteria. For instance, the critiquing criteria in Chapter 5 (p. 109) are as follows: The literature review identifies gaps and inconsistencies in the literature about a subject, concept, or problem; and all of the concepts and variables are included in the review. These two criteria relate to critiquing the research question and the literature review components of the research process. The Practical Application box shows several examples in which Wong and associates (2010) identified gaps in the literature and how they intended to fill these gaps by conducting a study for the stated objective and purpose (see Appendix B for the complete study). Remember that when you are doing a critique, you are pointing out strengths, as well as weaknesses. Developing critical reading skills will enable you to complete a critique successfully. To review the appraisal strategies that facilitate the understanding gained by reading for analysis, see Box 3-1. Standardized critical appraisal tools, such as the Critical Appraisal Skills Programme (CASP; http://www.phru.nhs.uk/Pages/PHD/CASP.htm), can also be used by students and clinicians to systematically appraise the strength and quality of evidence provided in research articles (see Chapter 20).

Critiquing can be thought of as looking at a completed jigsaw puzzle. Does it form a comprehensive picture, or is a piece out of place? What is the level of evidence provided by the study and its findings? What is the balance between the risks and benefits of the findings that contribute to clinical decisions? How can the evidence be applied in the treatment of a patient or a patient population or in a specific setting? In the case of reading several studies for synthesis, you need to consider how interrelated each of the studies are and determine the overall strength and quality of evidence and its applicability to practice. Reading for synthesis is essential in critiquing research studies.

OVERCOMING BARRIERS: USEFUL CRITIQUING STRATEGIES

Throughout this text, you will find special features that will help refine and develop your competence as a research consumer. A *critical thinking decision path* related to each step of the research process will sharpen your decision-making skills as you critique research articles. Look for *Internet* resources in chapters that will enhance your research consumer skills. *Critical thinking challenges*, which appear at the end of each chapter, are designed to reinforce your critical thinking and critical reading skills in relation to the steps of the research process. *Helpful hints*, designed to reinforce your understanding and critical thinking, appear at various points throughout the chapters. *Evidence-informed practice tips*, which will help you apply evidence-informed practice strategies in your clinical practice, are also provided in each chapter. Finally, *Practical Application boxes* offer examples of translating principles and methods of nursing research into real-life nursing situations and interventions.

Once you complete a research critique or two, you will be ready to discuss your critique with your fellow students and professor. Best of all, you can enjoy discussing the points of your appraisal because your critique will be based on objective data, not just personal opinion. As you continue to use and perfect critical analysis skills by critiquing studies, remember that these very skills are an expected clinical competency for delivering evidence-informed nursing care.

EVIDENCE-INFORMED PRACTICE AND RESEARCH

Along with gaining confidence while reading and critiquing research studies, you must undertake a final step of reading and appraising the research literature: deciding how, when, and whether to apply a study or studies to your practice so that your practice is evidence informed. Evidence-informed practice allows you to systematically use the best available evidence with the integration of individual clinical expertise, as well as the patient's values and preferences, in making clinical decisions (Sackett, Straus, Richardson, Rosenburg, & Hayes, 2000). Evidence-informed practice has processes and steps that are followed, as does the research process. These steps are presented throughout the text.

When you use evidence-informed practice strategies, the first step is to be able to read a research article and understand how each section is linked to each step of the research process. The

following section introduces you to the steps of the research process as presented in published articles.

Once you read an article, you will need to decide which level of evidence a research article provides and how well the study was designed and executed. Figure 3-1 depicts a model for determining the levels of evidence associated with the design of a study, ranging from systematic reviews of randomized clinical trials to expert opinions. The rating system or evidence hierarchy model presented here is just one of many. Many

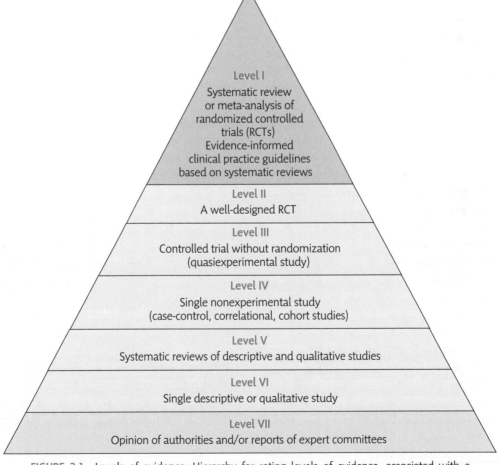

FIGURE 3-1 Levels of evidence: Hierarchy for rating levels of evidence, associated with a study's design. Evidence is assessed at a level according to its source.
From Melnyk, B. M., & Fincoult-Overholt, E. (2005). *Evidence-based practice in nursing & literature:* A guide to best practice. Philadelphia, PA: Lippincott, Williams & Wilkins.

hierarchies for assessing the relative worth of different types of research literature for both the qualitative and quantitative research literature are available.

You will note from Figure 3-1 that research evidence is traditionally categorized from weakest to strongest, with an emphasis on support for the effectiveness of interventions. The concept of levels of evidence tends to dominate the evidence-informed practice literature, rendering unclear the merit of qualitative studies. Chapter 2 suggests that different research methods provide different types and levels of evidence, all of which inform practice.

Although evidence provided by qualitative studies seems to rank lower in the hierarchy of evidence presented (that is, levels V and VI), Sandelowski (2004) noted that hierarchies are used under the assumption that randomized clinical trials are the "gold standard" of research; this assumption devalues qualitative research. However, qualitative research has increased and thrived over the years. Thousands of reports of well-conducted qualitative studies exist on topics such as (1) personal and cultural constructions of disease, prevention, treatment, and risk; (2) living with disease and managing the physical, psychological, and social effects of multiple diseases and their treatment; (3) decision-making experiences with beginning and end of life, as well as assistive and life-extending, technological interventions; and (4) contextual factors favouring and mitigating against quality care, health promotion, prevention of disease, and reduction of health disparities (Sandelowski, 2004). The answers provided by qualitative data reflect important evidence that may offer valuable insights about a particular phenomenon, patient population, or clinical situation. It is important to remember that researchers, in choosing which research methodology to use, base their decision primarily on the question they are trying to answer.

The meaningfulness of an evidence rating system will become clearer to you as you read the chapters on quantitative research. For example, Wong and associates' (2010) study (see Appendix B) is level IV because of its descriptive design, whereas the study by Seneviratne and colleagues (2009; see Appendix A) is level VI because of its qualitative design. Remember, as discussed earlier, that the level by itself does not reveal the full worth of a study but is another tool that helps you think about the strengths and weaknesses of a study and the nature of the evidence provided in the findings and conclusions. The chapters on qualitative research provide an understanding of how qualitative studies can be assessed for use in practice. You will use the evidence hierarchy presented in Figure 3-1 throughout the book as you develop your research consumer skills, and so it is important to become familiar with its content.

This rating system represents an evidence hierarchy for judging the strength of a study's design, which is just one level of assessment that influences how confident the reader is about the conclusions drawn by the researcher. Assessing the strength of scientific evidence or potential research bias provides a vehicle to guide nurses in evaluating research studies for their applicability in clinical decision-making. In addition to identifying the level of evidence needed to grade the strength of a body of evidence, there are the three domains of quality, quantity, and consistency (Agency for Healthcare Research and Quality, 2002):

- *Quality:* the extent to which a study's design, implementation, and analysis minimizes bias
- *Quantity:* the number of studies in which the research question has been evaluated, including overall sample size across studies, as well as the strength of the findings from the data analyses
- *Consistency:* the degree to which similar findings are reported from investigations of the same research question in studies that have similar and different designs

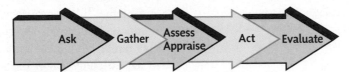

FIGURE 3-2   Evidence-informed practice steps.

Evidence-informed practice has specific processes and steps that are followed, as does the research process. The steps of the process are to ask, gather, assess and appraise, act, and evaluate (Figure 3-2). Chapter 20 provides an overview of evidence-informed practice and introduces you to the steps and strategies associated with evidence-informed practice.

RESEARCH ARTICLES: FORMAT AND STYLE

Before you consider reading research articles, it is important to have a sense of their organization and format. Many journals publish either only research articles or research in addition to clinical or theoretical articles. Although many journals have some common features, they also have unique characteristics. All journals have guidelines for manuscript preparation and submission; these guidelines are published by each journal. A review of these guidelines will give you an idea of the format of articles that appear in specific journals.

It is important to remember that even though each step of the research process is discussed at length in this text, you may find only a short paragraph or a sentence in the research article that gives the details of the step in a specific study. Because of the journal's publishing guidelines, the published study that appears in a journal is a shortened version of the complete work carried out by the researcher or researchers. You will also find that some researchers devote more space in an article to the results, whereas others present a longer discussion of the methods and procedures. Since the 1990s, most authors have given more

emphasis to the method, results, and discussion of implications than to the details of assumptions, hypotheses, or definitions of terms. Decisions about the amount of material presented for each step of the research process are constrained by the following:

- A journal's space limitations
- A journal's author guidelines
- The type or nature of the study
- An individual researcher's evaluation of what is the most important component of the study

The following discussion provides a brief overview of each step of the research process and how it might appear in an article (refer to Tables 3-1 and 3-2). It is important to remember that the format of a quantitative research article will differ from that of a qualitative research article.

Abstract

An **abstract** is a short, comprehensive synopsis or summary of a study at the beginning of an article. An abstract quickly focuses the reader on the main points of a study. A well-presented abstract is accurate, self-contained, concise, specific, nonevaluative, coherent, and readable.

Abstracts vary in length from 50 to 250 words. The length and format of an abstract are dictated by the journal's style. Both quantitative and qualitative research studies have abstracts that provide a succinct overview of the study. An example of an abstract can be found at the beginning of the study by Sobieraj and colleagues (2009; see Appendix C). Their abstract follows an outline format that highlights the major steps of the study. It reads in part as follows:

The purpose of this quasi-experimental study was to test an intervention on the use of music during simple laceration repair to promote parent-led distraction in children aged 1 to 5.

The remainder of the abstract provides a synopsis of the background of the study and the methods, results, and conclusions. All of the other studies in the appendixes have abstracts.

 Helpful Hint _____

A journal abstract is usually a single paragraph that provides a general reference to the research purpose, research questions, or hypothesis, or a combination of these aspects, and highlights the methodology and results, as well as the implications for future practice or research.

Introduction

Early in a research article, in a section that may or may not be titled "Introduction," the researcher presents a background picture of the area researched and its significance to practice. In the study by Thorne and associates (2009; see Appendix D) on communication during the cancer diagnostic period, the reader can find the basis of the research question early in the report:

Although it is well known that communication will have a strong impact on both the experience and psychosocial outcomes of cancer . . . poor communication remains a significant problem facing cancer patients across the spectrum of service. . . . In part, this is because of the complexity of communication and the variability of the human experience of cancer, both of which create significant challenges for the development of a solid empirical science within this field.

Another example is found in the study by Seneviratne and associates (2009; see Appendix A):

Nurses have long believed that they play an essential role in stroke care, but they remain uncertain about the nature of their contributions.

Definition of the Purpose

The purpose of the study is defined either at the end of the researcher's initial introduction or at the end of the "Literature Review" or "Conceptual Framework" section. The study's purpose may or may not be labelled as such, or it may be referred to as the study's aim or objective. Thorne and associates (2009; see Appendix D) described the purpose of the study in the last paragraph in the section on background to the literature:

The general problem that this article addresses is the continuing prevalence of poor communication during the diagnostic window of time within the cancer experience. Specifically, we report findings associated with those communication encounters that patients experience as problematic during the diagnostic period within the context of a longitudinal cohort study of patient perspectives of cancer communication across the illness trajectory.

In contrast, Seneviratne and colleagues (2009) had a section titled "Aim" (see Appendix A):

The aim of the study was to uncover nurses' perceptions of the contexts of caring for acute stroke survivors.

In a section titled "Purpose," Sobieraj and colleagues (2009) stated, "The purpose of this study was to test an intervention [by] using children's songs to promote parent-led distraction during simple laceration repair in children aged 1 to 5" (see Appendix C).

Literature Review and Theoretical Framework

Authors of studies and journal articles present the literature review and theoretical framework in different ways. In many research articles, the literature review is merged with the discussion of the theoretical framework. The resulting section includes the main concepts investigated and may be titled "Review of the Literature," "Literature Review," "Theoretical Framework," "Related Literature," "Background," or "Conceptual Framework"; or it may not be a separate section at all. In reviewing Appendixes A through D, you will find differences in the headings used. Wong and associates (2010) had both a "Literature

Review" and a "Theoretical Framework" section (see Appendix B); in the articles in Appendixes A and D, headings that reflect the theoretical concepts of the study were used in the "Background" sections, but the authors did not call such discussion a literature review or a framework. Finally, Appendix C has a "Literature Review" section. One style is not better than another; all of the studies in the appendixes contain all of the critical elements but present the elements differently.

Hypothesis or Research Question

A study's research questions or hypotheses can also be presented in different ways. Research reports in journals often do not have separate headings for reporting the "Hypotheses" or "Research Question." They are often embedded in the "Introduction" or "Background" section or not labelled at all (e.g., as in the studies in the appendixes). Quantitative research studies have hypotheses or research questions. If a researcher uses hypotheses in a study, the researcher may report whether the hypotheses were or were not supported; such reporting occurs toward the end of the article, in the "Results" or "Findings" section. Wong and associates (2010; see Appendix B) list the hypotheses in a section titled "Hypotheses," and Sobieraj and colleagues (2009; see Appendix C) discuss the hypothesis in the "Purpose" section. Qualitative research studies do not have hypotheses but do have research questions and purposes.

Research Design

The type of research design can be found in the abstract, within the purpose statement, or in the introduction to the "Procedures" or "Methods" section, or it may not be stated at all. For example, the studies in Appendixes A, B, C, and D all identify the design type in both the abstract and the body of the study report.

One of your first objectives is to determine whether the study is qualitative or quantitative so that the appropriate criteria are used. Although

the rigour of the critiquing criteria addressed does not substantially change, some of the terminology of the questions differs for qualitative and quantitative studies. For instance, in regard to the study by Wong and associates (2010; see Appendix B), you might ask whether the hypotheses were generated from the theoretical framework or literature review and whether the design chosen was appropriate and consistent with the study's questions and purpose. With a qualitative study such as that by Thorne and associates (2009; see Appendix D), however, you might be asking whether the researchers conducted the study in a manner consistent with the principles of qualitative research and therefore focused on the identification of the themes of knowledge and choice.

Do not get discouraged if you cannot easily determine the design. More often than not, the specific design is not stated or, if an advanced design is used, the details are not spelled out. One of the best strategies is to review the chapters in this text that address designs and to ask your professors for assistance. The following tips will help you determine whether the study you are reading employs a quantitative design:

- Hypotheses are stated or implied.
- The terms *control* and *treatment group* appear.
- The term *survey, correlational,* or *ex post facto* is used.
- The term *random* or *convenience* is mentioned in relation to the sample.
- Variables are measured by instruments or scales.
- Reliability and validity of instruments are discussed.
- Statistical analyses are used.

In contrast, qualitative studies do not usually focus on "numbers." In some articles about qualitative studies, standard quantitative terms (e.g., *subjects*) may be used rather than qualitative terms (e.g., *informants* or *participants*). Deciding on the type of qualitative design can be confusing; one of the best strategies is to review this text's chapters on qualitative design, as well as to critique qualitative studies. Begin trying to link the study's design with the level of evidence associated with that design as illustrated in Figure 3-1. This will give you a context for evaluating the strength and consistency of the findings and their applicability to practice. Although many studies may not specify the particular design used, all studies inform the reader of the specific methodology used, which can help you decide the type of design used to guide the study.

Sampling

The population from which the sample was drawn is discussed in the section titled "Methods" or "Methodology" under the subheadings of "Subjects," "Participants," or "Sample." For example, Seneviratne and colleagues (2009) discuss the sample in a section titled "Participants and Setting" that was separate from "Methodology" (see Appendix A). However, Thorne and associates (2009) present the sample selection criteria in a section titled "Study Method" (see Appendix D). Researchers should describe both the population from which the sample was chosen and the number of participants who took part in the study, and they should also mention whether participants dropped out of the study. The authors of all of the studies in the appendixes discuss their samples in enough detail so that who the participants were and how they were selected are quite clear.

Reliability and Validity

The discussion related to instruments used to measure the variables of a study is usually included in a "Methods" subsection titled "Instruments" or "Measures." The researcher usually describes the particular measure (i.e., instrument or scale) used by discussing its reliability and validity. Wong and associates (2010; see Appendix B) describe the reliability of the instrument to measure participation in decision making in a "Methods" subsection titled "Instrument."

Helpful Hint

Remember that not all research articles include headings related to each step or component of the research process, but each step is presented at some point in the article.

In some cases, researchers do not report the reliability and validity of commonly used, established instruments in an article and may refer you to other references. Ask for assistance from your instructor if you are in doubt about the validity or reliability of a study's instruments. Qualitative researchers typically report on the validity of the findings and on how potential biases are acknowledged and worked with (see Chapter 7). For example, Seneviratne and colleagues (2009; see Appendix A) described how they dealt with potential biases in a section titled "Reflexivity."

Procedures and Data-Collection Methods

The procedures used to collect data or the step-by-step way in which the researcher used the measures (instruments or scales) is generally described in the "Procedures" section. In each of the studies in Appendixes A through D, the researchers indicated how they conducted the study in detail in subsections titled "Data Collection," "Sample and Data Collection Procedures," and "Study Method." Notice that the researchers in each study in Appendixes A through D also stated that the studies were approved by an institutional review board (see Chapter 6), thereby ensuring that each met ethical standards.

Data Analysis/Results

The data analysis procedures (i.e., the statistical tests used and the results of descriptive and inferential tests applied in quantitative studies) are presented in the section titled "Results" or "Findings." Although qualitative studies do not involve the use of statistical tests, the procedures for analyzing the themes, concepts, and observational or print data are usually described in the "Methods" or "Data Collection" section and reported in the "Results," "Findings," or "Data Analysis" section. Seneviratne and colleagues (2009) reported on the methods of qualitative data analysis in their "Data Analysis" section and the results of their analysis in their "Findings" sections (see Appendix A). The article by Wong and associates (2010) has several sections, one titled "Data Analysis," which describes how the data were analyzed, and four subsections under "Results," which describe the results of the hypotheses tested (see Appendix B).

Discussion

The last part of an article about a research study is the "Discussion" section. In this section, the researchers explain how all of the parts of the study are related and analyze the study as a whole. The researchers refer to the literature reviewed and discuss how their study is similar to or different from other studies. Researchers may report the results and discussion in one section but usually report their results in separate "Results" and "Discussion" sections (see Appendixes A, B, C, and D). One way is not better than another. Journal and space limitations determine how these sections are handled. Any new findings or unexpected findings are usually described in the "Discussion" section.

Recommendations and Implications

In some articles, a separate section titled "Conclusions" describes the implications of the findings for practice and education, as well as related limitations based on the findings, and future studies may be recommended (see Appendixes A, B, and D); in other articles, this information appears in several sections with such titles as "Discussion," "Limitations," "Nursing Implications," "Implications for Research and Practice," and "Summary." Sobieraj and colleagues (2009; see Appendix C) concluded their study with a discussion subsection titled "Practice Recommendations." Again, one way is not better than another—only different.

References

All of the references cited in a research article are included at the end of the article. The main purpose of the reference list is to support the material presented by identifying the sources in a manner that allows for easy retrieval by the reader. Journals have various referencing styles to organize references.

Communicating Results

Communicating the results of a study can take the form of a research article, poster, or paper presentation. All are valid ways of providing nurses with the data and the ability to provide high-quality patient care that is based on research findings. Evidence-informed nursing care plans and practice protocols, guidelines, or standards are outcome measures that effectively indicate communicated research.

As you develop critical thinking and reading skills by using the strategies presented in this chapter, you will become more familiar with the research and appraisal processes. Your ability to read and critique research articles will gradually improve. You will be well on your way to becoming a knowledgeable user of research from nursing and other scientific disciplines for application in nursing practice.

Helpful Hint

When writing a paper on a specific concept or topic that requires you to critique and synthesize the findings from several studies, you might find it useful to create an evidence table of the data. Include the following information: author, date, type of study, design, level of evidence, sample, data analysis, findings, and implications.

SYSTEMATIC REVIEWS: META-ANALYSES, INTEGRATIVE REVIEWS, AND META-SYNTHESES

Another variety of articles that is appearing more frequently in the literature and is very important for understanding evidence-informed practice are systematic reviews. Systematic reviews include meta-analyses, integrative reviews, and meta-syntheses. The authors of these articles investigate a number of studies related to a specific clinical question and, using a specific set of criteria and methods, evaluate those articles as a whole. The methods detailed here are not prescriptive but serve as a general outline of how you will find these articles formatted. Overall, although they vary somewhat in their approach, these reviews are intended, in essence, to better inform practice and develop evidence-informed practice.

The components of these types of articles are as follows:

- *Background:* The introduction covers content related to the background of the clinical question and clarifies the specific question that the review answers. The article's authors clarify the definitions of the concepts in the question so that the reader understand the concepts that were used in assessment.
- *Method:* The methods used for searching the literature are detailed. The exact electronic databases, the dates, and the key words used to conduct the search are provided. In addition, the article details the inclusion and exclusion criteria by which the literature was chosen to review and critique. If a number of articles were found and not used, the authors detail why articles were excluded from the review.
- *Appraisal of the literature:* The articles that are included in the literature review are discussed in the body of the article, and an evidence table is used to present the highlights of each article. The author uses the evidence table to compare and contrast the articles, critique them for scientific validity, and discuss how well they answer the clinical question. If the author uses a meta-analysis format, a summary of the data is presented.
- *Conclusions/summary:* In the conclusions or summary, the strength, quality, and consistency of the data are described as they apply to practice. This section contains recommendations about which aspects of practice are supported by the data in the articles and for which aspects further research is needed to more fully answer the question posed in the review.

For example, Purc-Stephenson and Thrasher (2010) reviewed qualitative studies on telephone triage and advice (1) to understand nurses' experiences with telephone triage and advice and (2) to identify factors that facilitate or impeded the nurses' decision-making processes. In searching the peer-reviewed research literature databases from 1980 to 2008, the authors found 144 potential studies. After the inclusion criteria were applied (to determine which studies were relevant) and a quality appraisal review, 16 studies were chosen for the final sample. Each of the reviewers then extracted key themes from each of the studies and then compared them with one another. Once the themes were refined, the researchers synthesized the findings to identify new interpretations.

CLINICAL GUIDELINES

Clinical guidelines are systematically developed statements or recommendations that serve as a guide for practitioners. Guidelines have been developed to assist in bridging practice and research. Guidelines are developed by professional organizations, government agencies, institutions, and convened expert panels. Guidelines provide clinicians with an algorithm for clinical management or for decision making with regard to specific diseases (e.g., colon cancer) or treatments (e.g., pain management). Not all guidelines are well developed and, like research, must be assessed before implementation. Clinical guidelines, although they are systematically developed and make explicit recommendations for practice, may be formatted differently. Guidelines should clearly present scope and purpose of the practice, detail who contributed to the development of the guidelines, demonstrate scientific rigour, demonstrate clinical applicability, and demonstrate editorial independence. The Appraisal of Guidelines Research and Evaluation (AGREE; http://www.agreecollaboration.org) has developed an instrument for assessing the quality of clinical guidelines.

As you venture through this textbook, you will be challenged to think about not only reading and understanding research studies but also applying the findings to your practice. Nursing has a rich legacy of research that has grown in depth and breadth. Producers of research and clinicians must engage in a joint effort to translate findings into practice that will make a difference in the care of patients and families.

CRITICAL THINKING CHALLENGES

- The critical reading of research articles may require a minimum of three or four readings. Is this always the case? What assumptions underlie this claim?
- Why is it necessary to reach an analysis stage of critical reading before you can critique a study?
- To synthesize a research article, what questions must you first be able to answer?
- If registered nurses are not expected to conduct research, how can nursing students be expected to critique each step of the nursing process, an entire study, or several studies?
- Discuss several strategies that might motivate practising nurses to critically appraise research articles.
- What level of evidence is presented in each of the articles that appear in Appendixes A, B, C, and D? Justify your answers.

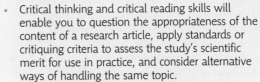

KEY POINTS

- Critical thinking and critical reading skills will enable you to question the appropriateness of the content of a research article, apply standards or critiquing criteria to assess the study's scientific merit for use in practice, and consider alternative ways of handling the same topic.
- Critical reading involves active interpretation and objective assessment of an article and searching for key concepts, ideas, and justifications.
- Critical reading requires four stages of understanding: preliminary (skimming), comprehensive, analysis, and synthesis. Each stage is characterized by specific strategies to increase your critical reading skills.
- Critically reading for preliminary understanding is accomplished by skimming or quickly and lightly reading an article in order to familiarize yourself with its content and to provide you with a general sense of the material.
- Critically reading for a comprehensive understanding is designed to increase your understanding both of the concepts and research terms in relation to the context and of the parts of the study in relation to the whole study, as presented in the article.
- Critically reading for analysis understanding is designed to divide the content into parts so that each part of the study is understood. The critiquing process begins at this stage.
- Critical reading to reach the goal of synthesis understanding combines the parts of a research study into a whole. During this final stage, the reader determines how each step of the research process relates to all the other steps, how well the study meets the critiquing criteria, and the usefulness of the study for practice.
- Critiquing is the process of objectively and critically evaluating the strengths and weaknesses of a research article for scientific merit and application to practice, theory, and education. The need for more research on the topic or clinical problem is also addressed at this stage.
- Each article should be reviewed for level of evidence as a means of judging the application of the findings to practice.
- Research articles have different formats and styles, depending on journal manuscript requirements and whether they are quantitative or qualitative studies.
- The basic steps of the research process are presented in journal articles in various ways. Detailed examples of such variations can be found in chapters throughout this text.
- Evidence-informed practice begins with the careful reading and understanding of research articles.

REFERENCES

Agency for Healthcare Research and Quality. (2002). *Systems to rate the strength of scientific evidence* (File inventory, Evidence Report/Technology Assessment No. 47, AHRQ Publication No. 02-E016). Rockville, MD: Author.

American Psychological Association. (2010). *Publication manual of the American Psychological Association* (6th ed.). Washington, DC: Author.

Paul, R., & Elder, L. (2008). *The miniature guide to critical thinking concepts and tools*. Dillon Beach, CA: Foundation for Critical Thinking Press.

Purc-Stephenson, R. J., & Thrasher, C. (2010). Telephone triage and advice: A meta-ethnography. *Journal of Advanced Nursing, 66*(3), 482-494. doi: 10.1111/j.1365-2648.2010.05275.x

Sackett, D. L., Straus, S. E., Richardson, W. S., Rosenburg, W., & Hayes, R. B. (2000). *Evidence-based medicine: How to practise and teach EBM*. London: Churchill Livingstone.

Sandelowski, M. (2004). Using qualitative research. *Qualitative health research, 14*(10), 1366-1386.

Seneviratne, C. C., Mather, C. M., & Then, K. L. (2009). Understanding nursing on an acute stroke unit: Perceptions of space, time and interprofessional practice. *Journal of Advanced Nursing, 65*(9), 1872-1881. doi: 10.1111/j.1365-2648.2009.05053.x

Sobieraj, G., Bhatt, M., LeMay, S., Rennick, J., & Johnston, C. (2009). The effect of music on parental participation during pediatric laceration repair. *Canadian Journal of Nursing Research, 41*(4), 68-82.

Thorne, S., Armstrong, E., Harris, S. R., Hislop, T. G., Kim-Sing, C., Oglova, V., . . . Stajduhar, K. L. (2009). Patient real-time and 12-month retrospective perceptions of difficult communications in the cancer diagnostic period. *Qualitative Health Research, 19*(10), 1983-1394. doi: 10.1177/1049732.309348382

Wong, C. A., Laschinger, H., Cummings, G. G., Vincent, L., & O'Connor, P. (2010). Decisional involvement of senior nurse leaders in Canadian acute care hospitals. *Journal of Nursing Management, 18*, 122-133. doi: 10.1111/j.1365-2834.2010.01053.x

FOR FURTHER STUDY

ⓔvolve   Go to Evolve at http://evolve.elsevier.com/Canada/LoBiondo/Research for Audio Glossary, how-to instructions for Writing Proposals for Funding, and additional research articles for practice in reviewing and critiquing.

CHAPTER 4

Developing Research Questions, Hypotheses, and Clinical Questions

Judith Haber | Cherylyn Cameron

LEARNING OUTCOMES

After reading this chapter, you will be able to do the following:

- Discuss the purpose of developing a research question.
- Describe how the research question and hypothesis are related to the other components of the research process.
- Describe the process of identifying and refining a research question.
- Identify the criteria for determining the significance of a research question.
- Discuss the appropriate use of the purpose, aim, or objective of a research study.
- Discuss how the purpose, research question, and hypothesis suggest which level of evidence is to be obtained from the findings of a research study.
- Identify the characteristics of research questions and hypotheses.
- Describe the advantages and disadvantages of directional and nondirectional hypotheses.
- Compare the use of statistical hypotheses with that of research hypotheses.
- Discuss the appropriate use of research questions versus hypotheses in a research study.
- Discuss the differences between a research question and a clinical question in relation to evidence-informed practice.
- Identify the criteria used for critiquing a research question and a hypothesis.
- Apply the critiquing criteria to the evaluation of a research question and a hypothesis in a research report.

KEY TERMS

clinical question	nondirectional hypothesis	research question
dependent variable	population	statistical hypothesis
directional hypothesis	problem statement	testability
hypothesis	purpose	testable
independent variable	research hypothesis	variable

STUDY RESOURCES

Go to Evolve at http://evolve.elsevier.com/Canada/LoBiondo/Research for Audio Glossary, how-to instructions for Writing Proposals for Funding, and additional research articles for practice in reviewing and critiquing.

AS YOU READ EACH CHAPTER, REMEMBER that each step of the research process is defined and discussed as to how that particular step relates to evidence-informed practice. All research studies begin with questions and/or hypotheses. The first step in developing evidence-informed practice is also to ask a question, but it is a clinical question. The purpose of research questions and hypotheses in a research study discussed in the beginning of this chapter are different from those of the clinical questions found in a project concerning evidence-informed practice. In a research study, the research question and hypothesis lead to the development of a research study, whereas in a project on evidence-informed practice, the clinical question is what leads to the study. At the beginning of this chapter, you will learn about research questions and hypotheses from the perspective of the researcher, which, in the second part of this chapter, will help you to generate your own clinical questions that you will use to guide the development of evidence-informed practice projects. From a clinician's perspective, you must understand how the research question and hypothesis align with the rest of the study. In your role as a practising nurse, the clinical questions you will develop (see Chapter 20) represent the first step of the evidence-informed practice process.

When nurses ask certain questions, they are often well on their way to developing a research question or hypothesis. Such questions include "What is happening in this situation?"; "What are the patient's experiences?"; "Why are things being done this way?"; "I wonder what would happen if . . . ?"; "What characteristics are associated with . . . ?"; and "What is the effect of . . . on patient outcomes?" Research questions are usually generated from situations or problems that emerge from practice. These are often articulated in a **problem statement** such as the following, posed by Thorne and associates (2009): "The general problem that this article addresses is the continuing prevalence of poor communication during the diagnostic window of time within the cancer experience" (see Appendix D).

For an investigator conducting a study, the research question or the hypothesis is a key preliminary step in the research process. The **research question** presents the idea that is to be examined in the study and is the foundation of the research study. Once the research question is clear, the researcher selects the most appropriate research design. If the research question is primarily explorative, descriptive, or theory generating, the researcher opts for qualitative methods. In these studies, a hypothesis is not formulated. For studies in which the researcher is seeking a specific answer to a research question, however, a hypothesis is generated and tested.

Hypotheses can be considered intelligent hunches, guesses, or predictions that help researchers seek the solution or answer to the research question. Hypotheses are a vehicle for testing the validity of the theoretical framework assumptions and provide a bridge between theory and actuality. In the scientific world, researchers derive hypotheses from theories and subject them to empirical testing. A theory's validity is not directly examined. Instead, through testing hypotheses, researchers can evaluate the merit of a theory.

For a clinician making an evidence-informed decision about a patient care issue, a clinical question—such as whether chlorhexidine or povidone-iodine is more effective in preventing infections in central catheters—would guide the nurse in searching for and retrieving the best available evidence. This evidence, combined with clinical expertise and patient preferences, would provide an answer on which to base the most effective decision about patient care for the affected population.

Research questions or hypotheses often appear at the beginning of research articles. However, because of space constraints or stylistic considerations in journal publications, the research question or hypothesis may be embedded in the purpose, aims, goals, or even the results section of the research report. Both the consumer and the producer of research need to understand the importance of research questions and hypotheses as the foundational elements of a research study. This chapter provides methods of developing research questions and hypotheses, the standards for writing them, and a set of criteria for evaluating them. It also highlights the importance of clinical questions and how to develop them.

DEVELOPING AND REFINING A RESEARCH QUESTION: STUDY PERSPECTIVE

A researcher spends a great deal of time refining a research idea or problem into a research question. Unfortunately, the evaluator of a research study is not privy to this creative process because it occurs during the study's conceptualization. The final research question usually does not appear in the research article unless the study is qualitative rather than quantitative. Although this section does not teach you how to formulate a research question, it does provide an important glimpse into the researcher's process of developing a research question.

Research questions or topics do not arise spontaneously. As shown in Table 4-1, research questions should indicate that practical experience, critical appraisal of the scientific literature, or interest in an untested theory was the basis for the generation of a research idea. The research question should reflect a refinement of the researcher's initial thinking. The evaluator of a nursing research study should be able to discern that the researcher has done the following:

1. Defined a specific topic area
2. Reviewed the relevant scientific literature
3. Examined the question's potential significance in nursing
4. Pragmatically examined the feasibility of studying the research question

Defining the Research Question

Brainstorming with teachers, advisers, or colleagues may provide valuable feedback to help the researcher focus on a specific question area. For example, suppose a researcher told a colleague that an area of interest was whether men and women recovered differently after cardiac surgery. The colleague may have said, "What is it about the topic that specifically interests you?" Such a conversation may have initiated a train of thought that resulted in a decision to explore the recovery processes and gender differences. Box 4-1 illustrates how a broad area of interest was narrowed to a specific research topic.

Evidence-Informed Practice Tip

A well-developed research question guides a focused search for scientific evidence about assessing, diagnosing, treating, or assisting patients with understanding their prognosis with regard to a specific health problem.

Beginning the Literature Review

The literature review should reveal a collection of relevant individual studies and systematic reviews that have been critically examined (see Chapter 5). Concluding sections in such articles— that is, the recommendations and implications for practice—often identify remaining gaps in the literature, the need for replication, or the need for extension of the knowledge base about a particular research focus.

Qualitative and quantitative researchers conduct literature reviews differently. For qualitative researchers, the value of the literature review

TABLE **4-1**

HOW PRACTICAL EXPERIENCE, SCIENTIFIC LITERATURE, AND UNTESTED THEORY INFLUENCE THE DEVELOPMENT OF A RESEARCH IDEA

AREA	INFLUENCE	EXAMPLE
Practical experience	Clinical practice provides a wealth of experience from which research problems can be derived. The nurse may observe the occurrence of a particular event or pattern and become curious about why it occurs, as well as its relationship to other factors in the patient's environment.	Of the 98,500 emergency visits by children, 25% are for the treatment of lacerations and open wounds. Although the treatment is relatively painless with the use of topical anaesthesia, the fear, anxiety, and distress associated with the experience is significant. Several techniques, such as distraction, have proved to have a positive effect on procedural distress. Can music be a useful tool to distract the child and involve the parent in positive behaviour (Sobieraj, Bhatt, LeMay, Rennick, & Johnston, 2009)?
Critical appraisal of the scientific literature	The critical appraisal of research studies that appear in journals may indirectly suggest a problem area by stimulating the reader's thinking. Nurses may observe the outcome data from a single study or a group of related studies that provide the basis for developing a pilot study or quality improvement project to determine the effectiveness of this intervention in their own practice.	Several studies have been conducted on the needs of family members of patients in the ICU. A subset focused on the informational needs of families. Families benefitted from informational interventions, as evidenced by improved comprehension, decreased anxiety, and increased satisfaction. The researchers recognized a need for better understanding of the family members' (1) perception of informational support, (2) anxiety levels, and (3) satisfaction with care and the relationships among these. The overall objective was to further refine the informational program and to initiate a formal evaluation program (Bailey, Sabbagh, Loiselle, Boileau, & McVey, 2010).
	A research idea may also be suggested by a critical appraisal of the literature that identifies gaps and suggests areas for future study. Research ideas also can be generated by research reports that suggest the value of replicating a particular study to extend or refine the existing body of scientific knowledge.	Workplace bullying is prevalent in Canada, affecting millions of women every year. Being bullied at work is a devastating life experience with many negative consequences particularly related to physical, emotional, social, and economic well-being. Although many of the consequences have been studied extensively, absence because of sickness has not been extensively explored (O'Donnell, MacIntosh, & Wuest, 2010).
	Verification of an untested nursing theory provides a relatively uncharted territory from which research questions can be derived. Inasmuch as theories themselves are not tested, a researcher may think about investigating a particular concept or set of concepts related to a particular nursing theory. The deductive process would be used to generate the research question. The researcher would pose questions such as, "If this theory is correct, what kind of behaviour will I expect to observe in particular patients and under which conditions?" or "If this theory is valid, what kind of supporting evidence will I find?"	Health care structuring in Canada has resulted in considerable role changes for senior nurse leaders (SNLs), providing the opportunity for nurse leaders to leverage their leadership skills and play a greater role in decision making at the senior level. Little is known about the patterns of SNL decision making. Using an adapted theoretical framework on health care professionals' participation in strategic decision making in health care organizations, Wong and associates (2010) described the scope and degree of involvement of SNLs in executive level decisions in acute care organizations across Canada (see Appendix B).

ICU, intensive care unit

DEVELOPMENT OF A RESEARCH HYPOTHESIS

IDEA EMERGES

- Senior nurse leaders' (SNLs') work post-restructuring

BRAINSTORMING

- Do the changes subsequent to the health care restructuring provide new opportunities for leadership and greater roles in decision making?
- Do the changes result in diminished authority and a decrease in representation at the policymaking level?
- What do nursing leaders perceive about their decision making?
- What are the organizational outcomes?

LITERATURE REVIEW

- In many cases the restructuring resulted in opportunities to provide leadership and to play a greater role in decision-making.
- However, in other organizations without discipline-based nursing service, SNLs reported decreased direct supervision of nurses.
- Decision-making involvement can be measured, and there is a connection between involvement in decision activities, perceived influence over decisions, and organizational outcomes.
- The scope and intensity of SNL involvement in strategic decision-making is related to their perceptions of influence in the organization.

VARIABLES

- Independent (predictor) variable
  - Scope (timing and breadth) and intensity of participation (number of decision activities)
- Dependent variable
  - Decision-making influence

RESEARCH QUESTION

- Does the scope and intensity of SNL participation in executive decision-making processes predict the degree of SNL decision influence?

From Wong, C. A., Laschinger, H., Cummings, G. G., Vincent, L., & O'Connor, P. (2010). Decisional involvement of senior nurse leaders in Canadian acute care hospitals. *Journal of Nursing Management, 18*, 122–133. doi; 10.1111/j.1365-2834.2010.01053.x
See Appendix B.

usually start with a very cursory or general review of the literature to help focus the study, whereas quantitative researchers begin their study with an extensive review of the literature on their research questions and related topics (Streubert & Carpenter, 2011). The literature review also helps researchers determine whether their study can contribute to the field of nursing. Qualitative researchers conduct a literature review during the data analysis or discussion of the findings to "tell the reader how the findings fit into what is already known about the phenomenon" (Streubert & Carpenter, 2011, p. 26).

The databases that researchers use for the literature review—for example, Cumulative Index to Nursing and Allied Health Literature (CINAHL), PsycINFO, MEDLINE, and PubMed—contain relevant articles that have been critically examined. Concluding sections in such articles (i.e., the recommendations and implications for practice) often identify remaining gaps in the literature, the need for replication, or the need for extension of the knowledge gleaned on a particular research focus.

In the example about decision making among senior nurse leaders (SNLs; see Box 4-1), the researchers may have conducted a preliminary review of books and journals for theories and research studies on the changes in the health care system, governance structures, and organizational models and factors related to decision making. These factors, termed *variables* in the language of research, should be potentially relevant, of interest, and measurable.

The search for relevant factors to SNL decision making that are mentioned in the literature might begin with an exploration of the scope and degree of SNLs' contributions to executive-level decisions in acute care organizations across Canada. Wong and associates (2010) investigated participation in strategic organizational decision making as a theoretical framework for describing such participation with the use of information processing and complexity science theories. The

is controversial. Many researchers believe that an extensive literature review causes investigators to develop biases or beliefs that limit their openness to exploring the phenomenon under study. As a general rule, qualitative researchers researcher can then use this information to further define the research question, to address a gap in the literature, and to extend the body of knowledge related to decision making among SNLs. At this point, the researcher could write the following tentative research question: "What is the scope and degree of SNL involvement after restructuring in acute care organizations across Canada?" After reading this question, you should be able to envision the interrelatedness of the initial definition of the research question, the literature review, and the refined research question. Readers of research reports examine the end product of this process in the form of a research question, hypothesis, or both. Thus, readers need an appreciation of how the researcher formulates the final research question directing the study.

Helpful Hint

Reading the literature review or theoretical framework section of a research article helps you trace the development of the implied research question, hypothesis, or both.

Examining Significance

When considering a research question, it is crucial that the researcher has examined the question's potential significance to nursing. The research question should have the potential to contribute to and extend the scientific body of nursing knowledge. Guidelines for selecting research questions should meet the following criteria:

- Patients, nurses, the medical community in general, and society will potentially benefit from the knowledge derived from the study.
- The results will be applicable for nursing practice, education, or administration.
- The results will be theoretically relevant.
- The findings will lend support to untested theoretical assumptions, extend or challenge an existing theory, or clarify a conflict in the literature.
- The findings will potentially enable professionals to formulate or alter nursing practices or policies.

If the research question has not met any of these criteria, the researcher needs to extensively revise the question or discard it. For example, in the research question "Does the scope and intensity of SNL participation in executive decision-making processes predict the degree of SNL decision influence?" (see Box 4-1), the significance of the question includes the following facts:

- Health care restructuring has contributed to significant changes in SNLs' roles.
- New governance structures and organizational models have radically changed nursing leadership structures.
- SNLs' participation in decision making is important for an organization's strategic decisions.
- Participation in organizations' strategic decisions is associated with reductions in hospital costs and improvement in patient outcomes.

Evidence-Informed Practice Tip

Without a well-developed research question, the researcher may search for incorrect, irrelevant, or unnecessary information. Such information is a barrier to identifying the potential significance of the study.

Determining Feasibility

The feasibility of a research question must be examined pragmatically. Regardless of how significant or researchable a question may be, pragmatic considerations—such as time; availability of participants, facilities, equipment, and money; experience of the researcher; and any ethical considerations—may render the question inappropriate because it lacks feasibility.

THE FULLY DEVELOPED RESEARCH QUESTION

As discussed previously, qualitative researchers develop and refine a research question that outlines a general topic area. Examples include the following:

- What is the impact of an education program about acquired immune deficiency syndrome (AIDS) on the lives of a group of Ugandan nurses and nurse-midwives? (Harrowing & Mill, 2010)
- What is the effect of a brief, focused educational intervention on the quality of verbal interactions between nursing staff and patients in a chronic care facility? (Boscart, 2009)
- What is it about immunizing children who strongly resist needle injection that is a problem for public health nurses? (Ives & Melrose, 2010)

As a quantitative researcher finalizes a research question, the following three characteristics should be evident:

1. The *variables* under consideration are clearly identified.
2. The *population* being investigated is specified.
3. The possibility of empirical *testing* is implied.

Because each of these elements is crucial in the formulation of a satisfactory research question, the criteria are discussed in greater detail in the following sections. These elements can often be found in the introduction of the published article; however, they are not always stated in an explicit manner.

Helpful Hint_____

Remember that research questions are used to guide all types of research studies, but they are most often used in exploratory, descriptive, qualitative, or hypothesis-generating studies.

Evidence-Informed Practice Tip _____

The answers to questions generated by qualitative data reflect evidence that may provide the first insights about a phenomenon that has not been studied previously.

Variables

Researchers call the properties that they study *variables*. Such properties take on different values. Thus, a **variable** is, as the name suggests, something that varies. Properties that differ from each other, such as age, weight, height, religion, and ethnicity, are examples of variables. Researchers attempt to understand how and why differences in one variable relate to differences in another variable. For example, a researcher may be concerned about the rate of pneumonia in postoperative patients on ventilators in critical care units. This rate is a variable because not all critically ill postoperative patients on ventilators have pneumonia. A researcher may also be interested in what other factors can be linked to ventilator-acquired pneumonia (VAP). Clinical evidence suggests that elevation of the head of the bed is also associated with VAP. You can see that these factors are also variables that need to be considered in relation to the development of VAP in postoperative patients.

When speaking of variables, the researcher is essentially asking, "Is X related to Y? What is the effect of X on Y? How are X_1 and X_2 related to Y?"* The researcher is asking a question about the relationship between one or more independent variables *(X)* and a dependent variable *(Y)*.

An **independent variable,** usually symbolized by X, is the variable that has the presumed effect on the dependent variable. In experimental research studies, the researcher manipulates the independent variable. For example, a nurse may

_____

*Note: In cases in which multiple independent or dependent variables are present, subscripts are used to indicate the number of variables under consideration.

study how different methods of administering pain medication affect the patient's perception of pain intensity. The researcher may manipulate the independent variable (i.e., the method of administering pain medication) by using nurse- versus patient-controlled administration of analgesics. In nonexperimental research, the independent variable is not manipulated and is assumed to have occurred naturally before or during the study. For example, the researcher may be studying the relationship between gender and the perception of pain intensity. The independent variable—gender—is not manipulated; it is presumed to exist and is observed and measured in relation to pain intensity.

The **dependent variable,** represented by Y, is often referred to as the consequence or the presumed effect that varies with a change in the independent variable. The dependent variable is not manipulated. It is observed and assumed to vary with changes in the independent variable. Predictions are based on how changes to the independent variable will affect the dependent variable. The researcher is interested in understanding, explaining, or predicting the response of the dependent variable. For example, a researcher might assume that the perception of pain (i.e., the dependent variable) will vary according to the person's gender (i.e., the independent variable). In this case, the researcher is trying to explain the perception of pain in relation to the gender: that is, male or female. Although variability in the dependent variable is assumed to depend on changes in the independent variable, this assumption does not imply that a causal relationship exists between X and Y or that changes in X cause Y to change.

In a study about nurses' attitudes toward patients with hepatitis C, the researcher discovered that older nurses had a more negative attitude about such patients than did younger nurses. The researcher did not conclude that the nurses' attitudes toward patients with hepatitis C were negative because of their age; however, it is apparent that there was a directional relationship between age and negative attitudes about patients with hepatitis C: that is, the older the nurses were, the more negative were their attitudes about patients with hepatitis C. This example highlights the fact that causal relationships are not necessarily implied by the independent and dependent variables; rather, only a relational statement with possible directionality is proposed.

Table 4-2 presents a number of examples to help you learn how to write research questions. Practise substituting other variables for the examples in the table. You will be surprised at the skill you develop in writing and critiquing research questions.

Although one independent variable and one dependent variable were used in the examples just given, there is no restriction on the number of variables that can be included in a research question. Remember, however, that questions should not be unnecessarily complex or unwieldy, particularly in beginning research efforts. Research questions that include more than one independent or dependent variable may be divided into more concise subquestions.

Finally, note that variables are not inherently independent or dependent. A variable that is classified as independent in one study may be considered dependent in another study. For example, a nurse may review an article about sexual behaviours that are predictive of the risk for HIV infection or AIDS. In this case, HIV/AIDS is the dependent variable. In another article in which the relationship between HIV/AIDS and maternal parenting practices is considered, HIV/AIDS status is the independent variable. Whether a variable is independent or dependent depends on the role it plays in a particular study.

Population

The **population** (a well-defined set that has certain properties) is either specified or implied in the research question. If the scope of the question has been narrowed to a specific focus and the variables have been clearly identified, the nature

TABLE **4-2**

RESEARCH QUESTION FORMAT

TYPE	FORMAT	EXAMPLE
QUANTITATIVE EXPERIMENTAL		
Correlational	Is there a relationship between X (independent variable) and Y (dependent variable) in the specified population?	Is there a relationship between the effectiveness of pain management strategies and quality of life?
Comparative	Is there a difference in Y (dependent variable) between people who have characteristic X (independent variable) and those who do not have characteristic X?	Is there a difference in prevention of osteoporosis in at-risk survivors of breast cancer who receive a combination of long-term progressive strength training exercises, alendronate, calcium, and vitamin D, in comparison with those who do not receive this treatment?
Quantitative	Is there a difference in Y (dependent variable) between Group A, which received X (independent variable), and Group B, which did not receive X?	What is the difference in physical, social, and emotional adjustment in women with breast cancer (and their partners) who have received phase-specific standardized education by video versus phase-specific telephone counselling?
QUALITATIVE		
Phenomenological	What is or was it like to have X?	How do older adults learn to live with early-stage dementia?

of the population is evident to the reader of the research report. For example, a research question may be "Is there a relationship between the type of discharge planning for older adults hospitalized with heart failure and the outcomes for participating patients and their caregivers?" This question suggests that the population under consideration includes older adults hospitalized for heart failure and their caregivers. The question also implies that some of the older adults and their caregivers were involved in a professional-patient partnership model of discharge planning, in contrast to other older adults who received the usual discharge planning. The researcher or reader will have an initial idea of the composition of the study population from the outset.

Evidence-Informed Practice Tip

Make sure that the population of interest and the setting have been clearly described so that if you plan to replicate the study, you will know exactly who the study population needs to be.

Testability

The research question must be phrased in such a way that there is a specific issue that needs to be answered. In many cases, the question is **testable:** that is, measurable by quantitative methods. For example, the research question "Should postoperative patients control how much pain medication they receive?" is stated incorrectly for a variety of reasons. One reason is that the question is not testable; it represents a value statement rather than a relational problem statement. A scientific or relational question must propose a relationship between an independent variable and a dependent variable in such a way that the variables can be measured. Many interesting and important questions are not valid research questions because they are not amenable to testing.

The question "Should postoperative patients control how much pain medication they receive?" could be revised from a philosophical question to a research question that implies testability. Examples of the revised research question are as follows:

- Is there a relationship between patient-controlled analgesia versus nurse-administered analgesia and the perception of postoperative pain?
- What is the effect of patient-controlled analgesia on pain ratings provided by post-operative patients?

These examples illustrate the relationship between the variables, identify the independent and dependent variables, and imply the testability of the research question.

Now that the elements of the formal research question have been presented in greater detail, this information can be integrated by formulating a formal research question. Earlier in this chapter, the following unrefined research question was formulated: "What is the scope and degree of SNL involvement after restructuring in acute care organizations across Canada?"

This research question was originally derived from a general area of interest: understanding the new role of SNLs in acute care organizations. The topic was more specifically defined by delineating a particular research question. The question crystallized further after a preliminary literature review and emerged in the unrefined form just given. It is now possible to propose a refined research question in which the problem is stated specifically in question form and the relationship of the key variables in the study, the population being studied, and the empirical testability of the question are specified: "Does the scope and intensity of SNL participation in executive decision-making processes predict the degree of SNL decision influence?" (see Appendix B).

As another example, Table 4-3 lists the components of the research question regarding variance in the perception of pain in relation to a person's race.

TABLE 4-3	
COMPONENTS OF THE RESEARCH QUESTION AND RELATED CRITERIA	
Testability	Differential effect of pain intensity and number of painful sites on functional disability (physical and social functioning)
Population	Black and white older adults
Variables	**Independent Variables:**
	Pain intensity
	Pain sites
	Race
	Health (number of limiting diagnoses)
	Dependent Variables:
	Management effectiveness
	Functional status

Helpful Hint

Remember that research questions are often not explicitly stated. The reader must infer the research question from the report's title, the abstract, the introduction, or the purpose.

Using your focused question, search the literature for the best available answer to your clinical questions.

STUDY PURPOSE, AIMS, OR OBJECTIVES

Once the research question is developed and the literature review is critiqued in terms of the level, strength, and quality of evidence available for the particular research question, the purpose, aims, or objectives of the study become focused, and the researcher can decide whether a hypothesis should be tested or a research question answered.

The **purpose** of the study encompasses the aims or objectives the investigator hopes to achieve with the research, not the question to be answered. *Purpose, aims,* and *objectives* are synonymous terms. For example, a nurse working with patients with bladder dysfunction who are in rehabilitation may be disturbed by the high incidence of urinary tract infections. The nurse may propose the following research question: "What is the optimum frequency of changing urinary drainage bags in patients with bladder dysfunction to reduce the incidence of urinary tract infection?" If this nurse were to design a study, its purpose might be to determine the differential effect of 1-week and 4-week schedules of changing urinary drainage bags on the incidence of urinary tract infections in patients with bladder dysfunction.

The purpose communicates more than just the nature of the question. Through the researcher's selection of verbs, the purpose statement suggests the manner in which the researcher sought to study the question. Verbs such as *discover, explore,* or *describe* suggest an investigation of a relatively underresearched topic that might be more appropriately guided by research questions than by hypotheses. In contrast, verbs such as *test* (testing the effectiveness of an intervention) or *compare* (comparing two alternative nursing strategies) suggest a study with a better-established body of knowledge that is hypothesis testing in nature. Box 4-2 provides other examples of purpose statements.

BOX **4-2**

EXAMPLES OF PURPOSE STATEMENTS

"The purpose of this study was to describe satisfactory and unsatisfactory experiences of postpartum nursing care from the perspective of adolescent mothers." (Peterson, Sword, Charles, & DiCenso, 2007, p. 201)

"The aim of this phenomenological study was to understand the meaning of living alone from the perspective of older people with Alzheimer disease or a related dementia." (de Witt, Ploeg, & Black, 2010, p. 1700)

"The aim of this meta-ethnography [a method used to synthesize qualitative research findings] was to explore nurses' experience with telephone triage and advice within the primary-care sector and to understand the factors that facilitate or impede their decision-making process." (Purc-Stephenson & Thrasher, 2010, p. 483)

"The purpose of this study was to test an intervention using children's songs to promote parent-led distraction during simple laceration repair in children aged 1 to 5?" (Sobieraj, Bhatt, LeMay, Rennick, & Johnston, 2009, p. 70)

"Specifically, this study set out to explore nurses' perceptions of the impact of the 15-minute interview on the hospital admission process and on their family nursing practice." (Martinez, D'Artois, & Rennick, 2007, p. 162)

Evidence-Informed Practice Tip ____

The purpose, aims, or objectives often provide the most information about the intent of the research question and hypotheses and suggest the level of evidence to be obtained from the findings of the study.

DEVELOPING THE RESEARCH HYPOTHESIS

Like the research question, hypotheses are often not stated explicitly in a research article. The hypotheses are often embedded in the data analysis, results, or discussion section of the research report. You then need to discern the nature of the hypotheses being tested. Similarly, the population may not be explicitly described but is identified in the background, significance, and literature review. It is then up to you to discern the nature of the hypotheses and population being tested. For example, in the study by Meneses and colleagues (2007), the hypotheses are embedded in the "Methods" section of the article: "the overall hypotheses are to determine the effect of the breast cancer psychoeducational intervention (BCEI) on overall quality of life . . . and on the individual quality of life . . . and to examine whether the effects of the intervention were durable over time." You must interpret this statement as representing the hypotheses that test the effect of the BCEI on quality of life in survivors of breast cancer. Therefore, it is important for you to be acquainted with the components of hypotheses, how they are developed, and the standards for writing and evaluating them.

Hypotheses flow from the research question, literature review, and theoretical framework. Figure 4-1 illustrates this flow. A **hypothesis** is a statement about the relationship between two or more variables that suggests an answer to the research question. A hypothesis converts the question posed by the research question into a declarative statement that predicts an expected outcome. It explains or predicts the relationship or differences between two or more variables in terms of the expected results or outcomes of a

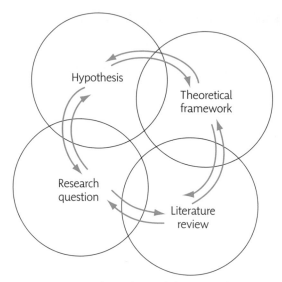

FIGURE 4-1 Interrelationships of the research question, literature review, theoretical framework, and hypothesis.

study. Hypotheses are formulated before the study is actually conducted; they provide direction for the collection, analysis, and interpretation of data.

Helpful Hint

When hypotheses are not explicitly stated by the author at the end of the "Introduction" section or before the "Methods" section, they are embedded or implied in the "Results" or "Discussion" section of a research article.

Characteristics

Nurses who are conducting research or critiquing published research studies must have a working knowledge of what constitutes a "good" hypothesis. Such knowledge provides a standard for evaluating their own work and the work of others. The following discussion about the characteristics of hypotheses presents criteria to be used when a hypothesis is formulated or evaluated.

Relationship Statement

The first characteristic of a hypothesis is that it is a declarative statement identifying the predicted relationship between two or more variables. This implies a systematic relationship between an independent variable *(X)* and a dependent variable *(Y)*. The direction of the predicted relationship is also specified in this statement. Phrases such as "greater than"; "less than"; "positively related," "negatively related," or "curvilinearly related"; and "difference in" connote the directionality that is proposed in the hypothesis. The following is an example of a directional hypothesis: "the rate of continuous smoking abstinence [dependent variable] at 6 months post partum, according to self-report and biochemical validation, will be significantly higher in the treatment group [receiving postpartum counselling intervention] than in the control group [independent variable]." The dependent and independent variables are explicitly identified, and the relational aspect of the prediction in the hypothesis is contained in the phrase "significantly higher than."

The nature of the relationship, either causal or associative, is also implied by the hypothesis. A causal relationship is one in which the researcher can predict that the independent variable *(X)* causes a change in the dependent variable *(Y)*. In research, it is rare that a definitive stand can be assumed about a cause-and-effect relationship. For example, a researcher might hypothesize that relaxation training would have a significant effect on the physical and psychological health status of patients who have suffered myocardial infarction. The researcher would have difficulty predicting a strong cause-and-effect relationship, however, because the multiple intervening variables (e.g., age, medication, and lifestyle changes) might also influence the participant's health status.

Variables are more commonly related in non-causal ways; that is, the variables are related but in an associative way. This means that variables change in relation to each other. For example, because strong evidence exists that asbestos exposure is related to lung cancer, a researcher may be tempted to state a causal relationship between asbestos exposure and lung cancer.

However, not all individuals exposed to asbestos develop lung cancer and, conversely, not all individuals who have lung cancer have been exposed to asbestos. Thus, a position advocating a causal relationship between these two variables would be scientifically unsound. Instead, only an associative relationship exists between the variables of asbestos exposure and lung cancer, with a strong systematic association between the two phenomena.

Testability

The second characteristic of a hypothesis is its **testability.** The variables of the study must lend themselves to observation, measurement, and analysis. The hypothesis is either supported or not supported after the data have been collected and analyzed. The predicted outcome proposed by the hypothesis is or is not congruent with the actual outcome when the hypothesis is tested. Hypotheses advance scientific knowledge by confirming or refuting theories.

A hypothesis may fail to meet the criteria of testability because the researcher has not made a prediction about the anticipated outcome, because the variables are not observable or measurable, or because the hypothesis is couched in terms that are value laden.

Helpful Hint

When a hypothesis is complex (i.e., contains more than one independent or dependent variable), it is difficult for the findings to indicate unequivocally that the hypothesis is supported or not supported. In such cases, the reader must infer which relationships are significant from the "Findings" or "Discussion" section.

Theory Base

A sound hypothesis is consistent with an existing body of theory and research findings. Whether a researcher arrives at a hypothesis inductively or deductively, the hypothesis must be based on a sound scientific rationale. Readers should be able to identify the flow of ideas from the research question to the literature review, to the theoretical

framework, and to the hypotheses. For example: The scope (timing and breadth) and intensity (number of decision activities) of SNLs' participation in executive decision-making processes is positively predictive of the degree of SNLs' influence on decisions (see Appendix B). This example makes clear that an explicitly developed, relevant body of scientific data provides the theoretical grounding for the study.

Wording the Hypothesis

As you become more familiar with the scientific literature, you will observe that a hypothesis can be worded in various ways. Regardless of the specific format used to state the hypothesis, the statement should be worded in clear, simple, and concise terms. If this criterion is met, the reader will understand the following:

- The variables of the hypothesis
- The population being studied
- The predicted outcome of the hypothesis

Information about hypotheses may be further clarified in the "Instruments," "Sample," or "Methods" section of a research report.

Statistical Versus Research Hypotheses

Readers of research reports may observe that a hypothesis is further categorized as either a research or statistical hypothesis. A **research hypothesis,** also known as a *scientific hypothesis,* consists of a statement about the expected relationship of the variables. A research hypothesis indicates what the outcome of the study is expected to be. A research hypothesis is also either directional or nondirectional. If the researcher obtains statistically significant findings for a research hypothesis, the hypothesis is supported. For example, in a study of the effectiveness of a home-based nursing intervention in reducing parenting stress in three groups of families with irritable infants, the research hypothesis was that "mothers who received the home-based nursing intervention (REST—reassurance, empathy, support, and time-out) for infant irritability will report less parenting stress than the mothers who did not receive the intervention" (Keefe, Kajrlsen, Lobo, Kotzer, & Dudley, 2006). Because the findings for this hypothesis were not statistically significant, the hypothesis was not supported, thereby indicating that the REST intervention did not significantly reduce parenting stress for parents with irritable infants. The examples in Table 4-4 represent research hypotheses.

According to a **statistical hypothesis** (also known as a *null hypothesis*), there is no relationship between the independent and dependent variables. The examples in Table 4-5 illustrate statistical hypotheses. If, in the data analysis, a statistically significant relationship emerges between the variables at a specified level of significance, the statistical hypothesis is rejected. Rejection of the statistical hypothesis is equivalent to acceptance of the research hypothesis. For example, Simonson and colleagues (2007) sought to identify differences in the rates of anaesthetic complications in hospitals whose obstetric anaesthesia is provided solely by certified registered nurse anaesthetists (CRNAs) in comparison with hospitals with only anaesthesiologists. The statistical hypothesis—that there would be no differences in anaesthetic complication rates between the hospitals that relied on different anaesthesia providers—was supported. Because the difference in outcomes was not greater than that expected by chance, the statistical hypothesis was accepted. To further differentiate between a statistical hypothesis and a research hypothesis, consider the following hypotheses:

> *Research hypothesis:* Hospitals with higher nurse-to-patient ratios will have fewer adverse patient events.
>
> *Statistical (null) hypothesis:* There is no difference in the number of adverse patient events in hospitals with higher nurse-to-patient ratios.

Some researchers refer to the statistical hypothesis as a statistical contrivance that obscures a straightforward prediction of the outcome. Others state that it is more exact and conservative statistically and that failure to reject the statistical hypothesis implies that the evidence to support the idea of a real difference is insufficient. You will note that research hypotheses are generally used more often than statistical hypotheses because they are more desirable for stating the researcher's expectation. Readers then have a more precise idea of the proposed outcome. In any study that involves statistical analysis, the underlying statistical hypothesis is usually assumed without being explicitly stated.

Directional versus Nondirectional Hypotheses

Hypotheses can be formulated directionally or nondirectionally. A **directional hypothesis** specifies the expected direction of the relationship between the independent and dependent variables. The reader of a directional hypothesis may observe not only that a relationship is proposed but also the nature or direction of that relationship. The following is an example of a directional hypothesis: "The scope (timing and breadth) and intensity (number of decision-making processes) *positively* predicts the degree of SNL decision influence" (Wong et al., 2010, p. 125; see Appendix B). Sobieraj and colleagues (2009) "hypothesized that parents in the intervention group would demonstrate a *greater* degree of parent-led distraction than those in the control group" (see Appendix C). Examples of directional hypotheses can also be found in examples 2 to 7 of Table 4-4.

Whereas a **nondirectional hypothesis** indicates the existence of a relationship between the variables, it does not specify the anticipated direction of the relationship. The following is an example of a nondirectional hypothesis "there will be a difference in the level of fatigue experienced by two groups of caregivers of preterm infants (infants on apnea monitors versus those not on apnea monitors) during three time periods: prior to discharge, 1 week after discharge and 1 month after discharge."

TABLE 4-4

EXAMPLES OF HOW TO WORD A HYPOTHESIS

VARIABLES	HYPOTHESIS	TYPE OF DESIGN; LEVEL OF EVIDENCE SUGGESTED

1. There are significant differences in self-reported cancer pain, symptoms accompanying pain, and functional status according to self-reported ethnic identity.

Independent	Nondirectional, research	Nonexperimental; level IV
Ethnic identity		
Dependent		
Self-reported cancer pain		
Symptoms accompanying pain		
Functional status		

2. Individuals who participate in usual care plus blood pressure telemonitoring will have a greater reduction in blood pressure from baseline to 12-month follow-up than would individuals who receive only usual care.

Independent	Directional, research	Experimental; level II
Telemonitoring		
Usual care		
Dependent		
Blood pressure		

3. There will be a greater decrease in state anxiety scores for patients receiving structured informational videos before abdominal or chest tube removal than for patients receiving standard information.

Independent	Directional, research	Experimental; level II
Preprocedure structured videotape information		
Standard information		
Dependent		
State anxiety		

4. The incidence and degree of severity of participants' discomfort will be lower after administration of medications by the Z-track intramuscular injection technique than after administration of medications by the standard intramuscular injection technique.

Independent	Directional, research	Experimental; level II
Z-track intramuscular injection technique		
Standard intramuscular injection technique		
Dependent		
Participant discomfort		

5. Nurses with high levels of social support from coworkers have low perceived job stress.

Independent	Directional, research	Nonexperimental; level IV
Social support		
Dependent		
Perceived job stress		

6. There will be no difference in rates of complications from anaesthetics between hospitals in which anaesthetics are administered primarily by certified registered nurse anaesthetists (CRNAs) and hospitals in which anaesthetics are administered primarily by anaesthesiologists (MDs).

Independent	Nondirectional; null	Nonexperimental; level IV
Type of anaesthesia provider (CRNA or MD)		
Dependent		
Anaesthesia complication rate		

7. There will be no significant difference in the duration of patency of a 24-gauge intravenous lock in a neonatal patient when flushed with 0.5 mL of heparinized saline (2 U/mL), standard practice, in comparison with 0.5 mL of 0.9% normal saline.

Independent	Nondirectional; null	Experimental; level II
Heparinized saline		
Normal saline		
Dependent		
Duration of patency of intravenous lock		

TABLE **4-5**

EXAMPLES OF STATISTICAL (NULL) HYPOTHESES		
HYPOTHESIS	**VARIABLES**	**TYPE OF DESIGN SUGGESTED**
Oxygen inhalation by nasal cannula of up to 6 L/min does not affect oral temperature measurement taken with an electronic thermometer.	Independent: Oxygen inhalation by nasal cannula Dependent: Oral temperature	Experimental
There will be no difference in performance accuracy between adult nurse practitioners (ANPs) and family nurse practitioners (FNPs) in formulating accurate diagnoses and acceptable interventions for suspected cases of domestic violence.	Independent: Nurse practitioner (ANP or FNP) category Dependent: Diagnosis and intervention performance accuracy	Nonexperimental

Nurses who are learning to critique research studies should be aware that both the directional and nondirectional forms of hypothesis statements are acceptable. There are definite advantages and disadvantages that pertain to each form.

Proponents of the directional hypothesis argue that researchers naturally have hunches, guesses, or expectations about the outcome of their research. It is the hunch, the curiosity, or the guess that initially leads them to speculate about the question. The literature review and the conceptual framework provide the theoretical foundation for deriving the hypothesis. For example, the theory (e.g., self-efficacy theory) provides a critical rationale for proposing that relationships between variables have particular outcomes. When there is no theory or related research on which to base a rationale, or when findings in previous research studies are ambivalent, a nondirectional hypothesis may be appropriate. As you read research articles, you will note that directional hypotheses are much more commonly used than nondirectional hypotheses.

In summary, when you evaluate a hypothesis, note that directional hypotheses have several advantages that make them appropriate for use in most studies:

- Directional hypotheses indicate that a theory base was used to derive the hypotheses and that the phenomena under investigation have been critically examined and interrelated.

You should note that nondirectional hypotheses may also be deduced from a theory base. Because of the exploratory nature of many studies for which the hypotheses are nondirectional, in contrast, the theory base may not be as developed.

- Directional hypotheses provide a specific theoretical frame of reference within which the study is being conducted.
- They suggest that the researcher believes that the evidence is indicative of a particular outcome, and as a result, the analyses of data can be accomplished in a statistically more sensitive way.

The important point about the directionality of the hypotheses is whether the rationale for the choice the researcher has proposed is sound.

RELATIONSHIP AMONG THE HYPOTHESIS, THE RESEARCH QUESTION, AND THE RESEARCH DESIGN

Regardless of whether the researcher uses a statistical or research hypothesis, there is a suggested relationship among the hypothesis, the research question, the research design of the study, and the level of evidence provided by the results of the study. The type of design, experimental or nonexperimental, influences the wording of the hypothesis. For example, when an experimental design is used, the research consumer would expect to see hypotheses that reflect relationship statements, such as the following:

- X_1 is more effective than X_2 on Y.
- The effect of X_1 on Y is greater than that of X_2 on Y.
- The incidence of Y will not differ in participants receiving X_1 and X_2 treatments.
- The incidence of Y will be greater in participants after X_1 than after X_2.

Such hypotheses indicate that an experimental treatment (i.e., independent variable X) will be used and that two groups of participants, experimental and control groups, are being used to test whether the difference in the outcome (i.e., dependent variable Y) predicted by the hypothesis exists. Hypotheses reflecting experimental designs also concern the effect of the experimental treatment (i.e., independent variable X) on the outcome (i.e., dependent variable Y).

In contrast, hypotheses related to nonexperimental designs reflect associative relationship statements such as the following:

- X will be negatively related to Y.
- A positive relationship will exist between X and Y.

Thus, in a study in which the hypotheses were associative relationship statements, the evidence provided by the results of that investigation have level IV strength (nonexperimental design).

The Critical Thinking Decision Path will help you determine both the type of hypothesis presented in a study and the study's readiness for a hypothesis-testing design.

Evidence-Informed Practice Tip

Think about the relationship between the wording of the hypothesis, the type of research design suggested, and the level of evidence provided by the findings of a study with each kind of hypothesis. The research consumer may want to consider which type of hypothesis potentially will yield the strongest results applicable to practice.

DEVELOPING AND REFINING A CLINICAL QUESTION: A CONSUMER'S PERSPECTIVE

Practising nurses, as well as students, are challenged to keep their practice up to date by searching for, retrieving, and critiquing research articles that apply to practice issues that they encounter in their clinical setting (Cullum, 2000). Practitioners strive to use the current best evidence from research in making clinical and health care decisions. Although research consumers are not conducting research studies, their search for information from practice is also converted into focused, structured clinical questions that are the foundation of evidence-informed practice. Clinical questions often arise from clinical situations for which there are no ready answers. You have probably had the experience of asking, "What is the most effective treatment for . . . ?" or "Why do we still do it this way?"

Framed according to criteria similar to those related to framing a research question, focused clinical questions are used as a basis for searching the literature to identify supporting evidence from research. A **clinical question** has five components:

1. Population
2. Intervention
3. Comparison
4. Outcome
5. Time

The five components, known as PICOT, constitute a format that is effective in helping nurses develop searchable clinical questions (Melnyk & Fineout-Overholt, 2011). Box 4-3 presents each component of the clinical question.

The significance of the clinical question becomes obvious as the research evidence from the literature is critiqued. The research evidence is used side by side with clinical expertise and the patient's perspective to develop or revise nursing standards, protocols, and policies that are used to plan and implement patient care (Cullum, 2000; Sackett, Straus, Richardson, Rosenberg, &

CRITICAL THINKING DECISION PATH

Determining the Type of Hypothesis or Readiness for Hypothesis Testing

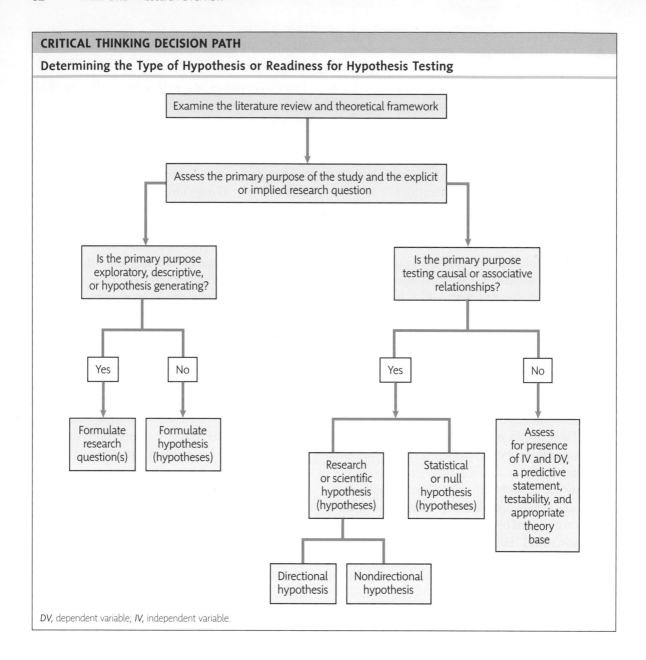

DV, dependent variable; *IV*, independent variable.

PICOT COMPONENTS OF A CLINICAL QUESTION

Population: The individual patient or group of patients with a particular condition or health care problem (e.g., adolescents aged 13 to 18 with type 1 insulin-dependent diabetes)

Intervention: The particular aspect of health care that is of interest to the nurse or the health team; for example, a therapeutic intervention (inhaler or nebulizer for treatment of asthma), a preventive intervention (pneumonia vaccine), a diagnostic intervention (measurement of blood pressure), or an organizational intervention (implementation of a bar coding system to reduce medication errors)

Comparison intervention: Standard care or no intervention (e.g., antibiotic or ibuprofen for children with otitis media); a comparison of two treatment settings (e.g., rehabilitation centre or home care)

Outcome: Improved outcome (e.g., improved glycemic control, decreased hospitalizations, decreased medication errors)

Time: time involved to demonstrate an outcome (e.g., weight loss maintained over a period of 2 years)

Practical Application

With regard to the example of pain, albeit from a different perspective, a nurse working in a palliative care setting wondered whether completing pain diaries was useful for patients with advanced cancer who were receiving palliative care. She wondered whether they were spending time developing something that had previously been shown to be useless or even harmful. After all, it is conceivable that monitoring one's pain in a diary actually heightens one's awareness and experience of pain. To focus her search of the literature, the nurse developed the following question: "Does the use of pain diaries in the palliative care of patients with cancer lead to improved pain control?"

Haynes, 2000; Thompson, Cullum, McCaughan, Sheldon, & Raynor, 2004). Issues or questions can arise from multiple clinical and managerial situations (see Practical Application box).

Sometimes it is helpful for nurses who develop clinical questions from a consumer's perspective to consider three elements—(1) the situation, (2) the intervention, and (3) the outcome—as they frame their focused question:

ELEMENTS OF A CLINICAL QUESTION

POPULATION	INTERVENTION	COMPARISON INTERVENTION	OUTCOME
People with advanced cancer	Pain diaries	No pain diaries	Increased pain control

- The situation is the patient or problem being addressed. This can be a single patient or a group of patients with a particular health problem (palliative care of patients with cancer).
- The intervention is the dimension of health care interest, and the question is often about whether a particular intervention (in this case, pain diaries) is a useful treatment.
- The outcome encompasses the effect of the treatment (intervention) for this patient or the patient population in terms of quality (e.g., decreased pain perception) and cost (low cost). It essentially answers whether the intervention makes a difference for the patient population.

The individual parts of the question are vital pieces of information to remember when you search for evidence in the literature. One of the easiest ways to do this is to use a table, such as Table 4-6. Examples of clinical questions are highlighted in Box 4-4. Chapter 5 provides examples of how to effectively search the literature to find answers to questions posed by researchers and research consumers.

Evidence-Informed Practice Tip

You should formulate clinical questions that arise from your clinical practice. Once you have developed a focused clinical question by using the PICOT format, search the literature for the best available evidence to answer your clinical question.

BOX 4-4

EXAMPLES OF CLINICAL QUESTIONS

- In overweight or obese people with type 2 diabetes, does an intensive lifestyle intervention reduce weight and cardiovascular disease risk factors? (Look AHEAD Research Group, Pi-Sunyer, Blackburn, et al., 2007)
- Is diet, exercise, or both effective for weight reduction in postpartum women? (Amorim, Linne, & Lourenco, 2007)
- In patients who require mechanical ventilation for longer than 48 hours, is oral decontamination with chlorhexidine or with chlorhexidine plus colistin effective for reducing the incidence of ventilator-associated pneumonia? (Koeman, van der Ven, Hak, Kaasjager, de Smet, Dormans, . . . Benton, 2006)

- What is the effect of arch supports on balance, functional mobility, back pain, and lower extremity joint pain in older adults? (Mulford, Taggart, Nivens, & Payrie, 2008)
- Is there a significant difference in the effect of different body positions on blood pressure in healthy young adults? (Eser, Korshid, Gunes, & Demir, 2007)
- In people with impaired glucose tolerance, do lifestyle or pharmacological interventions prevent or delay onset of type 2 diabetes? (Gillies, Abrams, Lambert, Cooper, Sutton, Hsu, & Khunti, 2007)
- What are the experiences of middle-aged people living with chronic heart failure? (Nordgren, Asp, & Fagerberg, 2007)

CRITIQUING THE RESEARCH QUESTION

The Critiquing Criteria box on p. 87 provides several criteria for evaluating this initial phase of the research process: the research question. Because the research question represents the basis for the study, it is usually introduced at the beginning of the research report to indicate the focus and direction of the study. Readers are then in a position to evaluate whether the rest of the study logically pertains to this basis. The author often begins by identifying the background and significance of the issue that led to crystallizing development of the unanswered question. The clinical and scientific background, significance, or both are summarized, and the purpose, aim, or objective of the study is identified. Finally, the research question and any related subquestions are proposed before or after the literature review.

The purpose of the introductory summary of the theoretical and scientific background is to provide the reader with a contextual glimpse of how the author critically thought about the development of the research question. The introduction to the research question places the study within an appropriate theoretical framework and begins the description of the study. This introductory section should also include the significance of the study (i.e., why the investigator is conducting the

study). For example, the significance may be to answer a question encountered in the clinical area and thereby improve patient care, to resolve a conflict in the literature regarding a clinical issue, or to provide data supporting an innovative form of nursing intervention that is more effective and is also cost effective.

Sometimes readers find that the research question is not clearly stated at the conclusion of the introduction. In some cases, the author only hints at the research question, and the reader is challenged to identify it. In other cases, the author embeds the research question in the introductory text or purpose statement. To some extent, where or whether the author states the research question depends on the style of the journal. Nevertheless, the evaluator must remember that the main research question should be implied if it is not clearly identified in the introductory section—even if the subquestions are not stated or implied.

When critiquing the research question, the reader looks for the presence of the three key elements described on p. 171:

- Does the research question express a relationship between two or more variables or, at least, between an independent variable and a dependent variable?
- Does the research question specify the nature of the population being studied?

- Does the research question imply the possibility of empirical testing?

You will use these three elements as criteria for judging the soundness of a stated research question. If the variables, the population, and the implications for testability are unclear, then the remainder of the study will probably falter. For example, a research study on anxiety during the perioperative period contained introductory material on anxiety in general, anxiety as it relates to the perioperative period, and the potentially beneficial influence of nursing care in relation to anxiety reduction. The author concluded that the purpose of the study was to determine whether selected measures of patient anxiety could be shown to vary when different approaches to nursing care were used during the perioperative period. The author did not state the research questions. A restatement of the problem in question form might be as follows:

$$(Y_1)\,(X_1, X_2, X_3)$$

What is the difference in patient anxiety level in relation to different approaches to nursing care during the perioperative period?

If this process of developing a research question is clarified at the outset of a research study, the report that follows can develop logically. Readers will have a clear idea of what the report should convey and can knowledgeably evaluate the material that is presented. When you critically appraise clinical questions, remember that they should be focused and specify the patient or problem being addressed, the intervention, and the outcome for a particular patient population. The author should provide evidence that the clinical question guided the literature search and that the question suggests the design and level of evidence to be obtained from the study findings.

CRITIQUING THE HYPOTHESES

As illustrated in the Critiquing Criteria box, several criteria for critiquing the hypotheses should be used as a standard for evaluating the strengths and weaknesses of the hypotheses in a research report:

1. When reading a research study, you may find the hypotheses clearly delineated in a separate hypothesis section of the research article (i.e., after the literature review or theoretical framework section or sections). In many cases, the hypotheses are not explicitly stated and are only implied in the results or discussion section of the article. In such cases, you must infer the hypotheses from the purpose statement and the type of analysis used. You should not assume that if hypotheses do not appear at the beginning of the article, they do not exist in the particular study. Even when hypotheses are stated at the beginning of an article, they are re-examined in the results or discussion section as the findings are presented and discussed.

2. If a hypothesis or set of hypotheses is presented, the data analysis should answer the hypotheses directly. Because the hypothesis should reflect the culmination and expression of this conceptual process, its placement in the research report logically follows the literature review and the theoretical framework discussion. It should be consistent with both the literature review and the theoretical framework.

3. Although a hypothesis can legitimately be nondirectional, it is preferable, and more common, for the researcher to indicate the direction of the relationship between the variables in the hypothesis. You will find that when data for the literature review are unavailable (i.e., the researcher has chosen to study a relatively undefined area of interest), a nondirectional hypothesis may be appropriate. Enough information simply may not be available for making a sound judgement about the direction of the proposed relationship. All that can be proposed is that there will be a relationship between

two variables. Essentially, you will want to determine the appropriateness of the researcher's choice regarding directionality of the hypothesis.

4. The notion of testability is central to the soundness of a hypothesis. One criterion related to testability is that the hypothesis should be stated in such a way that it can be clearly supported or dismissed. Although this criterion is very important to keep in mind, you should also understand that ultimately theories or hypotheses are never proved beyond a doubt through hypothesis testing. Claims that certain data have "proved" the validity of their hypothesis should be regarded with grave reservation. At best, findings that support a hypothesis are considered tentative. If repeated replication of a study yields the same results, more confidence can be placed in the conclusions advanced by the researchers. It is important to remember about testability that although hypotheses are more likely to be accepted with increasing evidence, they are ultimately never proved.

5. Another point about testability to consider is that the hypothesis should be objectively stated and devoid of any value-laden words. Value-laden hypotheses are not empirically testable. Quantifiable phrases—such as "greater than"; "less than"; "decrease"; "increase"; "positively related"; "negatively related"; and "related"—convey the idea of objectivity and testability. You should immediately be suspicious of hypotheses that are not stated objectively.

6. You should recognize that how the proposed relationship of the hypothesis is phrased suggests the type of research design that is appropriate for the study, as well as the level of evidence to be derived from the findings. For example, if a hypothesis proposes that treatment X_1 will have a greater effect on Y than treatment X_2, an experimental (level II evidence) or quasiexperimental design (level III evidence) is suggested. If a hypothesis proposes that there will be a positive relationship between variables X and Y, a nonexperimental design (level IV evidence) is suggested. Table 4-4 contains additional examples of hypotheses, the type of research design, and the level of evidence that is suggested by each hypothesis. The design and level of evidence have important implications for the remainder of the study in terms of the appropriateness of sample selection, data collection, data analysis, interpretation of findings, and—ultimately—the conclusions advanced by the researcher.

7. If the research report contains research questions rather than hypotheses, you will want to evaluate whether this is appropriate for the study. One criterion for making this decision, as presented earlier in this chapter, is whether the study is of an exploratory, a descriptive, or a qualitative nature. If it is, then it is appropriate to have research questions rather than hypotheses.

APPRAISING THE EVIDENCE

The Research Question and Hypotheses

The care taken by a researcher when developing the research question or hypothesis is often representative of the overall conceptualization and design of the study. A methodically formulated research question provides the basis for hypothesis development. In a quantitative research study, the remainder of the study revolves around testing the hypothesis or, in some cases, the research question. In a qualitative research study, the objective is to answer the research question. This task may be a time-consuming, sometimes frustrating endeavour for the researcher, but in the final analysis, the outcome, as evaluated by the consumer, is most often worth the struggle. Because this text focuses on the nurse as a critical consumer of research, the following sections pertain primarily to the evaluation of research questions and hypotheses in published research reports.

CRITIQUING CRITERIA

THE RESEARCH QUESTION

1. Is the research question introduced promptly?
2. Is the question stated clearly and unambiguously in declarative or question form?
3. Does the research question express a relationship between two or more variables or at least between an independent variable and a dependent variable, thereby implying its empirical testability?
4. Does the research question specify the nature of the population being studied?
5. Has the research question been substantiated by adequate experiential and scientific background material?
6. Has the research question been placed within the context of an appropriate theoretical framework?
7. Has the significance of the research question been identified?
8. Have pragmatic issues, such as feasibility, been addressed?
9. Have the purpose, aims, or goals of the study been identified?

THE HYPOTHESES

1. Is the hypothesis related directly to the research question?
2. Is the hypothesis stated concisely in a declarative form?
3. Are the independent and dependent variables identified in the statement of the hypothesis?
4. Are the variables measurable or potentially measurable?
5. Is each of the hypotheses specific to one relationship so that each hypothesis can be either supported or not supported?
6. Is the hypothesis stated in such a way that it is testable?
7. Is the hypothesis stated objectively, without value-laden words?
8. Is the direction of the relationship in each hypothesis clearly stated?
9. Is each hypothesis consistent with the literature review?
10. Is the theoretical rationale for the hypothesis explicit?
11. Are research questions appropriately used (i.e., for an exploratory, descriptive, or qualitative study or in relation to ancillary data analyses)?

CRITICAL THINKING CHALLENGES

- Discuss how the wording of a research question or hypothesis suggests the type of research design and level of evidence that will be provided.
- Using the study about decisional involvement of senior nurse leaders by Wong and associates (2010) in Appendix B, diagram how the hypotheses flow from the theoretical framework and literature review.
- Using Sobieraj and colleagues' (2009) study in Appendix C, describe how the significance of the research problem and purpose of the study are linked to the research objectives.
- A nurse is caring for patients in a clinical situation that produces a clinical question that has no ready answer. The nurse wants to develop and refine this clinical question by using the PICOT approach so that it becomes the basis for an evidence-informed practice project. How can the nurse accomplish that objective?

KEY POINTS

- Formulation of the research question and stating the hypothesis are key preliminary steps in the research process.
- The research question is refined through a process that proceeds from the identification of a general idea of interest to the definition of a more specific and circumscribed topic.
- A preliminary literature review reveals related factors that appear to be critical for the research topic of interest and helps further define the research questions.
- The significance of the research question must be identified in terms of its potential contribution to patients, nurses, the medical community in general, and society. The applicability of the question for nursing practice and its theoretical relevance must be established. The findings should also have the potential for formulating or altering nursing practices or policies.
- The feasibility of a research question must be examined in light of pragmatic considerations: for example, time; the availability of participants, money, facilities, and equipment; the nurse's experience; and ethical issues.

Continued

- The final research question consists of a statement about the relationship of two or more variables. The question clearly identifies the relationship between the independent variables and dependent variables, specifies the nature of the population being studied, and implies the possibility of empirical testing.
- Focused clinical questions arise from clinical practice and guide the literature search for the best available evidence to answer the clinical question.
- A hypothesis is an attempt to answer the research question. When the validity of the assumptions of the theoretical framework is tested, the hypothesis connects the theory and reality.
- A hypothesis is a declarative statement about the relationship between two or more variables in which an expected outcome is predicted. The characteristics of a hypothesis include a relationship statement, implications regarding testability, and consistency with a defined theory base.
- Hypotheses can be formulated directionally or nondirectionally. Hypotheses can be further categorized as either research or statistical (null) hypotheses.
- Research questions may be used instead of hypotheses in exploratory, descriptive, or qualitative research studies. Research questions may also be formulated in addition to hypotheses to answer questions related to ancillary data.
- The purpose, research question, or hypothesis provides information about the intent of the research question and hypothesis and suggests the level of evidence to be obtained from the study findings.
- The critiquing criteria are a set of guidelines for evaluating the strengths and weaknesses of the research question and hypotheses as they appear in a research report.
- In critiquing, the reader assesses the clarity of the research question and the related subquestions, the specificity of the population, and the implications for testability.
- The interrelatedness of the research question, the literature review, the theoretical framework, and the hypotheses should be apparent.
- The appropriateness of the research design suggested by the research question is also evaluated.
- The purpose of the study (i.e., why the researcher is conducting the study) should be differentiated from the research question.
- The reader evaluates the wording of the hypothesis in terms of the clarity of the relational statement, its implications for testability, and its congruence

with theory. The appropriateness of the hypothesis in relation to the type of research design is also examined. In addition, the appropriate use of research questions is evaluated in relation to the type of study conducted.

REFERENCES

Amorim, A. R., Linne, Y. M., & Lourenco, P. M. C. (2007). Diet or exercise or both, for weight reduction in women after childbirth. *Cochrane Database of Systematic Reviews*, (*3*), CD005627

Bailey, J. J., Sabbagh, M., Loiselle, C. G., Boileu, J., & McVey, L. (2010). Supporting families in the ICU: A descriptive correlational study of informational support, anxiety, and satisfaction with care. *Intensive & Critical Care Nursing*, *26*(2), 114-122.

Boscart, V. M. (2009). A communication intervention for nursing staff in chronic care. *Journal of Advanced Nursing*, *65*(9), 1823-1832. doi: 10.1111/j.1365-2648.2009.05035.x

Cullum, N. (2000). User's guides to the nursing literature: An introduction. *Evidence-Based Nursing*, *3*(2):71-72.

de Witt, L., Ploeg, J., & Black, M. (2010). Living alone with dementia: An interpretative phenomenological study with older women. *Journal of Advanced Nursing*, *66*(8), 1698-1707. doi: 10.1111/j.1365-2648.2010.05295.x

Eser, I., Korshid, L., Gunes, U. Y., & Demir, Y. (2007). The effect of different body positions on blood pressure. *Journal of Clinical Nursing*, *16*(1):137-140.

Gillies, C. L., Abrams, K. R., Lambert, P. C., Cooper, N. J., Sutton, A. J., Hsu, R. T., & Khunti, K. (2007). Pharmacological and lifestyle interventions to prevent or delay type 2 diabetes in people with impaired glucose tolerance: Systematic review and meta-analysis. *British Medical Journal*, *334*(7588), 299. doi: 10.1136/bmj.39063.689375.55

Harrowing, J. N., & Mill, J. (2010). Moral distress among Ugandan nurses providing HIV care: A critical ethnography. *International Journal of Nursing Studies*, *47*, 723-731.

Ives, M., & Melrose, S. (2010). Immunizing children who fear and resist needles: Is it a problem for nurses? *Nursing Forum*, *45*(1), 29-39.

Keefe, M. R., Kajrlsen, K. A., Lobo, M. L., Kotzer, A. M., & Dudley, W. N. (2006). Reducing parenting stress in families with irritable infants. *Nursing Research*, *55*(3), 198-205.

Koeman, M., van der Ven, A. J., Hak, E., Kaasjager, K., de Smet, A. G. A., Dormans, T. P. J., . . . Bonton, M. J. M. (2006). Oral decontamination with chlorhexidine reduces the incidence of ventilator-associated pneumonia. *American Journal of Respiratory and Critical Care*, *173*, 1348-1355.

Look AHEAD Research Group, Pi-Sunyer, X., Blackburn, G., et al. (2007). Reduction in weight and cardiovascular risk factors in overweight and obese people with type 2 diabetes: One-year results of the Look AHEAD trial. *Diabetes Care*, *30*, 1374-1383.

Martinez, A. M., D'Artois, D., & Rennick, J. E. (2007). Does the 15-minute (or less) family interview influence family nursing practice? *Journal of Family Nursing*, *13*(2), 157-178.

Melnyk, B. M., & Fineout-Overholt, E. (2011). *Evidence-based practice in nursing and healthcare: A guide to best practice* (2nd ed). New York: Wolters Kluwer.

Meneses, K. D., McNees, P., Loerzei, V. W., Su, X., Zhang, Y., & Hassey, L. A. (2007). Transition from treatment to survivorship: Effects of a psychoeducational intervention on quality of life in breast cancer survivors. *Oncology Nursing Forum*, *34*(5), 1007-1016.

Mulford, D., Taggart, H. M., Nivens, A., & Payrie, C. (2008). Arch support use for improving balance and reducing pain in older adults. *Applied Nursing Research*, *21*(3), 153-158.

Nordgren, L., Asp, M., & Fagerberg, I. (2007). Living with moderate-severe chronic heart failure as a middle-aged person. *Qualitative Health Research*, *17*(1), 4-13.

O'Donnell, S., MacIntosh, J., & Wuest, J. (2010). A theoretical understanding of sickness absences among women who have experienced workplace bullying. *Qualitative Health Research 20*(4), 439-452.

Peterson, W. E., Sword, W., Charles, C., & DiCenso, A. (2007). Adolescents' perceptions of inpatient postpartum nursing care. *Qualitative Health Research*, *17*(2), 201-212.

Purc-Stephenson, R. J., & Thrasher, C. (2010). Telephone triage and advice: A meta-ethnography. *Journal of Advanced Nursing*, *66*(3), 482-494. doi: 10.1111/j.1365-2648.2010.05275.x

Sackett, D. L., Straus, S. E., Richardson, W. S., Rosenberg, W., & Haynes, R. B. (2000). *Evidence-based medicine: How to practise and teach EBM*. London: Churchill Livingstone.

Simonson, D. C., Ahern, M. M., & Hendryx, M. S. (2007). Anesthesia staffing and anesthetic complications during cesarean delivery: A retrospective analysis. *Nursing Research*, *56*(1), 9-17.

Sobieraj, G., Bhatt, M., LeMay, S., Rennick, J., & Johnston, C. (2009). The effect of music on parental participation during pediatric laceration repair. *Canadian Journal of Nursing Research*, *41*(4), 68-82.

Streubert, H. J., & Carpenter, D. R. (2011). *Qualitative research in nursing: Advancing the humanistic imperative* (5th ed.). Philadelphia: Wolters Kluwer.

Thompson, C., Cullum, N., McCaughan, D., Sheldon, T., & Raynor, P. (2004) Nurses, information use, and clinical decision making: The real world potential for evidence-based decisions in nursing. *Evidence-Based Nursing*, *7*(3):68-72. doi:10.1136/ebn.7.3.68

Thorne, S., Armstrong, E., Harris, S. R., et al. (2009). Patient real-time and 12-month retrospective perceptions of difficult communications in the cancer diagnostic period. *Qualitative Health Research*, *19*(10), 1983-1394. doi: 10.1177/1049732.309348382

Wong, C. A., Laschinger, H., Cummings, G. G., Vincent, L., & O'Connor, P. (2010). Decisional involvement of senior nurse leaders in Canadian acute care hospitals. *Journal of Nursing Management*, *18*, 122-133. doi: 10.1111/j.1365-2834.2010.01053.x

FOR FURTHER STUDY

evolve Go to Evolve at http://evolve.elsevier.com/ Canada/LoBiondo/Research for Audio Glossary, how-to instructions for Writing Proposals for Funding, and additional research articles for practice in reviewing and critiquing.

CHAPTER 5

Finding and Appraising the Literature

Stephanie Fulton | Barbara Krainovich-Miller | Cherylyn Cameron

LEARNING OUTCOMES

After reading this chapter, you will be able to do the following:

- Discuss the relationship of the literature review to nursing theory, research, education, and practice.
- Discuss the purposes of the literature review from the perspective of the research investigator and the research consumer.
- Discuss the use of the literature review for quantitative designs and qualitative methods.
- Discuss the purpose of reviewing the literature in development of evidence-informed practice.
- Differentiate between primary and secondary sources.
- Compare the advantages and disadvantages of the most commonly used online databases for conducting a literature review.
- Identify the characteristics of an effective electronic search of the literature.
- Critically read, appraise, and synthesize primary and secondary sources used for the development of a literature review.
- Apply critiquing criteria to the evaluation of literature reviews in selected research studies.

KEY TERMS

Boolean operator	literature review	refereed (peer-reviewed) journal
citation management software	online database	secondary sources
concept	operational definition	theory
conceptual definition	primary sources	Web browser
controlled vocabulary	print indexes	

STUDY RESOURCES

Go to Evolve at http://evolve.elsevier.com/Canada/LoBiondo/Research for Audio Glossary, how-to instructions for Writing Proposals for Funding, and additional research articles for practice in reviewing and critiquing.

YOU MAY WONDER WHY AN ENTIRE chapter of a research text is devoted to finding and appraising the literature. The main reason is that searching for, retrieving, and critically appraising the literature is a key step in the research process for researchers and also for nurses involved in evidence-informed practice. A more personal question you might ask is "Will knowing more about how to critically appraise and gather the literature really help me as a student or later as a practising nurse?" The answer is that it most certainly will! Your ability to locate and retrieve research studies, critically appraise them, and decide that you have the best available evidence to inform your clinical decision making is a skill essential for your current role as a student and your future role as a nurse who is a competent research consumer.

Your critical appraisal, also called a *critique of the literature,* is an organized systematic approach to evaluating a research study or group of research studies. It involves the use of a set of established critical appraisal criteria to objectively determine the strength, quality, and consistency of evidence; these characteristics help you determine the applicability of the evidence to research, education, or practice. As a research consumer, you will become skilled at critically appraising research studies, combining the evidence with your clinical experience and the patient population that you are caring for, to make an evidence-informed decision about the applicability of a particular nursing intervention for your patient or for the patient population in your practice setting.

The section of a published research report titled "Literature Review" generally appears near the beginning of the report. It provides an abbreviated version of the complete literature review conducted by a researcher and represents the foundation for the study. Therefore, the **literature review,** a systematic and critical appraisal of the most important literature on a topic, is a key step in the research process that provides the basis of a research study.

The conceptual framework, or theoretical framework, of a research report is a structure of concepts or theories pulled together as a map for the study; this map provides rationale for the development of research questions or hypotheses. This section of a research report is often a titled subsection of the literature review and may be accompanied by a diagram illustrating the proposed relationships between and among the concepts. Alternatively, the conceptual/theoretical framework may not be separately identified; it may be embedded in the literature review section of an article or simply not included. The links between theory, research, education, and practice are intricately connected; together they create the knowledge base for the nursing discipline, as shown in Figure 5-1.

The purpose of this chapter is to introduce you to the literature review as it is used in research and evidence-informed practice projects. It provides you with the systematic tools to (1) consider how the theoretical or conceptual framework guides development of a research study; (2) critically appraise a research study or group of research studies; (3) locate, search for, and retrieve research studies, systematic reviews, documents, and statistical reports; and (4) differentiate between a research article and a conceptual article or book. This set of tools will help you develop your research consumer

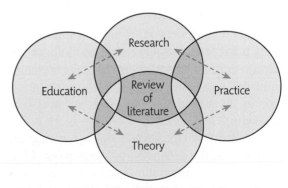

FIGURE 5-1 Relationship of the literature review to theory, research, education, and practice.

competencies and prepare your academic papers and evidence-informed practice projects.

THE CONCEPTUAL OR THEORETICAL FRAMEWORK

As discussed in Chapter 2, the conceptual framework, or theoretical framework, of a research report is a structure of concepts or theories that provides the basis for development of research questions or hypotheses. A **concept** is an image or a symbolic representation of an abstract idea. The researcher uses a concept, a set of concepts, or a particular theory or set of theories to build the theoretical framework of the study. Concepts are the major components of theory and convey the abstract ideas within a theory. A **theory** is a set of interrelated concepts, definitions, and propositions that convey a systematic view of phenomena for the purpose of explaining and making predictions about those phenomena. A **conceptual definition** includes the general meaning of a concept. An **operational definition** is a description of the method used to measure the concept; once the concept is linked to a measurement method or instrument, it is regarded as a variable.

For example, Wong and colleagues (2010), "investigating the scope and degree of involvement of senior nurse leaders in executive level decisions in acute care organizations across Canada" (p. 122), used a theoretical framework adapted from previous work on strategic decision making in health care organizations to guide the development of the study. The content related to the theoretical framework is identified in a separately titled section of the article and follows the presentation and critical appraisal of the literature on senior nurse role changes with restructuring and in organizational decision making (see Appendix B).

As described in the introduction to this chapter, the theoretical or conceptual framework of a research study is often illustrated with a diagram. For example, in the study by Wong and colleagues (2010) (see Appendix B), Figure B-1 (see p. 530 [in Appendix B]) of this article is a conceptual framework diagram that depicts the participation in organizational decision making and identifies the major variables of the study.

As you can see, theory, practice, and research are interconnected: Practice enables testing of theory and generates research questions; research contributes to theory building and provides supporting evidence for effective nursing interventions in clinical practice. Therefore, what is learned through practice, theory, and research is combined to create the knowledge of the discipline of nursing, which you are then taught in your nursing courses.

REVIEW OF THE LITERATURE

The Literature Review: The Researcher's Perspective

The overall purpose of the literature review in a research study is to present a strong knowledge base for the conduct of the research study. Specific objectives 1 through 7 listed in Box 5-1 reflect the purposes of a literature review for the conduct of quantitative research and most qualitative research. It is important to understand when you read a research article that the researcher's main goal when developing the literature review was to develop the knowledge foundation for a sound study and to generate research questions and hypotheses.

An extensive literature review is essential for all steps of the quantitative research process and for some qualitative methods. From this perspective, the review is broad and systematic, as well as in-depth. It is a critical collection and evaluation of the important published literature in journals, monographs, books, and book chapters, as well as unpublished research print and online materials (e.g., doctoral dissertations and masters' theses), audiovisual materials (e.g., audiotapes and videotapes), and sometimes personal communications (e.g., conference presentations and one-on-one interviews).

BOX 5-1

OVERALL PURPOSES OF A LITERATURE REVIEW

MAJOR GOAL

To develop a strong knowledge base to carry out a research study or an evidence-informed practice project

OBJECTIVES

A review of the literature helps you do the following:

1. Determine what is known and unknown about a subject, concept, or problem
2. Determine gaps, consistencies, and inconsistencies in the literature about a subject, concept, or problem
3. Discover conceptual traditions used to examine problems
4. Generate useful research questions and hypotheses
5. Determine an appropriate research design, methodology, and analysis for answering the research questions or hypotheses on the basis of an assessment of the strengths and weaknesses of earlier works
6. Determine the need for replication of a study or refinement of a study
7. Synthesize the strengths and weaknesses and findings of available studies on a topic or problem
8. Uncover one or more new practice interventions or obtain supporting evidence for revising or maintaining current interventions, protocols, and policies
9. Promote evidence-informed revision and development of new practice protocols, policies, and projects or activities related to nursing practice
10. Generate clinical questions that guide development of evidence-informed practice projects

From a researcher's perspective, the objectives in Box 5-1 direct the questions the researcher asks while reading the literature to determine one or more useful research questions or hypotheses and how best to design a particular study.

The following brief overview about the use of the literature review in relation to the steps of the quantitative and qualitative research process will help you to understand the researcher's focus. A critical review of relevant literature affects the steps of the quantitative research process as follows:

- *Theoretical or conceptual framework:* A literature review reveals conceptual traditions, concepts, theories, or conceptual models from nursing and other related disciplines that can be used to examine problems. This framework presents the context for studying the problem and can be viewed as a map for understanding the relationships between or among the variables in quantitative studies. The literature review provides rationale for the variables and explains concepts, definitions, and relationships between or among the independent and dependent variables used in the theoretical framework of the study.

- *Primary and secondary sources:* The author of a literature review should use mainly **primary sources:** that is, articles and books by the original author. Sometimes it is appropriate to use **secondary sources,** which are published articles or books that are written by persons other than the individual who developed the theory or conducted the research study. The studies selected for the literature review should offer the strongest and most consistent level of evidence available on the topic (Table 5-1 lists examples).

- *Research question and hypothesis:* The literature review helps you determine what is known and not known; uncover gaps, consistencies, or inconsistencies; or to disclose unanswered questions in the literature about a subject, concept, theory, or problem that generate or allow for refinement of research questions, hypotheses, or both.

- *Design and method:* The literature review exposes the strengths and weaknesses of previous studies in terms of designs and methods and helps the researcher choose an appropriate new, replicated, or refined design, including data-collection method,

TABLE 5-1

PRIMARY AND SECONDARY SOURCES

PRIMARY: ESSENTIAL	SECONDARY: USEFUL
Material written by the original person who conducted the study, developed the theory (model), or prepared the scholarly discussion on a concept, topic, or issue of interest (i.e., the original author).	Material written by one or more individuals other than the person who conducted the research study or developed a theory; the author is someone other than the original author who writes about or presents the original author's work. The material is usually in the form of a summary or critique (i.e., analysis and synthesis) of someone else's scholarly work or body of literature.
Primary sources can be published or unpublished.	Secondary sources can be published or unpublished.
Research example: An investigator's report of his or her research study (e.g., articles in Appendixes A through D).	Secondary source examples are the following: response, commentary, or critique articles of a research study, a theory or model, or a professional view of an issue; review of literature article published in a refereed scholarly journal; abstracts of a published work written by someone other than the original author; examples: a biography or a systematic review.
Theoretical example: Senior nurse leaders' participation in organizational decision making is the theoretical framework used by Wong et al. (2010) in their study of the scope and degree of senior nurse leaders' contributions to executive-level decisions. The theoretical framework used in this study was adapted from the work of Ashmos, Huonker, and McDaniel (1998) and Anderson and McDaniel (1998) and cited as such in the research report (see Appendix B).	*Hint:* Use secondary sources sparingly; however, secondary sources—especially of studies that include a research critique—are a valuable learning tool for a beginning research consumer.
Other primary source examples include autobiographies, diaries, films, letters, artifacts, periodicals, and tapes.	
Hint: Critical evaluation of mainly primary sources is essential in a thorough and relevant review of the literature.	

sampling strategy and size, valid and reliable measurement instruments, an effective data analysis method, and appropriate informed consent forms. Often, because of journal space limitations, researchers only include abbreviated information about these aspects in their journal article.

- *Outcome of the analysis (i.e., findings, discussion, implications, and recommendations):* The literature review is used to help the researcher accurately interpret and discuss the results/findings of a study. In the discussion section of a research article, the researcher refers to the research studies and

theoretical articles or books described earlier in the article in the literature review and uses this conceptual and research literature to interpret and explain the study's findings. For example, in the Discussion section of their article, Wong and colleagues (2010) commented that "Although there is some indication in the healthcare literature that increased involvement in organizational decision-making by physicians and registered nurses was associated with outcomes such as lower costs in hospitals (Ashmos, Huonker, & McDaniel, 1998) and improved resident outcomes in nursing

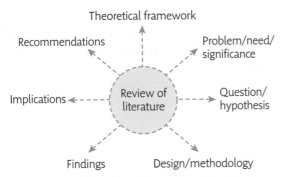

FIGURE 5-2   Relationship of the review of the literature to the steps of the quantitative research process.

homes (Anderson & McDaniel, 1999), we found that SNL decision involvement (timing, breadth and number of activities) and influence in decision-making did not predict their perceived quality of organizational decisions" (p. 130). Figure 5-2 relates the literature review to all aspects of the quantitative research process.

The Literature Review: The Consumers Perspective

From the perspective of the research consumer rather than that of a researcher, you review a number of studies to answer a clinical question or to solve a clinical problem. Therefore, you search the literature widely and gather multiple resources to answer your question by using an evidence-informed practice approach. This process includes (1) asking clinical questions; (2) identifying and gathering the evidence; (3) critically appraising and synthesizing the evidence or literature; (4) acting to change practice by using the best available evidence, coupled with your clinical experience and patient preferences (values, setting, and resources); and (5) evaluating the use of the research evidence found to assess applicability of the research findings to the practice change. In addition to objectives 1 through 7 in Box 5-1, objectives 7, 8, and 9 specifically reflect the purposes of a literature review

for nurses involved in evidence-informed practice projects.

As a student or practising nurse, you may be asked to generate a clinical question for an evidence-informed practice project and search for, retrieve, review, and critically appraise the literature to identify the "best available evidence" that provides the answer to a clinical question and informs your clinical decision making. A clear and precise articulation of a question is crucial for finding the best evidence. Evidence-informed questions may sound like research questions, but they are questions used to search the existing literature for answers. The evidence-informed practice process follows the PICOT format to generate clinical questions. For example, students in an adult health course were asked to generate a clinical question related to health care promotion for older women by using the PICOT format. As discussed in Chapter 4, The PICOT format is as follows:

P: Problem/patient population; specifically defined group

I: Intervention; what intervention or event will be studied

C: Comparison of intervention; with what the intervention will be compared

O: Outcome; the effect of the intervention

T: Time; the time frame

An example of its use is given in the following Practical Application box.

As a practising nurse you may be called on to revise or continue current evidence-informed practice protocols, practice standards, or policies in your health care organization or to develop new ones. This requires that you know how to retrieve and critically appraise research articles, systematic reviews, and practice guidelines to determine the degree of support or lack of support found in the literature. A critical appraisal of the literature related to a specific clinical question uncovers data that contribute evidence to support current practice and clinical decision making, as well as for making changes in practice.

Practical Application

One group of students was interested in whether regular exercise prevented osteoporosis for postmenopausal women who had osteopenia. The PICOT format for the clinical question that guided their search was as follows:

P: Postmenopausal women with osteopenia
I: Regular exercise program
C: No regular exercise program
O: Prevention of osteoporosis
T: After 1 year

Their assignment required that the students do the following:

- Search the literature by using electronic databases (e.g., Cumulative Index to Nursing and Allied Health Literature [CINAHL], via EBSCO; MEDLINE; Scopus; and Cochrane Database of Systematic Reviews) for the background information that enabled them to identify the significance of osteopenia and osteoporosis as a health problem in women.
- Identify systematic reviews, practice guidelines, and individual research studies that provided the "best available evidence" related to the effectiveness of regular exercise programs on prevention of osteoporosis.
- Critically appraise systematic reviews, practice guidelines, and research studies in accordance with standardized critical appraisal criteria (see Chapter 20).
- Synthesize the overall strengths and weaknesses of the evidence provided by the literature.
- Establish a conclusion about the strength, quality, and consistency of the evidence.
- Make recommendations about applicability of the evidence to clinical nursing practice that guides development of a health promotion project about osteoporosis risk reduction for postmenopausal women with osteopenia.

Research Conduct and Consumer of Research Purposes: Differences and Similarities

How does the literature review differ when it is used for research purposes versus for a consumer of research purposes? The literature review in a research study is used to develop a sound research proposal for a research study that will generate knowledge. From a broader perspective, the major focus of reviewing the literature as a consumer is to uncover multiple sources of evidence on a given topic that have been generated by researchers in their research studies that can potentially be used to improve clinical practice and patient outcomes.

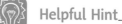

Helpful Hint

Remember that the findings of one study on a topic do not usually provide sufficient evidence to support a change in practice; be cautious when a nurse colleague tells you to change your practice on the basis of the results of one study.

From a student perspective, the ability to critically appraise the literature is essential to acquiring a skill set for successfully completing scholarly papers, presentations, debates, and evidence-informed practice projects. Both types of literature reviews are similar in that both should be framed in the context of previous research and theoretical literature and pertinent to the objectives presented in Box 5-1.

Evidence-Informed Practice Tip

For a research consumer, formulating a clinical question provides a focus that guides the literature review.

SEARCHING FOR EVIDENCE

In your student role, when you are preparing an academic paper, you read the required course materials, as well as additional literature retrieved from the library. Students often state, "I know how to do research." Perhaps you have thought the same thing because you "researched" a topic for a paper in the library. In that situation, however, it would be more accurate for you to say that you have been "searching" the literature to uncover research and conceptual information to prepare an academic term paper on a certain topic. You search for primary sources, which are articles, books, or other documents written by the person who conducted the study, developed the theory, or prepared the scholarly discussion on a concept, topic, problem, or issue of interest. You also search for secondary sources, which are materials written by persons other than the individuals who conducted a research study or developed a particular theory. Table 5-1 provides more extensive definitions and examples of primary and secondary sources.

Although reviewing the literature for research purposes and research consumer activities

requires the same critical thinking and reading skills, a literature review for a research proposal is usually much more extensive and comprehensive, and the critiquing process is more in-depth. From an academic standpoint, requirements for a literature review for a particular assignment differ, depending on the level and type of course, as well as the specific objective of the assignment. These factors determine whether a student's literature search requires a limited, selective review or a major or extensive review. Regardless

TABLE **5-2**

STEPS AND STRATEGIES FOR CONDUCTING A LITERATURE SEARCH

STEPS OF LITERATURE REVIEW	STRATEGY
Step 1: Determine the clinical question or research topic.	Keep focused on the characteristics of patients you deal with in your work setting. You know what works and does not work in the delivery of nursing care. In your student role, keep focused on the assignment's objective; use the literature to support opinions or develop a concept under discussion.
Step 2: Identify the key variables/terms.	Ask your reference librarian for help, and read research guidebooks, which are usually found near the computers that are used for student searches; include "research" as one of your variables.
Step 3: Conduct a computer search by using at least two recognized online databases.	Conduct the search yourself or with the help of your librarian; it is essential to use at least two health-related databases, such as CINAHL via EBSCO, MEDLINE, PsycINFO, or ERIC.
Step 4: Review abstracts online and disregard irrelevant articles.	Scan through your search, read the abstracts provided, and make a note of only those that fit your topic; select "references," as well as "search history" and "full-text articles" if available, before printing, saving, or e-mailing your search.
Step 5: Retrieve relevant sources.	Organize by article type or study design and year and reread the abstracts to determine whether the articles chosen are relevant and worth retrieving.
Step 6: Print or download articles; if you are unable to print directly from the database, you can order them through interlibrary loan.	Save yourself time and money: Buy a library copying card ahead of time or bring plenty of change so that you avoid wasting time midway to secure change; you can also bring a thumb drive to download PDF versions of your articles.
Step 7: Conduct preliminary reading and disregard irrelevant sources.	Review critical reading strategies (see Chapter 3; e.g., read the abstract at the beginning of the articles, and see the example in this chapter).
Step 8: Critically read each source (summarize and critique each source).	Use the critical appraisal strategies from Chapter 1 (e.g., use a standardized critiquing tool), take time to type up each summary and critical appraisal (no more than one page long), include the references in APA style at the top or bottom of each abstract, and attach the original article.
	Invest time in learning a citation management software tool. This will save you the hassle of formatting all of your citations.
Step 9: Synthesize critical summaries of each article.	Decide how you will present your synthesis of overall strengths and weaknesses of the reviewed articles (e.g., chronologically or according to type: research or conceptual) and type up the synthesized material and a reference list.

APA, American Psychological Association; *CINAHL*, Cumulative Index to Nursing and Allied Health Literature; *ERIC*, Education Resources Information Center.

of extent, discovering knowledge is the goal of any search; therefore, a consumer of research must know how to search the literature. Reference librarians can provide excellent help in searching for various sources of scholarly literature. If you are unfamiliar with the process of conducting a scholarly computer search, your reference librarian can help. Table 5-2 provides you with steps and strategies for conducting a literature search.

Prioritizing the Search for Evidence

In Chapter 3, an evidence hierarchy is presented for grading the strength and quality of evidence provided by individual studies or resources located during a search. In this chapter, an evidence-informed model, called the "6S" pyramid, is used to help you identify the highest-level information resource to facilitate your search for the best evidence about your clinical question or problem (DiCenso, Bayley, & Haynes, 2009). This model, as illustrated in Figure 5-3, suggests that when searching the literature, consider prioritizing your search strategy and begin by looking for the highest-level information resource available. For example, individual original studies such as those found in MEDLINE or CINAHL (e.g., a randomized clinical trial) are at the lowest level of the information resource pyramid. The next information resource levels of the 6S pyramid are *synopses of studies* (e.g., a brief summary of a high-quality study), then *syntheses* (e.g., Cochrane Library), followed by *synopses of syntheses* (comprehensive summary of all the research related to a clinical question), and *summaries*

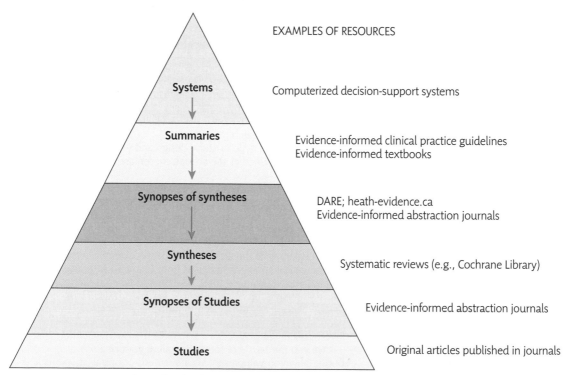

FIGURE 5-3   The 6S levels of organization of evidence from health care research.
Adapted by permission from BMJ Publishing Group Limited. Alba DiCenso, Liz Bayley, R Brian Haynes. (2009). "Accessing pre-appraised evidence: fine-tuning the 5S model into a 6S model." *Evidence Based Nursing.* Copyright © 2009, BMJ Publishing Group Ltd and the RCN Publishing Company Ltd.

(e.g., evidence-informed clinical practice guidelines and textbooks.

The highest information resource level pertains to computerized decision support systems, a resource built into an electronic medical record that links your patient's distinctive needs with current evidence-informed practice guidelines. These computerized systems are under development, but this does not mean that the information found within the other information resource levels is not useful or appropriate. The 6S model is a tool that can help guide your search for the strongest and most relevant evidence-informed information; however, it does not replace the importance of critically reading each piece of evidence and assessing its quality and applicability for current practice.

Helpful Hint_____
- Make an appointment with your educational institution's reference librarian so you can take advantage of his or her expertise in accessing electronic databases.
- Take the time to set up your computer for electronic library access.
- If the full text of an article is unavailable through your electronic search, read the abstract to determine whether you want to order the article through interlibrary loan.

Performing an Online Database Search

Why Use an Online Database?

Perhaps you are still not convinced that online database searches are the best way to acquire information for a review of the literature. Maybe you have searched by using Google or Yahoo and found relevant information. This is an understandable temptation, especially if your assignment requires you to use only five articles. Try to think about it from another perspective, and ask yourself the following question: "Is this the most appropriate and efficient way to find out what is the latest and strongest research on a topic that

affects patient care?" If you take the time to learn how to perform a sound database search, you will have the essential competency needed for your career in nursing. The Critical Thinking Decision Path illustrates a method for locating evidence to support your research or clinical question.

TYPES OF RESOURCES

Print: Books, Journals, and Indexes

Most college and university libraries have an online card catalog to find print and online books, journals (titles only), videos and other media items, scripts, monographs, conference proceedings, masters' theses, dissertations, archival materials, and more.

Before the 1980s, a search was usually done manually with **print indexes,** which were listings of published material. This was a tedious and time-consuming process. The print indexes are useful today for finding sources that have not been entered into electronic (online) databases. Some of your professors might talk about the "Red Books" in referring to print versions of what is now CINAHL. The print index started in 1956 but is no longer produced. Print resources are still necessary if a search requires materials not entered into an electronic database before a certain year.

Print: Refereed Journals

A major portion of most literature reviews consists of journal articles. In contrast to books and textbooks, which take much longer to publish, journals are a ready source of up-to-date information on almost any subject. Therefore, journals are the preferred mode of communicating the most recent theory or results of a research study. For you as a beginning research consumer, refereed journals should be your first choice when looking for theoretical, clinical, or research articles. A **refereed (peer-reviewed) journal** has a panel of internal and external reviewers who review submitted manuscripts for possible

CRITICAL THINKING DECISION PATH

Search for Evidence Thought Flow

Ask an answerable question with PICOT elements

↓

Select best source for evidence →

Synthesized or Summarized Sources
ACP PIER
BMJ Clinical Evidence
Cochrane Systematic Review
Evidence-informed nursing journal Government guidelines

↓

Find answer?

Yes → Appraise and summarize your findings

No ↓

Select next source to locate evidence →

Primary Sources
CINAHL
MEDLINE
PsycINFO

↓

Find answer?

Yes → Appraise and summarize your findings

No ↓

Consult your librarian and faculty. You may need to consider research project

Based on Kendall, S. American College of Physicians (ACP), ©2001, 2003, 2004, as found in Kendall, S. (2008). Evidence-based resources simplified. *Canadian Family Physician, 54*(2), 241–243.
BMJ, British Medical Journal; CINAHL, Cumulative Index to Nursing and Allied Health Literature; *PICOT,* population, intervention, comparison, outcome, time; *PIER,* Physicians' Information and Education Resource.

publication. The external reviewers are drawn from a pool of nurse scholars, and possibly scholars from other related disciplines, who are experts in various specialties. In most cases, the reviews are "blind"; that is, the reviewers do not know who the authors of manuscript are. The reviewers use a set of scholarly criteria to judge whether a manuscript meets the publication standards of the journal. These criteria are similar to those that you use when you are critically appraising the strengths and weaknesses of a study. The credibility of a published theoretical or research article is strengthened by the peer review process. Most refereed journals are available in print and accessible electronically through your library's online resources. If you cannot access some research articles from your library, consider the use of Google Scholar as a search engine to locate them.

Internet: Online Bibliographic and Abstract Databases

An **online database** is used to find journal sources (periodicals) of research and conceptual articles on a variety of topics (e.g., doctoral dissertations), as well as the publications of professional organizations and various governmental agencies. These sources contain bibliographic citation information such as the author, title, journal, date, and indexed terms for each record. Some also include the abstract. Box 5-2 lists examples of the more commonly used online databases.

Your college or university probably enables you to access such databases from your residence, whether it is or is not on campus. The most relevant and frequently used source for nursing literature remains CINAHL. Full text has been added to this database; thus, in many cases you can find the full article. Another premier resource is MEDLINE, which is produced by the National Library of Medicine. MEDLINE focuses on the life sciences, and its sources dates back to the early 1950s.

Internet: Online Secondary or Summary Databases

Some databases contain more than just journal article information. These online resources contain either summaries or synopses of studies, overviews of diseases or conditions, or a summary of the most recent evidence to support a particular treatment. For example, the Cochrane Library is an online resource that consists of six databases, including the Cochrane Database of Systematic Reviews. Using at least two electronic health-related databases such as CINAHL and MEDLINE (see Box 5-2) is recommended.

Internet: Online Search Engines

You are probably familiar with accessing a **Web browser** (a software program used to connect to or search the World Wide Web; e.g., Internet Explorer, Mozilla Firefox, or Safari) to conduct searches for music or other entities and using search engines such as Google to find information or articles. However, "surfing" the Web is not a good use of your time for scholarly literature searches. Table 5-3 lists sources of free online information. Review the table carefully to determine whether it is a good source of primary research studies. Note that it includes government Web sites for such U.S. organizations as the Health Resources and Services Administration and the National Institutes of Health, which are sources of health information, and some clinical guidelines based on systematic reviews of the literature, but most Web sites are not a primary source of research studies. Less common and less used sources of scholarly material are audiotapes, videos, personal communications (e.g., letters or telephone or in-person interviews), unpublished doctoral dissertations, master's theses, and conference proceedings.

Most searches with electronic databases include not only citation information but also the abstract of the article and options for obtaining the full text. When possible, print or copy the full

BOX 5-2

ONLINE DATABASES

AMERICAN COLLEGE OF PHYSICIANS: THE PHYSICIANS' INFORMATION AND EDUCATION RESOURCE (PIER)

- Produced by the American College of Physicians (ACP)
- Designed to be a point-of-care evidence-informed resource for 300 types of disease
- Available online from ACP (n.d.) or through StatRef

CLINICAL EVIDENCE FROM THE *BRITISH MEDICAL JOURNAL*

- Produced by the *British Medical Journal*
- Systematic reviews that summarize the current state of knowledge, or lack thereof, of medical conditions
- Provides evidence reviews for more than 250 conditions
- Available online from the *British Medical Journal* and Ovid Technologies

COCHRANE LIBRARY

- Collection of databases that contain high-quality evidence
- Includes the Cochrane Database of Systematic Reviews
- Full Cochrane Library available from Wiley Online Library other databases that make up the Cochrane Library available from other vendors, including Ovid Technologies
- Cochrane systematic reviews are indexed and searchable in both CINAHL and MEDLINE

CUMULATIVE INDEX TO NURSING AND ALLIED HEALTH LITERATURE (CINAHL)

- Initially called Cumulative Index to Nursing Literature
- Produced by CINAHL
- Electronic version available as part of the EBSCO online service
- Over 1,800 journals indexed for inclusion in database
- Citations in CINAHL are assigned index terms from a controlled vocabulary

EDUCATION RESOURCE INFORMATION CENTER (ERIC)

- Sponsored by the Institute of Education and the U.S. Department of Education
- Focuses on education research and information
- Currently indexes more than 600 journals and also includes references to books, conference papers, and technical reports

- References date from 1966
- Available from the ERIC Web site and by subscription from EBSCO, OCLC, and Ovid Technologies

EXCERPTA MEDICA

- Biomedical database
- More than 24 million indexed records
- Approximately 7,500 current, mostly peer-reviewed journals

MEDLINE (MEDICAL LITERATURE ANALYSIS AND RETRIEVAL SYSTEM ONLINE)

- Produced by the National Library of Medicine
- Premier bibliographic database for journal articles in life sciences
- References date from 1950, and approximately 5,200 worldwide journals are indexed
- Indexed with MeSH (Medical Subject Headings)
- MEDLINE is available for free through PubMed and by subscription from EBSCO, OCLC, and Ovid Technologies

PROQUEST DISSERTATIONS AND THESES

- Produced by ProQuest
- Earliest records from 1637
- PDF downloads available for over 1 million dissertations
- Available from ProQuest (n.d.)

PSYCINFO

- Produced by the American Psychological Association (APA, n.d.)
- An abstract database of the psychosocial literature beginning with citations dating back to 1800
- Covers more than 2,150 journals
- Of the journals covered, 98% are peer reviewed
- Also includes book chapters and dissertations
- Indexed with the Thesaurus of Psychological Index Terms
- Available through APA PsycNET, EBSCO, Ovid Technologies, and ProQuest

SCOPUS

- Largest abstract and citation database of peer-reviewed science literature and quality Web sources
- Provides 100% MEDLINE coverage
- Offers sophisticated tools to track, analyze, and visualize research

OCLC, Online Computer Library Center.

TABLE **5-3**

SELECTED EXAMPLES OF WEB SITES AND OUTCOMES FOR LITERATURE SEARCHES

WEB SITE	SCOPE	NOTES
Virginia Henderson International Nursing Library: http://www.nursinglibrary.org	Access to the Registry of Nursing Research database, which contains nearly 30,000 abstracts of research studies and conference papers.	Service offered without charge; locate conference abstracts and research study abstracts. This library is supported by Sigma Theta Tau International, honour society of nursing.
National Guideline Clearinghouse: http://www.guidelines.gov	Public resource for evidence-informed clinical practice guidelines. It contains more than 1,900 guidelines, including non–U.S. publications.	Offers a useful online feature of side-by-side comparison of guidelines.
National Institute of Nursing Research: http://www.nih.gov/ninr	Promotes science for nursing practice, funding for nursing and interdisciplinary research, and nurse scientist training programs. Provides links to many nursing organizations and search sites. Excellent site for graduate students.	Able to link to Computer Retrieval of Information on Scientific Projects (CRISP) and PubMed (search service of the National Library of Medicine), which accesses literature via MEDLINE and PreMEDLINE and other related material from online journals; however, this site has limited utility for the beginning consumer of research for conducting scholarly review of nursing research literature because MEDLINE alone does not include all nursing literature; searching CINAHL and MEDLINE on your own would be your first choice. Useful site for graduate students in addition to CINAHL and MEDLINE and as third database related to topic.
Turning Research into Practice (TRIP): http://www.tripdatabase.com	Content from a wide variety of free online resources, including synopses, guidelines, medical images, electronic textbooks, and systematic reviews; accessed together by the TRIP search engine.	Provides a wide sampling of available evidence.
Cochrane Collaboration: http://www.cochrane.org	Provides free access to abstracts from the Cochrane Database of Systematic Reviews. Full text of reviews and access to the databases that are part of the Cochrane Library—Database of Abstracts of Reviews of Effectiveness, Cochrane Controlled Trials Register, Cochrane Methodology Register, Health Technology Assessment database (HTA), and National Health Service (NHS) Economic Evaluation Database (EED)—are accessible through Wiley Online library	Abstracts of Cochrane Reviews are available without charge and can be browsed or searched; many databases are used in its reviews, including CINAHL via EBSCO and MEDLINE; some are primary sources (e.g., systematic reviews/meta-analyses); others (if commentaries of single studies) are a secondary source. Important source for clinical evidence but limited as a provider of primary documents for literature reviews.
Statistics Canada: http://www.statcan.gc.ca	Collects data on the Canadian population that are related to demographic trends, labour, health, trade, and education. Data on health trends are useful in identifying populations at risk and suggest associations among health determinants, health status, and population characteristics. Research papers on a variety of topics are also published.	Free source of primary data essential for comprehensive demographic data and socioeconomic trends; updated daily.

text, which of course will include the abstract and the complete references. If the text is not available, choose the option "complete reference," which will include the abstract. Reading the abstract is critical for determining whether you need to retrieve the article through another mechanism. Both the CINAHL and MEDLINE electronic databases will facilitate all steps of critically reviewing the literature, especially the gaps.

Evidence-Informed Practice Tip ____

Reading systematic reviews, if they are available, on your clinical question or topic will enhance your ability to implement evidence-informed nursing practice because they generally offer the strongest and most consistent level of evidence.

How Far Back Must the Search Go?

Students often ask questions such as the following: "How many articles do I need?"; "How much is enough?"; and "How far back in the literature do I need to go?" When conducting a search, you should use a rigorous focusing process; otherwise, you may end up with hundreds or thousands of citations. Retrieving too many citations is usually a sign that there was something wrong with your search technique or that you may have not sufficiently narrowed your clinical question.

Each online database offers an explanation of each feature; it is worth your time to click on each icon and explore the explanations offered because this will increase your confidence. Also keep in mind the types of articles you are retrieving. Many online resources allow you to limit your search to randomized controlled trials or systematic reviews. In CINAHL, there is a limit for "Research" that will restrict the number of citations you retrieve to research articles. Figure 5-4 shows an outcome of using the "Research" limit to locate Wong and colleagues' (2010) article on senior nurse leaders (see Appendix B).

A general timeline for most academic or evidenced-informed practice papers and projects

is to go back in the literature at least 3 years, but preferably 5 years, although some research projects may warrant going back 10 years or more until the researcher is satisfied that he or she has found literature that accurately represents the body of knowledge. In some cases, seminal research or research that has had a huge effect in the field should be reviewed regardless of publication date. For example, conducting a literature review on the effects of stress would not be complete without reading Hans Selye's (1955) pioneering work on stress. Extensive literature reviews on particular topics or a concept clarification methodology study helps you limit the length of your search.

Helpful Hint_____

Ask your instructor for guidance if you are uncertain how far back you need to conduct your search. If you come across a systematic review on your specific clinical topic, scan it to see what years the review covers; then begin your search from the last year to the present.

As you scroll through and mark the citations you wish to include in your downloaded or printed search, make sure you include all relevant fields when you save or print the publications. In addition to indicating which citations you want and choosing which fields to print or save, you can indicate whether you want the "search history" included. It is always a good idea to include this information because if your instructor suggests that some citations were missed, you can replicate your search and together figure out what variable or variables you omitted so that you do not make the same error again. This is also your opportunity to indicate whether you want to e-mail the search to yourself. If you are writing a paper and need to produce a bibliography, you can export your citations to **citation management software,** which is a software program that formats and stores your citations so that they are available for electronic retrieval when they must be inserted in a paper you are writing. Quite a few of these

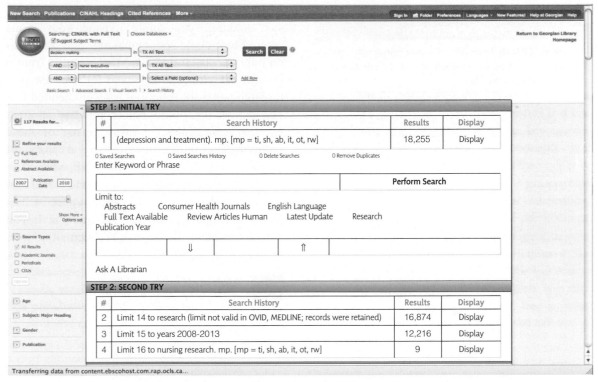

FIGURE 5-4 Illustration of a search screen obtained when the Cumulative Index to Nursing and Allied Health Literature (CINAHL) via EBSCO interface is used to locate Wong and colleagues' (2010) article on the decisional involvement of senior nurse leaders.

programs are available; some, such as Zotero, are free, and others, including EndNote and RefWorks, must be purchased, by either you or your institution.

What Do I Need to Know?

Each database usually has a specific search guide that provides information on the organization of the entries and the terminology used. The following suggestions and strategies, as listed in Box 5-3, incorporate general search strategies, as well as those related to CINAHL and MEDLINE. Finding the right terms to "plug in" as key words for a computer search is an important aspect of conducting a search. When it is possible, you want to match the words that you use to describe your question with the terms that indexers have assigned to the articles. In many online databases,

you can browse the **controlled vocabulary** terms and search. Used to conduct searches in databases, controlled vocabulary terms are carefully selected list of words and phrases that are applied to similar pieces of information units. If you are still having difficulty, ask your reference librarian for help.

Figure 5-4 is an illustration of a screenshot of search results with CINAHL via EBSCO. As noted, you have the option of searching by using the controlled vocabulary of CINAHL or a key word search. In this example, key word terms ("nurse leadership") and controlled vocabulary ("decision making") were used. Also note that these two concepts are connected with the **Boolean operator,** which defines the relationships between words or groups of words in your literature search. Examples of Boolean operators

TIPS: USING CINAHL VIA EBSCO

- Locate CINAHL from your library's home page. It may be located under databases, online resources, or nursing resources.
- In the "Advanced" tab, type in your key word or phrase (e.g., decision making, nurse executives, leadership). Do not use complete sentences. (Ask your librarian for the manual guide for each database or use feature in the database.)
- Before you choose "Search," make sure you mark "Research Articles," to ensure that you have retrieved only articles that are actually about research. See the results in Figure 5-4.
- Note that in the "Limit Your Results" section, you can limit by year, age group, clinical queries, and other specific characteristics.
- To narrow your search, use the Boolean connector "and" between each of the key words you wish to use and between additional variables. To broaden your search, use the Boolean connector "or."
- Note in Figure 5-4 that you can set up an RSS feed so that you are notified whenever new citations are added to the CINAHL database.
- Once the search results appear and you determine that they are manageable, you can decide whether to review them online; print, save, or export them; or e-mail them to yourself.

CINAHL, Cumulative Index to Nursing and Allied Health Literature; *RSS,* Really simple syndication (syndicates content from the Internet and sends it out [feeds] it to a subscriber)..

are conjunctions such as "and" and "or" and adverbs such as "not" and "near." To restrict the retrieval to research articles, the "Research Article" limit has been applied.

For further reading, a series in *Journal of Emergency Nursing* outlined the steps for embarking on an evidence-informed search (Bernardo, 2008; Engberg & Schlenk, 2007; Klem & Northcutt, 2008), which covers the stages of evidence-informed practice and basic search hints. This search was aimed at locating a known article to demonstrate some of the features of CINAHL. Lawrence (2007) presented a step-by-step approach for conducting a search in CINAHL. She described the controlled vocabulary, Boolean operators, and tips for narrowing results in the EBSCO interface.

To broaden this search for information on decision making, you might expand your terms entered to include "policymaking" and not focus on only "decision making." If the results from a broader search are to be saved for later use in a research paper for school, it is recommended that you export the bibliographic information to a *citation management software;* many of these programs have online interfaces so you can export directly from CINAHL, MEDLINE, and other databases. This software is designed to create bibliographies that conform to various styles such as the American Psychological Association. If you have not used a package such as Zotero, EndNote, or RefWorks, consult your librarian.

Helpful Hint

Look for useful tools within the search interfaces of online databases to make your searching more efficient. For example, when you search for a particular age group, use the built-in limits of the database instead of relying on a key word search. Other shortcuts include the "Clinical Queries" in CINAHL and MEDLINE that retrieve articles about therapy or diagnosis.

How Do I Complete the Search?

Now the truly important aspect of your searching begins: your critical reading of the retrieved materials. Critically reading scholarly material, especially research articles, requires several readings and the use of critiquing criteria. Do not be discouraged if not all of the retrieved articles are as useful as you first thought; this happens with the most experienced reviewers of literature. If most of the articles are not useful, be prepared to perform another search, but discuss with your instructor, the reference librarian, or both, the search terms that you will use next time; you may want to add a third database. In the previous example of a psychoeducational intervention for women who are survivors of breast cancer, the third database of choice may be PsycINFO (see Box 5-2). Remind yourself how quickly you will be able to perform the search, now that you have experience with searching.

Helpful Hint_____

Read the abstract carefully (review the discussion on critical reading strategies in Chapter 3) to determine whether the article is about research. It is also a good idea to review the references of the articles; if any seem relevant, you can retrieve them.

LITERATURE REVIEW FORMAT: WHAT TO EXPECT

Familiarity with the format of the literature review helps research consumers use critiquing criteria to evaluate the review. To decide which style you will use so that your review is presented in a logical and organized manner, you must consider the following:

- The research or clinical question or topic
- The number of retrieved sources reviewed
- The number and type of research materials versus conceptual materials

Some reviews are written according to the variables being studied and presented chronologically in the discussion of each variable. In others, the entire material is presented chronologically, and subcategories or variables are discussed within each time period. In still others, the variables are presented and the subcategories are related to the study's type or designs or related variables.

An example of a literature review, although brief, that was presented logically according to the variables under study was that of Sobieraj and colleagues (2009; see Appendix C). The researchers stated that the purpose of their study was to "test an intervention using children's songs to promote parent-led distraction during simple laceration repair in children aged 1 to 5." In the "Literature Review," the researchers indicated that there was extensive research on the undertreatment of pain in children and the long-term negative effects. Establishing the importance of the study, the authors identified age as a significant variable in the literature. The literature review then focused on psychological interventions and coping strategies by parents. The authors concluded that distraction is an effective means of decreasing distress in children. Music was chosen in those studies to provide distraction because, as Sobieraj and colleagues noted, it is recommended for the treatment of pain; however, this recommendation was not supported in the literature review. Sobieraj and colleagues further reported that parents who actively sing during a procedure may experience less anxiety. The research question and subsequent hypothesis were then formulated on the basis of the relationship between the conceptual areas: "Does music broadcast via speakers have a measurable effect on parent-led distraction during simple laceration repair in children aged 1 to 5"?

In contrast to the styles of previous quantitative studies, the literature reviews of qualitative studies are usually handled in a different manner. Little is often known about the topic under study. The literature review may be conducted at the beginning of the study or after the data analysis is completed. The researchers always compare the literature review with their findings. In some cases, the reviewed literature is used during the analysis process as well. In the study by Seneviratne and associates (2009) on understanding nursing on an acute stroke unit, the background section included a literature review that focused on the role of nurses in stroke rehabilitation, attitudes and perceptions of their role in stroke care, and observations of nurses in acute and rehabilitative care settings. After the data analysis, Seneviratne and associates returned to the literature to help explain and discuss the findings. For example, they compared the literature on space limitations and time constraints to further explore the challenges faced by nurses in the study (see Appendix A).

Evidence-Informed Practice Tip _____

Sort the research articles you retrieve according to the model of levels of evidence in Chapter 3. Remember that articles that are systematic reviews, especially meta-analyses, generally provide the strongest and most consistent evidence to include in a literature review.

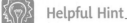

Helpful Hint_____

When you write up your literature review, include enough information so that your professor or fellow students could re-create your search path and come up with the same results. This means specifying the databases searched, the date you searched, years of coverage, terms used, and any limits or restrictions that you used.

Helpful Hint_____

- Use standardized critical appraisal criteria to evaluate your research articles.
- Make a table to represent the components of your study, and fill in your evaluation to help you see the "big picture" of your analysis.
- Synthesize the results of your analysis to try to determine what was similar or different among and between these studies in relation to your topic or clinical question, and then draw a conclusion.

APPRAISING THE EVIDENCE

Review of the Literature

Whether you are a researcher writing the literature review for the research study you are planning to conduct or a nurse writing a literature review for an evidence-informed practice project, you need to critically appraise individual research reports by using appropriate criteria. If you are appraising an individual research study that is to be included in a literature review, it must be evaluated in terms of critical appraisal criteria that are related to each step of the research process so that the strengths and weaknesses of each study can be identified. Standardized critical appraisal tools (e.g., CASP Tools and AGREE Guidelines) available for specific types of research designs (e.g., clinical trials, cohort studies, systematic reviews) can also be used to critically appraise an individual research study.

Critiquing the literature review of research or conceptual reports is a challenging task for seasoned consumers of research, so do not be surprised if you feel a little intimidated by the prospect of critiquing the published research. The important issue is to determine the overall value of the literature review, including both the research and theoretical materials. The purposes of a literature review (see Box 5-1) and the characteristics of a well-written literature review (Box 5-4) provide the framework for developing the evaluation criteria for a literature review.

The literature review should be presented in an organized manner. The theoretical and research literature can be presented chronologically from earliest studies to most recent; sometimes the theoretical literature that provided the foundation for the existing research is presented first, followed by the research studies that were derived from this theoretical base. Other times, the literature can be clustered by concept, grouped according to supportive or nonsupportive positions, or categorized by evidence that highlights differences in theoretical and/or research findings. The overall question to be answered is "Does the review of the literature develop and present a knowledge base for a research study or an evidence-informed

practice project that builds on previous research, identifies a conflict or gap in the literature, or proposes to extend the current knowledge base?" (see Box 5-1).

Regardless of how the literature review is organized, it should provide a strong knowledge base for carrying out the research, educational, or clinical practice project. Questions related to the logical organization and presentation of the reviewed studies are somewhat more challenging for beginning research consumers. The more you read research studies, the more competent you become at differentiating a well-organized literature review from one that has no organizing framework.

Whenever possible, read both qualitative (meta-syntheses) and quantitative (meta-analyses) systematic reviews that pertain to a clinical question and provide level I evidence. Systematic reviews are considered examples of secondary sources because they represent a body of completed research studies that have been critically appraised and synthesized by a team other than the original researchers; however, they often represent the best available evidence on a particular clinical issue. The article by Cummings and associates (2010) is an example of a quantitative systematic review in which the authors critically appraised and synthesized the evidence from research studies related to the leadership behaviours and outcomes for nurses and organizations. After reviewing and synthesizing 53 studies, Cummings and associates concluded that "transformational and relational leadership are needed to enhance nurse satisfaction, recruitment, retention and health work environments" (p. 363). In her article "Becoming a nurse: a meta-study of early professional socialization and career choice in nursing," Price (2009) gathered 10 primary qualitative studies on professional socialization in nursing and nurses' career choice decisions. After synthesizing the studies, Price reported "that nursing socialization is strongly associated with a person's preconceived notions and expectations of nursing" (p. 14).

APPRAISING THE EVIDENCE

Review of the Literature—cont'd

The Critiquing Criteria box summarizes general critiquing criteria for a review of the literature. In other sets of critiquing criteria, these questions may be phrased differently or more broadly. For instance, questions may be the following: "Does the literature search seem adequate?" and "Does the report demonstrate scholarly writing?" You may have difficulty answering these questions; you may begin, however, by determining whether the source is a refereed journal. It is reasonable to assume that the manuscripts published in a scholarly refereed journal are adequately searched, are based mainly on primary sources, and are written in a scholarly manner. This does not mean, however, that every study reported in a refereed journal meets all the critiquing criteria for a literature review and other components of the study in an equal manner. Because of style differences and space constraints, each citation summarized is often very brief, or related citations may be summarized as a group and lack a critique. You still must answer the critiquing questions. Consultation with a faculty adviser may be necessary to develop skill in answering the two questions.

The key to a strong literature review is a careful search of the published and unpublished literature. Whether you write or critically appraise a literature review written for a published research study, it should reflect a synthesis or compilation of the main points or value of all of the sources reviewed in relation to the study's research question or hypothesis (see Box 5-1). The relationship between and among these studies must be explained. The synthesis of a written review of the literature usually appears at the end of the review section before the section about the research question or hypothesis.

Searching the literature, like critiquing the literature, is an acquired skill. Practising your search and critical appraisal skills on a regular basis will make a huge difference. Seeking guidance from faculty is essential for developing critical appraisal skills. Synthesizing the body of literature you have critiqued is even more challenging. Critiquing the literature will help you apply new knowledge to practice. This process is vital to the "survival and growth of the nursing profession and is essential to evidence-based practice" (Pravikoff & Donaldson, 2001).

CRITIQUING CRITERIA

1. Are all the relevant concepts and variables included in the review?
2. Does the search strategy include an appropriate and adequate number of databases and other resources to identify key published and unpublished research and theoretical sources?
3. Are both theoretical literature and research literature included?
4. Does an appropriate theoretical or conceptual framework guide the development of the research study?
5. Are mainly primary sources used?
6. What gaps or inconsistencies in knowledge does the literature review uncover?
7. Does the literature review build on the findings of earlier studies?
8. Does the summary of each reviewed study reflect the essential components of the study design (e.g., type and size of sample, reliability and validity of instruments, consistency of data-collection procedures, appropriate data analysis, identification of limitations)?
9. Does the critique of each reviewed study mention strengths, weaknesses, or limitations of the design; conflicts; and gaps in information related to the area of interest?
10. Does the synthesis summary follow a logical sequence in which the overall strengths and weaknesses of the reviewed studies are presented and a logical conclusion is established?
11. Is the literature review presented in an organized format that flows logically (e.g., chronologically, clustered by concept or variables), enhancing the reader's ability to evaluate the need for the particular research study or evidence-informed practice project?
12. Does the literature review follow the proposed purpose of the research study or evidence-informed practice project?
13. Does the literature review generate research questions or hypotheses or answer a clinical question?

BOX 5-4

CHARACTERISTICS OF A WELL-WRITTEN REVIEW OF THE LITERATURE

Each reviewed source of information reflects critical thinking and scholarly writing and is relevant to the study, topic, or project, and the content satisfies the following criteria:

- The literature review is organized in a systematic approach.
- Each research or conceptual article is summarized succinctly and with appropriate references.
- Established critical appraisal criteria are used for specific study designs to evaluate the study for strengths, weaknesses, or limitations, as well as for conflicts or gaps in information that relate directly or indirectly to the area of interest.
- Evidence of a synthesis of the critiques is provided to highlight the overall strengths and weaknesses of the studies reviewed.
- The review consists of mainly primary sources; there are a sufficient number of research sources.
- The review concludes with a synthesis of the reviewed material that reflects why the study or project should be implemented.
- Research questions and hypotheses are identified, or clinical questions are answered.

CRITICAL THINKING CHALLENGES

- Using the PICOT format, generate a clinical question related to health promotion for children in elementary school.
- How does a research article's theoretical or conceptual framework interrelate concepts, theories, conceptual definitions, and operational definitions?
- A general guideline for a literature search is to use a timeline of 3 to 5 years. When would a nurse researcher need to search beyond this timeline?
- What is the relationship of the research article's literature review to the theoretical or conceptual framework?

KEY POINTS

- The review of the literature is defined as a broad, comprehensive, in-depth, systematic critique and synthesis of scholarly publications, unpublished scholarly print and online materials, audiovisual materials, and personal communications.
- The review of the literature is used for development of research studies, as well as other activities for consumers of research, such as development of evidence-informed practice projects.
- With regard to conducting and writing a literature review, the main objectives for the consumer of research are to acquire the abilities to accomplish the following: (1) conduct an appropriate search of electronic or print research on a topic; (2) efficiently retrieve a sufficient amount of materials for a literature review in relation to the topic and scope of project; (3) critically appraise (i.e., critique) research and theoretical material in accordance with accepted critiquing criteria; (4) critically evaluate published reviews of the literature in accordance with accepted standardized critiquing criteria; (5) synthesize the findings of the critiqued materials for relevance to the purpose of the selected scholarly project; and (6) determine applicability of the findings to practice.
- Primary research and theoretical resources are essential for literature reviews.
- The use of secondary sources, such as commentaries on research articles from peer-reviewed journals, is part of a learning strategy for developing critical critiquing skills.
- It is more efficient to use electronic rather than print databases for retrieving scholarly materials.
- Strategies for efficiently retrieving scholarly nursing literature include consulting the reference librarian and using at least two online sources (e.g., CINAHL and MEDLINE).
- Literature reviews are usually organized according to variables, as well as chronologically.
- Critiquing and synthesizing a number of research articles, including systematic reviews, is essential for implementing evidence-informed nursing practice.

REFERENCES

American College of Physicians. (n.d.). *ACP PIER overview*. Retrieved from http://pier.acponline.org/index.html

American Psychological Association. (n.d.) *PsycINFO*. Retrieved from http://www.apa.org/pubs/databases/psycinfo/index.aspx

Anderson, R. A., & McDaniel, R. R. (1998). Intensity of registered nurse participation in nursing home decision-making. *The Gerontologist*, *38*(1), 90-100.

Anderson, R. A., & McDaniel, R. R. (1999). RN participation in organizational decision-making and improvements in resident outcomes. *Health Care Management Review*, *24*(10), 7-16.

Ashmos, D. P., Huonker, J. W., & McDaniel, R. R. (1998). Participation as a complicating mechanism: The effect of clinical professional and middle manager participation on hospital performance. *Health Care Management Review*, *23*(4), 7-20.

Bernardo, L. M. (2008). Finding the best evidence, part 1: Understanding electronic databases. *Journal of Emergency Nursing*, *34*(1), 59-60.

Cummings, G. G., MacGregor, T., Davey, M., Lee, H., Wong, C., Lo, E., . . . Stafford, E. (2010). Leadership styles and outcome patterns for the nursing workforce and work environment: A systematic review. *International Journal of Nursing Studies*, *47*, 363-385. doi: 10.1016/j.ijnurstu.2009.08.006

DiCenso, A., Bayley, L., & Haynes, R. B. (2009). Accessing pre-appraised evidence: Fine-tuning the 5S model into a 6S model. *Evidence Based Nursing*, *12*(4), 99-101. doi:

Engberg, S., & Schlenk, E. A. (2007). Asking the right question. *Journal of Emergency Nursing*, *33*(6), 571-573.

Haynes, B. (2007). Of studies, syntheses, synopses, summaries, and systems: The "5S" evolution of information services for evidence-based healthcare decisions. *Evidence-Based Nursing*, *10*(1), 6-7.

Kendall, S. (2008). Evidence-based resources simplified. *Canadian Family Physician*, *54*(2), 241-243.

Klem, M. L., & Northcutt, T. (2008). Finding the best evidence part 2: The basics of literature searches. *Journal of Emergency Nursing*, *34*(2), 151-158.

Lawrence, J. C. (2007). Techniques for searching the CINAHL database using the EBSCO interface. *AORN Journal*, *85*(4), 779-780, 782-788, 790-791.

National Library of Medicine. (n.d.). Retrieved from http://www.nlm.nih.gov/bsd/disted/pubmedtutorial/010_050.html

Pravikoff, D., & Donaldson, N. (2001). Special section: Online journal publication. *Online Journal of Issues in Nursing*, *6*(2). Retrieved from http://www.nursingworld.org/MainMenuCategories/ANAMarketplace/ANAPeriodicals/OJIN/TableofContents/Volume62001/No2May01/ArticlePreviousTopic/ClinicalInnovations.aspx

Price, S. L. (2009). Becoming a nurse: A meta-study of early professional socialization and career choice in nursing. *Journal of Advanced Nursing*, *65*(1), 11-19. doi: 10.1111/j.1365-2648.2008.04839.x

ProQuest. (n.d.). *ProQuest dissertations and theses database: Key facts*. Retrieved from http://www.il.proquest.com/products_pq/descriptions/pqdt.shtml

Selye, H. (1955). Stress and disease. *Science*, *122*, 625-631.

Seneviratne, C. C., Mather, C. M., & Then, K. L. (2009). Understanding nursing on an acute stroke unit: Perceptions of space, time and interprofessional practice. *Journal of Advanced Nursing 65(*9), 1872-1881. doi: 10.1111/j.1365-2648.2009.05053.x

Sobieraj, G., Bhatt, M., LeMay, S., Rennick, J., & Johnston, C. (2009). The effect of music on parental participation during pediatric laceration repair. *Canadian Journal of Nursing Research*, *41*, 68-82.

Turning Research into Practice [TRIP]. (n.d.). *Introduction and background—TRIP database, 2011*. Retrieved from http://www.tripdatabase.com/about

Wiley Interface. (n.d.). *Reference works, 2011. The Cochrane Library 2011, Issue 3*. Retrieved from http://www.thecochranelibrary.com/view/0/index.html

Wong, C. A., Laschinger, H., Cummings, G. G., Vincent, L., & O'Connor, P. (2010). Decisional involvement of senior nurse leaders in Canadian acute care hospitals. *Journal of Nursing Management*, *18*, 122-133. doi: 10.1111/j.1365-2834.2010.01053.x

FOR FURTHER STUDY

⊖volve Go to Evolve at http://evolve.elsevier.com/Canada/LoBiondo/Research for Audio Glossary, how-to instructions for Writing Proposals for Funding, and additional research articles for practice in reviewing and critiquing.

CHAPTER 6

Legal and Ethical Issues

Judith Haber | Mina D. Singh

LEARNING OUTCOMES

After reading this chapter, you will be able to do the following:

- Describe the historical background that led to the development of ethical guidelines for the use of human participants in research.
- Identify the essential elements of an informed consent form.
- Evaluate the adequacy of an informed consent form.
- Describe the role of the research ethics board in the research review process.
- Identify populations of participants who require special legal and ethical research considerations.
- Appreciate the nurse researcher's obligations to conduct and report research in an ethical manner.
- Describe the nurse's role as patient advocate in research situations.
- Discuss the nurse's role in ensuring that Health Canada guidelines for testing of medical devices are followed.
- Discuss animal rights in research situations.
- Critique the ethical aspects of a research study.

KEY TERMS

animal rights	consent	research ethics board
anonymity	ethics	respect for persons
assent	informed consent	risk-benefit ratio
beneficence	justice	risks
benefits	process consent	
confidentiality	product testing	

STUDY RESOURCES

Go to Evolve at http://evolve.elsevier.com/Canada/LoBiondo/Research for Audio Glossary, how-to instructions for Writing Proposals for Funding, and additional research articles for practice in reviewing and critiquing.

NURSES ARE IN AN IDEAL POSITION to promote patients' awareness of the role played by research in the advancement of science and improvement in patient care. In Canada, the professional code of ethics (Canadian Nurses Association [CNA], 2008) outlines the ethical standards for practice, which can include research and patients' rights with regard to research. Not only do the standards represent rules and regulations regarding practice, but when research becomes the domain of a nurse, these standards can be applied to the participation of human research participants to ensure that nursing research is conducted legally and ethically. The code states that nurses must strive to uphold human rights and call attention to any violations of these rights. The *Code of Ethics for Registered Nurses,* originally published in 1983, was revised in 2008, and the revision was released that June. The revised CNA code includes clarification of the meanings of social justice, health, and well-being, with a stronger focus on human rights. These rights can also be translated to patients' or participants' rights in research, and nurses can be advocates to ensure that ethical concepts in nursing research are upheld.

Researchers and caregivers of patients who are research participants must be fully committed to the tenets of informed consent and patients' rights. The principle "the ends justify the means" must never be tolerated. Researchers and caregivers of research participants must take every precaution to protect people being studied from physical or mental harm or discomfort (although it is not always clear what constitutes harm or discomfort).

The focus of this chapter is the legal and ethical considerations that must be addressed before, during, and after the conduct of research to ensure that the research does not harm the patient. Informed consent, research ethics boards (REBs), and research involving vulnerable populations—older adults, pregnant women, children, prisoners, Aboriginal people, and persons with acquired immune deficiency syndrome (AIDS), as well as animals—are discussed. The nurse's role as patient advocate, whether functioning as researcher, caregiver, or research consumer, is addressed.

ETHICAL AND LEGAL CONSIDERATIONS IN RESEARCH: A HISTORICAL PERSPECTIVE

Past Ethical Dilemmas in Research

Ethical and legal considerations regarding medical research first arose in the United States and received focused attention after World War II. Lawyers defending war criminals intended to justify the atrocities committed by Nazi physicians by claiming their actions were in the name of "medical research." On learning of this defence, the U.S. Secretary of State and the Secretary of War asked the American Medical Association to appoint a group to develop a code of ethics for research to serve as a standard for judging the medical experiments committed by physicians on concentration camp prisoners. These experiments included the sterilization of people considered enemies of the state (Benedict & Georges, 2006).

The code of ethics developed as 10 rules that became known as the *Nuremberg Code* (Box 6-1). The Nuremberg Code's definitions of the terms *voluntary, legal capacity, sufficient understanding,* and *enlightened decision* have been the subject of numerous court cases and U.S. presidential commissions involved in setting ethical standards in research (Creighton, 1977). The code that was developed requires informed consent in all cases but makes no provisions for any special treatment of children, older adults, or people who are mentally incompetent. Several other international standards have followed; the most notable is the Declaration of Helsinki, which was adopted in 1964 by the World Medical Assembly and revised in 1975 (Levine, 1979).

The research heritage in the United States and Canada is well documented and is used here to

BOX 6-1

ARTICLES OF THE NUREMBERG CODE

1. The voluntary consent of the human subject is absolutely essential.
2. The study should be conducted so as to yield fruitful results for the good of society, unprocurable by other means of study, and not random and unnecessary in nature.
3. The experiment should be so designed and based on the results of animal experimentation and knowledge of the natural history of the disease or other problems under study that the anticipated results will justify the performance of the experiment.
4. The experiment should be conducted to avoid all unnecessary physical and mental suffering and injury.
5. No experiment should be conducted where there is an *a priori* reason to believe that death or disabling injury will occur. . . .
6. The degree of risk to be taken should never exceed that determined by the humanitarian importance of the problem to be solved by the experiment.
7. Proper preparations should be made and adequate facilities provided to protect the subject against even remote possibilities of injury, disability, or death.
8. The experiment should be conducted only by scientifically qualified persons. . . .
9. . . . The human subject should be at liberty to bring the experiment to an end. . . .
10. During the course of the experiment the scientist in charge must be prepared to terminate the experiment at any stage, if he [or she] has probable cause to believe . . . that a continuation of the experiment is likely to result in injury, disability, or death to the experimental subject.

From United States Government Printing Office. (2008). The medical case. In *Trials of war criminals before the Nuernberg Military Tribunals under Control Council Law No. 10* (Vol. 2, pp. 181-182). Washington, DC: Author, 1949. Retrieved from http://www.loc.gov/rr/frd/Military_Law/pdf/NT_war-criminals_Vol-II.pdf.

BOX 6-2

BASIC ETHICAL PRINCIPLES RELEVANT TO THE CONDUCT OF RESEARCH

RESPECT FOR PERSONS

People have the right to self-determination and to treatment as autonomous agents. Thus they have the freedom to participate or not participate in research. Persons with diminished autonomy are entitled to protection.

BENEFICENCE

Beneficence is an obligation to do no harm and maximize possible benefits. Persons are treated in an ethical manner when their decisions are respected, they are protected from harm, and efforts are made to secure their well-being.

JUSTICE

Human subjects should be treated fairly. An injustice occurs when benefit to which a person is entitled is denied without good reason or when a burden is imposed unduly.

From Elder, G. (1981). Social history & life experience. In D. H. Eichorn, J. A. Clausen, N. Haan, & P. H. Mussen (Eds.), *Present and past in middle life* (pp. 3-31). New York: Academic Press. Copyright 1981 Academic Press.

illustrate the human consequences of not adhering to ethical standards when conducting research. Some examples are highlighted in Table 6-1 and incorporated into Table 6-2 to show the violation of human rights that occurred in these studies.

In the United States, under the National Research Act of 1974 (Public Law 93-348), the National Commission for the Protection of Human Subjects of Biomedical and Behavioral Research was created. A major charge of the commission was to identify the basic principles that should underlie the conduct of biomedical and behavioural research involving human participants and to develop guidelines to ensure that research is conducted in accordance with those principles (Levine, 1986). Three ethical principles were identified as relevant to the conduct of research involving human participants: **respect for persons** (the idea that people have the freedom to participate or not participate in research), **beneficence** (obligation to do no harm and maximize possible benefits), and **justice** (the principle that human subjects should be treated fairly; Box 6-2). These three principles have formed the basis of many ethical guidelines in Canada.

In Canada, for the protection of human participants in all types of research, Health

TABLE 6-1

HIGHLIGHTS OF UNETHICAL RESEARCH STUDIES CONDUCTED IN THE UNITED STATES AND CANADA

RESEARCH STUDY	DATE OF STUDY	FOCUS OF STUDY	ETHICAL PRINCIPLE VIOLATED
Tuskegee syphilis study, Tuskegee, Alabama	1932–1973	For 40 years, the U.S. Public Health Service conducted a study using two groups of poor black male share-croppers. One group consisted of men with untreated syphilis; the other group was judged to be free of the disease. Treatment was withheld from the group with syphilis even after penicillin became generally available and accepted as effective treatment for syphilis in the 1950s. Steps were even taken to prevent the research participants from obtaining penicillin. The researcher wanted to study the untreated disease.	Many of the research participants who consented to participate in the study were not informed about the purpose and procedures of the research. Others were unaware that they were participants. The degree of risk outweighed the potential benefit. Withholding of known effective treatment violates the participants' right to fair treatment and protection from harm (Levine, 1986).
Sterilization experiments in Auschwitz concentration camp, Germany	1940–1944	Sterilization experiments	Basic human rights and rights to fair and ethical treatment were violated, and the research participants did not give informed consent. Nurses who were prisoners were forced to participate in the experiments, which was against their prima facie duty to protect (Benedict & Georges, 2006).
Dr. Ewen Cameron's psychiatric experiments, Allan Memorial Psychiatric Institute, Montreal, Quebec	1950s–1960s	The U.S. Central Intelligence Agency (CIA) funded psychic driving, or brain-washing, experiments on patients with psychiatric illnesses (Collins, 1988, cited by Charron, 2000). Psychic driving is a psychiatric procedure pioneered by Dr. Cameron in which electroconvulsive therapy (ECT) and psychedelic drugs, such as lysergic acid (LSD), are used in an attempt at mind control. To develop the psychic driving, increasingly higher levels of ECT were applied to patients as often as three times a day. This treatment would continue for 30 days. Considerable damage was done to patients after such severe treatment. Patients were unable to walk or feed themselves and were incontinent (Gillmor, 1987, cited by Charron, 2000).	The ethical principles of respect for persons and beneficence were severely violated. Dr. Cameron used patients with diminished autonomy (patients with psychiatric illnesses), even though, as a physician, he was obliged to protect them. The ECT treatments did more harm than good.
Hyman v. Jewish Chronic Disease Hospital, Jewish Chronic Disease study, New York City	1965	Doctors injected aged, senile patients with cancer cells to study the patients' response to injection of the cells.	Informed consent was not obtained, and no indication was given that the study had been reviewed and approved by an ethics committee. The two physicians involved claimed that they did not wish to evoke emotional reactions or New York City refusals to participate by informing the research participants of the nature of the study (Hershey & Miller, 1976).

Continued

TABLE 6-1

HIGHLIGHTS OF UNETHICAL RESEARCH STUDIES CONDUCTED IN THE UNITED STATES AND CANADA—*cont'd*

RESEARCH STUDY	DATE OF STUDY	FOCUS OF STUDY	ETHICAL PRINCIPLE VIOLATED
Milledgeville, Georgia, study	1969	Researchers administered investigational drugs to mentally disabled children without first obtaining the opinion of a psychiatrist.	The study protocol or institutional approval of the program was not reviewed before implementation (Levine, 1986).
San Antonio contraceptive study, San Antonio, Texas	1969	In a study of the side effects of oral contraceptives, 76 impoverished Mexican American women were randomly assigned to an experimental group receiving birth control pills or a control group receiving placebos. Research participants were not informed about the placebo and the attendant risk of pregnancy. Of the participants, 11 became pregnant; 10 of these women were in the placebo control group.	Principles of informed consent were violated; full disclosure of the potential risk, harm, results, and side effects was not evident in the informed consent document. The potential risk outweighed the benefits of the study. The participants' right to fair treatment and protection from harm was violated (Levine, 1986).
Willowbrook Hospital study, New York State	1972	Children with mental incompetence ($N = 350$) were not admitted to Willowbrook Hospital, a residential treatment facility, unless parents consented to their children's being research participants in a study of the natural history of infectious hepatitis and the effect of γ-globulin. The children were deliberately infected with the hepatitis virus under various conditions; some received γ-globulin, whereas others did not.	The principle of voluntary consent was violated. Parents were coerced into consenting to their children's participation for the research. Participants or their guardians have a right to self-determination; in other words, they should be free of constraint, coercion, and undue influence of any kind. Many participants feel pressured to participate in studies if they are in powerless, dependent positions (Rothman, 1982).
Schizophrenia medication study, University of California, Los Angeles	1983	In a study of the effects of withdrawing psychotropic medications in 50 patients receiving treatment for schizophrenia, 23 research participants suffered severe relapses after their medication was stopped. The goal of the study was to determine whether some patients with schizophrenia might do better without medications that had deleterious side effects.	Although all participants signed informed consent documents, they were not informed about how severe their relapses might be or that they could suffer worsening symptoms with each recurrence. Principles of informed consent were violated; full disclosure of the potential risk, harm, results, and side effects was not evident in the informed consent document. The potential risk outweighed the benefits of the study. The participants' right to fair treatment and protection from harm was violated (Hilts, 1995).
Côte d'Ivoire, Africa, AIDS/AZT case	1994	In research supported by the U.S. government and conducted in the Côte d'Ivoire, Dominican Republic, and Thailand, some pregnant women infected with HIV were given placebo pills rather than AZT, a drug known to prevent mothers from passing the virus to their babies. Babies born to these mothers were in danger of contracting a fatal disease.	Research participants who consented to participate and who were randomly assigned to the control group were denied access to a medication regimen with a known benefit. This denial violate the participants' right to fair treatment and protection (French, 1997; Wheeler, 1997).

AIDS, acquired immune deficiency syndrome; *AZT,* azidothymidine; *HIV,* human immunodeficiency virus.

TABLE **6-2**

PROTECTION OF HUMAN RIGHTS

BASIC HUMAN RIGHT	DEFINITION
Right to self-determination	This right is based on the ethical principle of respect for persons; people should be treated as autonomous agents who have the freedom to choose without external controls. An autonomous agent is one who is informed about a proposed study and is allowed to choose to participate or not to participate (Brink, 1992). Moreover, research participants have the right to withdraw from a study without penalty.
Right to privacy and dignity	This right is based on the ethical principle of respect for persons; privacy is the freedom of a person to determine the time, extent, and circumstances under which private information is shared or withheld from other people.
Right to anonymity and confidentiality	This right is based on the ethical principle of respect for persons; anonymity exists when the participant's identity cannot be discerned, even by the researcher, from his or her individual responses (American Nurses Association, 1985). Confidentiality means that the individual identities of participants will not be linked to the information they provide and will not be publicly divulged.

VIOLATION OF BASIC HUMAN RIGHT	EXAMPLE

A participant's right to self-determination is violated through the use of coercion, deception, and covert data collection.
- In coercion, an overt threat of harm or excessive reward is presented to ensure participants' compliance.
- In deception, participants are misinformed about the purpose of the research.
- In covert data collection, people become research participants and are exposed to research treatments without knowing it.
- The potential for violation of the right to self-determination is greater for research participants with diminished autonomy, who have decreased ability to give informed consent and are vulnerable.

The U.S. Privacy Act of 1974 was instituted to protect participants from privacy violations. These violations occur most frequently during data collection, when responses to invasive questions might result in the loss of a job, friendships, or dignity or might create embarrassment and mental distress. These violations also may occur when participants are unaware that information is being shared with other people.
Anonymity is violated when the participants' responses can be linked to their identity.

Confidentiality is breached when a researcher, by accident or direct action, allows an unauthorized person to gain access to study data that contain information about the participant's identity or responses, which creates a potentially harmful situation for the participant.

Participants may believe that their care will be adversely affected if they refuse to participate in research. The Willowbrook Hospital Study (see Table 6-1) is an example of how coercion was used to obtain the consent of parents of vulnerable children with mental retardation, who would not be admitted to the institution unless they participated in a study in which they were deliberately injected with the hepatitis virus.
The Jewish Chronic Disease Hospital Study (see Table 6-1) is an example of a study in which patients and their personal physicians did not know that cancer cells were being injected.
In Milgram's (1963) study, research participants were deceived when asked to administer electric shocks to another person, who was an actor pretending to suffer from the shocks. Participants administering the shocks were very distressed by participating in this study, although they were not administering shocks at all. This study is an example of deception.
Research participants may be asked personal questions such as "Were you sexually abused as a child?"; "Do you use drugs?"; and "What are your sexual preferences?" When questions are asked in the presence of hidden microphones or hidden recording devices, the participants' privacy is invaded because they have no knowledge that the data are being shared with other people. Participants' right to control access of other people to their records is also violated.
Researchers who choose to identify data by using the participant's name are breaching the basic human right of anonymity. Instead, researchers should assign participants a code number that is used for identification purposes. Research participants' names are never used in the reporting of findings.
Breaches of confidentiality with regard to sexual preference, income, drug use, prejudice, or person personality variables can be harmful to research participants. Data should be analyzed as group data so that participants cannot be identified by their responses.

Continued

TABLE 6-2

PROTECTION OF HUMAN RIGHTS—cont'd

BASIC HUMAN RIGHT	DEFINITION
Right to fair treatment	This right is based on the ethical principle of justice; people should be treated fairly and should receive what they are due or owed. "Fair treatment" refers to the equitable selection of research participants and their treatment during the research study. This treatment includes selection of participants for reasons directly related to the problem studied, as opposed to selection of participants because of convenience, the compromised position of the participants, or their vulnerability. Fair treatment also extends to the treatment of participants during the study, including fair distribution of risks and benefits of the research regardless of age, race, or socioeconomic status.
Right to protection from discomfort and harm	This right is based on the ethical principle of beneficence; people must take an active role in promoting good and preventing harm both in the world around them and in research studies. Discomfort and harm can be physical, psychological, social, or economic in nature. The five levels of harm and discomfort are as follows: 1. No anticipated effects 2. Temporary discomfort 3. Unusual level of temporary discomfort 4. Risk of permanent damage 5. Certainty of permanent damage Participants with diminished autonomy are entitled to protection. They are more vulnerable because of age, legal or mental incompetence, terminal illness, or confinement to an institution. A justification for the use of vulnerable participants must be provided.

VIOLATION OF BASIC HUMAN RIGHT	EXAMPLE
Injustices with regard to participant selection have occurred as a result of social, cultural, racial, and gender biases in society.	The Tuskegee Syphilis Study that ended in 1973 (Levine, 1986), the Jewish Chronic Disease Study of 1965 (Hershey & Miller, 1976), the San Antonio Contraceptive Study of 1969 (Levine, 1986), and the Willowbrook Hospital Study of 1972 (Rothman, 1982) (see Table 6-1) all are examples of unfair participant selection and the use of vulnerable populations.
Historically, research participants were often recruited from groups of people who were regarded as having less "social value," such as people living in poverty, prisoners, slaves, people who are mentally incompetent, and people who are dying. Participants were often treated carelessly, without consideration of physical or psychological harm.	Investigators should not be late for data collection appointments, should terminate data collection on time, should not change agreed-upon procedures or activities without consent, and should provide agreed-upon benefits, such as a copy of the study findings or a participation fee.

TABLE 6-2

PROTECTION OF HUMAN RIGHTS—*cont'd*	
VIOLATION OF BASIC HUMAN RIGHT	**EXAMPLE**
Research participants' right to be protected is violated when discomfort or disabling injury will occur and, thus, the benefits do not outweigh the risks.	Temporary physical discomfort involving minimal risk includes fatigue or headache; emotional discomfort includes the expense involved in travelling to and from the data collection site.
	Studies of sensitive issues (such as rape, incest, or spouse abuse) might cause unusual levels of temporary discomfort by increasing participants' awareness of current or past traumatic experiences. In these situations, researchers assess distress levels and provide debriefing sessions, during which the participant may express feelings and ask questions. The researcher has the opportunity to make referrals for professional intervention.
	Studies with the potential to cause permanent damage are more likely to be medical in nature rather than nursing in nature, inasmuch as physiological damage may be permanent. One clinical trial of a new drug, a recombinant activated protein C (Zovan) for treatment of sepsis, was halted when interim findings from the phase III clinical trials revealed that the rate of mortality among the patients receiving treatment was lower than that among those receiving the placebo. Evaluation of the data led to termination of the trial to make a known beneficial treatment available more quickly to all patients.
	In some research, such as the Tuskegee Syphilis Study or Nazi medical experiments, participants experienced permanent damage or died. In Dr. Cameron's study (see Table 6-1), the continued electroconvulsive therapy increased the damage.

Canada has adopted the *Good Clinical Practice: Consolidated Guidelines* (Health Canada, 1997). The collaboration of the three major funding agencies—the Canadian Institutes of Health Research (CIHR), the Natural Sciences and Engineering Research Council of Canada (NSERC), and the Social Sciences and Humanities Research Council of Canada (SSHRC)—has led to a joint statement for the protection of human participants. The revision of this document, the *Tri-Council Policy Statement: Ethical Conduct for Research Involving Humans* (CIHR et al., 2010), offers a more inclusive approach to delineating current trends in ethical issues. This revised document, sometimes called the Tri-Council Policy Statement-2, is henceforth referred to as TCPS2.

The original statement listed eight guiding principles, which are now subsumed under the three core principles "respect for person," "concern for welfare," and "justice." Of the others, "respect for human dignity" is articulated through these three core principles; "respect for free and informed consent" and "respect for vulnerable persons" are now reflected in the principle of "respect for persons," and "respect for vulnerable persons" is also reflected in the principle of "justice"; "respect for privacy and confidentiality" is part of "concern for welfare"; and "respect for justice and inclusiveness" is in the core principle of "justice." The core principle "concern for welfare" now also includes "balancing harms and benefits," "minimizing harm," and "maximizing benefit."

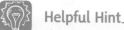

Helpful Hint

The qualitative researcher must be especially diligent in protecting the privacy and confidentiality of participants. When the participants' verbatim quotations are used in the "Results" or "Findings" section of the research report to highlight the findings, the smallness of the sample size may make it easy to identify an individual participant. Moreover, when researchers and REBs are engaging in naturalistic observation, the TCPS2 indicates that these boards "and researchers need to consider the methodological requirements of the proposed research project and the ethical implications associated with observational approaches, such as the possible infringement of privacy. They should pay close attention to the ethical implications of such factors as the nature of the activities to be observed, the environment in which the activities are to be observed, whether the activities are staged for the purpose of the research, the expectations of privacy that prospective participants might have, the means of recording the observations, whether the research records or published reports involve identification of the participants, and any means by which those participants may give permission to be identified" (CIHR et al., 2010, p. 142).

Current and Future Ethical Dilemmas in Research

Ethics is the theory or discipline dealing with principles of moral values and moral conduct. The ethical dilemmas in research for the twenty-first century concern biotechnology, the use of animals for research, and the creation of an organizational culture that values and nurtures research ethics and the rights of people who engage in research either as investigators or as participants (Pranulis, 1996). For example, in only 12 years, the Human Genome Project, an international research project launched by the United States in 1988, provided a vast amount of data on DNA, including the molecular details about the DNA of more than 26 organisms. Since then, the focus has been on studying (1) groups of genes rather than single genes; (2) functions of genes rather than structures of genes; and (3) proteomes, the proteins based on genes (Wheeler, 1999). To engage in genome research, genetic engineering and genetic information must exist

(Carroll & Ciaffa, 2008), which can raise ethical concerns about to the purpose of the engineering. If the purpose is to treat a disease, then the research is ethically acceptable, but the existence of germline intervention raises "more significant ethical concerns, because risks will extend across generations, magnifying the impact of unforeseen consequences" (Carroll & Ciaffa, 2008). Ethical concerns also arise with regard to the privacy of genetic information, mandatory testing of newborns, and mandatory genetic screening.

Other areas of research that engender much discussion and controversy are fetal tissue research and the use of women who are of childbearing potential as participants in drug or therapeutic studies. The Tri-Council (i.e., the CIHR, the NSERC, and the SSHRC) worked over a period of several years to make stem cell research a reality in Canada, with the appropriate ethical guidelines for the use of embryos, fetuses, gametes, and pluripotent stems cells. These guidelines are detailed in the TCPS2 (CIHR et al., 2010).

Of note is the following information (CIHR et al., 2010, p. 182, Article 13.2):

Researchers conducting genetic research shall:

(a) in their research proposal, develop a plan for managing information that may be revealed through their genetic research;
(b) submit their plan to the REB; and
(c) advise prospective participants of the plan for managing information revealed through the research. (p. 182, Article 13.2)

In the past, women of childbearing potential were denied participation in studies of a drug or potential therapy because of the unknown, potentially teratogenic effects of drugs and other therapies that were in various stages of testing. Guidelines related to the inclusion of pregnant women as research participants have been even more stringent than previous guidelines; as a result, women have been excluded from many important drug and research studies over the years. Similarly, inclusion of ethnic minorities in federally funded research studies is also a priority area for consideration in research ethics (Julion, Gross, & Barclay-McLaughlin, 2000).

The TCPS2 also has a well-articulated policy on the ethical guidelines for research with the Aboriginal population to ensure protection of the rights of that community (CIHR, 2007). This guideline comprises 15 principles, which include the need for research when benefit is mutual, incorporating the role of community elders in consent and the responsibilities of the researcher to understand and protect sacred knowledge. The inclusion of a separate chapter in TCPS2 outlining how to engage with and honour First Nations, Inuit, and Métis communities reflects the work that was accomplished over several years to advance the need for equitable partnerships and to provide safeguards with these communities. It is noted that "Aboriginal entities at local, regional and national levels have published and implemented principles and codes governing research practice—including ethical protections—that emphasize collective rights, interests and responsibilities" (CIHR, 2007, p. 106).

THE EVOLUTION OF ETHICS IN NURSING RESEARCH

The evolution of ethics in nursing research can be traced back to 1897 and the constitution of the Nurses' Associated Alumnae Organization in the United States. One of the first purposes of this organization was to establish a code of ethics for the nursing profession. In 1900, Isabel Hampton Robb wrote *Nursing Ethics: For Hospital and Private Use.* In describing the moral laws by which people must abide, she stated the following:

> Etiquette, speaking broadly, means a form of behavior or manners expressly or tacitly required on particular occasions. It makes up the code of polite life and includes forms of ceremony to be observed, so that we invariably find in societies that certain etiquette is required and observed either tacitly or by expressed agreement.

Although Robb's comments reflect the norms of Victorian society, they also highlight a historical concern for ethical actions by nurses as health care professionals (Robb, 1900).

In Canada, most disciplines have developed their own code of ethics with guidelines for research. The CNA's first document on ethical principles related to nursing research, *Ethical Guidelines for Nurses in Research Involving Human Participants,* was released in 1983. It was revised in 1994 and 2002 and is now titled *Ethical Research Guidelines for Registered Nurses* (CNA, 2002).

Clearly, ignorance and naïveté with regard to ethical and legal guidelines for the conduct of research is never an excuse for a nurse's failure to be familiar with and act on behalf of patients, whose human rights must be safeguarded at all times. Nurse researchers are often among the most responsible and conscientious investigators in respecting the rights of human participants. All nurses should be aware that in addition to the ethical research guidelines of the CNA, universities and hospitals may also have supplemental sets of ethical guidelines to follow.

PROTECTION OF HUMAN RIGHTS

Human rights are the claims and demands that have been justified according to an individual or by a group of individuals. The term *human rights* is applied to the following five rights outlined in the CNA's (2002) guidelines and linked to the Tri-Council's principles of respect for research participants:

1. Right to self-determination
2. Right to privacy and dignity
3. Right to anonymity and confidentiality
4. Right to fair treatment
5. Right to protection from discomfort and harm

These rights apply to everyone involved in a research project, including research team members involved in data collection, practising nurses involved in the research setting, and people participating in the study. As consumers of research read a research article, they must realize that any issues highlighted in Table 6-2 should have been addressed and resolved before a research study is approved for implementation.

Procedures for Protecting Basic Human Rights

Informed Consent

Informed consent, illustrated by the ethical principles of respect and the related right to self-determination, is outlined in Box 6-3. Nurses need to understand the elements of informed consent to be knowledgeable participants when either obtaining informed consent from patients or critiquing this process as it is presented in research articles.

Informed consent is the legal principle that requires a researcher to inform individuals about the potential benefits and risks of a study before the individuals can participate voluntarily. In theory, this principle governs the patient's ability to accept or reject individual medical interventions designed to diagnose or treat an illness. According to the TCPS2 (CIHR et al., 2010), free and informed consent is at the heart of ethical research and is a process of dialogue and information sharing to allow participants the choice to participate in research. Free and informed consent must be given without manipulation, undue influence, or coercion.

For example, Akhtar-Danesh and associates (2010) developed a learning needs assessment questionnaire for community health nurses. Approval for the use of human participants was obtained from appropriate ethics review boards before the data collection. The informed consent form described risks and benefits of the study and the participants' responsibilities, and it mentioned that their information would be confidential and anonymous. Confidentiality was ensured by the use of study identification numbers rather than

> **BOX 6-3**
>
> ## ELEMENTS OF INFORMED CONSENT
>
> 1. A statement that the study involves research
> 2. An explanation of the purposes of the research, delineating the expected duration of the subject's participation
> 3. A description of the procedures to be followed and identification of any procedures that are experimental
> 4. A description of any reasonably foreseeable risks or discomforts to the subject
> 5. A description of any benefits to the subject or to others that may reasonably be expected from the research
> 6. A disclosure of appropriate alternative procedures or course of treatment, if any, that might be advantageous to the subject
> 7. A statement describing the extent to which the anonymity and confidentiality of the records identifying the subject will be maintained
> 8. For research involving more than minimal risk, an explanation as to whether any medical treatments are available if injury occurs and, if so, what they consist of or where further information may be obtained
> 9. An explanation about whom to contact for answers to questions about the research and researcher subjects' rights and whom to contact in the event of a research-related injury to the subject
> 10. A statement that participation is voluntary, that refusal to participate will not involve any penalty or less benefit to which the subject is otherwise entitled, and that the subject may discontinue participation at any time without penalty or loss of otherwise entitled benefits
>
> From Code of Federal Regulations: Protection of human subjects, 45 CFR 46, *OPRR Reports*, revised March 8, 1983.

the addition of any private information on mailed documents.

No investigator may involve a human being as a research participant until the legally effective informed consent has been obtained from either the participant or a legally authorized representative of the participant, and prospective participants must have time to decide whether to take part in a study. The researcher must not coerce the participant into taking part in the study, nor may researchers collect data on participants who have explicitly refused to take part in a study.

An ethical violation of this principle is illustrated by the case of *Halushka v. University of Saskatchewan et al.* (1965). In this landmark case, a university student volunteered for a study testing a new anaesthetic, for which he would be paid $50.00. He consented to be in the study based on the following information disclosed to him: the test would last a few hours, the test was safe and had been conducted many times before, and the student had nothing to worry about. He was informed that the procedure would include placement of electrodes on his arms, legs, and head and insertion of a catheter into a vein in his arm. He signed a consent form releasing the physicians and the university from liability for any untoward effects or accidents, which were explained to him as "falling down at home after the test" (McLean, 1996, p. 49). The test proceeded with administration of an *untested* anaesthetic, and the student suffered a cardiac arrest. He was unconscious for four days in hospital and left with a residual inability to concentrate. The physicians and the university were found negligent for failing to "disclose that there was risk involved with the use of an anaesthetic and that this particular drug had not been previously tested by them" (McLean, 1996, p. 49).

When composing an informed consent form, researchers must ensure that the language is understandable. For example, the reading level should be no higher than grade 8 for adults, and the use of technical research language should be avoided (Rempusheski, 1991). The elements that need to be contained in an informed consent are listed in Box 6-3. Note that many institutions require additional elements. Figure 6-1 is an example of an informed consent form for a quantitative study, whereas Figure 6-2 is an example of an informed consent form for a qualitative study. Note that in each consent form, the elements of participation, risk and benefits, withdrawal, confidentiality, and whom to contact for further queries are clearly outlined.

In a qualitative research study of perceptions of space, time, and interprofessional practice on an acute stroke unit (see Appendix A), Seneviratne and associates (2009) obtained ethics approval from the appropriate REB. They "used several information sessions and interviews to introduce the study to members in the stroke unit. During these sessions and interviews, the researchers informed stroke unit members about client confidentiality. They obtained written consent only from observation and interview participants and verbal assent from clients when participants were providing direct care" (p. 1874).

Helpful Hint

Remember that research reports rarely provide readers with detailed information regarding the degree to which the researcher adhered to ethical principles, such as informed consent; this is because of space limitations in journals, which make it impossible to describe all aspects of a study. Failure to mention procedures to safeguard participants' rights does not necessarily mean that such precautions were not taken.

Most investigators obtain **consent** (agreement to participate in a study) through personal discussion with potential participants. This process allows the person who is the potential participant to obtain immediate answers to questions. However, consent forms, written in narrative or outline form, highlight elements that both inform and remind participants of the nature of the study and their participation (Dubler & Post, 1998; Haggerty & Hawkins, 2000). When one participant is scheduled to participate in many interviews, the participant must give **process consent** (voluntary continued participation in a study, which can be verbal) for each data collection point.

Assurance of anonymity and confidentiality (defined in Table 6-2), which is conveyed in writing, is sometimes difficult in unique research situations that capture the public's attention. For example, when physicians at Loma Linda University Hospital in California transplanted a

Text continued on p. 128

CONSENT TO PARTICIPATE IN A RESEARCH STUDY

Title
VISUAL DIFFERENTIATION IN LOOK-ALIKE MEDICATION NAMES

University Health Network Principal Investigator
Tasmine Halevy, Clinical Director of Pharmacy, UHN, 416-XXX-XXXX

Study Principal Investigator
Monica Blum, Associate Professor, Reed University, 416-XXX-XXXX

Co-Investigators
Joyce Davis, Vice President, ISMP Canada
Dr. Mina D. Singh, Associate Professor, York University, Faculty of Health, School of Nursing
Ravinder Sharma, Human Factors Engineer, Red Forest Consulting
Dr. Irmgard Mirren, Psychiatrist, Child and Parent Resource Institute
Evan Ross, Chief Pharmacist, Child and Parent Resource Institute

Collaborator
Jude Hartman

Sponsors
Canadian Patient Safety Institute, ISMP Canada; Red Forest Consulting; Child and Parent Resource Institute; York University Faculty of Graduate Studies, Department of Design and Faculty of Health

Introduction
You are being asked to take part in a research study. Please read this explanation about the study and its risks and benefits before you decide if you would like to take part. You should take as much time as you need to make your decision. You should ask the Principal Investigator or Research Assistants to explain anything that you do not understand and make sure that all of your questions have been answered before signing this consent form. Before you make your decision, feel free to talk about this study with anyone you wish. Participation in this study is voluntary.

Background and Purpose
This study will look at the visual display of look-alike medication names. It is hoped that this research will contribute to the design of shelf labelling, packaging, and computer displays to help reduce instances of medication errors due to look-alike medication names. The results from this research are intended to support health care workers in the safe delivery of health care. You have been asked to take part in this research study because you have or may come into contact with look-alike medications. A total of 130 to 135 nursing staff and 10 pharmacy staff from Princess Margaret Hospital, Toronto General Hospital, Toronto Western Hospital will participate in this study.

Study Design
You will help us evaluate the best ways to display look-alike names for ease and accuracy in recognition and selection of medications. If you choose to participate in this study, you will be asked to answer a short questionnaire to establish your demographic information and to ask you your opinion of current practices related to the display of look-alike medication names. You will participate in three experiments that emulate the selection of medications. The first two experiments are screen based, and you will be asked to identify look-alike names on a laptop display. For the third experiment, you will be asked to select medications from a series of baskets. The tasks will be explained thoroughly before each experiment. Your commitment for this study will be one session lasting approximately 45 to 60 minutes.

FIGURE 6-1   Example of an informed consent form for a quantitative study. *ISMP,* Institute for Safe Medication Practices; *UHN,* University Health Network.

CONSENT TO PARTICIPATE IN A RESEARCH STUDY—cont'd

Risks Related to Being in the Study
There are no known risks if you take part in this study, but you may refuse to answer questions or stop the experiments at any time if there is any discomfort. Your responses to the questionnaires will not have an impact on your employment, nor will they be shared with your supervisors or managers.

Benefits to Being in the Study
You will not receive any direct benefit from being in this study. Information learned from this study may help in the safe delivery of health care.

Voluntary Participation
Your participation in this study is voluntary. You may decide not to be in this study, or to be in the study now and then change your mind later. You may leave the study at any time without affecting your employment status. You may refuse to answer any question you do not want to answer on the questionnaire by writing "pass," or stop participating in the experiment at any time.

Confidentiality
The information that is collected for the study will be kept in a locked and secure area at York University by the study Principal Investigator for 10 years. Only the study team and the people or groups listed below will be allowed to look at the data. All information collected during this study will be kept confidential and will not be shared with anyone outside the study unless required by law. Any information about you that is collected for the study will have a code and will not show your name or address, or any information that directly identifies you. You will not be named in any reports, publications, or presentations that may come from this study. If you decide to leave the study, the information about you that was collected before you left the study will still be used. No new information will be collected without your permission. Representatives of the University Health Network Research Ethics Board may look at the study records to check that the information collected for the study is correct and to make sure the study followed proper laws and guidelines.

Questions about the Study
If you have any questions or concerns, or would like to speak to the study team for any reason, please call: Tasmine Halevy, University Health Network, at **416-XXX- XXXX** or Monica Blum, Reed University, **416-XXX-XXXX**.

The research has been reviewed and approved by the University Health Network Research Ethics Board (REB) and the Human Participants Review Committee (HPRC) at Reed University for compliance with senate ethics policy. If you have any questions about your rights as a research participant or have concerns about this study, call the Chair of the UHN (REB) or the Research Ethics office number at 416-XXX-XXXX or Manager, Research Ethics—Alicia Collins-Walker: 309 Elsevier Lanes, Reed University, 416-XXX-XXXX. The HPRC and REB are groups of people who oversee the ethical conduct of research studies. These people are not part of the study team. Everything that you discuss will be kept confidential.

Consent
This study has been explained to me and any questions I had have been answered. I know that I may leave the study at any time. I agree to take part in this study.

_____   _____   _____
Print Study Participant's Name   Signature   Date

(You will be given a signed copy of this consent form)

My signature means that I have explained the study to the participant named above. I have answered all questions

_____   _____   _____
Print Name of Person Obtaining Consent   Signature   Date

FIGURE 6-1, *cont'd*   Example of an informed consent form for a quantitative study.

INFORMATION AND INFORMED CONSENT STATEMENT: INTERVIEW

Title
BETTER UNDERSTANDING HOW COUPLES COPE WITH A CHILD'S LIFE-THREATENING ILLNESS

Principal Investigator
Dr. Susan Cadell, Associate Professor; Director, Manulife Centre for Healthy Living; Lyle S. Hallman Faculty of Social Work, Wilfrid Laurier University, 519-XXX-XXXX

Co-Investigators
Dr. Rosemary Stiles, School of Nursing, York University
Dr. Anna DeLaurentis, The Centre for Health and Coping Studies, University of British Columbia

Research Assistants
Matilde Negrini, Faculty of Social Work, Wilfrid Laurier University
Julian Millman, Faculty of Social Work, Wilfrid Laurier University
Nella Leone, Faculty of Social Work, Wilfrid Laurier University

Contact Person
Matthew Philips, Research Coordinator: 1-800-XXX-XXXX

We are inviting couples to participate in the next phase of this research study. The purpose of this study is to discover the experience of spouses/partners who are together caring for a child with a life-limiting illness. This study is being conducted by Dr. Susan Cadell, Associate Professor and Director of the Centre for Healthy Living at Wilfrid Laurier University, and Co-Investigator on the Canadian Institutes for Health Research's New Emerging Team (NET): *Transitions in Pediatric Palliative and End-of-Life Care.*

Information
During the interview, you and your spouse/partner will be interviewed together. You will be asked questions about your personal experience of caring for a child with a life-limiting condition, as well as questions about the role that each spouse/partner plays in the coping of the other. The interview will take approximately 1.5 to 2 hours. The interview will be conducted by a trained, sensitive interviewer and will take place at a location convenient to you. In order to make sure that we have an accurate record of what you have shared during the interview, your interview will be recorded and transcribed. All identifying information will be removed from the transcripts and only the investigators and research staff will have access to them. The recordings and transcripts will be identified only by code number and stored in a locked filing cabinet or secured information system. They will be stored for 5 years after the publication of the results from this study. After 5 years, the recordings and the transcripts will be destroyed. The recordings will not be used for any other purposes without your additional permission.

Phase Two of this study will involve the participation of approximately 15 to 20 couples who are together caring for their child. Due to the nature of this study, it is possible that quotes from your interview may be used in publication. To maintain confidentiality, all identifying information will be removed from the quotations. If a specific family or disease characteristic is rare and could potentially be identifying, the information will be changed in the quote. Please indicate your preference below regarding the use of your quotations.

Name: _____   Name: _____
☐ Yes – I can be quoted with no identifying information.   ☐ Yes – I can be quoted with no identifying information.
☐ No – Please do not use quotes.   ☐ No – Please do not use quotes.

FIGURE 6-2   Example of an informed consent form for a qualitative study.

INFORMATION AND INFORMED CONSENT STATEMENT: INTERVIEW—cont'd

Risk
This research project deals with a sensitive topic. The interviewer will monitor your distress level and will stop the interviewing process if you become upset. The interviewer will then ensure that you are aware of your right not to answer any questions asked and your right to terminate the interview at any time. If necessary, the interviewer will refer you to appropriate services and resources to ensure your support needs are met.

Benefits
You may benefit from the ability to communicate your experiences of pediatric palliative care in a safe, nonjudgemental setting. In addition, your participation may benefit other families, researchers, and policy makers in pediatric palliative care by providing a better understanding of the caregiver experience.

Confidentiality
Confidentiality will be provided to the fullest extent possible by law. Your identity and the identity of all family members will be kept strictly confidential. All identifying information will be removed from the data. All documents and recordings will be identified only by code number and the information will be retained in a secured information system and locked filing cabinet. All identifying information will be kept separate from the data. All documents that are kept on a computer will be password protected. Identifying information will not be emailed to anyone at any time. You will not be identified by name in any reports of the completed study. Only study personnel will have access to the study data.

Compensation
For participating in this study you and your spouse/partner will each receive $30 at the beginning of the interview. If you withdraw from the study after this point, you will still receive the full amount.

Participation
Your participation in this study is voluntary; you may decline to participate without penalty. If you decide to participate, you may withdraw from the study at any time without penalty and without loss of benefits to which you are otherwise entitled. If you withdraw from the study before data collection is completed, your data will be destroyed. You have the right to omit any question(s)/procedure(s) you choose.

Feedback and publication
It is expected that the results of this study will be presented and published as a journal article. If you would like to be notified of the results of the study, please indicate below.

Name: _____   Name: _____
☐ Yes – I would like to be notified of results.   ☐ Yes – I would like to be notified of results.

Contact
If you have questions at any time about the study or the procedures, or if you experience adverse effects as a result of participating in this study, you may contact the Research Coordinator, Matthew Philips, at 1-800-XXX- XXXX. This project has been reviewed and approved by the University Research Ethics Board at Wilfrid Laurier University. If you feel you have not been treated according to the descriptions in this form, or your rights as a participant in research have been violated during the course of this project, you may contact Dr. Mark Billingsley, Chair, University Research Ethics Board, Wilfrid Laurier University, 519-XXX-XXXX.

Consent
I have read and understand the above information. I have received a copy of this form. I agree to participate in this study.

_____   _____
Participant's signature   Date

_____   _____
Participant's signature   Date

_____   _____
Investigator's signature   Date

FIGURE 6-2, *cont'd* Example of an informed consent form for a qualitative study.

baboon's heart into a 2-week-old infant, her identity was hidden **(anonymity)** as she was known only as Baby Fae, and **confidentiality** was ensured in that the reports could not be linked to her and her family. Maintaining anonymity and confidentiality is particularly important for qualitative researchers because the researcher often functions as the data collection "instrument" and meets the participant. The consent form must be signed and dated by the participant. The presence of witnesses is not always necessary but does constitute evidence that the participant concerned actually signed the form. In cases in which the participant is a minor or is physically or mentally incapable of signing the consent, the signature must be obtained from a legal guardian or representative. The investigator also signs the form to indicate commitment to the agreement of anonymity and confidentiality.

In Jack and associates' (2005) study, the participants' anonymity and confidentiality were guaranteed, but in cases in which the researcher suspected child abuse or neglect, the participants were clearly informed that the researcher has a legal responsibility to report any suspicions to the child welfare agency. Another strategy that can be used to ensure confidentiality is to ask the transcribers in a qualitative study to sign a confidentiality agreement, as Heaman and colleagues (2007) did in their study of relationship work in an early childhood home-visiting program.

In general, the signed informed consent form is given to the participant. The researcher should also keep a copy. Some research, such as a retrospective chart audit, may require only institutional approval, not informed consent. In some cases, when minimal risk is involved, the investigator may have to provide the participant only with an information sheet and a verbal explanation. In other cases, such as a volunteer convenience sample, completion and return of research instruments constitute evidence of consent. The REB advises on exceptions to these guidelines, as in cases in which the REB might grant waivers

or amend its guidelines in other ways. The REB makes the final determination regarding the most appropriate documentation format. Research consumers should note whether and what kind of evidence of informed consent has been provided in a research article.

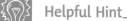 **Helpful Hint**_____

Note that researchers often do not obtain written informed consent when the major means of data collection is through self-administered questionnaires. Implied consent is usually assumed in such cases; in other words, the return of the completed questionnaire reflects the respondent's voluntary consent to participate.

Research Ethics Boards

Research ethics boards (REBs) are panels that review research projects to assess whether ethical standards are met in relation to the protection of the rights of human participants. Such boards are established in agencies to review biomedical and behavioural research involving human subjects within the agency or in programs sponsored by the agency. Universities, hospitals, and other health agencies applying for a grant or contract for any project or program that involves the conduct of biomedical or behavioural research with human participants are required by the Tri-Council and most funding agencies to submit with their application assurances that they have established an REB that reviews the research projects and protects the rights of the human participants (CIHR et al., 2010). The Tri-Council also requires that the REB have at least five members, including both men and women. Membership must include at least two professionals who have expertise in relevant research disciplines, fields, and methodologies covered by the REB; at least one who is knowledgeable in ethics; at least one who is knowledgeable in the relevant law (but that member should not be the institution's legal counsel or risk manager); and at least one who is a community member and has no affiliation with the institution but is recruited from the community served by the institution (CIHR et al., 2010).

The REB is responsible for protecting participants from undue risk and loss of personal rights and dignity. For a research proposal to be eligible for consideration by an REB, it must already have been approved by a departmental review group, such as a nursing research committee, that attests to the proposal's scientific merit and congruence with institutional policies, procedures, and mission. The REB reviews the study's protocol to ensure that it meets the requirements of ethical research that appear in Box 6-4. Most boards provide guidelines or instructions for researchers that include steps to be taken to receive REB approval. For example, guidelines for writing a standard consent form or criteria for qualifying for an expedited rather than a full REB review may be available. The REB has the authority to approve research, require modifications, or disapprove a research study, on the basis of the guidelines outlined in Box 6-5. A researcher must receive REB approval before beginning to conduct research. REBs have the authority to suspend or terminate approval of research that is not conducted in accordance with REB requirements or that has been associated with unexpected serious harm to participants. REB approval was obtained from the University of British Columbia and from the British Columbia Women's Hospital for a study to understand breast-feeding and infant health in Canada (Chen, 2010).

REBs in Canada also provide for reviewing research in an expedited manner when the risk to research participants is minimal. An expedited review usually shortens the length of the review process. Although a researcher may determine that a project involves minimal risk, however, the research cannot be conducted until the REB makes the final determination. Many qualitative research projects are eligible for an expedited review because the research is noninvasive and involves methods such as observation, interviews, and questionnaires. An expedited review does not automatically exempt the researcher from obtaining informed consent.

Not all research requires an ethical review. To follow protocol, researchers can submit a proposal to their own REB; however, according to the TCPS2 (CIHR et al., 2010), this step is not necessary when the research relies exclusively on information that is legally accessible to the public and appropriately protected by law or that is publicly accessible and there is no reasonable expectation of privacy. Legally accessible information includes registries of deaths, court judgements, or public archives and publicly available statistics (e.g., Statistics Canada public use files).

REB review is also not required when researchers use exclusively publicly available information that may contain identifiable information and for which there is no reasonable expectation of privacy. For example, identifiable information may be disseminated in the public domain through print or electronic publications; film, audio, or digital recordings; press accounts; official publications of private or public institutions; artistic installations, exhibitions, or literary events freely open to the public; or publications accessible in public libraries. Research that is nonintrusive and does not involve direct interaction between the researcher and individuals through the Internet also does not require REB review. Online material such as documents, records, performances, online archival materials, or published third-party interviews to which the public is given uncontrolled access on the Internet and for which there is no expectation of privacy is considered to be publicly available information.

Adapted from Canadian Institutes of Health Research, Natural Sciences and Engineering Research Council of Canada, & Social Sciences and Humanities Research Council of Canada. (2010, December). *Tri-Council policy statement: Ethical conduct for research involving humans.* Chapter 2, "Scope and approach." Retrieved from http://www.pre.ethics.gc.ca/pdf/eng/tcps2/TCPS_2_FINAL_Web.pdf

BOX 6-4

CANADIAN NURSES ASSOCIATION'S ETHICAL RESEARCH GUIDELINES FOR REGISTERED NURSES

These guidelines are the primary values in the Canadian Nurses Association's (2008) *Code of Ethics for Registered Nurses,* and they form the structural framework for the *Ethical Research Guidelines for Registered Nurses* (Canadian Nurses Association [CNA], 2002). Below each guideline are examples of principles for implementation.

GUIDELINE 1: PROMOTING SAFE, COMPASSIONATE, COMPETENT, AND ETHICAL CARE
Implementation

Nurses engaged in research must comply with the *Code of Ethics for Registered Nurses* (CNA, 2008) and conduct themselves with honesty and integrity in all their interactions with research subjects and research colleagues (CNA, 2002, p. 6).

Nurses involved as principal investigators, clinical research coordinators or research assistants must base their research on relevant knowledge of research methods and continue to acquire new skills and knowledge to develop and maintain their level of competence in research (CNA, 2002, p. 6).

GUIDELINE 2: PROMOTING HEALTH AND WELL-BEING
Implementation

Nurses engaged in nursing practice must hold people's optimum health and well-being as first and foremost in their interactions with all those they serve (CNA, 2002, p. 7).

Nurses should recognize the importance of bringing a nursing perspective to health research and engage with other health professionals in interdisciplinary health research promoting health and well-being (CNA, 2002, p. 8).

GUIDELINE 3: PROMOTING AND RESPECTING INFORMED DECISION MAKING
Implementation

Nurses caring for people involved in research should do their part in ensuring that consent is free and informed. The investigator, or the individual designated by the investigator, should fully inform the subject of all pertinent aspects of the study, including the type and level of commitment required and potential benefits and risks (CNA, 2002, p. 9).

Nurses caring for persons must be alert to any signs that these individuals feel pressured or coerced into participating in a research study. If they suspect that these individuals feel pressured or coerced, nurses must advise the investigator and/or the agency's REB (CNA, 2002, p. 9).

GUIDELINE 4: PRESERVING DIGNITY
Implementation

Nurses demonstrate equal respect for persons who choose to become research subjects and for those who choose not to participate (CNA, 2002, p. 12).

Nurse should respect the process by which communities determine whether and under what conditions research can be conducted (e.g., First Nations communities) (CNA, 2002, p. 13).

GUIDELINE 5: MAINTAINING PRIVACY AND CONFIDENTIALITY
Implementation

Nurses caring for persons involved in research must be attentive to the subject's privacy and exercise caution in use, access, collection, and disclosure of information. They should be aware of relevant provincial legislation about the confidentiality of health and research information (CNA, 2002, p. 14).

In all cases where research data must be released, nurses should release only the minimum amount of data required and restrict the number of people to whom data is released (CNA, 2002, p. 14).

GUIDELINE 6: PROMOTING JUSTICE
Implementation

Nurses must seek to ensure that all persons have access to opportunities, subject to availability, to be involved as research subjects (CNA, 2002, p. 15).

Nurses should promote participatory research where research subjects can work in partnerships with researchers in design, implementation and dissemination of research (CNA, 2002, p. 15).

GUIDELINE 7: BEING ACCOUNTABLE
Implementation

Nurses engaged in research must conduct the research within their own level of competence. Even if others assume that nurses know and should be able to perform certain research interventions required in the study, nurses must advise researchers and clinical staff if they do not feel they have the level of competence needed to perform these tasks. If placed in such a position, they should seek information and help from investigators and other knowledgeable researchers (CNA, 2002, p. 17).

Nurses engaged in research and nurse educators should seek to ensure their students learn about research design, research ethics and the need for ethics approval. They should also help students be aware of their level of competence in conducting research (CNA, 2002, p. 17).

BOX 6-5

PARTIAL GUIDELINES FOR RESEARCH ETHICS BOARD APPROVAL OF RESEARCH STUDIES

To approve research, the REB must determine that the following guidelines have been satisfied:
1. There is an analysis of balance and distribution of harms and benefits.
2. There is a proportionate approach based on the general principle that the level of review is determined by the level of risk presented by the research: the lower the level of risk, the lower the level of scrutiny (delegated review); the higher the level of risk, the higher the level of scrutiny (full board review).
3. There is a formal informed consent process.

From Canadian Institutes of Health Research, Natural Sciences and Engineering Research Council of Canada, & Social Sciences and Humanities Research Council of Canada. (2010, December). *Tri-Council policy statement: Ethical conduct for research involving humans.* Retrieved from http://www.pre.ethics.gc.ca/pdf/eng/tcps2/TCPS_2_FINAL_Web.pdf
REB, research ethics board.

The CIHR Web site has a complete listing of updated information concerning ethical guidelines involving human participants. In addition, all researchers should consult their agency's research offices to ensure that the application being prepared for REB approval adheres to the most current requirements. Nurses who are critiquing published research should be familiar with current regulations to determine whether ethical standards have been met. The Critical Thinking Decision Path illustrates the ethical decision-making process an REB might use in evaluating the risk-benefit ratio of a research study.

Protecting the Basic Human Rights of Vulnerable Groups

Researchers are advised to consult their agency's REB for the most recent guidelines when considering research involving vulnerable groups, such as older adults, children, pregnant women, unborn children, persons who are emotionally or physically disabled, prisoners, deceased persons, students, and persons with AIDS. In addition, researchers should consult the REB before planning research that potentially involves an oversubscribed research population, such as patients who have undergone organ transplantation, patients with AIDS, or "captive" and convenient research populations, such as prisoners. The use of special populations does not preclude undertaking research; safeguards must be undertaken, however, to protect the rights of these participants (CIHR et al., 2010). Davis (1981) reminded us that a society can be judged by the way it treats its most vulnerable people; this point is worth remembering in research that involves children, older adults, and other vulnerable groups.

Pediatric research can be particularly problematic. Mitchell (1984) discussed the U.S. National Commission's concept of assent versus consent in regard to pediatric research. **Assent**—an aspect of informed consent that pertains to protecting the rights of children as research subjects—is composed of the following three fundamental elements:
1. A basic understanding by the child of what the child will be expected to do and what will be done to the child
2. A comprehension by the child of the basic purpose of the research
3. An ability of the child to express a preference regarding participation

An example of research in a pediatric group in which assent was used is the study of Rennick and colleagues (2004). These researchers were interested in identifying children at high risk for psychological problems after hospitalization in a pediatric intensive care unit. The children were categorized as being at either high or low risk for developing persistent psychological sequelae on the basis of illness severity and the number of invasive procedures that they underwent. The children gave assent verbally or in writing, and their parents provided written consent for their children to participate.

In contrast to assent, consent requires a relatively advanced level of cognitive ability.

CRITICAL THINKING DECISION PATH

Evaluating the Risk-Benefit Ratio of a Research Study

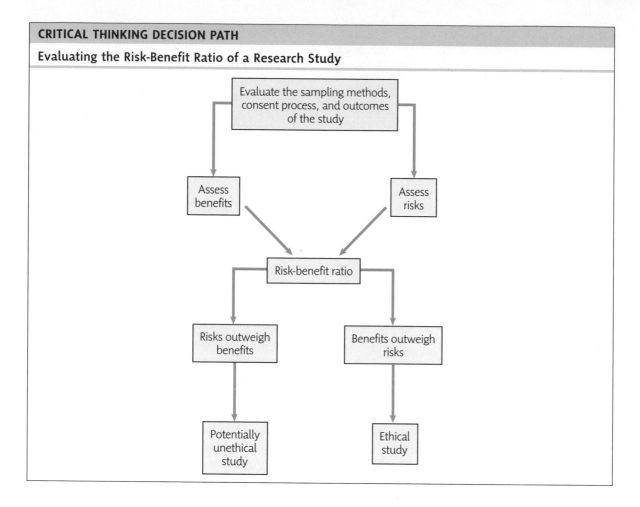

Informed consent reflects competency standards requiring abstract appreciation of and reasoning about the information provided. The issue of assent versus consent is an interesting one. For example, at what age can children be expected to make meaningful decisions about participating in research? In terms of the work by Jean Piaget about cognitive ability, children aged 6 years and older can participate in giving assent. Children age 14 years and older, although not legally authorized to give sole consent unless they are emancipated minors, can make such decisions as capably as adults (Mitchell, 1984; Piaget, 1937/1954).

If the research involves more than minimal risk and does not offer a direct benefit to the individual child, then both parents must grant permission. When children reach maturity, usually at 18 years of age in the case of research, they may render their own consent. They may do so at a younger age if they have been legally declared emancipated minors. Questions regarding assent, consent, and the age of the individual should be addressed by the REB or research administration office and not left to the discretion of the researcher to answer.

Special ethical considerations also exist when research is conducted with older adults. As an advocate for vulnerable older adults who are increasingly dependent on other people for care and whose cognitive ability is declining, the American Geriatrics Society Ethics Committee (1998) stated that older adults are precisely the class of persons who were historically and are potentially vulnerable to abuse and for whom specific legal protection is needed. The issue of the legal competence of older adults is often raised (Flaskerud & Winslow, 1998), but no issue exists if the potential participant can supply legally effective informed consent. Competence is not clearly measurable. The complexity of the study may affect an individual's ability to consent to participate. The capacity to give informed consent should be assessed in each individual for each research protocol being considered (American Geriatrics Society Ethics Committee, 1998). For example, an older person may be able to consent to participate in a simple observation study but not in a clinical drug trial.

The issue of the necessity of requiring the older adult to provide consent often arises. N. N. Dubler (personal communication, 1993) referred to research regulations that indicate that some or all of the elements of informed consent may be waived for the following reasons:

1. The research involves no more than minimal risk to the participants.
2. The waiver or alteration will not adversely affect the rights and welfare of the participants.
3. The research could not feasibly be carried out without the waiver or alteration.

No vulnerable population may be singled out for study merely for convenience. For example, neither people with mental illness nor prisoners may be studied simply because they are available and their presence is convenient. Prisoners may be studied if the study pertains to them; for example, studies concerning the effects and processes of incarceration. Similarly, people with mental illness may participate in studies that focus on expanding knowledge about psychiatric disorders and treatments. Students also are often a conveniently available group. They must not, however, be singled out as research participants because of convenience; the research questions must have some bearing on their status as students.

Researchers and patient caregivers involved in research with vulnerable people are well advised to seek advice from appropriate REBs, clinicians, lawyers, ethicists, and other professionals. In all cases, the burden should be on the investigator to show the REB that it is appropriate to involve vulnerable participants in research.

Helpful Hint

Keep in mind that researchers rarely mention explicitly that the study participants were vulnerable participants or that special precautions were taken to appropriately safeguard the human rights of this vulnerable group. Research consumers need to be attentive to the special needs of individuals who may be unable to act as their own advocates or are unable to adequately assess the risk-benefit ratio of a research study.

RESEARCH INVOLVING ABORIGINAL PEOPLE

When developing ethical guidelines, attention is paid to the culture and traditions of Aboriginal people in Canada. To this end, the Tri-Council (CIHR et al., 2010) developed the following "good practices" for researchers and REBs to consider when engaged in research (CIHR, 2007, Section 6):

- To respect the culture, traditions, and knowledge of the Aboriginal group
- To conceptualize and conduct research with the Aboriginal group as a partnership
- To consult members of the group who have relevant expertise
- To involve the group in the design of the project
- To examine how the research may be shaped to address the needs and concerns of the group
- To make best efforts to ensure that the emphasis of the research, and the ways chosen to conduct it, respect the many viewpoints of different segments of the group in question
- To provide the group with information respecting the following:

- Protection of the Aboriginal group's cultural estate and other property
- The availability of a preliminary report for comment
- The potential employment by researchers of members of the community appropriate and without prejudice
- Researchers' willingness to cooperate with community institutions
- Researchers' willingness to deposit data, working papers and related materials in an agreed-upon repository
- To acknowledge in the publication of the research results the various viewpoints of the community on the topics researched
- To afford the community an opportunity to react and respond to the research findings before the completion of the final report, in the final report or even in all relevant publications

Smith and colleagues (2006), in using a participatory action research approach, were able to acknowledge many of the aforementioned considerations by involving leaders of the community and other key informants in the research design. In some cases, however, these "good practices" are not fully implemented. For example, Smylie and associates (2005) raised concerns about ethical issues in certain studies in which community members were not consulted during the formulation of the study and cautioned researchers that using "Aboriginality" as a social construct is not paying attention to the heterogeneity in the various groups.

To understand the evidence being collected, and to make informed choices about what First Nations leaders need to improve the social and economic conditions of their people, an ethical framework, "Ownership, Control, Access, and Possession" (OCAP), was developed by the First Nations Statistics Initiative. This initiative is important because a perceived mistrust exists between First Nations people and researchers, and researchers choose participants and studies on the basis of their own interests rather than the needs of the participants ("'Ownership, control, access, and possession'" 2003).

SCIENTIFIC FRAUD AND MISCONDUCT

Fraud

Periodically, articles reporting the unethical actions of researchers appear in the professional and lay literature. Data may have been falsified or fabricated, or participants may have been coerced into participating in a research study (Kevles, 1996; Office of Research Integrity, U.S. Department of Health and Human Services, 2011; Tilden, 2000). In a climate of "publish or perish" in academic and scientific settings and declining research dollars, academics and scientists are under increasing pressure to produce significant research findings. Job security and professional recognition are coveted, essential, and often predicated on being a productive scientist and a prolific writer. These pressures have been known to overpower some people, who then take shortcuts, fabricate data, and falsify findings to advance their positions (Rankin & Esteves, 1997; Tilden, 2000).

The risks of engaging in fraudulent research are many, including harming research participants or basing clinical practice on false data. As advocates of patient welfare and professional practice, nurses should be aware that sometimes they might observe or suspect a researcher's misconduct. In such cases, nurses must contact the appropriate group, such as the REB, to ensure that this matter receives appropriate attention and review.

Misconduct

Of equal importance is the issue of basing nursing practice on reports that appear in journals when subsequent research and reports on those participants change the scientific basis for practice. Corrections or further research in follow-up reports may be buried, obscure, or underreported. As patient advocates and research consumers, nurses must keep up to date on scientific reports related to nursing practice and must adjust their practice as directed by ever-evolving, evidence-informed research findings. In addition, researchers have a responsibility to keep current with federal compliance regulations on prevention, detection, investigation, and adjudication of scientific misconduct.

Unauthorized Research

At times, ad hoc or informal and unauthorized research is conducted, including **product testing** (the testing of medical devices). Although the testing may seem harmless, it is, again, not the purview of the investigator to make that determination. Nurses must carefully avoid being involved in unauthorized research for a number of reasons, including the following (Raybuck, 1997):

- These treatments or methods of care are usually not monitored as closely for untoward effects; hence, the patient may be exposed to unwarranted risk.
- Patients' rights to informed consent in clinical trials are not protected.
- The success or failure of these unrecorded trials contributes nothing to the organized scientific knowledge of the efficacy or complications of the treatment.
- The lack of independent quality supervision allows deviations from the adopted experimental program that may eliminate the program's effectiveness.

Product Testing

Nurses are often approached by manufacturers to test products on patients. Often, nurses assume the role of research coordinator in clinical drug or product trials (Raybuck, 1997). Consequently, nurses should be aware of the Health Products branch guidelines (see Health Canada, n.d.) and regulations for testing of medical devices before they initiate any form of clinical testing. Medical devices are classified according to the extent of control necessary to ensure the safety and effectiveness of each device.

LEGAL AND ETHICAL ASPECTS OF ANIMAL EXPERIMENTATION

The laws that have been written regarding **animal rights**—guidelines used to protect the rights of animals in the conduct of research—in research emanate from an interesting history of attitudes toward animals and the value that people place on them. In 1963, the Medical Research Council of Canada (now CIHR) requested that a committee be established to investigate the care and use of experimental animals. The Canadian Council on Animal Care (CCAC) was formed and became a nonprofit, autonomous, and independent body in 1982 (CCAC, 2005). It is now funded by the CIHR and the NSERC and conducts assessment visits to each institution every 3 years, often unannounced. The CCAC requires that institutions conducting animal-based research, teaching, or testing establish an animal care committee and that this committee be functionally active. The CCAC has a detailed guide regarding developing terms of reference for animal care committees (CCAC, 2006).

The CIHR scrutinized the proposed amendments to the Cruelty to Animal Provisions of the *Criminal Code of Canada,* Bill-C15. The objective of these changes is to strengthen but simplify the existing penal code and "to enhance the effectiveness of the offence provisions for clearly abusive, brutal and cruel treatment of animals." The CIHR supported this objective in principle and, with the NSERC, prepared a joint submission to the House of Commons Standing Committee on Justice and Human Rights in the fall of 2001, recommending amendments to clarify certain provisions of the bill with regard to their application to health research.

This section serves only as an introduction to the concept of legal and ethical issues related to animal experimentation. Principles of protection of animal rights in research have evolved over time. Animals, unlike humans, cannot give informed consent, but other conditions related to their welfare must not be ignored. Nurses who encounter the use of animals in research should be alert to their rights.

RESEARCH INVOLVING HUMAN GAMETES, EMBRYOS, OR FETUSES

Research on the human genome and other reproductive issues have caused much ethical debate and concern; thus, the Tri-Council (CIHR et al., 2010) developed pertinent guidelines, as demonstrated by these examples:

- Materials related to human reproduction for research use shall not be obtained through commercial transaction, including exchange for services (Article 12.6).
- Research on in vitro embryos already created and intended for implantation to achieve pregnancy is acceptable if:
  - The research is intended to benefit the embryo
  - Research interventions will not compromise the care of the woman or the subsequent fetus
  - Researchers closely monitor the safety and comfort of the woman and the safety of the embryo
  - Consent was provided by the gamete donors (Article 12.7)
- Research involving embryos that have been created for reproductive or other purposes permitted in Canada under the Assisted Human Reproduction Act (Assisted Human Reproduction Canada, 2004), but are no longer required for these purposes, may be ethically acceptable if:
  - The ova and sperm from which they are formed were obtained in accordance with Article 12.7

- Consent was provided by the gamete donors
- Embryos exposed to manipulations not directed specifically to their ongoing normal development will not be transferred for continuing pregnancy
- Research involving embryos will take place only during the first 14 days after their formation by combination of the gametes, excluding any time during which embryonic development has been suspended (Article 12.8)
- Research involving a fetus or fetal tissue:
  - Requires the consent of the woman
  - Should not compromise the woman's ability to decide whether to continue her pregnancy (Article 12.9)

Nurses working in labour rooms, especially those being required to assist with embryonic research, should be aware of these ethical issues.

To protect participant and institutional privacy, the locale of the study frequently is described in general terms in the report's subsection on the sample. For example, the article might state that data were collected at a 500-bed tertiary care centre in Ontario, without mentioning the centre's name. Protection of participant privacy may be explicitly addressed by statements indicating that the anonymity or confidentiality of the data was maintained or that grouped data were used in the data analysis.

Determining whether participants were subjected to physical or emotional risk is often accomplished indirectly by evaluating the study's "Methods" section. The reader evaluates the **risk-benefit ratio:** that is, the extent to which the **benefits** of the study—the potential positive outcomes of participation in a research study—are maximized and the **risks**—the potential negative outcomes of participation in a research study—are minimized, so that participants are protected from harm during the study (Dubler & Post, 1998; Pruchino & Hayden, 2000). The Practical Application boxes list examples of how researchers attempt to protect study participants from harm.

APPRAISING THE EVIDENCE

The Legal and Ethical Aspects of a Research Study

Research articles and reports often do not contain detailed information regarding either the degree to which or all of the ways in which the investigator adhered to the legal and ethical principles presented in this chapter. Space considerations in articles preclude extensive documentation of all legal and ethical aspects of a research study. Lack of written evidence regarding the protection of human rights does not imply that appropriate steps were not taken.

The Critiquing Criteria box provides guidelines for evaluating the legal and ethical aspects of a research report. Although research consumers reading a research report will not see all areas explicitly addressed in the research article, they should be aware of them and should determine that the researcher has addressed them before gaining REB approval to conduct the study. A nurse who is asked to serve as a member of an REB will find the critiquing criteria useful in evaluating the legal and ethical aspects of the research proposal.

Information about the legal and ethical considerations of a study is usually presented in the "Methods" section of a research report, probably in the subsection on the sample or data collection methods. The author most often indicates in a few sentences that informed consent was obtained and that approval from an REB or similar committee was granted. A manuscript without such a discussion will probably not be accepted for publication; thus, it is almost impossible for unauthorized research to be published. Therefore, when a research article provides evidence of having been approved by an external review committee, the reader can feel confident that the ethical issues raised by the study have been thoroughly reviewed and resolved.

CRITIQUING CRITERIA

1. Was the study approved by an REB or other agency committee members?
2. Is there evidence that informed consent was obtained from all participants or their representatives? How was it obtained?
3. Were the participants protected from physical or emotional harm?
4. Were the participants or their representatives informed about the purpose and nature of the study?
5. Were the participants or their representatives informed about any potential risks that might result from participation in the study?
6. Was the research study designed to maximize the benefit or benefits and to minimize the risks to human participants?
7. Were participants coerced or unduly influenced to participate in this study? Did they have the right to refuse to participate or withdraw without penalty? Were vulnerable participants used?
8. Were appropriate steps taken to safeguard the privacy of participants? How have data been kept anonymous or confidential?

Practical Application

Chalmers and colleagues (2002) reported the attitudes, beliefs, and personal behaviours of baccalaureate students in regard to tobacco use. The researchers adhered to the principles of informed consent and confidentiality and ensured that the team remained sensitive to the issues of power differences between the students and the faculty engaged in the study. In addition, the students were reassured that their participation or nonparticipation in the study would not affect their education.

Practical Application

Morse and associates (2000) investigated the efficiency and effectiveness of approaches to nasogastric tube insertion during trauma care. To conduct this study, the procedure was videotaped. Approval was granted by the local REB, and all staff, patients, and visiting support individuals were approached for consent to participate. Extra care was taken for the preservation of anonymity; all identifying information was removed, and any mentions of names, addresses, or other identification were erased from the videotapes.

The obligation to balance the risks and benefits of a study is the responsibility of the researcher. However, the research consumer reading a research report also should be confident that participants have been protected from harm.

When considering the special needs of vulnerable participants, research consumers should be sensitive to whether the investigators have addressed the special needs of individuals who are unable to act on their own behalf. For example, has the right of self-determination been addressed by the informed consent protocol identified in the research report? Schell and associates (2010) conducted a study to compare upper arm and calf automatic blood pressures in a convenience sample of 221 children, aged 1 to 8 years, admitted to a pediatric intensive care unit of a 180-bed teaching hospital. Informed consent was obtained from the parent or guardian for all enrolled participants. Informed assent was obtained from children aged 7 and 8 years, if appropriate.

When qualitative studies are reported, verbatim quotations from informants often are incorporated into the "Findings" section of the article. In such cases, the reader will evaluate how effectively the author protected the informant's identity, either by using a fictitious name or by withholding information such as age, gender, occupation, or other potentially identifying data.

Although the need for guidelines for the use of human and animal participants in research is evident and the principles themselves are clear, many instances arise in which nurses must use their best judgement, as both patient advocates and researchers, when evaluating the ethical nature of a research project. In any research situation, the basic guiding principle of protecting the patient's human rights must always apply. When conflicts arise, nurses must feel free to raise suitable questions with appropriate resources and personnel. In an institution, raising questions may include contacting the researcher first; then, if there is no resolution, the matter must be raised with the director of nursing research and the chairperson of the REB. In cases in which ethical considerations in a research article are in question, clarification from a colleague, agency, or the researcher's REB is indicated. Nurses should pursue their concerns until they are satisfied that the patient's rights and their rights as professionals are protected.

CRITICAL THINKING CHALLENGES

- As part of a needs assessment for future health care delivery planning, the Ministry of Health is interested in determining the number of babies infected with the human immunodeficiency virus (HIV). A province-wide study is funded that will include the testing of all newborns for HIV, but the mothers will not be told that the test is being done, nor will they be told the results. Using the basic ethical principles found in Box 6-2, defend or refute this practice.
- The REB of your health care agency does not include a nurse, and you think it should. You discuss this matter with your supervisor, who states that including a nurse is not necessary because the REB uses strict guidelines. What essential arguments and explanations should your proposal address for including a nurse on your institution's REB?
- A qualitative researcher intends to conduct a phenomenological study on caring and to recruit informants who are severely and persistently mentally ill and attend an outpatient clinic. The REB denies the study, indicating that informed consent cannot be obtained and that these patients will not be able to tolerate an interview. What assumptions have the members of this REB made? If you were the researcher and you were given the opportunity to address their concerns, what would you say? Include information from Table 6-2.
- How do you see computer electronic databases and Web sites assisting researchers in conducting ethical studies? Do you think that REBs can use this technology to assist them in their goals?

KEY POINTS

- Ethical and legal considerations in research first received attention after World War II, during the Nuremberg trials, which resulted in the development of the Nuremberg code. This code became the standard for research guidelines protecting the human rights of research participants.
- The U.S. National Research Act, passed in 1974, created the National Commission for the Protection of Human Subjects of Biomedical and Behavioral Research. The findings, contained in the Belmont Report (National Commission for the Protection of Human Subjects of Biomedical and Behavioral Research, 1978), are discussed with regard to the three basic ethical principles of respect for persons, beneficence, and justice that underlie the conduct of research involving human participants. U.S. federal regulations developed in response to the Commission's report provide guidelines for informed consent and REB protocols.
- Protection of human rights includes the rights to (1) self-determination, (2) privacy and dignity, (3) anonymity and confidentiality, (4) fair treatment, and (5) protection from discomfort and harm.
- Procedures for protecting basic human rights include obtaining informed consent, which illustrates the ethical principle of respect, and obtaining REB approval, which illustrates the ethical principles of respect, beneficence, and justice.
- Special consideration of ethics should addressed in studies involving vulnerable populations, such as children, older adults, prisoners, and those who are mentally or physically disabled.
- Scientific fraud or misconduct represents unethical conduct, and professional responsibility must include monitoring for such conduct. Informal, ad hoc, or unauthorized research may expose patients to unwarranted risk and may not protect participants' rights adequately.
- Nurses who are asked to be involved in product testing should be aware of Health Canada guidelines and regulations for testing medical devices before becoming involved in product testing and, perhaps, violating guidelines for ethical research.
- Animal rights need to be protected, and regulations for animal research have evolved over time. Nurses who encounter the use of animals in research should be alert to their rights.
- As consumers of research, nurses must be knowledgeable about the legal and ethical components of a research study so that they can evaluate whether a researcher has ensured appropriate protection of human or animal rights.

REFERENCES

Akhtar-Danesh, N., Valaitis, R. K., Schofieled, R., Underwood, J., Martin-Misener, R., Baumann, A., & Kolotylo, C. (2010). A questionnaire for assessing community health nurses' learning needs. *Western Journal of Nursing Research, 32*(8), 1055-1072.

American Geriatrics Society Ethics Committee. (1998). Informed consent for research on human subjects with dementia. *Journal of the American Geriatric Society, 46,* 1308-1310.

American Nurses Association. (1985). *Code for nurses with interpretive statements*. Kansas City, MO: Author.

Assisted Human Reproduction Canada. (2004). *The Assisted Human Reproduction Act (AHR Act)*. Retrieved from http://www.ahrc-pac.gc.ca/v2/aaa-app/wwr-qnr/ahra-alpa/ahra-lspa-eng.php.

Benedict, S., & Georges, J. M. (2006). Nurses and the sterilization experiments of Auschwitz: A postmodernist perspective. *Nursing Inquiry, 13,* 277-288.

Brink, P. J. (1992). Autonomy versus do no harm. *Western Journal of Nursing Research, 14,* 264-266.

Canadian Council on Animal Care. (2005). *About the Canadian Council on Animal Care*. Retrieved from http://www.ccac.ca/en/CCAC_Main.htm.

Canadian Council on Animal Care. (2006). *Terms of reference for animal care committees*. Retrieved from http://www.ccac.ca/Documents/Standards/Policies/Terms_of_reference_for_ACC.pdf.

Canadian Institutes of Health Research. (2007). *CIHR guidelines for health research involving Aboriginal people*. Retrieved from http://www.cihr-irsc.gc.ca/e/29134.html.

Canadian Institutes of Health Research, Natural Sciences and Engineering Research Council of Canada, & Social Sciences and Humanities Research Council of Canada. (2010, December). *Tri-Council policy statement: Ethical conduct for research involving humans*. Retrieved from http://www.pre.ethics.gc.ca/pdf/eng/tcps2/TCPS_2_FINAL_Web.pdf.

Canadian Nurses Association. (1983). *Ethical research guidelines for nurses in research involving human participants*. Ottawa: Author.

Canadian Nurses Association. (2002). *Ethical research guidelines for registered nurses*. Ottawa: Author.

Canadian Nurses Association. (2008). *Code of ethics for registered nurses: 2008 centennial edition*. Ottawa: Author. Retrieved from http://www.cna-nurses.ca/CNA/documents/pdf/publications/Code_of_Ethics_2008_e.pdf.

Carroll, M. L., & Ciaffa, J. (2008). *The human genome project: A scientific and ethical overview*. Retrieved from http://www.actionbioscience.org/genomic/carroll_ciaffa.html.

Chalmers, K., Squire, M., & Brown, J. (2002). Tobacco use and baccalaureate nursing students: A study of their attitudes, beliefs and personal behaviours. *Journal of Advanced Nursing, 40*(1), 17-24.

Charron, M. (2000). *Ewen Cameron and the Allan Memorial Psychiatric Institute: A study in research and treatment ethics*. Retrieved from http://www.sfu.ca/~wwwpsyb/issues/2000/summer/charron.htm

Chen, W. (2010). Understanding the cultural context of Chinese mothers' perceptions of breastfeeding and infant health in Canada. *Journal of Clinical Nursing, 19*, 1021-1029.

Code of Federal Regulations. (1983). Protection of human subjects, 45 CFR 46, OPRR Reports, revised.

Collins, A. (1988). *In the sleep room: The story of the CIA brainwashing experiments in Canada*. Toronto: Lester & Orpen Dennys.

Creighton, H. (1977). Legal concerns of nursing research. *Nursing Research, 26*, 337-340.

Davis, A. (1981). Ethical issues in gerontological nursing research. *Geriatric Nursing, 2*, 267-272.

Dubler, N. N., & Post, L. F. (1998). Truth telling and informed consent. In J. C. Holland (Ed.), *Textbook of psycho-oncology* (pp. 1085-1095). New York: Oxford Press.

Elder, G. (1981). Social history and life experience. In D. H. Eichorn, J. A. Clausen, N. Haan, & P. H. Mussen (Ed.), *Present and past in middle life* (pp. 3-31). New York: Academic Press.

Flaskerud, J. H., & Winslow, B. J. (1998). Conceptualizing vulnerable populations' health-related research. *Nursing Research, 47*, 69-78.

French, H. W. (1997, October 9). AIDS research in Africa: Juggling risks and hopes. *New York Times*, pp. A1, A12.

Gillmor, D. (1987). *I swear by Apollo: Dr. Ewen Cameron and the CIA-brainwashing experiments*. Montreal: Eden Press.

Haggerty, L. A., & Hawkins, J. (2000). Informed consent and the limits of confidentiality. *Western Journal of Nursing Research, 22*, 508-514

Halushka v. University of Saskatchewan et al., 53 D.L.R. (2nd) 436, 52 W.W.R. 608 (Sask. CA. 1965).

Health Canada. (n.d.). *Health Products and Food Branch Inspectorate—Recall Policy* (POL-0016). Retrieved from http://www.hc-sc.gc.ca/dhp-mps/compli-conform/info-prod/drugs-drogues/pol_0016_recall_policy-politique_retrait_ltr-doc-eng.php#a2)

Health Canada. (1997, revised 2004). *ICH Guidance E6: Good clinical practice: Consolidated guideline*. Ottawa: Health Products and Food Branch. Retrieved from http://www.hc-sc.gc.ca/dhp-mps/prodpharma/applic-demande/guide-ld/ich/efficac/e6-eng.php

Heaman, M., Chalmers, K., Woodgate, R., & Brown, J. (2007). Relationship work in an early childhood home visiting program. *Journal of Pediatric Nursing, 22*, 319-330.

Hershey, N., & Miller, R. D. (1976). *Human experimentation and the law*. Germantown, MD: Aspen.

Hilts, P. J. (1995, March 9). Agency faults a UCLA study for suffering of mental patients. *New York Times*, pp. A1, A11.

Jack, S. M., DiCenso, A., & Lohfeld, L. (2005). A theory of maternal engagement with public health nurses and family visitors. *Journal of Advanced Nursing, 49*, 182-190.

Julion, W., Gross, D., & Barclay-McLaughlin, G. (2000). Recruiting families of color from the inner city: Insights from the recruiters. *Nursing Outlook, 48*, 230-237.

Kevles, D. J. (1996, July 5). An injustice to a scientist is reversed, and we learn some lessons. *Chronicle of Higher Education*, pp. B1-BB2.

Levine, R. J. (1979). Clarifying the concepts of research ethics. *Hastings Center Report, 93*(3), 21-26.

Levine, R. J. (1986). *Ethics and regulation of clinical research* (2nd ed.). Baltimore: Urban and Schwartzenberg.

McLean, P. (1996, November). Biomedical research and the law of informed consent. *The Canadian Nurse, 92*, 49-50.

Milgram, S. (1963). Behavioral study of obedience. *Journal of Abnormal and Social Psychology, 67*, 371-378.

Mitchell, K. (1984). Protecting children's rights during research. *Pediatric Nursing, 10*, 9-10.

Morse, J. M., Penrod, J., Kassab, C., & Dellasega, C. (2000). Evaluating the efficiency and effectiveness of approaches to nasogastric tube insertion during trauma care. *American Journal of Critical Care, 9*, 325-333.

National Commission for the Protection of Human Subjects of Biomedical and Behavioral Research. (1978). *Belmont report: Ethical principles and guidelines for research involving human subjects* (DHEW Pub. No. [OS] 78-0012). Washington, DC: U.S. Government Printing Office.

Office of Research Integrity, U.S. Department of Health and Human Services. (2011). Retrieved from http://www.ori.dhhs.gov/misconduct/cases/.

"Ownership, control, access and possession" and research ethics. (2003). *The Aboriginal Nurse, 18,* 10-11.

Piaget, J. (1937/1954). *La construction du réel chez l'enfant / The construction of reality in the child.* New York: Basic Books.

Pranulis, M. F. (1996). Protecting rights of human subjects. *Western Journal of Nursing Research, 18,* 474-478.

Pruchino, R. A., & Hayden, J. M. (2000). Interview modality: Effects on costs and data quality in a sample of older women. *Journal of Aging and Health, 12*(1), 3-24.

Rankin, M., & Esteves, M. D. (1997). Perceptions of scientific misconduct in nursing. *Nursing Research, 46,* 270-276.

Raybuck, J. A. (1997). The clinical nurse specialist as research coordinator in clinical drug trials. *Clinical Nurse Specialist, 11*(1), 15-19.

Rempusheski, V. F. (1991). Elements, perceptions, and issues of informed consent. *Applied Nursing Research, 4,* 201-204.

Rennick, J. E., Morin, I., Kim, D., Johnston, C., Dougherty, G., & Platt, R. (2004). Identifying children at risk for psychological sequelae after pediatric intensive care unit hospitalisation. *Pediatric Critical Care Medicine, 5,* 358-363.

Robb, I. H. (1900). *Nursing ethics: For hospital and private use.* Milwaukee: GN Gaspar.

Rothman, D. J. (1982). Were Tuskegee and Willowbrook studies in nature? *Hastings Centre Report, 12*(2), 5-7.

Schell, K., Brienning, E., Lebet, R., Pruden, K., Pawheiser, S., & Jackson, B. (2010). Comparison of arm and calf automatic non-invasive blood pressures in pediatric intensive care patients. *Journal of Pediatric Nursing, 26,* 3-12.

Seneviratne, C. C., Mather, C. M., & Then, K. L. (2009). Understanding nursing on an acute stroke unit: perceptions of space, time and interprofessional practice. *Journal of Advanced Nursing, 17,* 1872-1881.

Smith, D., Edwards, N., Varcoe, C., Martens, P. J., & Davies, B. (2006). Bringing safety and responsiveness into the forefront of care for pregnant and parenting Aboriginal people. *Advances in Nursing Science, 29*(2), E27-E44.

Smylie, J., Tonelli, M., Hemmelgarn, B., Yeates, W. M., Joffres, M. R., Tataryn, I. V., et al. (2005). The ethics of research involving Canada's Aboriginal populations. *Canadian Medical Association Journal, 172,* 977-979.

Tilden, V. P. (2000). Preventing scientific misconduct— Times have changed. *Nursing Research, 49,* 243.

United States Government Printing Office. (2008). The medical case. In *Trials of war criminals before the Nuremberg Military tribunals under Control Council Law No. 10* (Vol. 2, pp. 181-182). Washington, DC: Author, 1949. Retrieved from http://www.loc.gov/rr/frd/Military_Law/pdf/NT_war-criminals_Vol-II.pdf

Wheeler, D. L. (1997, December 12). Three medical organizations embroiled in controversy over use of placebos in AIDS studies abroad. *Chronicle of Higher Education,* A15-A16.

Wheeler, D. L. (1999, August 13). For biologists, the postgenomic world promises vast and thrilling new knowledge. *Chronicle of Higher Education,* A17-A18.

FOR FURTHER STUDY

evolve Go to Evolve at http://evolve.elsevier.com/Canada/LoBiondo/Research for Audio Glossary, how-to instructions for Writing Proposals for Funding, and additional research articles for practice in reviewing and critiquing.

Qualitative Research

RESEARCH **VIGNETTE**

Creating Qualitatively Derived Knowledge for a Practice Discipline

Sally Thorne RN, PhD, FCAHS
Professor
School of Nursing
University of British Columbia
Vancouver, British Columbia

To build knowledge for a practice discipline with the complexity and dynamism of nursing, ideas must be drawn from a wide variety of perspectives, disciplines, and inquiry approaches. In the practice arena, nurses universally recognize the patient's perspective as among the fundamentally important aspects that must be considered when decisions are made. Beyond what can be gleaned from individual patient-centred approaches, general knowledge about how patient perspectives are constituted and expressed is needed to guide that individualized assessment, to help nurses understand what they are looking for and then how to interpret and make sense of what they find. The primacy of this patient perspective knowledge as a foundational core of disciplinary practice creates the intellectual climate within which nurse researchers have led the way among the applied health disciplines to develop groundbreaking qualitative, methodological innovations for understanding health phenomena.

Many techniques used in qualitative research actually originated in the social sciences, in which the study of human complexity has been active for generations. Since nurse scholars began to adopt these methods in the 1980s, they have appreciated that the needs of this applied health discipline are quite distinct from those of the more theoretical social sciences; thus, qualitative nursing research approaches have been evolving from being primarily theoretical and toward being more practically applicable. The kind of knowledge that is desirable is not concerned simply with building theories; it is about translating what is known into what nurse researchers can potentially use.

For example, nurses have become increasingly dissatisfied with research that merely describes something; instead, they are seeking knowledge that both describes and interprets: telling not only what seems to be happening but also why that is important. Because they understand that their knowledge products are most valuable when they contribute to the evidentiary basis on which health practice and policy are constructed, nurses increasingly orient their questions and the methods by which they seek to answer them to the most pressing and hard-to-solve clinical challenges. Nurses who engage in a qualitative study are doing so not merely out of curiosity or theoretical inclination, but rather with a desire to add to the knowledge that will help practising nurses and real patients in some meaningful way.

I happened to enter graduate studies just at the time when the worldview of qualitative approaches was emerging as an alternative to the more conventional scientific methods with which nurse scholars had been struggling. The prevailing assumption was that qualitative researchers were entirely different thinkers than their quantitative colleagues, and the two kinds of research products were completely incommensurate. Thus, my entry into a nursing research career coincided with a time of tension and transition in the methodological universe we inhabited. As time passed, I was fortunate enough to be part of the emerging explorations in methodology; for example, the systematic and rigorous integration of the unique insights derived from both measurement and interpretation into robust knowledge "platforms." Instead of arguing the merits of the various ways of studying phenomena, nurse researchers have increasingly joined together in solving the complex problems faced by health care planners, policymakers, and clinicians. By applying the best parts of all of our different perspectives in a thoughtful and rational manner, we are trying to build and implement systems of care that provide the best possible conditions for our patients. It is an exciting time to be involved in nursing scholarship!

The kinds of studies that most attract my interest these days are those addressing aspects of health care in which usual nursing practice is not yet as effective as it ought to be and meaningful improvements can be envisioned. For me, professional-patient communication is one such complex challenge. Although all nurses experientially know how powerful human communication can be in the thoughts, feelings, and behavioral responses to critical events in life, it is extraordinarily difficult to articulate and enforce evidence-informed best practices in this regard.

In cancer care, communication ought to be a priority, in view of what nurses know of its power to nurture or deflate, to inform or misinform, to discourage or encourage hope. Because communication is so nuanced, complex, and various, it is not particularly amenable to conventional quantitative inquiry methods. Although a few things may be quantifiable in relation to communication, much of what we learn from quantification is rather irrelevant to the overall subjective experience of being in a communicative encounter, and the quantitative evidence provides very little guidance for improving patient experience. Therefore, communication is an ideal phenomenon to be studying from multiple angles, including— of most importance—the perspective of those involved in the communication encounter. One might argue that interpersonal communication about difficult issues such as a cancer diagnosis is so complex that it ought not to be possible; however, nurses know that patients truly benefit from skilled and competent communication and experience harm from miscommunications. Patients ought not to launch their cancer journeys with levels of confusion, fear, anxiety, or emotional distress that are caused directly by how nurses interact with them, and there is much to be gained from studying as wide a range of human experience as possible to keep refining the sense of how to communicate well.

In a topic such as cancer communication, although I orient my research questions from the perspective of how a nurse sees the problem, I also recognize the inherent interdisciplinarity of the challenge. I therefore thrive on working with strong interprofessional and interdisciplinary research teams. In the cancer communication work, about half of my team is composed of nurses, and the other half represents epidemiology, physical therapy, radiation oncology, and social work. In our program of research, we have chosen to focus attention on the patient perspective, acknowledging that what we can glean is not in and of itself a "truth" but rather a detectable pattern of subjective material that—together with material we can obtain from other angles of vision—creates an evolving body of understanding. Although we recognize the possibility that patient reports could be skewed in particular directions, we have found over many years in this field that they are remarkably authentic to the perceptions that clinicians hold about what goes on in the practice context. Furthermore, they provide a rich and varied contextual understanding to the trends that can be detected quantitatively: why certain kinds of information exchange are more satisfying to some kinds of patients and not others, why particular forms of communication trigger frustration and despair, and so on.

Interpretive description, which is the applied qualitative research approach that nurse scholars use, is derived from a clinician's perspective on what kinds of knowledge are likely to be most useful. Nurse researchers read and consider social theoretical perspectives, but they do not believe that one theoretical perspective ought to ground or frame their studies. Rather, they believe that a clinical logic is the most appropriate intellectual scaffolding on which to base design decisions, including all aspects of research orientation and data collection, analysis, and interpretation. Nurse scholars try to design studies that will not only illuminate common patterns but also guide them in detecting and making sense of predictable and even infrequent variations, since nursing never deals with standardization in the absence of individualization.

What nurses aspire to is the kind of research report that will elucidate the relationship between practice elements that may not have been well aligned previously, so that thoughtful clinicians can "see" directionality in practice more clearly and be more confident in their practice improvements. Nurses also aim to help teachers of communication competencies look beyond generalities and into more finely tuned expert practices, understand how to nurture and support those practices, and to challenge poor practices when they exist.

I genuinely believe that nurses have a pivotal role in shaping the communicative environment in which patients with cancer are informed, guided, supported, and connected throughout their cancer services. I am also convinced that qualitative research provides nurses with some insight that would otherwise be missing in the evidentiary base that allows them to advocate on behalf of patients.

As you read this book and familiarize yourself with the wonderful world of nursing research, I hope that your imagination will be inspired with directions that you might take your own inquiries on behalf of our profession. Great research really can be a powerful tool for practice! ■

CHAPTER 7

Introduction to Qualitative Research

Julie Barroso | Cherylyn Cameron

LEARNING OUTCOMES

After reading this chapter, you will be able to do the following:

- Differentiate between qualitative and quantitative research paradigms.
- Describe the beliefs generally held by qualitative researchers.
- Describe the components of a qualitative research report.
- Identify the links between qualitative research and evidence-informed practice.
- Identify four ways in which qualitative findings can be used in evidence-informed practice.
- Discuss significant issues that arise in conducting qualitative research.

KEY TERMS

bracketing	"grand tour" question	purposive sample
context dependent	inclusion criteria	qualitative research
data saturation	inductive	reflexivity
deductive	metasynthesis	text
exclusion criteria	naturalistic setting	triangulation
focus group		

STUDY RESOURCES

Go to Evolve at http://evolve.elsevier.com/Canada/LoBiondo/Research for Audio Glossary, how-to instructions for Writing Proposals for Funding, and additional research articles for practice in reviewing and critiquing.

LET'S SAY THAT YOU ARE READING an article that reports findings that men infected with the human immunodeficiency virus (HIV) are more adherent to their antiretroviral regimens than are HIV-infected women. You wonder why that is so: Why would women be less adherent in taking their medications? Certainly, it is not solely because they are women. Or you are working on a post-partum unit and have just discharged a new mother who has debilitating rheumatoid arthritis. You wonder what the process is by which disabled women decide to have children: How do they go about making that decision? These, like so many other questions that nurses have, can be best answered through research conducted with qualitative methods. Qualitative research yields the answers to those difficult questions. Although qualitative methods can be used at many different points in a program of research, you can most often use them to answer questions that nurses have when a particular phenomenon in nursing is not well understood.

In this chapter, the basic tenets of qualitative research are reviewed; the components of a qualitative report, qualitative research, and evidence-informed practice are explored; and the issues in qualitative research are examined.

WHAT IS QUALITATIVE RESEARCH?

Qualitative research is a systematic, interactive, and subjective research method used to describe and give meaning to human experiences. This broad term encompasses several methodologies that share many similarities in the conduct of such research. According to Denzin and Lincoln (1994), "qualitative researchers study things in their natural settings, attempting to make sense of, or interpret, phenomena in terms of the meanings people bring to them" (p. 2). A **naturalistic setting** is one that people live in every day. Therefore, the researcher conducting qualitative research goes wherever the participants are: in their homes, schools, communities, and, sometimes, in the hospital or an outpatient setting.

Qualitative studies most often help researchers begin to formulate an understanding of a phenomenon. Although qualitative research has a long history in the social sciences, it is only since 1990 that it has become more accepted in nursing research. For many years, doctoral nursing students were dissuaded from conducting qualitative studies; the push was for the traditional quantitative approach, which was viewed by many authorities in the "hard" sciences as being more credible. Thus, as nursing gained its foothold in academics, doctoral students were urged to conduct research by using the quantitative paradigm, or worldview (beliefs and practices, shared by communities of researchers), to help nursing gain legitimacy in academe. However, as academe and research evolved along two different but parallel channels, qualitative research received greater acceptance; today's generation of nurse scholars are trained in qualitative methods and encourage students to use the method that best answers their research questions, as opposed to using methods that might add a veneer of scientific legitimacy to its conduct but do not answer the research question at hand.

Qualitative research is discovery oriented; it is explanatory, descriptive in nature. Words, as opposed to numbers, are used to explain a phenomenon. The data gathered in qualitative research come from the text. The term **text** used in this context means that data are in textual form: that is, narrative or words written from interviews that were recorded and then transcribed or notes written from the researcher's observations. Qualitative research lets us see the world through the eyes of another: the woman who struggles to take her antiretroviral medication or the woman with a debilitating illness who has nonetheless carefully thought through what it might be like to have a baby. Qualitative researchers assume that nurses can understand these experiences only if they consider the context in which the experiences take place, and this is why most qualitative research takes place in naturalistic settings.

Qualitative studies make the world of an individual visible to the other people. Qualitative research "encompasses modes of inquiry oriented toward how the social world is interpreted, understood, experienced, produced, or constituted" (Mason, 2002, p. 3). Refer to the Critical Thinking Decision Path in Chapter 2 (p. 32) to see an illustration of the different views and approaches within the qualitative and quantitative research processes. This decision algorithm shows that different beliefs lead to different questions, which lead to selecting different research approaches.

WHAT DO QUALITATIVE RESEARCHERS BELIEVE?

Qualitative researchers believe that there are multiple realities; for example, they believe that the experience of having a baby, although some aspects are common to all deliveries, is not the same for any two women and is definitely different for a disabled mother. Qualitative researchers believe that reality is socially constructed and **context dependent**—that is, the meaning of an observation is defined by its circumstance or the environment. For example, even the experience of reading this book is different for any two students; one may be completely engrossed by the content, while another is reading but is worrying about whether her financial aid application will be approved soon. Figure 7-1 is an illustration of

context dependence; what an individual sees depends on who that individual is and what experiences the individual brings to the situation. Qualitative researchers believe that the discovery of meaning is the basis for knowledge. Qualitative researchers know that they must describe the phenomenon under study well; ideally, the reader, if even slightly acquainted with the phenomenon, would have an "Aha!" moment in reading a well-written qualitative report.

You may now be saying, "Wow! This sounds great! Qualitative research is for me!" Many nurses do feel very comfortable with this approach because they are educated in how to talk to people about the health issues concerning them; they are used to listening and listening well. The most important consideration for any research study, however, is whether the methodology fits the question. It must fit, or else the study will contribute little to they scientific knowledge base for practice. This is also the first question you should ask yourself when you read studies and are considering them as evidence on which to base your practice: Does the methodology fit with the research question under study?

Helpful Hint

All research is based on a paradigm, but the paradigm is seldom specifically identified in a research report.

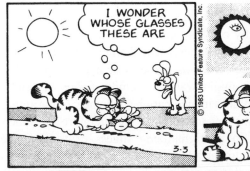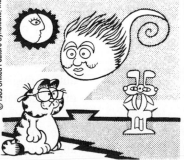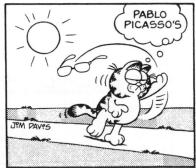

FIGURE 7-1 Shifting perspectives: seeing the world as others see it.

DOES THE METHODOLOGY FIT WITH THE RESEARCH QUESTION BEING ASKED?

As stated before, qualitative methods are often best for helping researchers determine the nature of a phenomenon. Sometimes, authors state that they are using qualitative methods because little is known about a phenomenon; that alone is not a good reason for conducting a study, however. Little may be known about a phenomenon because it does not matter! Before researchers ask people to participate in a study, to reveal themselves and their lives to them, the researchers should be asking about things that will help make a difference in people's lives, in how professionals provide nursing care. You should be able to articulate a valid reason for conducting a study, beyond "little is known about…." In the first example at the start of this chapter, researchers need to know why HIV-infected women are less adherent to their medication regimens so that the researchers can work to change these barriers and can anticipate these barriers when a woman is ready to start taking these pills. In the second example, when researchers learn about the decision-making processes that disabled women use to decide whether to have a child, researchers can better answer the questions of the next woman who is going through this process.

The parts of a qualitative research study are discussed next. Box 7-1 outlines the steps of a qualitative study.

BOX 7-1

STEPS IN THE QUALITATIVE RESEARCH PROCESS

Review of the literature
Study design
Sample
Setting: recruitment and data collection
Data collection
Data analysis
Findings
Conclusions

COMPONENTS OF A QUALITATIVE RESEARCH REPORT

Review of the Literature

The first step has already been discussed: being clear that a qualitative approach is the best way to answer the research question. Next, the author presents a quick review of the relevant literature. This may require creativity on the author's part because published research on the phenomenon in question may not exist. However, there are likely to be studies on similar participants, with the same patient population, or on a closely related concept. For example, the author may want to research how women who have a disabling illness make decisions about becoming pregnant. Although no other studies in this particular area may have been conducted, there may be some on decision making in pregnancy when a woman does not have a disabling illness. These would be important inclusions in the review of the literature to show readers that the author is familiar with the research on this process in a nondisabled woman. Or there may be literature on decision making in pregnancy when a woman has a different but not disabling illness, such as cancer or HIV infection. Reading all of this related literature will help you discern whether the author really seems to know the field and thus the kinds of questions they asked the participants.

Assume that the author wanted to examine HIV-infected women's adherence to regimens of antiretroviral therapy. If there is no research directly on this topic, the author might examine research on adherence to therapy for other chronic illnesses, such as diabetes or hypertension. The author might want to include studies of gender differences in medication adherence; or the author might want to examine the literature on adherence in a stigmatizing illness or to examine appointment adherence for women, to see what facilitates or acts as a barrier to attending health care appointments. The major point is that even though no literature on the author's exact subject may exist, the author should review the literature. In fact, it usually is more challenging to write the review of the literature for a qualitative study because the authors must be creative and think of all of the other comparisons they need to make, whether it is on the study subject, relevant study concepts, or similar/dissimilar patient groups.

At the conclusion of the review, the most important points that you have learned should be clear, and you should be able to articulate the problem to be studied and the purpose for studying it. As discussed in previous chapters, some qualitative researchers conduct a very limited review because they want to be amenable to discovering and learning about the phenomenon under study and not be swayed or otherwise influenced by previous findings in the field.

Study Design

In the next part of the report, the authors should explain the study design. In qualitative research, there may simply be a descriptive or naturalistic design, in which the researchers adhere to the general tenets of qualitative research but do not commit to a particular method. However, there are different types of qualitative methods, which are discussed in Chapter 8. What is important, as you read from this point forward, is that the study design is congruent with the philosophical beliefs that qualitative researchers hold. In other words, you would not expect to read about a random sample, a battery of questionnaires administered in a hospital outpatient clinic, or a complicated statistical analysis. Usually, the researchers also indicate that they have received ethical approval from the appropriate research ethics board.

You may read about a pilot study in the opening of the design section; this is work that the researchers performed before undertaking the main study to make sure that the logistics of the proposed study were reasonable: Were they able to recruit participants? Did the questions they asked of participants yield the information

they needed? Lack of a pilot study is not a deficit, however.

Sample

The next part of the report is the description of the sample and setting. This section contains critical information that enables you to understand how qualitative research differs from quantitative research. In qualitative studies, the researchers are usually looking for a **purposive sample:** a group consisting of particular people who can elucidate the phenomenon they want to study. Therefore, their recruitment materials must be very specific so that when people read their recruitment flyers, they know whether they satisfy the criteria. Thus, if the researchers want to talk to HIV-infected women about adherence, they may distribute flyers recruiting for women who are adherent and those who are not. Or they may want to talk to women who qualify for only one of those categories. The researchers who are examining decision making in pregnancy among women with disabling conditions would clearly list the conditions they want to study. For example, they may describe wanting to talk to women with multiple sclerosis or those with rheumatoid arthritis.

Researchers may impose other parameters as well, such as requiring that participants be older than 18 years, or not using illicit drugs, or deciding about a first pregnancy (as opposed to subsequent pregnancies). These parameters are known as **inclusion criteria** (criteria that people must satisfy to participate in a study) and **exclusion criteria** (criteria used to exclude people from participating in a study). It is critical that the authors make these criteria transparent to the reader, so the reader can judge the abilities of the participants to shed light on the phenomenon in question.

Often the researchers make decisions such as how to define a "long-term survivor" of a certain illness. In this case, they need to tell you, the reader, why and how they decided who would qualify this category. Is a long-term survivor someone who has had an illness for 5 years? For 10 years? What is the median survival time for people with this diagnosis? The researchers' decisions should be based on sound scientific rationale. Then the researchers need to describe how they found these participants. In the example of finding HIV-infected women who are having difficulties adhering to a medical regimen, they may report distributing flyers describing the study at acquired immune deficiency syndrome (AIDS) service organizations, support groups for HIV-infected women, clinics, and other places where people with HIV may seek services. Again, this is one of the most critical parts of the qualitative research process, and you should read it with great care.

In qualitative research, there is no set sample size as there is in a quantitative study (see Chapter 12). Qualitative researchers gather participants until data saturation occurs. **Data saturation** is the point in a qualitative study when the information being shared with the researcher from participants become repetitive; in other words, the ideas shared by the participants have been shared by previous participants and no new ideas emerge.

Setting: Recruitment and Data Collection

The setting section may actually describe two settings: the setting in which participants were recruited and the setting in which data were collected. As already discussed, the settings in which data were collected are another area of critical difference between quantitative and qualitative studies. In a qualitative study, data is usually collected in a naturalistic setting; the participants are not usually brought into a clinic interview room. The setting for data collection is often the participant's home, which can be an incredible window into other aspects of the participant's life. To be in someone else's home is a great privilege and helps the researcher understand what that participant values. For example, those who are ill may have everything they could need to get through a day clustered around a favorite chair: The

researcher might see an oxygen tank, a glass of water, medications, telephone, television, a box of tissues, and so on. This may be an indicator that the participant is someone for whom getting around is tremendously difficult. In any event, a good qualitative researcher considers this setting as additional data to help complete the complex, rich scenario that is being rendered in the study.

Data Collection

Data collection is another part of the process in which the two research paradigms differ tremendously. In a qualitative study, the data to be collected are usually words: The researcher may interview an individual, interview a group of people in what is called a **focus group,** or observe an individual as she or he goes about a task such as sorting medications into a pill minder. In each of these cases, however, the data collected are expressed in words. The researcher asks the participant about the phenomenon of interest and then listens. However, the researcher does not have to do this without some technical assistance. Most qualitative researchers use audio recorders to ensure that they have captured the participant's exact words. This also takes some of the pressure off of researchers to write down every single word, and it frees them up to listen fully. The recordings are usually transcribed verbatim, and then the researcher who conducted the interviews listens to the recordings for accuracy.

The data collection section should also describe details such as whether informed consent was obtained and the steps from when a participant contacted the researcher to the end of the study visit. It is important to also know how long each interview or focus group lasted and how much time overall the researcher spent "in the field" collecting data.

Another important component in this section is the description of when the researcher decided that the sample was sufficient. In qualitative studies, researchers generally continue to recruit participants until they have reached data saturation: that is, when no new information is emerging from the interviews. As stated earlier, the number of participants to be selected is usually not predetermined as in quantitative studies; rather, the researchers keep recruiting until they have the data they need. One important exception to this is a study in which a researcher is very interested in getting different types of people in the study; for example, in the study of HIV-infected women and medication adherence, the researchers may want to interview some women who were very adherent in the beginning but then became less so over time, women who were not adherent in the beginning but then became adherent, or women with children and those without children to determine the influence of being a mother on adherence. However, sample sizes tend to be fairly small (fewer than 30 participants) because of the enormous amounts of written text that need to be analyzed by the researcher.

Finally, you should read in this section about the kinds of questions the researchers asked the participants. These are different from the research question or questions, which should be broad and perhaps written in fairly esoteric language. The interview questions should be clear, be plain, and elicit exactly what the researcher wants to know.

In qualitative studies, there may be a broad overview or **"grand tour" question,** such as "Tell me about taking your medications: the things that make it easier and the things that make it harder," or "Tell me what you were thinking about when you decided to get pregnant." Along with this overview question, there are usually a series of prompts (additional questions) that were derived from the literature; these are areas that the researcher believes are important to cover and that the participant will probably cover, but they are available to remind the researcher in case the material is not mentioned. For example, with regard to medication adherence, the researcher may have read in other studies that motherhood can influence adherence in two very different ways: children can become a reason to live, which would facilitate taking antiretroviral medication,

and children can be all-demanding, leaving the mother with little to no time to take care of herself. Therefore, a neutrally worded question about the influence of children would be a prompt if the participants do not mention it spontaneously.

The sample may be described in the data collection section or in the "Findings" section. In any event, besides the typical demographic data collected in any study, a qualitative researcher should also report on key areas of difference in the sample: In a sample of HIV-infected women, there should be information about stage of illness, what kind/how many medications they must take, how many children they have, and so on. This information helps you, the reader, place the data into some context.

Data Analysis

Next in the report is the description of data analysis, in which the researcher describes how he or she handled the raw data, which are usually transcripts of the recorded interviews in a qualitative study. Many qualitative researchers use computer-assisted data analysis programs to help with this task, which can seem overwhelming because of the sheer quantity of data to be dealt with. However, other researchers analyze the data themselves. In either situation, the goal is to find commonalities and differences in the interviews, and then to group these into broader, more abstract, overarching categories of meaning that capture much of the data. For example, in the case regarding pregnancy for disabled women, one woman might talk about having discussed the need for assistance with her friends and found that they were willing and able to help her with the baby. Another woman might talk about how she discussed the decision with her mother and sisters and found them to be a ready source of aid. A third woman may say that she talked about this with her church study group, and they told her that they could arrange to bring meals and help with housework during the pregnancy and afterward. On a more abstract level, these women are all talking about social support. Thus, it is possible to find a term that is all-encompassing for these descriptions. In an ideal situation, the authors might even describe an example such as the one you just read, but the page limitations of most journals do not permit this level of detail. Chapter 15 includes a more in-depth exploration on qualitative data analysis methods.

Evidence-Informed Practice Tip

Qualitative researchers use more flexible procedures than do quantitative researchers. While collecting data for a project, they consider all of the experiences that may occur.

Findings

At last, we come to the results! First, the authors should discuss whether they are describing a process (as in the decision-making example) or a list of circumstances that are functioning in some way (such as a list of barriers to and facilitators for taking medications), a set of conditions that must be present for something to occur (what parents state they need to care for a ventilator-dependent child at home), or a description of what it is like to go through some health-related transition (what it is like to become the caretaker of a parent with dementia). This is by no means an all-inclusive list but rather examples to help you know what you should be looking for.

After the description, the author presents the results, usually by breaking them down into units of meaning that help the data cohere and tell a story. It is very useful if the author describes the logic for breaking down the units as they are: Are they discussing the themes from most prevalent to least prevalent? Are they describing a process in temporal terms? Are they starting with topics that were most important to the participant and then moving to less important topics?

After describing how the story will be told, the author should proceed with a thorough description of the phenomenon, defining each of

the themes and fleshing out each theme with a thorough explanation of the role that it plays in the question under study. The author should also provide quotations that support each of the themes. Ideally, the quotation will be staged, which gives you some information about the participant from whom it came: Was it a woman of colour with newly diagnosed HIV infection who did not have children? Was it a disabled woman who has chosen to become pregnant but has suffered two miscarriages? Staging of quotes allows you to put the information into some social context.

In a really good report of qualitative research, some of the quotations will give you an "Aha!" feeling: you will have a sense that the researcher has done an excellent job of getting to the core of the problem. Quotations are as critical to qualitative reports as numbers are to a quantitative study; you would not have a great deal of confidence in a quantitative report in which the author asks you to believe some finding without giving you some statistical findings to back it up.

At the end of the report is the conclusion. The researcher should summarize the results and should compare the findings with those in the existing literature. How are these findings similar to and different from those in the existing literature? The author can also describe new findings or new conceptual conclusions in this section because the findings may have revealed areas that were not anticipated at the beginning of the study. This is one of the great contributions of qualitative research: opening up new venues of discovery that were not heretofore anticipated. The researcher also makes suggestions regarding how to use the findings in practice and offers further directions for future research.

Helpful Hint

Values are involved in all research. It is important, however, that they not influence the results of the research.

EVIDENCE-INFORMED PRACTICE

Because nursing is a practice discipline, the most important purpose of nursing research is to use research findings to improve the care of patients. The best way to start to answer questions that have not been addressed or when a new perspective is needed in practice is through the use of qualitative methods. The answers to questions provided by qualitative data reflect important evidence that may offer the first systematic insights about a phenomenon and the setting in which it occurs. Therefore, broadening evidence models beyond a narrow hierarchical perspective is imperative.

Unfortunately, qualitative research studies do not fare well in the typical systematic reviews on which evidence-informed practice recommendations are based. Randomized clinical trials and other types of intervention studies traditionally have been the major focus of evidence-informed practice, as exemplified by the systematic reviews conducted by groups such as the Cochrane Collaboration. Typically, the selection of studies to be included in systematic reviews is guided by evidence hierarchies (see Chapter 3) that focus on the effectiveness of interventions according to their strength and consistency. Because evidence models are hierarchical in nature, which perpetuates the use of intervention studies—for example, randomized controlled studies (RCTs) are the "gold standard" of research design—the value of qualitative studies and the evidence offered by their results have remained unclear. Qualitative studies historically have been ranked lower in a hierarchy of evidence, as a "weaker" form of research design.

Kearney (2001) developed a useful typology of levels and applications of qualitative research evidence (Table 7-1). She described five categories of qualitative findings that are distinguished from one another in their levels of complexity and discovery: those restricted by a priori (existing theory) frameworks, descriptive categories,

shared pathway or meaning, depiction of experiential variation, and dense explanatory description. From these, Kearney proposed four modes of clinical application: (1) insight or empathy, (2) assessment of status or progress, (3) anticipatory guidance, and (4) coaching. She argued that the greater the complexity and discovery within qualitative findings, the stronger is the potential for clinical application. The evidence that qualitative studies provide is used conceptually by the nurse: Qualitative studies let nurses gain access to the experiences of patients and help nurses expand their ability to understand, which should lead to more helpful approaches to care (Kearney, 2001; see Table 7-1).

Kearney (2001) argued that findings restricted by an existing set of ideas or a priori frameworks provide little or no evidence for practice; no new discoveries can be made when the analyst has used an existing theory to explain the findings. Descriptive categories can portray a high level of discovery when a phenomenon is vividly portrayed from a new perspective. For evidence-informed nursing practice, these findings can serve as maps of previously uncharted territory in human experience. The third category, shared pathway or meaning, is more complex in that these reports are syntheses of a shared process or experience. The integration of concepts or themes results in a logical, complex portrayal of the phenomenon. The researcher's ideas at this level reveal how discrete bits of data can be organized in a meaningful whole. For nursing practice, these syntheses represent the bigger picture and what it means for the human experience (Kearney, 2001).

Research on depiction of experiential variation is even more complex than that on shared pathways or meaning; it describes the main essence of an experience but goes on to show how this experience varies, depending on the individual or context. For nursing practice, these studies reveal a variety of viewpoints and realizations of a human experience and the contextual sources of

TABLE 7-1

KEARNEY'S CATEGORIES OF QUALITATIVE FINDINGS,* FROM LEAST TO MOST COMPLEX

CATEGORY	DEFINITION	EXAMPLE
Restricted by a priori (existing theory) frameworks	Discovery is aborted because researcher has obscured the findings with an existing theory	Use of the theory of "relatedness" to describe women's relationships without substantiation in the data and when an alternative explanation may describe how women exist in relationship to others; the data seem to point to another explanation other than "relatedness"
Descriptive categories	Phenomenon is vividly portrayed from a new perspective; provides a map into previously uncharted territory in the human experience of health and illness	Children's descriptions of pain, including descriptors, attributed causes, and what constitutes good care during a painful episode
Shared pathway or meaning	Synthesis of a shared experience or process; integration of concepts that provides a complex picture of a phenomenon	Description of women's process of recovery from depression; each category was fully described, and the conditions for progression were laid out; the origins of a phase are discernible in the previous phase
Depiction of experiential variation	Description of the main essence of an experience, but also demonstration of how the experience varies, depending on the individual or context	Description of how pregnant women recovering from cocaine addiction might or might not move forward to create a new life, depending on the amount of structure they imposed on their behavior and their desire to give up drugs and change their lives
Dense explanatory description	Rich, situated understanding of a multifaceted and varied human phenomenon in a unique situation; portrayal of the full range and depth of complex influences; findings are densely interwoven in a cohesive structure	Unique cultural conditions and familial breakdown and hopelessness led young people to deliberately expose themselves to HIV infection in order to find meaning and purpose in life; description of loss of social structure and demands of adolescents caring for their diseased or drugged parents who were unable to function as adults

HIV, human immunodeficiency virus.
*Information from Kearney, M. H. (2001). Levels and applications of qualitative research evidence. *Research in Nursing Health, 21,* 45-153.

that variety. Conditional models that explain how different variables can produce different consequences broaden nurses' thinking about a phenomenon. Finally, dense explanatory description is the highest level of complexity and discovery, and is a rich, situated understanding of a multi-faceted and varied human phenomenon in a unique situation. Such studies portray the full depth and range of complex influences that propel people to make decisions. Physical and social context are fully accounted for. In these studies,

the findings are densely interwoven in a cohesive structure that provides a rich fund of clinically and theoretically useful information for nursing practice, in which the layers of detail interconnect to increase understanding of human choices and responses in particular contexts (Kearney, 2001).

How can nurses further use qualitative evidence? The simplest mode, according to Kearney (2001), is to use the information to better understand the experiences of patients, which in turn helps nurses offer more sensitive support.

Qualitative findings can also help nurses assess the patient's status or progress, through descriptions of trajectories of illness or through offering a different perspective on a health condition. They enable nurses to consider a range of possible responses from patients. Nurses can then determine the fit of a category to a particular patient or try to locate the patient's condition on an illness trajectory.

Anticipatory guidance includes sharing qualitative findings directly with patients. Patients can learn about others with a similar condition and what to anticipate in the future. This enables them to better obtain resources for future events or to look for markers of improvement. Anticipatory guidance can also be tremendously comforting because sharing research results can help patients realize that they are not alone, that other people have been through a similar experience. Finally, Kearney (2001) argued that coaching is a way of using qualitative findings; in this instance, nurses can advise patients of steps they can take to reduce distress, improve symptoms, or monitor trajectories of illness. Table 7-2 is an overview of clinical applications of qualitative research. Sandelowski and Barroso (2003) also suggested a typology of qualitative research. Grace and Powers (2009), building on the work of Kearney (2001) and Sandelowski and Barroso (2003), suggested a method of assessing qualitative studies for evidence-informed practice that is based not on a hierarchical model but on a pyramid. The use of a pyramid removes the focus from a hierarchical design perspective to acknowledging the importance of the question, not the design.

The definition of evidence-informed practice has three components: clinically relevant evidence, clinical expertise, and patient preferences. Qualitative research does not test interventions but does require researchers to apply their clinical expertise to the choice of the research question and study design, as well as getting a solid understanding of the patient's experience. Although qualitative research entails the use of different

TABLE 7-2

KEARNEY'S MODES OF CLINICAL APPLICATION FOR QUALITATIVE RESEARCH*

MODE OF CLINICAL APPLICATION	EXAMPLE
Insight or empathy: Nurses can better understand their patients and offer more sensitive support	Nurse is better able to understand the behaviors of a patient who is a woman recovering from depression
Assessment of status or progress: Descriptions of trajectories of illness	Nurse is able to describe the trajectory of recovery from depression and can assess how the patient is progressing through this trajectory
Anticipatory guidance: Sharing of qualitative findings with the patient	Nurse is able to explain the phases of recovery from depression to the patient and reassure her that she is not alone, that others have made it through a similar experience
Coaching: Advising patients of steps they can take to reduce distress or improve adjustment to an illness, according to the evidence in the study	Nurse describes the six stages of recovery from depression to the patient and, in ongoing contact, points out the patient's progress through the stages, coaching her to recognize signs that her condition is improving

*Information from Kearney, M. H. (2001). Levels and applications of qualitative research evidence. *Research in Nursing Health, 21,* 45-153.

methods and has different goals, it is important to explore how and when to use the evidence provided by findings of qualitative studies in practice. Remember too that when knowledge about a particular patient care situation is scarce, the data provided by qualitative studies may provide the best available evidence that informs a clinical question or decision about a patient population or patient care.

QUALITATIVE APPROACH AND NURSING SCIENCE

Qualitative research is particularly well suited to studying the human experience of health, a central concern of nursing science. Because qualitative methods focus on the whole of human experience and the meaning ascribed by individuals living the experience, these methods extend understanding of health beyond traditionally measured units to include the complexity of the human health experience as it occurs in everyday life. This closeness to what is "real" and "everyday" hold the promise of guidance for nursing practice; it is also important for instrument and theory development. In Figure 7-2, three examples are cited to emphasize the capacity of qualitative research methods to (1) guide nursing practice, (2) contribute to instrument development, and (3) develop nursing theory.

ISSUES IN QUALITATIVE RESEARCH

Ethics

Inherent in all research is the protection of human participants. This requirement exists for both quantitative and qualitative research approaches and is discussed in Chapter 6. The basic tenets of ethical practice hold true for the qualitative approach. However, several characteristics of qualitative methods, outlined in Table 7-3, generate unique concerns and necessitate expanding the protection of human participants.

Naturalistic Setting

The central concern that arises when research is conducted in naturalistic settings focuses on the need to obtain consent. Obtaining informed consent is a basic responsibility of the researcher,

TABLE 7-3

CHARACTERISTICS OF QUALITATIVE RESEARCH THAT GENERATE ETHICAL CONCERNS

CHARACTERISTICS	ETHICAL CONCERNS
Naturalistic setting	Some researchers using methods that rely on participant observation may believe that consent is not always possible or necessary.
Emergent nature of the design	Planning for questioning and observation emerges over the duration of the study. Thus, it is difficult to inform participants precisely of all potential threats before they agree to participate.
Researcher-participant interaction	Relationships developed between the researcher and the participant may blur the focus of the interaction.
Researcher as instrument	In collecting data, the researcher may misinterpret the participant's reality.

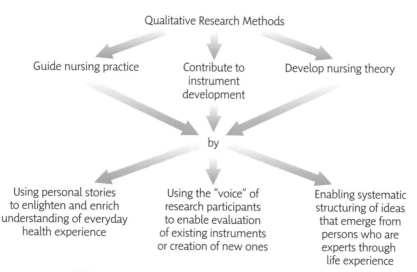

FIGURE 7-2   Qualitative approach and nursing science.

but it is not always easy in naturalistic settings. For example, when research methods include observing groups of people interacting over time, the complexity of obtaining consent is apparent. These complexities generate controversy and debate among qualitative researchers. The balance between respect for human participants and efforts to collect meaningful data must be continuously negotiated. The reader should look for evidence that the researcher has addressed this issue of balance by recording attention to the protection of human participants.

Emergent Nature of the Design

The emergent nature of the research design emphasizes the necessity for ongoing negotiation of consent with the participant. During the course of a study, situations change, and what was agreeable at the beginning may become intrusive. Sometimes, as data collection proceeds and new information emerges, the study shifts direction in a way that is not acceptable to the participant.

For example, if the researcher is present in a family's home during a time in which marital discord arises, the family may choose to renegotiate the consent. From another perspective, Morse (1998) discussed the increasing involvement of participants in the research process, which sometimes resulted in participants' request to have their names published in the findings or be included as coauthors. Morse suggested that if the participant originally signed a consent form and then chose an active identified role, the participant should then sign a "release for publication" form.

The underlying point of this discussion is that the emergent qualitative research process mandates ongoing negotiating of researcher-participant relationships, including the consent relationship. The opportunity to renegotiate consent establishes a relationship of trust and respect, characteristic of the ethical conduct of research.

Researcher-Participant Interaction

The nature of the researcher-participant interaction over time introduces the possibility that the research experience may become therapeutic: a case of research becoming practice. Basic differences exist between the intention of the nurse when conducting research and when engaging in practice (Smith & Liehr, 2003). In practice, the nurse has caring-healing intentions. In research, the nurse intends to understand the perspective of the participant. Such understanding may be a therapeutic experience for the participant. Sometimes talking to a caring listener about things that matter energizes healing, even though this result was incidental. From an ethical perspective, the qualitative researcher is promising only to listen and to encourage the participant's story. If this experience is therapeutic for the participant, it becomes an unplanned benefit of the research.

Several ethical dilemmas may emerge from the qualitative researcher's interaction with participants. Glesne (2011) described several roles that the qualitative researcher may assume, such as exploiter, intervener or reformer, advocate, and friend. All researchers "use" participants to some extent to meet their own needs, such as status and recognition from ensuing publications, with no recognition of the participants. Furthermore, the researcher is in a position of power (researchers who conduct studies in collaboration with others share the power). Often, the "exploitation" is rationalized by the good that may come of sharing the knowledge obtained from the research. Issues of reciprocity are particularly troublesome for ethnographic researchers, who are immersed in fieldwork for long periods of time (Lipson, 1994).

Other dilemmas are faced when the researcher attempts to intervene in a situation. For example, if the researcher becomes aware of potentially dangerous drug abuse among a group of young adults, should the researcher intervene, with the possible consequence of breaching the confidentiality and, ultimately, the trust of the participants? Finally, as trust and respect are established, researchers may find themselves in the role of confidant, which may, in some cases, lead to friendship. Although some qualitative researchers find the role of friend acceptable if it is based on trust, caring, and collaboration, an inherent danger exists that the data are given in the context of friendship and not for the purposes of research (Glesne, 2011). Investigators may also find it difficult to end the relationship and say goodbye to participants. Fournier and colleagues (2006) indicated that more attention needs to be given to psychological preparation, focused on exiting the relationship. In participatory action research, the researcher also needs to consider whether there are any long-term obligations to sustain the project (Fournier et al., 2006).

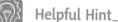 Helpful Hint_____

Researchers are privileged to enter the lives of other people and must treat the ensuing relationship with the utmost respect.

Researcher as Instrument

Qualitative research mandates that the researcher become immersed in the field. Understanding how other people think, act, and feel is paramount (Patton, 2002). Because researchers are interpreting what they observe and experience, their own personal history, experiences, knowledge, and bias may distort the data. The responsibility to remain true to the data requires that the researchers acknowledge any personal bias and interpret findings in a way that accurately reflects the participant's reality. Researchers need to become aware of and monitor their own subjectivity to decrease any distortion of the data. This responsibility is a serious ethical obligation. To accomplish this, researchers should prepare for differences in other cultures and groups by reading, interacting, and seeking out experiences outside of their own norms (Roper & Shapira, 2000). Qualitative researchers frequently write in personal journals during their research activity to

monitor and become aware of their personal biases and feelings (Glesne, 2011). Through this process of **reflexivity** in qualitative research, researchers constantly challenge themselves to understand how their perspective may be shaping the method, interviews, analysis, and interpretations. In addition, many researchers may return to the participants at critical interpretive points and ask for clarification or validation. Patton (2002) advocated the stance of neutrality; in other words, the researcher does not enter the field with predisposed notions but is open to understanding "the world as it unfolds" (p. 51).

Streubert and Carpenter (2011) recommended that researchers identify their own thoughts, feelings, and perceptions by compartmentalizing them in the process referred to as **bracketing,** in which personal biases about the phenomenon of interest are identified in order to clarify how personal experience and beliefs may influence what is heard and reported. Bracketing is important in both the descriptive phenomenological and the ethnographic traditions and is necessary for the researcher to be "open" and receptive to the phenomenon under study. Bracketing is based on the assumption that people can separate their personal knowledge about a specific phenomenon from their experiences and background. For this reason, bracketing may not always be possible, but, at a minimum, researchers should be aware as much as possible of their own assumptions and how those assumptions may affect their observations and interpretations and thus influence the results of the study.

Triangulation

Triangulation has become a buzzword in qualitative research. The view of triangulation has progressed from merely a strategy for ensuring data accuracy (more than one data source presents the same findings) to an opportunity to more fully address the complex nature of the human experience. From this perspective, **triangulation** can be defined as the expansion of research strategies in a single study or multiple studies to enhance diversity, enrich understanding, and accomplish specific goals. Richardson (2000) suggested that the triangle be replaced by the crystal as a more appropriate metaphor for the multimethod approach.

Five basic types of triangulation were described (Denzin, 1978; Janesick, 1994):

1. Data triangulation: the use of a variety of data sources in a study. For example, the researcher collects data at different times, in different settings, and from different groups of people.
2. Investigator triangulation: the collaboration of several different researchers or evaluators from divergent backgrounds.
3. Theory triangulation: the use of multiple perspectives to interpret a single set of data.
4. Methodological triangulation: the use of multiple methods to study a single problem.
5. Interdisciplinary triangulation: the use of other disciplines to increase understanding of the phenomenon (e.g., nursing and sociology).

Although support exists for the use of multiple research methods, controversies surround the appropriateness of combining qualitative and quantitative research approaches and of combining multiple qualitative methods in one study (Barbour, 1998; Giddings & Grant, 2007). Mixed methods research can take two approaches: the mixing of different research methodologies (defined as the theoretical assumptions underlying the research approach) or the mixing of different research methods (defined as the tools for collecting and analyzing data; Giddings & Grant, 2007). Mixing methodologies can be more difficult if the assumptions and values underlying the research approaches (i.e., the methodologies being mixed) are from different paradigms. Giddings and Grant (2007) also argued that because most mixed-methods studies favour the forms of analysis associated with positivism, this form of research is a "Trojan horse" for positivism. In other words, results from mixed-methods research are more likely to be associated with post-positivism. Remember that post-positivism, as discussed in Chapter 2, is the assumption that a "reality" exists that can be observed, measured, and understood.

In spite of the dangers of mixing methodologies and methods, serious readers of nursing research do not take long to determine that approaches and methods are being combined to contribute to theory building, to guide practice, and to facilitate instrument development. Several mixed-methodology research designs have been developed, many from the seminal work of nurse researchers such as Morgan (1998) and Morse (1991). Note that researchers need to determine the primary method (qualitative or quantitative). For example, if the purpose of the study is to describe, discover, or explore, then the theoretical drive is **inductive** (generalizing from specific data), with principal methods that are qualitative. Observations lead to the development of generalizations and in some cases. theory to explain the phenomenon. However, if the purpose of the research is to confirm a theory or hypothesis, the underpinning of the research is **deductive** (concluded from data) and, subsequently, a quantitative drive will be used. Theory is tested by the development of a hypothesis and the gathering of data to accept or reject it. This recognition is imperative because it drives the design of the study from the size of the sample to the analysis of the data.

Morgan (1998) identified several models: for example, (1) small, preliminary, qualitative data providing information useful in the development of a larger quantitative study; (2) limited use of quantitative methods to guide the researcher in decisions pertaining to the larger qualitative project; (3) qualitative methods used to interpret results from a quantitative study; and (4) quantitative methods used to confirm results from the qualitative study. Morse (2003) identified eight different types of multimethod designs with simultaneous or sequential use of qualitative and quantitative methods (Table 7-4).

Mixed-methods research provides researchers with a wider range of tools and options to study phenomena. The variety of methods provides different views and different levels of data.

Table 7-5 synthesizes three studies reporting multimethod analyses. The table notes the conceptual focus of the work, the study purposes, and whether the study suggests implications for theory, practice, and instrument development.

Swanson's (1999) work is a good example of a research program. Utilizing a variety of methodologies and analysis (see Table 7-5), she addressed implications for practice, instrument development, and theory building focused on the issue of caring for women who have had a miscarriage. Her research program included an initial theory-building phase (studies 1 and 2), an instrument development phase (studies 3, 4, and 5), and a phase of testing a practice intervention (study 6). Swanson used the phenomenological method for studies 1 and 2 and quantitative methods for each of her other studies. She did not use more than one method in any of her studies, but her use

of multiple methods during the course of her 15-year research program can be likened to examining different facets of one crystal: in this case, the experience of miscarrying. The crystallization process has contributed to theory building, nursing practice, and instrument development. Her practice contribution is highlighted by a case exemplar (Swanson, 1999), which synthesized her years of work with women living through the experience of miscarriage.

Both Cameron (2003) and Covell and Ritchie (2009) used mixed methodology; the quantitative portion elicited data about a sample, and providing the qualitative portion consisted of interview questions. Cameron (2003) combined qualitative (interviews) and quantitative (questionnaire) methods to explore the lived experience of transfer students in a collaborative baccalaureate nursing program in Ontario (see Table 7-5). Data from the quantitative survey supported the findings emerging from the qualitative methods. The qualitative methods provided depth and substance to the findings from the questionnaire—again, like differing facets of a crystal. Covell and Ritchie (2009; see Table 7-5) studied how nurses

TABLE **7-4**

TYPES OF MULTIMETHOD DESIGNS

DESIGN	ORDER	COMMENTS
INDUCTIVE PARADIGM		
Qualitative + qualitative	Simultaneous	One method is dominant and forms the basis for the study; paradigm is used when more than one perspective is required
Qualitative → qualitative	Sequential	One method is dominant and forms the basis for the study; the second supplements the first
Qualitative + quantitative	Simultaneous	Inductive drive; paradigm is used when some portion of the phenomenon can be measured
Qualitative → quantitative	Sequential	Inductive drive; paradigm can confirm earlier qualitative findings
DEDUCTIVE PARADIGM		
Quantitative + quantitative	Simultaneous	One method is dominant and forms the basis for the study; paradigm validates the finding of each instrument used
Quantitative → quantitative	Sequential	One method is dominant and forms the basis for the study; paradigm is used to elicit further details
Quantitative + qualitative	Simultaneous	Deductive theoretical drive; paradigm is used when some aspect of the phenomenon is not measurable
Quantitative → qualitative	Sequential	Deductive theoretical drive; paradigm is often used when the findings are unexpected, and the qualitative method is used to find explanations

TABLE 7-5

RESEARCH USING MULTIMETHOD APPROACHES

AUTHOR, YEAR	CONCEPTUAL FOCUS	MULTIMETHOD APPROACH	STUDY PURPOSE	THEORY-BUILDING IMPLICATIONS	PRACTICE IMPLICATIONS	INSTRUMENT DEVELOPMENT IMPLICATIONS
Swanson, 1999	Miscarriage and caring	Six studies, each involving the use of one method	Study 1: To define common themes for women who had recently miscarried	Yes	Yes	—
			Study 2: To describe the human experience of miscarriage and the meaning of caring	Yes	Yes	—
			Study 3: To use descriptive data to create a survey instrument that is based on women's experience of miscarriage	—	—	Yes
			Study 4: To evaluate the relevance of the survey items to create a miscarriage scale	—	—	Yes
			Study 5: To assess the reliability and validity of the miscarriage scale			Yes
			Study 6: To test the effects of caring, measurement, and time on women's wellbeing in the first year after miscarriage	Yes	Yes	Yes
Cameron, 2003	Transition resilience	One study involving the use of multiple methods	To explore the lived experience of students transferring from college to university in a collaborative nursing program	Yes	Yes	Yes
Covell & Ritchie, 2009	Medication errors	One study involving the use of multiple methods	To determine the types of medication errors nurses report, why errors are or are not reported, and the strategies believed to improve reporting	Yes	Yes	—

handle medication errors. The data were collected concurrently with semistructured interviews (qualitative) and questionnaires (quantitative). The interviews focused on the story of the medication error, whereas the questionnaire focused on barriers to reporting medication errors.

The studies of Swanson (1999), Cameron (2003), and Covell and Ritchie (2009) constitute a range of approaches for combining methods in research studies (see Table 7-5). The mixed methods field continues to evolve as nurse researchers strive to determine which research combinations promise an enhanced understanding of human complexity and a substantial contribution to nursing science. Consumers of nursing research are encouraged to follow this ongoing discussion.

Synthesizing Qualitative Evidence: Metasynthesis

The depth and breadth of qualitative research has grown over the years. It has become important to qualitative researchers to synthesize critical amounts of qualitative findings. Qualitative **metasynthesis** is a type of systematic review applied to qualitative research. Unlike quantitative research, in which statistical approaches are used to aggregate or average data by means of meta-analysis, metasynthesis involves integrating qualitative research findings on a topic and is based on comparative analysis and interpretative synthesis of qualitative research findings, whereby the researcher seeks to retain the essence and unique contribution of each study (Sandelowski & Barroso, 2007).

Sandelowski and Barroso (2005) reported the results of a qualitative metasynthesis and metasummary that integrated the findings of qualitative studies of expectant parents who received a prenatal diagnosis of a fetal abnormality. Using the methods of qualitative research synthesis (meta-analysis and metasummary (see Sandelowski & Barroso, 2007), they analytically reviewed 17 qualitative studies retrieved from multiple databases. On the basis of the synthesis

process detailed in the article, clinical implications and the need for further research in the area were identified.

Essentially, metasynthesis provides a way for researchers to build up a critical amount of qualitative research evidence that is relevant to clinical practice. Sandelowski (2004) cautioned that the use of qualitative metasynthesis is laudable and necessary but that researchers who use metasynthesis methods must clearly understand qualitative methodologies, as well as the nuances of the various qualitative methods. It will be interesting for research consumers to follow the progress of researchers who seek to develop criteria for appraising a set of qualitative studies and to use those criteria to guide the incorporation of these studies into systematic literature reviews.

Evidence-Informed Practice Tip

Qualitative research findings can be used in many ways, including improving ways clinicians communicate with patients and with each other.

Foundation of Qualitative Research

A final example illustrates the differences in the methods discussed in this chapter and provides you with the beginning skills of how to critique qualitative research. The information in this chapter, coupled with the information presented in Chapter 8, provides the underpinnings of critical appraisal of qualitative research (see Critiquing Criteria box, Chapter 8). Consider the question of nursing students learning how to conduct research. The empirical analytical approach (quantitative research) might be used in an experiment to see whether one teaching method led to better learning outcomes than did another. The students' knowledge might be tested with a pretest, the teaching conducted, and then a posttest of knowledge given. Scores on these tests would be analyzed statistically to determine whether the different methods produced a difference in the results.

In contrast, a qualitative researcher may be interested in the process of learning research. The researcher might attend the class to see what occurs and then interview students to ask them to describe how their learning changed over time. They might be asked to describe the experience of becoming researchers or becoming more knowledgeable about research. The goal would be to describe the stages or process of this learning. Or a qualitative researcher might consider the class as a culture and could join to observe and interview students. Questions would be directed at the students' values, behaviours, and beliefs in learning research. The goal would be to understand and describe the group members' shared meanings. Either of these examples are ways of viewing a question with a qualitative perspective. The specific qualitative methodologies are described in Chapter 8.

Many other research methods exist. Although it is important to be aware of the basis of the qualitative research methods used, it is most important that the method chosen is the one that will provide the best approach to answering the question being asked.

A helpful metaphor about the need to use a variety of research methods was used by Seymour Kety, a key figure in the development of biological research in psychiatry, who was the scientific director to the U.S. National Institute of Mental Health (NIMH) for many years. He invited readers to think about a civilization whose inhabitants, although very intelligent, had never seen a book (Kety, 1960). On discovering a library, they set up a scientific institute for studying books, which included anatomists, physical chemists, molecular biologists, behavioural scientists, and psychoanalysts. Each discipline discovered important facts, such as the structure of cellulose and the frequency of collections of letters of varying length. However, the meaning of a "book" continued to escape them. As he put it, "We do not always get closer to the truth as we slice and homogenize and isolate." He argued that a truer picture of a topic under study would emerge only from research by a variety of disciplines and techniques, each with its own virtues and particular

limitations. Qualitative research methods could be added to understand how books are used by different groups and to understand the meaning of books to the inhabitants.

This idea provides an important point for qualitative research. One research method does not rank higher than another. Instead, various methods based on different paradigms are essential for the development of a well-informed and comprehensive approach to evidence-informed nursing practice.

CRITICAL THINKING CHALLENGES

- Discuss how a researcher's values could influence the results of a study. Include an example in your answer.
- Can the metaphor "We do not always get closer to the truth as we slice and homogenize and isolate [it]" be applied to both qualitative and quantitative methods? Justify your answer.
- What is the value of qualitative research in evidence-informed practice? Give an example.
- Using the model in Figure 7-2, discuss how you could apply the findings of a qualitative research study about coping with a miscarriage.

KEY POINTS

- All research is based on philosophical beliefs, a worldview, or a paradigm.
- Qualitative research encompasses different methodologies.
- Qualitative researchers believe that reality is socially constructed and is context dependent.
- Researchers' values should be kept as separate as possible from the conduct of research.
- Qualitative research, like quantitative research, follows a process, but the components of the process vary.
- Qualitative research contributes to evidence-informed practice.
- Ethical issues in qualitative research involve issues related to the naturalistic setting, the emergent nature of the design, researcher-participant interaction, and the researcher as instrument.

REFERENCES

Barbour, R. S. (1998). Mixing qualitative methods: Quality assurance or qualitative quagmire? *Qualitative Health Research, 8*, 352-361.

Cameron, C. (2003). *The lived experience of transfer students in a collaborative baccalaureate nursing program*. Unpublished doctoral dissertation, University of Toronto.

Covell, C. & Ritchie, J. A. (2009). Nurses' responses to medication errors. *Journal of Nursing Care Quality, 24*(4), 287-292.

Denzin, N. K. (1978). *The research act: A theoretical introduction to sociological methods*. New York: McGraw-Hill.

Denzin, N. K., &Lincoln, Y. (Eds.). (1994). *Handbook of qualitative research*. Thousand Oaks, CA: Sage.

Fournier, B., Mill, J., Kipp, W., & Walusimbi, M. (2006). Discovering voice: A participatory action research study with nurses in Uganda. *International Journal of Qualitative Methods, 6*(2). Retrieved from http://www.ualberta.ca/~iiqm/backissues/6_2/fournier.pdf

Giddings, L. S., & Grant, B. M. (2007). A Trojan horse of positivism? A critique of mixed methods research. *Advances in Nursing Science, 30*, 52-60.

Glesne, C. (2011). *Becoming qualitative researchers: An introduction* (4th ed.). Toronto: Pearson.

Grace, G. T., & Powers, B. A. (2009). Claiming our core: Appraising qualitative evidence for nursing questions about human response and meaning. *Nursing Outlook, 57*, 27-34.

Janesick, V. J. (1994) The dance of qualitative research design. In Denzin, N. K., & Lincoln, Y. S. (Eds.), *Handbook of qualitative research* (pp. 209-219). Thousand Oaks, CA: Sage.

Kearney, M. H. (2001). Levels and applications of qualitative research evidence. *Research in Nursing Health, 21*, 45-153.

Kety, S. (1960). A biologist examines mind and behavior. *Science, 132*, 1861-1870, 1960.

Lipson, G. L. (1994). Ethical issues in ethnography. In Morse, J. (Ed.), *Critical issues in qualitative research methods* (pp. 333-355). Thousand Oaks, CA: Sage.

Mason, J. (2002). *Qualitative researching* (2nd ed.). Thousand Oaks, CA: Sage.

Morgan, D. (1998). Practical strategies for combining qualitative and quantitative methods: Applications to health research. *Qualitative Health Research, 8*, 362-377.

Morse, J. M. (1991). Approaches to qualitative-quantitative research methodological triangulation. *Nursing Research, 40*, 120-123.

Morse, J. M. (1998). The contracted relationship: Ensuring protection of anonymity and confidentiality. *Qualitative Health Research, 8*(3), 301-303.

Morse, J. M. (2003). Principles of mixed methods and multimethod research design. In Tashakkori, A., & Teddlie, C. (Eds.), *Handbook of mixed methods in social & behavioural research* (pp. 189-208). Thousand Oaks, CA: Sage.

Patton, M. (2002). *Qualitative research & evaluation methods* (3rd ed.). Thousand Oaks, CA: Sage.

Richardson, L. (2000) Writing: A method of inquiry. In N. K. Denzin & Y. S. Lincoln (Eds). *Handbook of qualitative research* (2nd ed., pp. 923-948). Thousand Oaks, CA: Sage.

Roper, J., & Shapira, J. (2000). *Ethnography in nursing research*. Thousand Oaks, CA: Sage.

Sandelowski, M. (2004). Using qualitative research. *Qualitative Health Research, 14*(10), 1366-1386.

Sandelowski, M., & Barroso, J. (2003) Classifying the findings in qualitative studies. *Qualitative Health Research, 13*, 905-923.

Sandelowski, M., & Barroso, J. (2005). The travesty of choosing after positive prenatal diagnosis. *Journal of Obstetrical, Gynecologic & Neonatal Nursing, 34*(4), 307-318.

Sandelowski, M., & Barroso, J. (2007). *Handbook for synthesizing qualitative research*. Philadelphia: Springer.

Smith, M. J., & Liehr, P. (2003). The theory of attentively embracing story. In Smith, M. J., & Liehr, P. (Eds.), *Middle range theory for nursing*. (pp 167-187. New York: Springer.

Streubert, H. J., Carpenter, D. (2011). *Qualitative research in nursing: Advancing the humanistic imperative* (5th ed.). New York: Wolters Kluwer.

Swanson, K. M. (1999). Research-based practice with women who have had miscarriages. *Image Journal of Nursing Scholarship, 31*(4), 339-345.

FOR FURTHER STUDY

ⓔvolve Go to Evolve at http://evolve.elsevier.com/Canada/LoBiondo/Research for Audio Glossary, how-to instructions for Writing Proposals for Funding, and additional research articles for practice in reviewing and critiquing.

CHAPTER 8

Qualitative Approaches to Research

Julie Barroso | Cherylyn Cameron

LEARNING OUTCOMES

After reading this chapter, you will be able to do the following:

- Identify the processes of phenomenological, grounded theory, ethnographic, and case study methods.
- Recognize the appropriate use of historical methods.
- Recognize the appropriate use of community-based participatory research methods.
- Apply critiquing criteria to evaluate a report of qualitative research.

KEY TERMS

behavioural/materialist perspective	emic perspective	intrinsic case study
case study method	ethnographic method	key informants
cognitive perspective	ethnography	lived experience
community-based participatory research	etic perspective	narrative inquiry
	external criticism	orientational qualitative inquiry
constant comparative method	grounded theory method	participatory action research
context	hermeneutics	phenomenological method
culture	historical research method	phenomenology
data saturation	instrumental case study	propositions
domains	internal criticism	snowball sampling
	intersubjectivity	theoretical sampling

STUDY RESOURCES

Go to Evolve at http://evolve.elsevier.com/Canada/LoBiondo/Research for Audio Glossary, how-to instructions for Writing Proposals for Funding, and additional research articles for practice in reviewing and critiquing.

CHAPTER 3 DESCRIBES HOW RESEARCH EVIDENCE is categorized, according to traditional hierarchies of research evidence, from strongest to weakest, with an emphasis on support for the effectiveness of interventions. This perspective does not take into account the ways that qualitative research can support practice, as discussed in Chapter 7. There is no doubt about the merit of qualitative studies; the problem is that no one has developed a satisfactory method for including them in the evidence hierarchies. In addition, qualitative studies can answer the critical "why?" questions that result from many evidence-informed practice summaries; a research question may have been answered, but how the answer operates in the caring for people is not explained. You as a research consumer should know that qualitative methods are the best way to start to answer clinical and research questions about what little is known or when a new perspective is needed in practice. The very fact that the number of qualitative research studies has increased exponentially in nursing and other social sciences reflects the urgent need of clinicians to better understand the experience of illness. Thousands of reports of well-conducted qualitative studies exist on topics such as the following (Sandelowski, 2004; Sandelowski & Barroso, 2007):

- Personal and cultural constructions of disease, prevention, treatment, and risk.
- Living with disease and managing the physical, psychological, and social effects of multiple diseases and their treatment.
- Decision-making experiences with technological interventions involving the beginning and end of life, as well as assistive and life-extending care.
- Contextual factors favouring and mitigating against quality care, health promotion, prevention of disease, and reduction of health disparities. The answers provided by qualitative data reflect important evidence that provides valuable insights about a particular phenomenon, patient population, or clinical situation.

This chapter describes a variety of qualitative research methods, including phenomenological, grounded theory, ethnographic, participatory action research, historical, and case study methods. You are encouraged to use the researcher's standpoint as each method is introduced: to imagine how it would be to study an issue of interest from the perspective of each of these methods. No matter which method a researcher uses, there is a demand to embrace the wholeness of humans, focusing on the human experience in natural settings.

The researcher using these methods believes that each unique human being attributes meaning to his or her experience, and experience evolves from his or her social and historical context. Thus, one person's experience of pain is distinct from another's and can be known by the individual's subjective description of it. For example, for the adolescent with rheumatoid arthritis, the researcher interested in studying the child's lived experience of pain spends time in the child's natural settings, such as the home and school. Efforts are directed at uncovering the meaning of pain as it extends beyond the number of medications taken or a rating on a pain scale. Qualitative methods are grounded in the belief that objective data do not capture the whole of the human experience; rather, the meaning of the adolescent's pain emerges within the context of personal history, current relationships, and future plans as the adolescent lives daily life in dynamic interaction with the environment.

The researcher using qualitative methods begins collecting bits of information and piecing them together, building a mosaic or a picture of the human experience being studied. As with a mosaic, when one steps away from the work, the whole picture emerges. This whole picture transcends the bits and pieces and cannot be known from any one bit or piece. In presenting study findings, the researcher strives to capture the human experience and present it so that other people can understand it.

QUALITATIVE RESEARCH METHODS

Thus far, the overview of the qualitative research approach (see Chapter 7) has focused on the importance of evidence offered by qualitative research for nursing science. This overview has highlighted how choice of a qualitative approach is reflective of a researcher's worldview and the research question. These topics provide a foundation for examining the qualitative methods discussed in this chapter. The Critical Thinking Decision Path introduces you to a process for recognizing differing qualitative methods by distinguishing areas of interest for each method and noting how the research question might be introduced for each distinct method. The phenomenological, grounded theory, ethnographic, case study, and participatory action research methods are described in detail. Each of these research traditions is discussed as shown in Figure 8-1 and are based on views along a continuum from post-positivist to constructivist to social critical theory. The constructivist paradigm (multiple realities) is the basis of most qualitative research, and the positivist or contemporary empiricist paradigm (single reality) is the basis of most empirical analytical or quantitative research. The philosophical foundation and assumptions of qualitative research are discussed in Chapter 2. You may wish to quickly review pp. 26 to 31 to refresh your memory. Make sure that you can differentiate between post-positivism and constructivism. In addition, several other qualitative research methods are briefly described here.

Phenomenological Method

"**Phenomenology** is a science whose purpose is to describe particular phenomena, or the appearance of things, as lived experience" (Streubert & Carpenter, 2011, p. 73). Phenomenological research is used to answer questions of personal meaning. This method is most useful when the task is to understand an experience in the way that people having the experience understand it and is well suited to the study of phenomena important to nursing. For example, what is the experience of men facing prostate surgery? What is the meaning of pain for people with chronic arthritis? Phenomenological research is an important method with which to begin studying a new topic or a topic that has been studied but needs a fresh perspective.

Phenomenological research is based on phenomenological philosophy, which has changed over time and with different philosophers. Various phenomenological methods exist, including the following:

1. Descriptive phenomenology, which focuses on rich detailed descriptions of the lived world and is based on Edmund Husserl's philosophy.

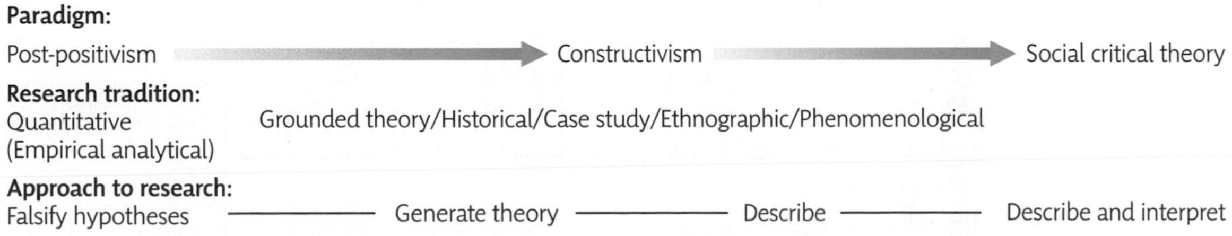

Paradigm:

Post-positivism ➡ Constructivism ➡ Social critical theory

Research tradition:
Quantitative   Grounded theory/Historical/Case study/Ethnographic/Phenomenological
(Empirical analytical)

Approach to research:
Falsify hypotheses ———— Generate theory ———— Describe ———— Describe and interpret

FIGURE 8-1 Continuum of philosophical foundations and qualitative research methods.

CRITICAL THINKING DECISION PATH

Selecting a Qualitative Research Method

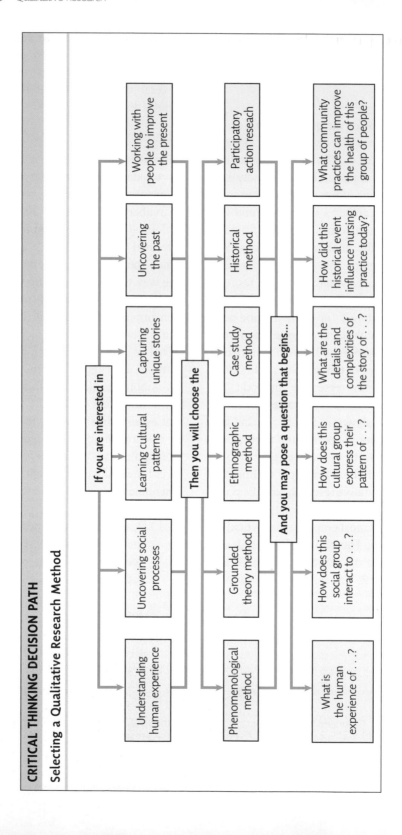

2. Heideggerian phenomenology, which expands description to understanding achieved through searching for the relationships and meanings of phenomena.

3. Hermeneutic philosophy, which focuses on interpretation of phenomena.

Derived from the Greek word *hermeneuein,* the term **hermeneutics** refers to a theoretical framework in which to understand or interpret human phenomena. Hermeneutic researchers believe that interpretation cannot be absolutely correct or true but must be viewed from the perspective of the historical or cultural context and the original purpose of the text. Researchers "use qualitative methods to establish context and meaning for what people do," and hermeneutists are much clearer about the fact that they are "constructing the reality on the basis of their interpretations of data with the help of the participants who provided data in the study" (Patton, 2002, p. 115). Hermeneutic researchers clearly outline their own perspectives and how they may influence the interpretation and analysis of the data. In many nursing studies, the hermeneutic approach is used to understand a particular phenomenon and scientifically interpret phenomena from text or the written word (Streubert & Carpenter, 2011).

Patton (2002) described many of the different phenomenological approaches in his text, *Qualitative Research & Evaluation Methods.* Although he acknowledged the complexity and differing traditions of these approaches, he also stated their similarities:

> What these various phenomenological and phenomenographic approaches share in common is a focus on exploring how human beings make sense of experience and transform experience into consciousness, both as individuals and as shared meaning. This requires methodologically, carefully, and thoroughly capturing and describing how people experience some phenomenon—how they perceive it, describe it, feel about it, judge it, remember it, make sense of it, and talk about it with others. To gather such data, one must take undertake in-depth interviews with people who have directly experienced the phenomenon of interest; that is, they have "lived experience" as opposed to second-hand experience. (p. 104)

The five important concepts or values in phenomenological research (Cohen, 1987) are as follows:

1. The **phenomenological method** is a process of learning and constructing the meaning of human experience through intensive dialogue with persons who are living the experience. This method was developed to understand meanings. The goal was to develop a rigorous science in the service of humanity. The goal of this science is to uncover the roots or foundations of a topic in order to clarify the basic concepts and what their meanings.

2. Phenomenology was based on a critique of positivism, or the positivist view, which was seen as inappropriate in the study of some human concerns.

3. The object of study is the "life world" *(Lebenswelt),* or lived experience, not contrived situations. In other words, as the philosopher Husserl said, researchers are concerned with the appearance of things *(phenomena)* rather than the things themselves *(noumena).* For example, think about a desk in a classroom. The desk is a real physical object, the noumena, which people can see. If it were not visible, people would bump into the desk every time they passed it. In addition, your view of that desk, the phenomenon, changes as you move in the room. If you sit at the desk, you see only the top of it. However, as you move away, you can see the desk's legs, and so on. Nurses are often interested in various aspects of people's experiences or views of health, illness, and treatment.

4. **Intersubjectivity**—a person's belief that other people share a common world with him or her—is an important tenet in

phenomenology. Although phenomena differ, they also share similarities that are based on the similarities in people. The most fundamental of those similarities is that every person has a body in space and time. In other words, the physical body and historical sense lead to similarities in how people experience phenomena. The basic elements, or an essence, of the shared experience are common among people or members of a specific society.

5. The phenomenological reduction, also called *bracketing,* is controversial and more important in some phenomenological approaches than in others (e.g., descriptive methods). Phenomenological reduction means that researchers must be aware of and examine their prejudices or values.

Whatever the form of phenomenological research, you will find the researcher asking a question about the lived experience.

Identifying the Phenomenon

Because the focus of the phenomenological method is the **lived experience**—the undergoing of events and circumstances, as opposed to thinking about these events and circumstances—the researcher is likely to choose this method when studying some dimension of day-to-day existence for a particular group of people. The example used in this chapter is an article by de Witt and colleagues (2010) about the meaning of living alone from the perspective of older people with dementia.

Structuring the Study

For the purpose of describing structuring, the following topics are addressed: the research question, the researcher's perspective, and sample selection. The issue of human participants' protection has been suggested as a dimension of structuring (Parse, Coyne, & Smith, 1985); this issue is discussed generally with ethics in Chapter 7.

RESEARCH QUESTION. The question that guides phenomenological research always concerns some human experience. It guides the researcher to ask the participant about some past or present experience. The research question is not exactly the same as the question used to initiate dialogue with the participant, but often the research question and the question used to begin dialogue are very similar. de Witt and colleagues (2010) were interested in understanding the meaning of living alone from the perspective of older people with Alzheimer's disease or a related dementia.

RESEARCHER'S PERSPECTIVE. When using the phenomenological method, the researcher's perspective is bracketed; that is, the researcher identifies personal biases about the phenomenon of interest to clarify how personal experience and beliefs may influence what is heard and reported. The researcher is expected to set aside personal biases—to bracket them—when engaging with the participants. By becoming aware of personal biases, the researcher is more likely to be able to pursue issues of importance introduced by the participant, rather than leading the participant to issues the researcher deems important.

Helpful Hint

Managing personal bias is an expectation of researchers who use all the methods discussed in this chapter.

The use of phenomenological methods always entails some strategy to identify personal biases and hold them in abeyance while the participant is interviewed. The reader may find it difficult to identify bracketing strategies because they are seldom explicitly identified in a research manuscript. Sometimes, the researcher's worldview or assumptions provide insight into biases that have been considered and bracketed. Bracketing is not mentioned in de Witt and colleagues' (2010) study; again, this is not unusual and does not detract from the quality of the report. Usually, you will find some mention about bracketing if such an issue exists, but not if there are no bracketing issues.

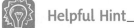

Helpful Hint_____
Although the research question may not always be explicitly reported, you may identify it by evaluating the study's purpose or the question/statement posed to the participants.

SAMPLE SELECTION. As you read a report of a phenomenological study, you will find that the selected participant is either living the experience the researcher is querying about or has lived the experience in their past. Because phenomenologists believe that each individual's history is a dimension of the present, a past experience exists in the present moment. Even when a participant is describing an experience occurring in the present, remembered information is being gathered. The participants in the study by de Witt and colleagues (2010) were eight women aged 58 to 87 years old. All of the participants recruited through purposive sampling were white women of European descent and fit the following inclusion criteria: they (1) had mild to moderate dementia, (2) had discussed their diagnosis with a physician, (3) lived alone, (4) spent the night alone, (5) were English speaking, and (6) were 55 years of age or older.

Helpful Hint_____
Qualitative studies often involve the use of purposive sampling (see Chapter 7).

Data Gathering

Written or oral data may be collected when the phenomenological method is used. The researcher may pose the query in writing and ask for a written response or may schedule a time to interview the participant and record the interaction. In either case, the researcher may return to ask for clarification of written or recorded transcripts. To some extent, the particular data-collection procedure is guided by the choice of a specific analysis technique. Various analysis techniques require different numbers of interviews. In general, open-ended questions—such as "What comes to mind when you think of . . . ?"—guide the participants to describe their lived experience. During the interview, the researcher attempts to gather more information by asking clarifying questions. Data saturation usually guides decisions regarding how many interviews are enough. As described in Chapter 7, **data saturation** is the point in a qualitative study when the information from the participants becomes repetitive, so that in interviews of additional participants, no new data emerge.

de Witt and colleagues (2010) conducted 14 interviews in which the participants were asked to share their thoughts on (1) what it was like to live alone with memory loss, (2) continuing to live alone, (3) safety and living alone with memory loss, (4) what it was like to need and ask for help, and (5) the future. The researcher was able to conduct a second interview, 8 to 10 weeks later, with six of the participants; of the others, two were unable to participate further because of worsening of the disease process. In addition to the interview data, other sources of data included a socioeconomic questionnaire, notes written during and after the interviews by the researcher, de Witt and colleagues' reflexive journal, and a letter received from one of the participants.

Data Analysis

As data are collected, data analysis begins. Several techniques are available for data analysis when the phenomenological method is used. Detailed information about specific techniques is available in the original sources (Colaizzi, 1978; Giorgi, Fischer, & Murray, 1975; Spiegelberg,

1976; van Kaam, 1969). Although the techniques are slightly different from each other, there is a general pattern of moving from the participant's description to the researcher's synthesis of all participants' descriptions. The steps generally include the following:

1. Thorough and sensitive reading of presence with the entire transcription of the participant's description
2. Identification of shifts in participant thought, resulting in division of the transcription into thought segments
3. Specification of significant phrases in each thought segment, in the participant's own words
4. Distillation of each significant phrase to express the central meaning of the segment in the researcher's words
5. Grouping together of segments that contain similar central meanings for each participant
6. Preliminary synthesis of grouped segments for each participant with a focus on the essence of the phenomenon being studied
7. Final synthesis of the essences that have surfaced in all participants' descriptions, resulting in an exhaustive description of the lived experience

de Witt and colleagues (2010) utilized three techniques developed by van Manen (1997) to isolate themes during their data analysis: (1) the "wholistic approach" of reading each transcript in its entirety to understand the overall meaning, (2) the "selective approach" to identify meaningful portions of transcript text, and (3) the "line-by-line approach" to discover what each line reveals about the participant's experience. The researchers then developed a summary paragraph from each of the first interviews and shared this with the participants during the second interview, in which the participants had the opportunity to make any changes. These summary paragraphs also guided the second interview. Each of the interview transcripts was then coded, individual

codes were grouped together into subthemes, and finally they were grouped together as overall themes.

Giving verbatim transcripts to participants can have unanticipated consequences. It is not unusual for people to deny that they said something in a certain way or that they said it at all. Even when the actual recording is played for them, they may have difficulty believing it. This is one of the more challenging aspects of any qualitative method: Every time a story is told, it changes for the participant. The participant may sincerely believe that the story-as-recorded is not the story as it is now after being described.

Describing the Findings

When using the phenomenological method, the nurse researcher constructs a path of information leading from the research question through samples of participants' words and the researcher's interpretation to the final synthesis that elaborates the lived experience. When reading the report of a phenomenological study, you should find that detailed descriptive language is used to convey the complex meaning of the lived experience. de Witt and colleagues (2010) provided numerous quotations from participants to support their findings. They identified a main theme of holding back time and four subthemes of (1) stored time, (2) dreaded time, (3) holding on to the present, and (4) limited time. These themes described the emotions, vulnerability, challenges, and issues experienced by these women. Direct quotations from participants enable you to evaluate the connection between what the participant said and how the researcher labelled it. For example, the subtheme of "dreaded time" describes how the participants chose to hold on to the present, because looking ahead to their own future of worsening dementia was framed by their past experiences of observing other people with dementia. Becoming worse is the dreaded time.

The following quotation expresses a participant's dread of the future.

Well, you saw other people (in the adult day program) in the worst stages and then you think 'I'm gonna be like that . . . it's almost the way you feel as if you've gone to the lowest end when you can't even go to the bathroom by yourself.

Evidence-Informed Practice Tip

Phenomenological research is an important approach for accumulating evidence when researchers study a new topic about which little is known.

Narrative Analysis

When **narrative inquiry** is used as a form of qualitative research, stories of people are collected and examined as the primary source of data (Duffy, 2011). The hermeneutic tradition is extended to include in-depth interview transcripts, memoirs, stories, and creative nonfiction. This discipline also draws from the phenomenological tradition in its interest in the lived experience and perceptions of experience. On the basis of the "stories" of people, at times including those of the researcher, researchers using narrative analysis attempt to interpret and understand experiences in terms of cultural and social meanings (Patton, 2002; see Practical Application box). As Lindsay (2006) noted, "Thinking narratively

Practical Application

Lapum and colleagues (2010) used narrative inquiry to examine patients' experiential accounts of technology in open-heart surgery and recovery. Data were collected from two interviews in which the participants were encouraged to tell their story through prompts and questions, such as "Tell me about waking up from surgery." The participants also documented their experiences in journals for several weeks after surgery. The researchers listened, heard, and felt through the stories what was happening to the participants. Although focus was placed on the content of the stories, emphasis was also placed on how the stories were put together: "We attended to facets of temporality, contextuality, plot, scene, and characters in order to understand processes and activities involved in narrative emplotment" (Lapum, Angus, Peter, & Watt-Watson, 2010, p. 756).

about experience by including the personal and social over time in particular places is personal, reflective and relational work that is autobiographically meaningful and socially significant" (p. 62).

Orientational Qualitative Inquiry

In **orientational qualitative inquiry,** an ideology or orientation is used to direct the investigation, including the research question, methodology, fieldwork, and analysis of the findings. Ideologies include feminist, queer, and critical theories (Patton, 2002). For example, a feminist researcher presumes that gender influences all relationships and societal processes. The researcher will attend to "women's ways of knowing" and include the participants throughout the research. Queer theory, which emerged from feminist theory, focuses on sexual orientation and activities. For example, Holmes and associates (2006, 2007) explored why gay men continue to have unprotected sex despite the associated health risks. Critical theory focuses on issues of power and justice and how injustice and subjugation shape people's experiences and their view of the world. Rather than studying to understand, the critical theorist attempts to critique society, name injustices, and change society. Nurses are particularly interested in addressing and changing oppressive practices that influence health and health care (Browne, 2000). Smith and colleagues (2006) took a critical postcolonial stance in their study on pregnancy and parenting experiences among Aboriginal peoples. In the postcolonial stance, issues of power are viewed in terms of the legacy of the colonialization of Aboriginal peoples and the neocolonial present.

Grounded Theory Method

In the **grounded theory method,** a systematic set of procedures is used to explore the social processes that guide human interaction and to inductively develop a theory on the basis of those observations. The philosophical spectrum of grounded theory ranges from the post-positivist view to the constructivist view (see Figure 8-1). The grounded theory method is based on the sociological tradition of the Chicago School of Symbolic Interactionism, a tradition that reflects on issues related to human behaviour. Glaser and Strauss (1967) developed the method of grounded theory and published the classic first text describing the methodology: *The Discovery of Grounded Theory.* According to Strauss and Corbin (1990), grounded theory

> is one that is inductively derived from the study of the phenomenon it represents. That is, it is discovered, developed, and provisionally verified through systematic data collection and analysis of data pertaining to that phenomenon. Therefore, data collection, analysis, and theory stand in reciprocal relationship with each other. One does not begin with a theory, then prove it. Rather one begins with an area of study and what is relevant to that area is allowed to emerge. (p. 23)

In many qualitative research traditions, explanatory models and theories are described and developed in relation to a human phenomenon under study; grounded theory is distinctive from the other traditional qualitative research methods because its primary focus is on generating theory about dominant social processes. The three major premises that continue to underlie grounded theory research are outlined in Box 8-1.

BOX 8-1

MAJOR PREMISES OF GROUNDED THEORY

1. Humans act toward objects on the basis of the meaning that those objects have for them. Meaning is embedded in context and, therefore, it cannot be separated from the context or from the consequences of the meanings in a particular setting.
2. Social meanings arise from social interactions with other people over time and are embedded socially, historically, culturally, and contextually. Therefore, the focus of grounded theory is on social interactions.
3. People use interpretive processes to handle and change meanings in dealing with their situations.

The purpose of grounded theory, as the name implies, is to generate a theory from data. Grounded theory has contributed substantively to the body of knowledge in the field of nursing. Often, the theories generated from grounded research are then tested empirically. Qualitative data are gathered through interviews and observation. Through analysis of the data, substantive codes are generated and then are clustered into categories. **Propositions** link the concepts to create a foundation that guides further data collection. Additional data that are thought likely to answer generated hypotheses are collected until all categories are "saturated"; that is, no new information is generated. The goal of generating a theory implies that laws drive at least some portion of reality. The truth is sought from relevant groups: for example, patients who are dying.

The context is very important, as was shown in a classic work by Glaser and Strauss (1965). They noted that, at the time of their work, patients were unwilling to talk openly about the process of their own dying, physicians were unwilling to disclose the imminence of death to patients, and nurses were expected not to make these disclosures. This lack of communication led Glaser and Strauss to their study of the problem of awareness of dying. They described various types of awareness contexts, problems of awareness, and practical uses of awareness theory. Their early fieldwork led to hypotheses and the gathering of additional data, and the framework was refined with further analysis until they formed a systematic substantive theory.

Identifying the Phenomenon

Researchers typically use the grounded theory method when they are interested either in social processes from the perspective of human interactions or in patterns of action and interaction between and among various types of social units (Denzin & Lincoln, 1998). The basic social process is sometimes expressed as a gerund, indicating change across time as social reality is negotiated. Schrieber and MacDonald (2010) explored the role and practice of nurse anaesthetists, with a focus on how the practice is part of the nursing domain.

Structuring the Study

RESEARCH QUESTION. Research questions appropriate for the grounded theory method are those that address basic social processes that shape human behaviour. In a grounded theory study, the research question can be a statement or a broad question that permits in-depth explanation of the phenomenon. For example, in Schrieber and MacDonald's (2010) study, the aim of the study was to explore and develop a theory of nurse anaesthetist practice. The researcher does not always need to identify a problem or research question but chooses an area of interest.

RESEARCHER'S PERSPECTIVE. In a grounded theory study, the researcher brings some knowledge of the literature to the study, but an exhaustive literature review is not performed (Streubert & Carpenter, 2011). Therefore, theory emerges directly from data and reflects the contextual values that are integral to the social processes being studied. Thus, the theory product that emerges is "grounded in" the data. This type of study was exemplified in Schrieber and MacDonald's (2010) article, in which a background or literature section was not included.

SAMPLE SELECTION. Sample selection involves (1) choosing participants for a purposive sample who are experiencing the circumstance and (2) selecting events and incidents that are related to the social process under investigation and "are judged to have good knowledge of the study domain" (Wuest, 2011, p. 235). As problems begin to emerge, the researchers may conduct **theoretical sampling,** a sampling method used to select experiences that helps the researchers test ideas and gather complete information about developing concepts. In this method, researchers seek participants who can further clarify the emerging concepts. Schrieber and MacDonald (2010) recruited participants at a general meeting for nurse anaesthetists through purposive and, secondarily, through snowball sampling. **Snowball sampling** occurs when a participants recommends other participants from their contacts. As more and more participants bring on new recruits, the sample appears to grow like a snowball.

Theoretical sampling occurs as key informants are sought to provide clarification on issues such as regulatory and legal issues. **Key informants** are individuals who have special knowledge, status, or communication skills and who are willing to teach the researcher about the phenomenon (Creswell, 1998).

Data Gathering

In the grounded theory method, data are collected through interviews and through skilled observations of individuals interacting in a social setting. Interviews are audio-recorded and then transcribed, and observations are recorded as field notes. Open-ended questions are used initially to identify concepts for further focus. Schrieber and MacDonald (2010) interviewed 18 nurse anaesthetic practitioners, leaders, and students. They gathered documentation and observed the conference sessions, convention rituals, and mentoring relationships. In addition, they interviewed key informants familiar with the regulatory and legal issues, scope of practice, and financial aspects. Field notes were also part of the data collection; they enabled the researchers to document and have a fuller understanding of their observations and conversations.

Data Analysis

A major feature of the grounded theory method is that data collection and analysis occur simultaneously. The process requires systematic, detailed record keeping through the use of field notes and transcribed interview recordings. Hunches about emerging patterns in the data are noted in memos, and the researcher directs activities in the field by pursuing these hunches. This technique of theoretical sampling is used to select participants whose experiences that will help the researcher test ideas and gather complete information about developing concepts. The researcher begins by noting indicators or actual events, actions, or words in the data. Concepts, or abstractions, are developed from the indicators (Charmaz, 2000; Strauss, 1987).

The initial analytical process is called *open coding* (Strauss, 1987). Data are examined carefully line by line, categorized into discrete parts, and compared for similarities and differences (Corbin & Strauss, 2008). Data are compared with other data continuously as they are acquired during research. This is a process called the **constant comparative method.** Codes in the data are clustered to form categories. The categories are expanded and developed, or they are collapsed into one another. Theory is constructed through this systematic process. As a result, data collection, analysis, and theory generation have a direct reciprocal relationship (Charmaz, 2000; Strauss & Corbin, 1990). Schrieber and MacDonald (2010) used the constant comparative method described earlier.

Describing the Findings

Grounded theory studies are reported in sufficient detail to provide the reader with the steps in the process, the logic of the method, and the theory that has emerged. In reports of grounded theory studies, descriptive language and diagrams of the process are used as evidence to ensure that the theory reported in the findings remains connected to the data. Instead of providing a description of people's experiences, the focus is to provide theoretical statements about the relationships between the concepts (Wuest, 2011). Schrieber and Mac-Donald (2010) described the key concept of keeping patients safe throughout surgical procedures. The nurse anaesthetists see themselves as "having a sacred trust to ensure the best outcomes

Evidence-Informed Practice Tip

When you think about the evidence generated by the grounded theory method, consider whether the theory is useful in explaining, interpreting, or predicting the study phenomenon of interest.

for patients, becoming patient surrogates and taking over vital body functions" (p. 554). They keep this vigil by using four interconnected strategies: engaging with patient, finessing the human-technology interface, "massaging the message," and foregrounding nursing. Figure 8-2 visually presents the interconnections among the strategies. The researchers also concluded that the nursing was clearly evident in nurse anaesthesia practice.

Helpful Hint

In a report of research in which the grounded theory method was used, you can expect to find a diagrammed model of a theory in which the researcher's findings are synthesized in a systematic way.

Ethnographic Method

Ethnographic research has a long history in the qualitative research tradition and is considered by some authorities to be the oldest of the traditions (Roberts, 2009). Anthropologists developed the **ethnographic method,** defined as a method of scientifically describing cultural groups. Scotch (1963) first described medical anthropology as the field of research that focuses on health and illness within a cultural system. Nurses also conduct medical ethnographic studies that focus on health and illness within a cultural system (Roper & Shapira, 2000). Although early work addressed the cultural patterns of village life, often in distant locations, nurses now often conduct focused ethnographic research: the study of distinct problems within a specific context among a small group of people, or the study of a group's social construction and understanding of a health or illness experience (Roper &

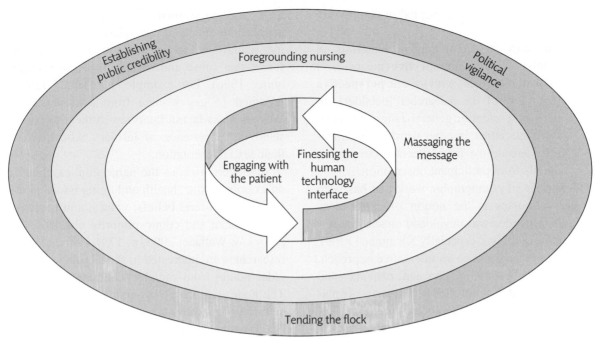

FIGURE 8-2   Keeping vigil over the patient.
From Schrieber, R., & MacDonald, M. (2010). Keeping vigil over the patient: A grounded theory of nurse anaethesia practice. *Journal of Advanced Nursing, 66,* 552–561. doi:10.1111/j.1365-2648.2009.05207.x. © 2010 Blackwell Publishing Ltd.

Shapira, 2000). Leininger (1985) developed an ethnographic research method called *ethnonursing,* which has since been redefined as "a rigourous, systematic, and in-depth method for studying multiple cultures and care factors within familiar environments of people and to focus on the interrelationships of care and culture to arrive at the goal of culturally congruent care services" (Leininger, 2006, p. 20).

Ethnography (ethnographic research) is the study of cognitive models or patterns of behaviour of people within a culture. Ethnographers seek to understand another way of life from the perspective of the people experiencing it. The following values underlie ethnography:

- Culture is fundamental to ethnographic studies. Culture includes behavioural/ materialist and cognitive perspectives. Through the **behavioural/materialist perspective,** culture is observed through a group's patterns of behaviour and customs, its way of life, and what it produces. The **cognitive perspective** is the view that culture consists of the beliefs, knowledge, and ideas people use as they live. **Culture** refers to the structures of meaning through which people shape experiences.

- Understanding culture requires a holistic perspective that captures the breadth of the beliefs, knowledge, and activities of the group being studied.

- **Context**—the personal, social, and political environment in which a phenomenon of interest (time, place, cultural beliefs, values, and practices) occurs—is important for an understanding of a culture. Understanding this context requires intensive face-to-face contact over an extended period of time. People are studied where they live, in their natural settings, or where an experience occurs, such as in a hospital or community setting.

- The aim of ethnographic research is to combine the **emic perspective** (the insider's view of the world) with the **etic perspective** (the view of the researcher [outsider]) to develop a scientific generalization about different societies. In other words, generalizations are drawn from special examples or details from participant observation.

An example of ethnographic work that has been useful to nurses is the notion of explanatory models. This idea was developed most by cognitive anthropologists, especially Kleinman (1980). Explanatory models use an interactive approach, emphasizing variations between patients' and practitioners' models of illness. They offer explanations of sickness and treatment, guide choices among available therapies and therapists, and give social meaning to the experience of sickness. These cognitive models vary over time and in response to a particular episode of illness.

Several ethnographic schools of thought exist, three of which are of particular interest to nurse researchers: critical, feminist, and ethnogeriatric. Critical ethnography does not entail the use of different methods; instead, it focuses on beliefs and practices that limit human freedom, justice, and democracy (Usher, 1996). Critical ethnographic researchers make their values explicit. In other words, they document tacit rules that govern human interaction and behaviour. They also explore how dominant social groups oppress those in the minority or those without power. For example, Pesut and Reimer-Kirkham (2010) conducted a critical ethnographic study to describe how religious and spiritual values and beliefs are negotiated in encounters between health care professionals and health care recipients. Finally, many critical ethnographers consider the study participants to be co-investigators and explore problems and possible solutions with them.

Feminist researchers, like critical ethnographers, focus on oppression and power but apply their work to women. They also consider and analyze the effects of race, class, culture, ethnicity, sexual preference, and other identities as forces that cause and sustain oppression (Macquire, 1996). For example, McDonald (2006) recruited 15 gay women from a university in Western Canada and interviewed them to understand the experience of lesbians who disclose their sexual orientation.

Ethnogeriatrics, as the name implies, focuses on examining the "health and aging issues in the context of cultural beliefs, values, and practices among racial and ethnic minority elders" (Fitzpatrick & Wallace, 2006, p. 179). Ethnogeriatric researchers are interested in the disparities facing older adults from racial and ethnic minorities. The hope is to develop nursing knowledge and culturally appropriate interventions to guide health care systems to be more inclusive of this patient population.

Identifying the Phenomenon

The phenomenon under investigation in an ethnographic study varies in scope from a long-term study of a very complex culture, such as that of the Aborigines (Mead, 1949), to a shorter-term study of a phenomenon within subunits of cultures. Kleinman (1992) notes the clinical utility of ethnography in describing the "local world" of groups of patients who are experiencing a particular phenomenon, such as suffering. The local worlds of patients have cultural, political, economical, institutional, and social-relational dimensions in much the same way as larger complex societies do. Seneviratne and associates' (2009) study on nurses' perceptions of the contexts of caring for acute stroke survivors (see Appendix A) provides an introduction to ethnography.

Structuring the Study

RESEARCH QUESTION. When you review a report of ethnographic research, notice that questions are asked about lifeways, or particular patterns of behaviour within the social context of a culture or subculture. Culture is viewed as the system of knowledge and linguistic expressions used by social groups that allows the researcher to interpret or make sense of the world of those groups (Aamodt, 1991). Ethnographic nursing studies address questions that concern how cultural knowledge, norms, values, and other contextual variables influence a person's health care experience. Ethnographers have a broader definition of culture, whereby a particular social context is conceptualized as a culture. In this case, in Seneviratne and associates' (2009) study on understanding nursing on an acute stroke unit, the acute stroke unit is seen as a culture appropriate for ethnographic study (see Appendix A).

RESEARCHER'S PERSPECTIVE. When a researcher uses the ethnographic method, the researcher's perspective is that of an interpreter entering an alien world and attempting to make sense of that world from the insider's point of view (Agar, 1986). Like phenomenologists and grounded theory researchers, ethnographers make their own beliefs explicit and bracket, or set aside, their personal biases as they interpret the findings and seek to understand the worldview of other people.

SAMPLE SELECTION. The ethnographer selects a cultural group that is experiencing the phenomenon under investigation. The researcher gathers information from general informants and from key informants. Seneviratne and associates' (2009) research took place in an 18-bed acute stroke unit that provided specialized interventions, management, and investigative care, located in a large tertiary medical centre in Canada. The staff included nurses; licensed practical nurses; patient care attendants; a nurse practitioner; physicians; and physical, occupational, and speech therapists (see Appendix A).

Data Gathering

Ethnographic data gathering involves participant observation or immersion in the setting, interviews of informants, and interpretation by the researcher of cultural patterns (Crabtree & Miller, 1992). According to Boyle (1991), ethnographic research in nursing, as in other disciplines, involves interviewing in the natural setting as the major data-collection method. Thus, fieldwork is a major focus of the method. Other techniques may include obtaining life histories and collecting material items reflective of the culture. Photographs and films of the informants in their world can be used as data sources. Spradley (1979) identified three categories of questions for ethnographic inquiry: descriptive, or broad, open-ended questions; structural, or in-depth, questions that expand and verify the unit of analysis; and contrast questions, which further clarify and provide criteria for exclusion.

In Seneviratne and associates' (2009) study, data were collected from observations obtained by monitoring the unit staff (20 individuals) and from interviews with nine of those staff. The fieldwork took place over a period of 8 months for an average of 2 to 3 hours three times a week. Initially, the fieldworker began with 3 months of general observation while located at the charting desk, located at the nursing station, and walking in the hall. After the field notes from each day were reviewed, a more focused approach was taken to fill in the gaps. To further explore work practices, participants were interviewed with "grand tour" questions such as "Can you walk me through your typical day?" Of importance is that although nurses were the focus of the study, four other health professionals were interviewed in order to contextualize interprofessional perspectives (see Appendix A).

Data Analysis

As with other qualitative methods, data are collected and analyzed simultaneously. Data analysis proceeds through several levels as the researcher looks for the meaning of cultural symbols in the informant's language. Analysis begins with a search for **domains,** or symbolic categories that include smaller categories. Language is analyzed for semantic relationships, and structural questions are formulated to expand and verify data. Analysis proceeds through increasing levels of complexity until the data, grounded in the informant's reality and synthesized by the researcher, lead to hypothetical propositions about the cultural phenomenon under investigation. Creswell (1998) provided a detailed description of the ethnographic analysis process. Seneviratne and associates (2009) described a three-step data-analysis plan. Initially, they identified three main themes and then further identified theme components. They then categorized the work activities into types on the basis of relationships between nurses and then between nurses and the other health care professionals. They cross-checked their findings by reading the field notes and interview transcripts and then returning to the field to make further observations (see Appendix A).

Describing the Findings

In ethnographic studies, field notes of observations, interview transcriptions, and sometimes other artifacts such as photographs yield large quantities of data. Charmaz (2000) provided guidelines for ethnographic writing that you can use when you wish to critique descriptions of ethnographic studies. The five techniques recommended in Charmaz's guidelines are pulling the reader in, re-creating experiential mood, adding surprising observations, reconstructing ethnographic experience, and creating closure for the study. When you critique, be aware that the report of findings usually provides examples from data, thorough descriptions of the analytical process, and statements of the hypothetical propositions and their relationship to the ethnographer's frame of reference.

Evidence provided by complete ethnographies may be published as monographs. Seneviratne and associates (2009) described three local domains that frame how nurses understand nursing on an acute care unit: perceptions of space, time, and interprofessional practice. Each of the three domains was further divided into theme units. For example, in the domain of space, nurses described "space" as a challenge to patient care with three themes: "nursing in a submarine," "nursing too close," and "nursing in a state of code burgundy"; a "code burgundy" referred to a lack of beds, so that nurses had to care for patients in the hallway, which resulted in increased workload and the ethical challenges associated with "hallway care" (see Appendix A).

> ### Evidence-Informed Practice Tip
> Evidence generated by ethnographic studies answers questions about how cultural knowledge, norms, values, and other contextual variables influence the health experience of a particular patient population in a specific setting.

Case Study Method

Case study as a research method involves an in-depth description of the essential dimensions and processes of the phenomenon being studied. Case study research, rooted in sociology, is described slightly differently by major thinkers who write about this method, such as Yin, Stake, Merriam, and Creswell (Aita & McIlvain, 1999). For the purpose of introducing you to this research method, Stake's view is emphasized. The **case study method** is about studying the peculiarities and the commonalities of a specific case over time to provide an in-depth description of the essential dimensions and processes of the phenomenon—familiar ground for practising nurses. Stake (2003) noted that case study is not a methodological choice but rather a choice of what to study. Case study can include quantitative or qualitative data, or both, but it is defined by its focus on uncovering an individual case. Stake (2003) distinguished intrinsic from instrumental case study. **Intrinsic case study** is research that is undertaken to have a better understanding of the case—nothing more or nothing less. "The researcher at least temporarily subordinates other curiosities so that the stories of those 'living the case' will be teased out" (Stake, 2003, p. 122). **Instrumental case study** is defined as research that is performed when the researcher is pursuing insight into an issue or wants to challenge some generalization.

Case studies can be used for a variety of purposes, including to present data gathered with another method, as a teaching device, or as a research method (Yin, 1994). Case studies have been used in various disciplines, including nursing, political science, sociology, business, social work, economics, and psychology. Nurses have a long and continuing tradition of using case studies for teaching and learning about patients (e.g., Parsons, 1911). Nightingale (1858/1969) stressed the importance of coming to know patients and of basing practice on experience. She noted that knowing how to provide care requires the nurse to learn about the patient's life. In case studies, these details are described, and the lessons that can be learned from the particular patient are made clear. Persons who have had a particular experience can provide insights that are both valuable and unavailable to those who have not had the experience. Obtaining these descriptions through the use of case studies can serve a variety of functions: making practitioners and researchers aware of patients' experiences; clarifying the concepts included in an experience or general label; policy decision making; and theory building by identifying hypotheses for testing with further research (Cohen & Saunders, 1996). Maddalena and colleagues (2010) examined the experiences and recollections of primary caregivers of African Canadians who died from cancer. The researchers were also interested in the use of complementary and alternative medicine and home remedies at the end of life.

Identifying the Phenomenon

Although some definitions of case study demand that the focus of research be contemporary,

Stake's (1995, 2003) defining criterion of attention to the single case broadens the scope of phenomenon for study. By using a single case, Stake designated a focus on an individual, a family, a community, an organization: some complex phenomenon that mandates close scrutiny for understanding. Maddalena and colleagues (2010) wanted to examine the experiences of caregivers of patients of African Canadian descent who died of cancer. They chose three case studies of families of African Canadian descent in Nova Scotia.

Structuring the Study

RESEARCH QUESTION. The research question for a case study is one that provokes the curiosity of the researcher. Stake (2003) suggested that research questions be developed around issues that serve as a foundation to uncover complexity and pursue understanding. Although researchers pose questions to begin discussion, the initial questions are never all-inclusive. Rather, the researcher uses an iterative process of "growing questions" in the field; that is, as data are collected to address these questions, other questions emerge to guide the researcher in the process of untangling the complex story. Therefore, research questions evolve over time and re-create themselves in case study research. Maddalena and colleagues (2010) were initially interested in the experiences and recollections of the caregivers of African Canadian patients with cancer at the end of life. Later, they also became interested in the use of complementary and alternative therapies and home remedies used at the end of life.

RESEARCHER'S PERSPECTIVE. When the researcher begins with questions developed around suspected issues of importance, the perspective of the researcher is reflected in the questions; this is sometimes referred to as an *etic perspective*. As the researcher begins engaging the phenomenon of interest, the story unfolds and leads the way, shifting from an etic (researcher-based) to an emic (story-based) perspective (Stake, 2003). The reader may recognize a shift from etic to emic perspective when stories spin off of the original questions posed by the researcher. Maddalena and colleagues (2010), with the exception of the first author, self-identified as African Canadian, which provided, at least initially, a strong etic perspective.

SAMPLE SELECTION. Sample selection is one of the areas of which scholars in the field present differing views, ranging from choosing only the most common cases to choosing only the most unusual cases (Aita & McIlvain, 1999). Stake (2003) advocated selecting cases that may offer the best opportunities for learning. For example, if several heart transplant recipients are available for the researcher to study, practical factors will influence the opinion of which patient offers the best opportunity for learning. It would be more practical to study patients who live in the area and can be easily visited at home or in the medical centre than to study someone living in another country. The researcher may want to choose someone who has an actively participating family, because most transplant recipients reside in a family setting. No choice is perfect when a case is selected. There is much to learn about any one individual, situation, or organization during case study research, regardless of the contextual factors influencing the unit of analysis. Using purposive sampling, Maddalena and colleagues (2010) followed specific inclusion criteria: (1) that the caregivers were African Canadian and (2) that they provided care for someone who had died in the previous 3 years. Three case studies were examined: one rural family, one urban family, and one recently arrived immigrant family. From these families, a total of seven participants—three primary and four secondary caregivers—were identified. The different experiences of the primary and secondary caregivers provided a richer understanding of the experience and validated the findings.

Data Gathering

Data are gathered through the use of interview, observation, document review, and any other methods by which researchers accumulate evidence that enables understanding of the complexity of the case. The researcher will do what is needed to get a sense of the environment and the relationships that provide the context for the case. Stake (1995) advocates development of a data-gathering plan to guide the progress of the study from definition of the case through decisions regarding reporting. You may find little explicit information about data gathering in the report of research. The primary source of data in Maddalena and colleagues' (2010) study was individual in-depth interviews with the primary caregivers. Secondary caregivers were also interviewed to provide more depth and thus facilitated triangulation. Follow-up interviews were also conducted to seek clarification of issues raised in the first interview.

Data Analysis and Describing Findings

Data analysis is closely tied to data gathering and description of findings as the case study story is generated: "Qualitative case study is characterized by researchers spending extended time, on site, personally in contact with activities and operations of the case, reflecting, revising descriptions and meanings of what is going on" (Stake, 2003, p. 450). Reflecting and revising meanings are the work of the case study researcher, who has recorded data, searched for patterns, linked data from multiple sources, and devised preliminary thoughts regarding the meaning of collected data. This reflective dynamic evolution is the iterative process of creating the case study story that can be thought of as the evidence. You may have difficulty determining how data analysis was conducted because the research report generally does not list research activities. Findings are embedded in (1) a chronological development of the case; (2) the researcher's story of coming to know the case; (3) the descriptions of individual case dimensions; and (4) vignettes that highlight case qualities (Stake, 1995). In Maddalena and colleagues' (2010) study, the verbatim-transcribed interviews were coded manually individually by four members of the research team. The team met to compare coding and engage in the analysis of the data. Once the team reached consensus, a thematic and discourse analysis was used to further analyze the data. As prevalent themes emerged, each was explored in the context of how culture influenced their experiences during the time from initial diagnosis through interactions with the health system to death and bereavement. With the researchers' etic view of the black community and culture, the team made sense of the data through the shared historical and cultural experiences of the black community. Using a discourse analysis approach, the researchers examined each of the themes in terms of their social, political, and historical contexts. The researchers found that the end of life for African Canadians was characterized by end-of-life care provided by family in the home setting, community involvement, a focus on spirituality, and a preference for home care over institutionalized care. In the home setting, the caregivers were faced with a myriad of challenges. Common among the three case studies was the use of complementary and alternative methods and home remedies. In each of the three case studies, the use of prayer was considered a complementary method.

Evidence-Informed Practice Tip

Case studies are a way of providing in-depth, evidence-informed discussion of clinical topics that can be used to guide practice.

Historical Research Method

The **historical research method** is a systematic approach for understanding the past through collection, organization, and critical appraisal of facts. One of the goals in historical methodology is to shed light on the past so that it can guide the present and the future: "Through historical research, we can better understand how nurses in the present can assume control of their practice, education, and roles in the contemporary healthcare system" (Lundy, 2011, p. 383). The attention in nursing to historical methodology was initiated by Teresa E. Christy, who elaborated the method (Christy, 1975) and the need (Christy, 1981) for historical research long before most nurse scholars accepted it as a legitimate research method. More recently, Lusk (1997) summarized important information for the nurse interested in understanding historical research. She provided guidance for choosing a topic, acquiring data, addressing ethical issues, analyzing data, and reporting findings.

When you appraise a study in which the historical method was used, expect to find the research question embedded in the phenomenon to be studied. The question is stated implicitly rather than explicitly.

The three theoretical frameworks that guide historical research are as follows (Streubert & Carpenter, 2011):

1. Biographical history: an exploration of the life of an individual to understand the effects of the time and culture on the person's life
2. Social history: an exploration of the prevailing values and beliefs in a particular period by examining everyday events
3. Intellectual history: an exploration of the ideas of a particular individual or a group of people

An example of biographical history is the book about Gertrude Richard Ladner (i.e., her family and nursing life), in which the authors presented new ideas about nursing and family life in the late nineteenth and early twentieth centuries in Western Canada (Zerr, Zilm, & Grant, 2006). Although the authors believed that Ladner represented the ordinary life of women and nurses in that time, they discovered that she was more than a handmaiden for the physicians with whom she worked. Many of the details included in the book were gathered from her personal journal, providing a record of the work of nurses, their day-to-day experiences, and nursing knowledge that informed their practice.

Reeves and associates (2010) applied a socio-historical analysis of historical documents to understand how modern health care professions emerged from sixteenth century craft guilds. Their analysis provides an understanding of how the historical practice of protecting and promoting one's own members of the guild is one of the roots of today's barriers to effective collaboration and interprofessional teamwork.

Data sources provide the sample for historical research. The more clearly a researcher delineates the historical event being studied, the more specifically data sources can be identified. Data may include written or video documents, interviews with persons who witnessed the event, photographs, and other materials that shed light on the subject. Sometimes pivotal information cannot be retrieved and must be eliminated from the list of possible sources. To determine which data sources were used when you review a published study, look at the reference list. Sources of data may be primary or secondary. Primary sources are eyewitness accounts provided by varying sorts of communication appropriate to the time. Secondary sources provide a view of the phenomenon from another person's perspective rather than a first-hand account.

Validity of documents is established by external criticism; reliability is established by internal criticism. In **external criticism,** the authenticity of the data source is judged. The researcher seeks to ensure that the data source is indeed what it seems to be. For instance, if the researcher is reviewing a handwritten letter of Florence Nightingale, some of the validity issues are the following:

- Are the ink, paper, and wax seal on the envelope representative of Nightingale's time?
- Is the wax seal one that Nightingale used in other authentic data sources?
- Is the writing truly Nightingale's?

Only if the data source passes the test of external criticism does the researcher begin internal criticism. **Internal criticism** is the process of judging the reliability or consistency of information within the historical document (Christy, 1975). To judge reliability, the researcher must become familiar with the time in which the data emerged. A sense of the context and language of the time is essential to understanding a document. The meaning of a word in one era may not be equivalent to the meaning in another era. Knowing the language, customs, and habits of the historical period is critical for judging reliability. The researcher assumes that a primary source provides a more reliable account than does a secondary source (Christy, 1975). The further a source is from an eyewitness account, the more questionable is its reliability. The researcher using historical methods attempts to establish fact, probability, or possibility (Box 8-2).

During the analytic stage, the researcher begins the process of interpretation of meaning. Often working with incomplete records, the historian researcher is reaching beyond the evidence to make inferences. The report usually contains extensive samples of the data, along with evidence of reliability and validity: "A critical description of historical evidence, an evaluation of its historical significance to contemporary society, and creative narratives are provided in the written research report, including the derived interferences" (Lundy, 2011, p. 391).

Helpful Hint

When you critique a study based on the historical method, expect not to find a report of data analysis but simply a description of findings synthesized into a continuous narrative.

BOX 8-2

ESTABLISHING FACT, PROBABILITY, AND POSSIBILITY WITH THE HISTORICAL METHOD

FACT

Two independent primary sources that agree with each other

or

One independent primary source that receives critical evaluation and one independent secondary source that is in agreement and receives critical evaluation and no substantive conflicting data

PROBABILITY

One primary source that receives critical evaluation and no substantive conflicting data

or

Two primary sources that disagree about particular points

POSSIBILITY

One primary source that provides information but is not adequate to receive critical evaluation

or

Only secondary or tertiary sources

Adapted from Christy, T. E. (1975). The methodology of historical research: A brief introduction. *Image, 24*(3), 189-192.

Evidence-Informed Practice Tip ___

The presentation of a historical study should be logical, consistent, and easy to follow.

Participatory Action Research

Based on orientational qualitative inquiry, **participatory action research** (PAR) is also a method in which a goal is to change society. According to the tenets of PAR, all forms of knowledge, including indigenous knowledge, are of value and can be applied to practical problems. The researcher studies a particular setting to identify areas in which improvements in practice are needed (Glesne, 2011). After possible solutions are identified, action is taken to implement changes in partnership with the "stakeholders." Careful attention is given to evaluating the process to ensure that the changes have the desired effect.

PAR requires careful collaboration with the research participants and focuses on practical problems that are particular to a practice setting or community (Streubert & Carpenter, 2011). Stringer and Genat (2004) defined action research as

> a systematic, participatory approach to inquiry that enables people to extend their understanding of problems or issues and to formulate actions directed towards the resolution of those problems or issues . . . action research seeks local understandings that are specifically relevant to the particular context of a study. (p. 4)

Community-based participatory research (CBPR) is a method by which the voice of a community is systematically accessed in order to plan context-appropriate action. CBPR "provides an alternative to traditional research approaches that assume a phenomenon may be separated from its context for purposes of study. . . . CBPR recognizes the importance of involving members of a study population as active and equal participants, in all phases of the research project, if the research process is to be a means of facilitating change" (Holkup, Tripp-Reimer, Salois, & Weinert, 2004, p. 162). Change or action is the intended outcome of CBPR, and action research is a term related to CBPR. Some scholars would consider CBPR a sort of action research and would group both action research and CBPR within the tradition of critical science (Fontana, 2004).

Evidence-Informed Practice Tip ___

Although qualitative in its approach to research, CBPR leads to an action component in which a nursing intervention is implemented and evaluated for its effectiveness in a specific patient population.

In his book *Action Research,* Stringer (1999) distilled the research process into three phases: "look," "think," and "act." Stringer defined the "look" as "building the picture" by getting to know stakeholders so that the problem is defined on their terms and the problem definition is reflective of the community context. The "think" phase addresses interpretation and analysis of what was learned in the "look" phase; the researcher is charged with connecting the ideas of the stakeholders so that they provide evidence that is understandable to the community group (Stringer, 1999). Finally, in the "act" phase, Stringer advocated for planning, implementing, and evaluating, on the basis of information collected and interpreted in the other phases of research.

Identifying the Phenomenon

PAR evolved from the work of Lewin (1948), who viewed action research as a means for solving practical social problems and for enacting change for the improvement of communities. PAR is heavily used as a research methodology in education, and in the health professions, PAR methods are used to improve health care services in communities. PAR has been applied to health and wellness programs, program evaluation, care plans, community nursing, and health care delivery and policy. Studies have ranged from issues and conditions stemming from chronic illness, pregnancy and childbirth, pain management, and incontinence to rehabilitation (Stringer & Genat, 2004). For example, Fournier, Mill, Kipp, and Walusimbi (2007) were interested in the experiences of Ugandan nurses and their role in caring for people with acquired immune deficiency syndrome (AIDS). Their study is used in the following section to illustrate PAR.

Structuring the Study

RESEARCH QUESTION. The first step in structuring the PAR study, as in other qualitative methods, is to frame the research question and to identify who is affected by or has an effect on the problem. Because of the emergent nature of PAR, researchers can begin with a tentative problem and questions and then refine or reframe them as they enter the field. Recall the look-think-act cycle of Stringer and Genat (2004) described earlier. In the "look" phase, the researcher explores the problem by "asking who is involved, what is happening, and how, where and when events and activities occur" (p. 36). Reflecting on their observations, researchers, in collaboration with the stakeholders, can fine-tune the final research question, which serves as a guide to the study. As mentioned earlier, Fournier and colleagues (2007) explored the experiences of nurses from Uganda who cared for people with human immunodeficiency virus (HIV) infection and AIDS. As part of the research project, they worked with the participants to define their issues, suggest solutions, and act on them and then to reflect on the process and outcomes.

RESEARCHER'S PERSPECTIVE. When using PAR methods, the researcher is no longer the expert but acts more as a consultant. In their case study of pregnant Aboriginal women and parenting Aboriginal families, in which participatory methodology was used, Smith and colleagues (2006) stated, "participatory research views all forms of knowledge as valuable" (p. E21). The participants are co-researchers and are engaged in the research process as it emerges. This involvement requires processes that are democratic, participatory, empowering, and life-enhancing (Stringer & Genat, 2004). PAR investigators, like ethnographers, immerse themselves in the field for deep understanding and to build trust and credibility. For example, Fournier, a faculty lecturer from the University of Alberta, spent 5 months during two trips on site in Uganda (Fournier et al., 2007).

SAMPLE SELECTION. Because it is not possible to include everyone who may have a "stake" or interest in the research question, researchers purposively select a sample of participants who represent varied perspectives, experiences, and backgrounds. Participants may be people who have the widest range of differences in their experiences, particularly interesting backgrounds or experiences; those who are typical; and those with particular knowledge of the phenomenon under study. For example, Fournier and colleagues (2007) selected nurses who worked in a variety of health care units and regularly cared for people with AIDS.

Data Gathering

In the "look" phase, data are gathered from a variety of sources; interviews are the principal means for understanding the experiences of the participants. PAR also includes observation in the field, gathering and reviewing of relevant documents, and the examination of relevant materials and equipment. A literature review may add information to enhance the understanding of the data emerging from the interviews and other sources. Fournier and colleagues (2007) used the photovoice method in their work with nurses in Uganda. Photovoice, developed by Caroline Wang and Maryann Burris is

> a participatory health promotion strategy in which people use cameras to document their health and work realities. As participants engage in a group process of critical reflection, they may advocate for change in their communities by using the power of their images and stories to communicate with policy makers. In public health initiatives from China to California, community people have used photovoice to carry out participatory needs assessment, conduct participatory evaluation, and reach policy makers to improve community health. (Wang & Redwood-Jones, 2001)

The participants took pictures of what they considered to be nurses' work. During photovoice meetings, the nurses shared stories about their pictures. Viewing their work from behind the camera and sharing stories allowed the nurses to critically assess their work. They discovered that they were not working at their fullest potential because the hospital administration did not value their input or opinions.

Data Analysis

In the "think" phase, the researchers think about and reflect on all of the data gathered. The purpose of data analysis is to distill and reduce the volumes of information into a manageable and organized set of concepts or ideas. The process in PAR must directly capture the experiences of the participants and be distilled in such a way "that it makes sense to them all" (Stringer & Genat, 2004).

Stringer and Genat (2004) identified two approaches to analysis. The first, based on "epiphanic moments" (Denzin, 1998), focuses on the significant experiences as the primary units of analysis, giving voice to the participants' experiences. A second process involves the categorization and coding of data to reveal patterns and themes. Regardless of the process used, PAR allows the participants to make sense of their experience and then to use the new understanding to make a positive change.

In Fournier and colleagues' (2007) study, the nurses participated fully in the analysis. Each nurse reviewed the stories and developed themes independently. A leader was selected to moderate a group meeting to develop broader themes from the input of each nurse. Fournier, the principal investigator, spent an additional 2 months further analyzing the data with the next two authors of the study.

Describing the Findings

In accordance with Stringer and Genat's (2004) look-think-act framework, the next step is to present the outcomes to the participants and other nonparticipant stakeholders so that they understand what is happening. Several dissemination mechanisms may be used because formal academic writing is not accessible for most lay participants. The results may be shared in written reports, oral presentations, or performances. Written narrative accounts and storytelling are often used to describe the findings. The next and most important step is to apply the findings to solve the research problem or issue that instigated the study. This action portion of PAR parallels the nursing process of identification of goals and objectives, intervention, and, finally, evaluation.

The action plans should include the following (Stringer & Genat, 2004):

Why: A statement of the overall purpose

What: A set of objectives to be obtained

How: A sequence of tasks and steps for each objective

Who: The people responsible for each task and activity

Where: The place where the tasks will be done

When: The time for initiation and completion

The researcher should also arrange for ongoing evaluation of the process. As with the exploratory phase, stakeholders are intimately involved in each step of the action plan, from identifying the plan to implementing it. The participants in Fournier and colleagues' (2007) study indicated that one of their issues was inadequate knowledge about antiviral medications. This finding resulted in an unexpected outcome: the researchers determined that they would develop a research proposal. These nurses, who formed supportive and strong bonds, began to take leadership roles in the hospital, particularly in addressing ethical issues.

QUALITATIVE APPROACH: NURSING METHODOLOGY

The qualitative methodologies elaborated throughout this chapter are derived from other disciplines, such as sociology, anthropology, and philosophy. In the discipline of nursing, these methodologies are used to conduct research. However, as the discipline matures, methodology based on nursing ontology (belief system) emerges. Madeleine Leininger (1996), Rosemarie Rizzo Parse (1997), and Margaret Newman (1997) are nurse theorists who have created research methods specific to their theories. In Table 8-1, the methodologies of these theorists are compared. Each method was developed over years and tested by other researchers. Each researcher has attempted to advance nursing knowledge through inquiry that is congruent with the specific nursing theory.

In this section of the chapter, we have explored several different traditions and methods of qualitative research; however, many researchers are now combining a number of related or different methods to frame their naturalistic study. Remember that qualitative inquiry is evolving and changing. As Glesne (2011) noted, "The open, emergent nature of qualitative inquiry means a lack of standardization; there are no clear criteria to package into neat research steps" (p. 25). As you read more qualitative research studies, you will note many interesting designs, all amenable to exploring the complexity of the human experience.

TABLE **8-1**

NURSING RESEARCH METHODOLOGIES

ASPECT	LEININGER (1996)	PARSE (1997)	NEWMAN (1997)
Theory	Culture care	Human becoming	Health as expanding consciousness
Research methodology	Ethnonursing is centred on learning from people about their beliefs, experiences, and culture care information	Parse's research methodology is the study of universal health experiences through true presence both with participants sharing life stories and with transcribed data to uncover meaning	Newman's method focuses on pattern recognition and uses multiple interviews, involving collaboration, to arrive at recognized life patterns
Research example	Use of culture care theory with Anglo-American and African American older persons in a long-term care setting (McFarland, 1997)	The lived experience of serenity: using Parse's research method (Kruse, 1999)	Pattern of expanding consciousness in women in creative movement and narrative as modes of expression (Picard, 2000)

Smith and colleagues' (2006) study on pregnant Aboriginal women and parenting Aboriginal families, for example, combines a postcolonial standpoint, participatory research principles, and a case study design. Ford-Gilboe and associates (2005) applied a feminist perspective to their grounded theory on the basic social processes of health promotion among single-parent families recovering from intimate family violence.

In summary, the term *qualitative research* is an overriding description of multiple methods with distinct origins and procedures. In spite of distinctions, each method shares a common nature that guides data collection from the perspective of the participants to create a story that synthesizes disparate pieces of data into a comprehensible whole that provides evidence and promises direction for building nursing knowledge.

APPRAISING THE EVIDENCE

Qualitative Research

Although general criteria for critiquing qualitative research are proposed in the following Critiquing Criteria box, each qualitative method has unique characteristics that influence what you may expect in the published research report, and journals often have page restrictions that penalize qualitative researchers because it is difficult at times to fully explain all of the steps in Chapter 4 in a few pages. The criteria for critiquing are formatted to evaluate the selection of the phenomenon, the structure of the study, data gathering, data analysis, and description of the findings. Each question of the criteria focuses on factors discussed throughout the chapter. Appraising qualitative research is a useful activity for learning the nuances of this research approach. You are encouraged to identify a qualitative study of interest and apply the criteria for critiquing. Keep in mind that qualitative methods are the best way to start answering clinical and research questions that previously have not been addressed in research studies or that do not lend themselves to a quantitative approach. The answers provided by qualitative data reflect important evidence that may provide the first insights into a patient population or clinical phenomenon.

CRITIQUING CRITERIA

Qualitative Approaches

IDENTIFYING THE PHENOMENON

1. Is the phenomenon focused on human experience within a natural setting?
2. Is the phenomenon relevant to nursing or health, or both?

STRUCTURING THE STUDY

Research Question

3. Does the question specify a distinct process to be studied?
4. Does the question identify the context (participant group/place) of the process that will be studied?
5. Does the choice of a specific qualitative method fit with the research question?

Researcher's Perspective

6. Are the biases of the researchers reported?
7. Do the researchers provide a structure of ideas that reflect their beliefs?

Sample Selection

8. Is it clear that the selected sample is experiencing the phenomenon of interest?

DATA GATHERING

9. Are data sources and methods for gathering data specified?
10. Is there evidence that participant consent is an integral part of the data-gathering process?

DATA ANALYSIS

11. Can the dimensions of data analysis be identified and logically followed?
12. Is the participant's reality clearly described?
13. Is there evidence that the researcher's interpretation captured the participant's meaning?
14. Have other professionals confirmed the researcher's interpretation?

DESCRIBING THE FINDINGS

15. Are examples provided to guide the reader from the raw data to the researcher's synthesis?
16. Does the researcher link the findings to existing theory or literature, or is a new theory generated?

CRITICAL THINKING CHALLENGES

- How does the researcher select a specific type of qualitative research method to answer the research question?
- Do findings from qualitative research studies need to be validated in subsequent studies?
- How can a nurse researcher select a qualitative research method when he or she is attempting to accumulate evidence regarding a new topic about which little is known?
- How can the case study approach to research be applied to evidence-informed practice?

KEY POINTS

- Qualitative research is the investigation of human experiences in naturalistic settings, pursuing meanings that inform theory, practice, instrument development, and further research.
- Qualitative research studies are guided by research questions.
- Data saturation occurs when the information being shared with the researcher becomes repetitive.
- Qualitative research methods include five basic elements: identifying the phenomenon, structuring the study, gathering the data, analyzing the data, and describing the findings.
- The phenomenological method is a process of learning and constructing the meaning of human experience through intensive dialogue with persons who are living the experience.
- The grounded theory method is an inductive approach that implements a systematic set of procedures to arrive at theory about basic social processes.
- The ethnographic method focuses on scientific descriptions of cultural groups.
- The case study method focuses on a selected phenomenon over a short or long time to provide an in-depth description of its essential dimensions and processes.
- The historical research method is the systematic compilation of data and the critical presentation, appraisal, and interpretation of facts regarding people, events, and occurrences of the past.
- CBPR is a method that systematically accesses the voice of a community to plan context-appropriate action.

REFERENCES

Aamodt, A. A. (1991). Ethnography and epistemology: Generating nursing knowledge. In J. M. Morse (Ed.), *Qualitative nursing research: A contemporary dialogue* (pp. 29-40). Newbury Park, CA: Sage.

Agar, M. H. (1986). *Speaking of ethnography.* Beverly Hills, CA: Sage.

Aita, V. A., & McIlvain, H. E. (1999). An armchair adventure in case study research. In B. Crabtree & W. L. Miller (Eds.), *Doing qualitative research* (2nd ed., pp. 253-268). Thousand Oaks, CA: Sage.

Boyle, J. S. (1991). Field research: A collaborative model for practice and research. In J. M. Morse (Ed.), *Qualitative nursing research: A contemporary dialogue.* Newbury Park, CA: Sage.

Browne, A. J. (2000). The potential contribution of critical social theory to nursing science. *Canadian Journal of Nursing Research, 32*(2), 35-55.

Charmaz, K. (2000). Grounded theory: Objectivist and constructivist methods. In N. K. Denzin & Y. S. Lincoln (Eds.), *Handbook of qualitative research* (2nd ed., pp. 509-535). Thousand Oaks, CA: Sage.

Christy, T. E. (1975). The methodology of historical research: A brief introduction. *Nursing Research, 24*(3), 189-192.

Christy, T. E. (1981). The need for historical research in nursing. *Research in Nursing & Health, 4*(2), 227-228.

Cohen, M.Z. (1987). A historical overview of the phenomenological movement. *Imae, 19*(1), 31-34.

Cohen, M. Z., & Saunders, J. (1996). Using qualitative research in advanced practice. *Advanced Practice Nursing Quarterly, 2*(3), 8-13.

Colaizzi, P. (1978). Psychological research as a phenomenologist views it. In R. S. Valle & M. King (Eds.), *Existential phenomenological alternatives for psychology* (pp. 48-71). New York: Oxford University Press.

Corbin, J., & Strauss, A. (2008). *Basics of qualitative research.* Los Angeles: Sage.

Crabtree, B. F., & Miller, W. L. (1992). *Doing qualitative research.* Newbury Park, CA: Sage.

Creswell, J. W. (1998). *Qualitative inquiry and research design: Choosing among five traditions.* Thousand Oaks, CA: Sage.

Denzin, N. K. (1998). The practices and politics of interpretation. In N. K. Denzin & Y. S. Lincoln (Eds.), *Collecting and interpreting qualitative materials* (pp. 458-498). Thousand Oaks, CA: Sage.

Denzin, N. K., & Lincoln, Y. S. (1998). *The landscape of qualitative research.* Thousand Oaks, CA: Sage.

de Witt, L., Ploeg, J., & Black, M. (2010). Living along with dementia: An interpretative phenomenological study with older women. *Journal of Advanced Nursing, 66*(8), 1698-1707. doi: 10.1111/j.1365-2648.2010.05295.x.

Duffy, M. (2011). Narrative inquiry: The method. In P. Munhall (Ed.), *Nursing research: A qualitative perspective* (5th ed., pp. 421-440). Mississauga, ON: Jones & Bartlett Learning.

Fitzpatrick, J. J., & Wallace, M. (Eds.). (2006). *Encyclopedia of nursing research* (2nd ed.). New York: Springer.

Fontana, J. S. (2004). A methodology for critical science in nursing. *Advances in Nursing Science, 27*, 93-101.

Ford-Gilboe, M., Wuest, J., & Merritt-Gray, M. (2005). Strengthening capacity to limit intrusion: Theorizing family health promotion in the aftermath of woman abuse. *Qualitative Health Research, 15*, 477-601.

Fournier, B., Mill, J., Kipp, W., & Walusimbi, M. (2007). Discovering voice: A participatory action research study with nurses in Uganda. *International Journal of Qualitative Methods, 6*(2). Retrieved from http://www.ualberta.ca/~iiqm/backissues/6_2/fournier.htm.

Giorgi, A., Fischer, C. L., & Murray, E. L. (Eds.). (1975). *Duquesne studies in phenomenological psychology*. Pittsburgh: Duquesne University Press.

Glaser, B., & Strauss, A. (1965). *Awareness of dying*. Chicago: Aldine de Gruyter.

Glaser, B. G., & Strauss, A. L. (1967). *The discovery of grounded theory: Strategies for qualitative research*. Chicago: Aldine.

Glesne, C. (2011). *Becoming qualitative researchers: An introduction* (4th ed.). Toronto: Pearson.

Holkup, P. A., Tripp-Reimer, T., Salois, E. M., & Weinert, C. (2004). Community-based participatory research: An approach to intervention research with a Native American community. *Advances in Nursing Science, 27*, 162-175.

Holmes, D., O'Byrne, P., & Gastaldo, D. (2006). Raw pleasure as limit experience: A Foucauldian analysis of unsafe anal sex between men. *Social Theory and Health, 4*, 319-333.

Holmes, D., O'Byrne, P., & Gastaldo, D. (2007). Setting the space for sex: Architecture, desire and health issues in gay bathhouses. *International Journal of Nursing Studies, 44*(2), 273-284.

Kleinman, A. (1980). *Patients and healers in the context of culture*. Berkeley: University of California Press.

Kleinman, A. (1992). Local worlds of suffering: An interpersonal focus for ethnographies of illness experience. *Qualitative Health Research, 2*, 127-134.

Kruse, B.G. (1999). The lived experience of serenity: Using Parse's research method. *Nursing Science Quarterly, 12*, 143-150.

Lapum, J., Angus, J. E., Peter, E., & Watt-Watson, J. (2010). Patients' narrative accounts of open-heart surgery and recovery: Authorial voice of technology. *Social Science & Medicine, 70*, 754-762. doi: 10.1016/j.socsimed.2009.11.021

Leininger, M. (1985). Life-health-care history: Purposes, methods and techniques. In M. M. Leininger (Ed.), *Qualitative research methods in nursing* (pp. 119-132). New York: Grune & Stratton.

Leininger, M. M. (1996). Culture care theory. *Nursing Science Quarterly, 9*, 71-78.

Leininger, M. M. (2006). *Culture care, diversity and universality: A worldwide nursing theory* (2nd ed). Mississauga, ON: Jones & Bartlett.

Lewin, K. (1948). *Resolving social conflicts*. New York: Harper.

Lindsay, G. (2006). Constructing a nursing identity: Reflecting on and reconstructing experience. *Reflective Practice, 7*, 59-72.

Lundy, K. S. (2011). Historical research. In P. Munhall (Ed.), *Nursing research: A qualitative perspective* (5th ed., pp. 381-397). Mississauga, ON: Jones & Bartlett Learning.

Lusk, B. (1997). Historical methodology for nursing research. *Image, 29*, 355-359.

Macquire, P. (1996). Considering more feminine participatory research: What's congruency got to do with it? *Qualitative Inquiry, 2*, 106-118.

Maddalena, V. J., Bernard, W. T., Etowa, J., Murdoch, S. D., Smith, D., & Jarvis, P. M. (2010). Cancer care experiences and the use of complementary and alternative medicine at the end of life in Nova Scotia's black communities. *Journal of Transcultural Nursing, 21*(2), 114-122. doi: 10.1177/1043659609357634

McDonald, C. (2006) Lesbian disclosure: Disrupting the taken for granted. *Canadian Journal of Nursing Research, 38*, 42-57.

McFarland, M.R. (1997). Use of culture care theory with Anglo and African American elders in long-term care settings. *Nursing Science Quarterly, 10*, 186-192.

Mead, M. (1949). *Coming of age in Samoa*. New York: New American Library/Mentor Books. (Original work published 1928).

Newman, M. A. (1997). Evolution of the theory of health as expanding consciousness. *Nursing Science Quarterly, 10*, 22-25.

Nightingale, F. (1969). *Notes on nursing: What it is and what it is not.* New York: Dover. (Original work published 1858).

Parse, R. R. (1997). Transforming research and practice with the human becoming theory. *Nursing Science Quarterly, 10,* 171-174.

Parse, R. R., Coyne, A. B., & Smith, M. J. (1985). *Nursing research: Qualitative and quantitative methods.* Bowie, MD: Brady.

Parsons, S. (1911). The case method of teaching nursing. *American Journal of Nursing, 11,* 1009-1011.

Patton, M. (2002). *Qualitative research & evaluation methods* (3rd ed.). Thousand Oaks, CA: Sage.

Pesut, B., & Reimer-Kirkham, S. (2010). Situated clinical encounters in the negotiations of religious and spiritual plurality: A critical ethnography. *International Journal of Nursing Studies, 47,* 815-825. doi: 10.1016/j.ijnurstu.2009.11.014.

Picard, C. (2000). Patterns of expanding consciousness in midlife women: Creative movement and narrative as modes of expression. *Nursing Science Quarterly, 13,* 150-157.

Reeves, S., Macmillan, K., & van Soeren, M. (2010). Leadership of interprofessional health and social care teams: A socio-historical analysis. *Journal of Nursing Management, 18,* 258-264. doi: 10.1111/j.1365-2834.2010.01077.x

Roberts, T. (2009). Understanding ethnography. *British Journal of Midwifery, 17*(5), 291-294.

Roper, J., & Shapira, J. (2000). *Ethnography in nursing research.* Thousand Oaks, CA: Sage.

Sandelowski, M. (2004). Using qualitative research. *Qualitative Health Research, 14,* 1366-1386.

Sandelowski, M., & Barroso, J. (2007). *Handbook for synthesizing qualitative research.* Philadelphia: Springer.

Schrieber, R., & MacDonald, M. (2010). Keeping vigil over the patient: A grounded theory of nurse anaethesia practice. *Journal of Advanced Nursing, 66*(3), 552-561. doi: 10.1111/j.1365-2648.2009.05207.x

Scotch, N. (1963). Medical anthropology. *Biennial Review of Anthropology, 3,* 30-68.

Seneviratne, C. C., Mather, C. M., & Then, K. L. (2009). Understanding nursing on an acute stroke unit: Perceptions of space, time and interprofessional practice. *Journal of Advanced Nursing, 65*(9), 1872-1881. doi: 10.1111/j.1365-2648.2009.05053.x

Smith, D., Edwards, N., Varcoe, C., Martens, P. J., & Davies, B. (2006). Bringing safety and responsiveness into the forefront of care for pregnant and parenting Aboriginal people. *Advances in Nursing Science, 29*(2), E27-E44.

Spiegelberg, H. (1976). *The phenomenological movement* (Vols. I and II). The Hague: Martinus Nijhoff.

Spradley, J. P. (1979). *The ethnographic interview.* New York: Holt, Rinehart, & Winston.

Stake, R. E. (1995). *The art of case study research.* Thousand Oaks, CA: Sage.

Stake, R. E. (2003). Case studies. In N. K. Denzin & Y. S. Lincoln (Eds.), *Strategies of qualitative inquiry* (2nd ed., pp. 134-164). Thousand Oaks, CA: Sage.

Strauss, A., & Corbin, J. (1990). *Basics of qualitative research: Grounded theory procedures and techniques.* Newbury Park, CA: Sage.

Strauss, A. L. (1987). *Qualitative analysis for social scientists.* New York: Cambridge University Press.

Streubert, H. J., & Carpenter, D. R. (2011). *Qualitative research in nursing: Advancing the humanistic imperative* (5th ed.). Philadelphia: Wolters Kluwer.

Stringer, E. T. (1999). *Action research* (2nd ed.). Thousand Oaks, CA: Sage.

Stringer, E. T., & Genat, W. J. (2004). *Action research in health.* Thousand Oaks, CA: Sage.

Usher, P. (1996). Feminist approaches to research. In D. Scott & R. Usher (Eds.), *Understanding educational research* (pp. 120-143). New York: Routledge.

van Kaam, A. (1969). *Existential foundations in psychology.* New York: Doubleday.

van Manen, M. (1997). *Researching lived experience: Human science for an action sensitive pedagogy* (2nd ed.). London, ON: Althouse Press.

Wang, C. & Redwood-Jones, Y. (2001). Photovoice Ethics: Perspective from Flint Photovoice. Retrieved from http://www.photovoice.org. *Health Education Behaviour, 28* (5), 560-572 doi: 10.1177/109019810102800504

Wuest, J. (2011). Grounded theory: The method. In P. Munhall (Ed.), *Nursing research: A qualitative perspective* (5th ed., pp. 225-256). Mississauga, ON: Jones & Bartlett Learning.

Yin, R. (1994). *Case study research: Design and methods* (2nd ed.). Thousand Oaks, CA: Sage.

Zerr, S. J., Zilm, G., & Grant, V. (2006). *Labor of love. A memoir of Gertrude Richards Ladner, 1879 to 1976.* Delta, BC: ZGZ.

FOR FURTHER STUDY

℮volve   Go to Evolve at http://evolve.elsevier.com/Canada/LoBiondo/Research for Audio Glossary, how-to instructions for Writing Proposals for Funding, and additional research articles for practice in reviewing and critiquing.

Quantitative Research

RESEARCH **VIGNETTE**

Tackling the Prevention of Falls Among Older Adults

Nancy C. Edwards, RN, BScN, MSc, PhD
Full Professor
Department of Epidemiology and
    Community Medicine
School of Nursing
University of Ottawa
Ottawa, Ontario

In the late 1980s, while working as a clinical nurse consultant at the Ottawa Public Health Department, I was asked to assist with a needs assessment of older adults living in low-income apartment buildings in Ottawa. The survey covered a wide range of topics, and at the last minute, the public health nurses decided to add a few questions about older adults' experiences with falls. The findings were startling: They revealed a high incidence of falls and injuries. Published epidemiological studies indicated that our findings were not spurious. Indeed, one third of all older adults fall annually, and approximately 25% of falls result in some sort of injury.

Soon after this survey was conducted, our then medical officer of health, Dr. Steve Corber, spoke to me about the possibility of setting up and evaluating a fall prevention initiative. Dr. Corber suggested that preventing falls should become a program focus within the health department. I was working with a senior nursing manager, Maureen Murphy, at the time, and we were interested in a more theoretical question: the relative contribution of self-care versus collective action initiatives to promote health. However, we decided to meld these two interests, and a randomized controlled trial was born!

With funding from the Ontario Ministry of Health and Long-Term Care, we compared the effect of fall prevention clinics and a community action strategy on the incidence of falls among older adults living in 48 apartment buildings. I worked closely with the fall prevention team as we piloted and implemented the two interventions. Although we did not detect a change in the rate of falls, we did note improvements in some behavioural outcomes for fall prevention among older adults in the community action buildings in comparison with the control buildings.

Many important issues surfaced during this trial and have become the basis of nearly a decade's worth of research. In particular, we became interested in the role of the built environment in falls. In some of our study buildings, older adults who had difficulties getting into and out of the bathtub described their failed efforts to persuade landlords to have grab bars installed. Landlords were refusing them permission because the installation of grab bars was thought to "lower property values." In essence, aesthetics trumped safety.

Several qualitative and quantitative studies ensued. Older adults described the embarrassment of using grab bars and other assistive devices. A survey of older adults in apartment buildings with and without universally installed grab bars identified barriers to access of grab bars. A comparison of low-income and public apartment buildings with private apartment buildings indicated that older adults living in low-income buildings were much more likely to have access to grab bars than were older adults living in private buildings.

Concerns about bathroom grab bars and safe stairs became a focus for our regional fall prevention coalition. We began to consider what research was necessary to inform changes to building codes in Canada. It became apparent that, to complement our community-based studies, we needed the expertise of researchers who were able to design and conduct laboratory studies to determine what grab bar configurations are optimal to assist transfers into and out of a bathtub.

From both the laboratory and the community studies, we were able to identify the configuration of grab bars that older adults find easiest to use. We determined that older adults are 2.8 times more likely to use universally installed grab bars consistently, in comparison with grab bars they had installed themselves, after other factors were adjusted. We also documented both the high proportion of falls in bathrooms and on stairs and the high rates of injury that result from these falls, in relation to falls occurring in other locations.

In a subsequent community study funded by the Canadian Institutes of Health Research, we identified stair hazards prevalent in private homes and public buildings. Older adults were asked to identify the most common locations of hazardous stairs. Churches and community centres were among the locations most frequently identified. Independent raters also assessed indoor and outdoor stairs, both those identified by older adults as hazardous in the community and the stairs that the raters used in their own homes or apartment buildings. The most common hazards were the lack of contrast marking on the edge of the stairs, inadequate tread length, risers that were too high, and nonuniform risers. Although older adults were able to identify hazardous stairs they had difficulty navigating, fewer than 25% of them had specific suggestions for ways to improve stair safety.

Our research findings on bathroom and stair falls are now being used to inform policy change. For example, I submitted a request to the National Research Council for an additional requirement to the building codes for the universal installation of grab bars in showers and bathtubs in all residential homes. Included with the submission was an estimate of the costs of such a requirement and the cost savings that would be incurred. These estimates are an important consideration for committee members who review code change requests. I have also been a member of several National Research Council task groups and subgroups reviewing potential code changes for stairs, handrails, ramps, and guards. Our research on stair falls is being reviewed as part of the evidence for changes to the building codes in the current cycle of building code changes.

Bridging the interface between research and policy is a critical knowledge translation strategy. Informing and influencing policy change require the engagement of an informed public, which led us to establish a networking infrastructure called CHNET-Works (http://www.chnet-works.ca). Using teleconference lines, conferencing software (Bridgit), and the support of a network animateur, we host weekly "fireside chats" for 9 months of the year. Our aim is to bring together academic researchers, front-line practitioners and managers, policymakers, and colleagues from the volunteer sector to address common issues. Participants consider how evidence might inform intersectoral practices and policies and how activities in the field and in policy arenas might inform research. We held a series of fireside chats on fall prevention and related changes to the building codes. An outcome of these chats was a series of resolutions on evidence-informed changes to building codes that pertain to bathtub grab bars and safe stairs. These resolutions were submitted for the consideration of various professional associations.

Our work on preventing falls has reinforced the importance of the role of interdisciplinary research in the design of community health interventions. Substantial health care changes in populations such as older adults will come about only through long-term research and policy change efforts. "Quick fixes" are rare. As a researcher, I need to be prepared to work actively with colleagues at the local, provincial, and national levels and to use a wide repertoire of knowledge translation strategies. ■

CHAPTER 9

Introduction to Quantitative Research

Geri LoBiondo-Wood | Mina D. Singh

LEARNING OUTCOMES

After reading this chapter, you will be able to do the following:

- Define research design.
- Identify the purpose of the research design.
- Define control as it affects the research design.
- Compare and contrast the elements that affect control.
- Begin to evaluate the degree of control that should be exercised in the design.
- Define internal validity.
- Identify the threats to internal validity.
- Define external validity.
- Identify the conditions that affect external validity.
- Identify the links between study design and evidence-informed practice.
- Evaluate the design by using the critiquing questions.

KEY TERMS

accuracy	feasibility	mortality
attrition	Hawthorne effect	objectivity
bias	history threat	pilot study
constancy	homogeneity	randomization
control	instrumentation threats	reactivity
control group	internal validity	selection bias
experimental group	maturation	selection effects
external validity	measurement effects	testing effect
extraneous variable		

STUDY RESOURCES

Go to Evolve at http://evolve.elsevier.com/Canada/LoBiondo/Research for Audio Glossary, how-to instructions for Writing Proposals for Funding, and additional research articles for practice in reviewing and critiquing.

THE WORD *DESIGN* IMPLIES THE ORGANIZATION of elements into a masterful work of art. In the world of art and fashion, the word conjures up images of processes and techniques that are used to express a total concept. When an individual creates, process and form are employed. The form, process, and degree of adherence to structure depend on the aims of the creator.

The same can be said of the research process. The research process does not need to be a sterile procedure, but it should be one in which the researcher develops a masterful work within the limits of a problem and the related theoretical basis. The framework that the researcher creates is the design. When reading a study, the research consumer should be able to recognize that the research problem, purpose, literature review, theoretical framework, and hypothesis all interrelate with, complement, and assist in the operationalization of the design (Figure 9-1). The degree to which a fit exists between these design elements determines the strength of the study and of the consumer's confidence in the evidence provided by the findings and their potential applicability to practice.

Nursing practice is concerned with a variety of activities that require varying degrees of process and form, such as the provision of quality care, cost-effective patient care, responses of patients to disease, and factors that affect caregivers. When nurses administer patient care, they draw on the nursing process. Previous chapters stressed the importance of theory and knowledge of subject matter to research. How a researcher structures, implements, or designs a study affects the results of a research project.

To grasp the implications and the use of research, you need to understand the central issues in the design of a research project. This chapter provides an overview of the meaning, purpose, and issues related to quantitative research design. Chapters 10 and 11 discuss specific types of quantitative designs.

PURPOSE OF THE RESEARCH DESIGN

The purpose of the research design is to provide the plan for answering research questions. These questions can result in research driven by a researcher's curiosity or interest in a theoretical question. This process is called *basic research,* and its motivation is to expand nursing knowledge. In contrast, applied research is designed to solve clinical problems rather than to acquire knowledge for knowledge's sake; thus, the goal is to improve the patient's health care condition.

The design in quantitative research then becomes the vehicle for hypothesis testing or answering research questions, whether they are basic or applied. The design involves a *plan,* a *structure,* and a *strategy.* These three design concepts guide a researcher in writing the hypothesis or research questions, conducting the project, and analyzing and evaluating the data. The overall purpose of the research design is twofold: to aid in the solution of research problems and to maintain control (see Practical Application box). All

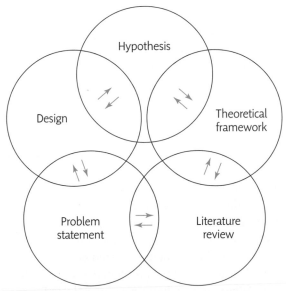

FIGURE 9-1   Interrelationships of design, problem statement, literature review, theoretical framework, and hypothesis.

research is an attempt to answer questions. The design, coupled with the methods and analysis, is the mechanism for finding solutions to research questions. **Control** is defined as the measures that the researcher uses to hold the conditions of the study uniform and avoid possible impingement of **bias** (distortion of the results) on the dependent variable or outcome.

> ### Practical Application
> A research example that demonstrates how the design can aid in answering a research question and maintain control is the study by Ireland and colleagues (2010). The main purpose of their study was to examine the extent to which selected demographic, social-psychological, physiological, and adherence characteristics were predictive of achievement of blood pressure and glucose targets in a group of patients referred to a stroke prevention clinic with either confirmed transient ischemic attack (TIA) or confirmed stroke and with hypertension or diabetes or both. To maintain control, the researchers had strict sample characteristics. Inclusion criteria were as follows: (1) TIA or stroke plus a documented history of hypertension, diabetes, or both; (2) age older than 18 years; (3) ability to speak English; and (4) ability to independently provide admission information to a clinic registration clerk. Exclusion criteria were as follows: severe hearing or visual impairment, severe aphasia, and confusion. By establishing the specific sample criteria and participant eligibility, the researchers were able to maintain control over the study's conditions and suggest an extension of the study's outcome with further research.

Various considerations, including the type of design, affect the accomplishment of the study. These considerations include **objectivity**—the use of facts without distortion by personal feelings or bias—in the conceptualization of the problem; accuracy; feasibility; control of the experiment; internal validity; and external validity. Statistical principles underlie the many forms of control, but it is more important that the research consumer have a clear conceptual understanding of statistics and how they inform the research questions.

The type of design used in a study also affects its application to practice. Chapters 10 and 11 present a number of experimental, quasiexperimental, and nonexperimental designs. The type of design used in a study is linked to the level of evidence, and, in turn, the contribution of a study's findings is linked to evidence-informed practice. As discussed in Chapter 1, the term *evidence-informed practice* is currently being used instead of *evidence-based practice* because it is more inclusive in that it encompasses many forms of evidence such as clinical experience and judgement with research utilization. As you critically appraise the design, take into account other aspects of a study's design, which are reviewed in this chapter.

OBJECTIVITY IN THE CONCEPTUALIZATION OF THE PROBLEM

In the conceptualization of the problem, objectivity is derived from a review of the literature and development of a theoretical framework (see Figure 9-1). Using the literature, the researcher assesses the depth and breadth of available knowledge about the problem. The literature review and theoretical framework should show that the researcher reviewed the literature critically and objectively (see Chapters 2 and 5) because this conceptualization of the problem affects the type of design chosen. For example, for a question about the relationship of the length of a breast-feeding education program, either an experimental or a correlational design may be recommended (see Chapters 10 and 11), whereas for a question regarding the physical changes in a woman's body during pregnancy and the maternal perception of the unborn child, a survey or correlation study may be advised (see Chapter 11). The literature review should reflect the following:

- When the problem was studied
- The aspects of the problem that were studied
- Where the problem was investigated
- By whom the problem was investigated
- The gaps or inconsistencies in the literature

ACCURACY

Accuracy in determining the appropriate design is also accomplished through the theoretical framework and review of the literature (see Chapters 2 and 5). **Accuracy** means that all aspects of a study systematically and logically follow from the research problem. The beginning researcher is wise to answer a question involving few variables that does not require the use of sophisticated designs. The simplicity of a research project does not render it useless or of a lesser value for practice. However, although the project is simple, the researcher should not forgo accuracy. The consumer should believe that the researcher chose a design that was consistent with the research problem and offered the maximum amount of control.

Many clinical problems have not yet been researched, so a preliminary, or pilot, study is a wise approach to testing the accuracy of a study design before a larger study is undertaken. A **pilot study** is a small, simple study conducted as a prelude to a larger study. The key is the accuracy, validity, and objectivity used by the researcher in attempting to answer the question. Accordingly, you should read various types of research reports and assess whether and how the criteria for each step of the research process were followed. Many nursing journals publish not only sophisticated clinical research projects but also smaller clinical studies whose results can be applied to practice.

FEASIBILITY

When you, as a consumer of research, critique the study design, you must also be aware of the pragmatic consideration of feasibility. **Feasibility** is the capability of the study to be successfully carried out. Sometimes, the reality of feasibility does not truly sink in until the researcher begins the study. When you review a study, you should consider feasibility, including availability of the participants, timing of the research, time required for the participants to take part in the study, costs, and analysis of the data (Table 9-1). Studies in which researchers are testing feasibility are also called *pilot studies* (see Practical Application box).

An example of a feasibility study is that conducted by McGilton and associates (2011), who examined the feasibility of a "patient care communication intervention." Before conducting a larger multicentre study, they wanted to know more about how staff perceptions of the intervention affected the implementation of the intervention. In addition, the researchers explored changes in patients' perceptions of care and psychosocial functioning and explored changes in nurses' knowledge of and attitude toward communication with patients. The results indicated that the nurses adhered to the intervention and the response rate was high.

Before a large experimental study (such as a randomized clinical trial) is conducted, it is helpful to first conduct a pilot study with a small number of participants to determine the feasibility of participant recruitment, the intervention, the data-collection protocol, the likelihood that participants

TABLE 9-1

PRAGMATIC CONSIDERATIONS IN DETERMINING THE FEASIBILITY OF A RESEARCH PROBLEM

FACTOR	PRAGMATIC CONSIDERATION
Time	The research problem must be able to be studied within a realistic period of time. All researchers have deadlines for completion of a project. The scope of the problem must be circumscribed enough to provide ample time for the completion of the entire project. Research studies generally take longer than anticipated to complete.
Participant availability	The researcher must determine whether a sufficient number of eligible participants will be available and willing to take part in the study. If a researcher has a "captive" audience (e.g., students in a classroom), it may be relatively easy to enlist their cooperation. When a study involves the participants' independent time and effort, they may be unwilling to participate when they will receive no apparent reward for doing so. Other potential participants may have fears about harm or confidentiality and be suspicious of the research process in general. Participants with unusual characteristics, such as rare diseases, are often difficult to locate. People are generally cooperative about taking part in a study, but a researcher must consider needing a larger participant pool than will actually participate. At times, when reading a research report, the researcher may note how the procedures were liberalized or the number of participants was altered— probably as a result of some unforeseen pragmatic consideration.
Facility and equipment availability	All research projects require some kind of equipment, such as questionnaires, telephones, stationery, stamps, technical equipment, or another apparatus. Most research projects also require the availability of a facility for the work, such as a hospital site for data collection, a laboratory space, or a computer centre for data analysis.
Money	Many research projects require some expenditure of money. Before embarking on a study, the researcher probably itemized the expenses and estimated the total cost of the project. This estimation of cost provides a clear picture of the budgetary needs for items such as books, stationery, postage, printing, technical equipment, telephone and computer charges, and salaries. These expenses can range from about $200 for a small-scale student project to hundreds of thousands of dollars for a large-scale federally funded project.
Researcher experience	The selection of the research problem should be based on the nurse's experience and interest. It is much easier to develop a research study related to a topic that is either theoretically or experientially familiar. Selecting a problem that is of interest to the researcher is essential for maintaining enthusiasm when the inevitable successes and failures occur.
Ethics	Research problems that place unethical demands on participants are not feasible for study. Researchers must take ethical considerations seriously. The consideration of ethics may affect the choice of the design and the methodology.

will complete the study, the reliability and validity of new measurement tools, and the costs of the study. Such a pilot study was conducted by Hayward and colleagues (2007), who investigated the feasibility of data collection (on the effects of co-bedding twins on parental self-efficacy) before beginning a larger multicentre study. The results were used to estimate effect size and the organization of staff and bedside care, evaluate the feasibility of data-collection measures, and identify issues related to recruitment and follow-up. Hayward and colleagues made revisions to the inclusion criteria: that is, they used infants' gestational age rather than weight. They found that blinding the data-collection procedure would strengthen the larger study. Redundancy in data collection was removed. The rate of response to the parental questionnaire was poor at 1 month; this led to adjustments in the follow-up study, in which a small compensation was mailed with the questionnaire and the research nurse conducted the 1-month discharge follow-up by phone interview.

These pragmatic considerations are not presented as a step in the research process, as are the theoretical framework and methods, but they do affect every step of the process and therefore should be considered when you assess a study. For example, the student researcher may or may not have monies or accessible services. When you critique a study, note the credentials of the author or authors and whether the investigation was part of either a student project or a fully funded grant project. If the project was a student project, the standards of critiquing are applied more liberally than for projects conducted by an experienced researcher or clinician with a doctoral degree. Finally, the pragmatic issues raised affect the scope and breadth of an investigation and therefore its generalizability.

CONTROL

A researcher attempts to use a design to maximize the degree of control over the tested variables. Control involves holding the conditions of the study constant and establishing specific sampling criteria, as described by Sobieraj and colleagues (2009; see Appendix C). An efficient design can maximize results, decrease errors, and control preexisting conditions that may affect outcome. To accomplish these tasks, the research design and methods should demonstrate the researcher's efforts at control.

For example, to test their hypothesis and apply control, Sobieraj and colleagues (2009) calculated a sample size (see Chapter 12) of a minimum of 25 participants per group. Thirty participants were recruited to compensate for those who dropped out. The intervention was controlled by asking the participants to demonstrate their massage technique to ensure proper administration. A registered nurse with a master's degree performed all of the teaching and demonstrations to avoid variance in the intervention from multiple teachers.

An efficient design can maximize results, decrease errors, and control preexisting conditions that may affect outcomes. To accomplish these tasks, the research design and methods should demonstrate the researcher's efforts at control, which is important in all designs. When various research designs are critiqued, the issue of control is always raised but with varying levels of flexibility. The issues discussed here will become clearer as you review the various types of designs.

Control is accomplished by ruling out extraneous variables that compete with the independent variables as an explanation for a study's outcome. An **extraneous variable** (also called a *mediating variable*) interferes with the operations of the phenomena being studied (e.g., age and gender). Means of controlling extraneous variables include the following:

- Use of a homogeneous sample
- Use of consistent data-collection procedures
- Manipulation of the independent variable
- Randomization

An investigator might be interested in how a new smoking cessation program (independent variable) affects smoking behaviour (dependent variable). The independent variable is assumed to affect the outcome or dependent variable. An investigator needs to be relatively sure that the decrease in smoking is truly related to the smoking cessation program rather than to another variable, such as motivation.

The following example illustrates and defines these concepts further. Ploeg and associates (2010) evaluated the effect of an intervention involving a provider-initiated primary care outreach program in comparison with usual care among older adults at risk of functional decline. To rule out the effects of extraneous variables on the quality of life (dependent variable) among the older adults, demographic information was collected, including gender, marital status, level of education, household income, whether the participant was living alone, and scores on the minimental state examination (MMSE). Although the design of the research study alone does not inherently provide control, an appropriately designed study with the necessary controls can increase an investigator's ability to answer a research question.

Evidence-Informed Practice Tip ____

As you read a report, assess whether the study includes a tested intervention and whether the report contains a clear description of the intervention and how it was controlled. If the details are not clear, the intervention may have been administered differently among the participants, which would affect the interpretation of the results.

Homogeneous Sampling

In the example of smoking cessation, extraneous variables may affect the dependent variable. The characteristics of a study's participants are common extraneous variables. Age, gender, length of time smoked, amount smoked, and even smoking rules may affect the outcome in the smoking cessation example, even though they are extraneous or outside the study's design. As a control for these and other similar problems, the researcher's participants should demonstrate **homogeneity,** or similarity with regard to the extraneous variables relevant to the particular study (see Chapter 13). Extraneous variables are not fixed but must be reviewed, and their inclusion in the analyses is based on the study's purpose and theoretical base. By using a sample of homogeneous participants, the researcher has used a straightforward step of control.

For example, Ploeg and associates (2010) ensured the homogeneity of the sample by using the following sampling criteria: Participants were aged 75 years or older, they or their proxy were able to answer questions in English, and they lived in Hamilton, Ontario. The sample was therefore homogeneous with regard to age, language, and location of home. This control step limits the generalizability or application of the outcomes to other populations when the outcomes are analyzed and discussed (see Chapter 17). The results can then be generalized only to a similar population of individuals. Homogeneity could be considered limiting, but not necessarily because no treatment or program is applicable to all populations, and educated consumers of research must take into consideration the differences in populations.

Helpful Hint_____

When reviewing studies, remember that it is better to have a "clean" study, whose results can be used to make generalizations about a specific population, than a "messy" study, whose results may be poorly or not at all generalizable.

If the researcher believes that one of the extraneous variables is important, it may be included in the design. In the smoking cessation example, if individuals are working in an area where smoking is not allowed and this condition is considered to be important to the study, the researcher could account for it in the design and set up a control condition for it. This condition can be established by comparing two different work areas: one where smoking is allowed and one where it is not. Of importance is that before the data are collected, the researcher should have identified, planned for, and controlled the important extraneous variables.

Constancy in Data Collection

Another basic but critical component of control is constancy in data-collection procedures. **Constancy** refers to the ability of the data-collection design to hold the conditions of the study to a cookbook-like recipe. In other words, for the purpose of collecting data for the study, each participant is exposed to the same environmental conditions, timing of data collection, data-collection instruments, and data-collection procedures (see Chapter 13).

An example of constancy in data collection is illustrated in the study by Doran and associates (2006). The objective of this study was to explore which nursing interventions provided during hospitalization are associated with patients' therapeutic self-care and functional health outcomes. Nurses collected data on patient outcomes using the Minimum Data Set and the Therapeutic Self-Care Scale. Chart audits were conducted by research assistants. Constancy was attained by training the research assistants in a half-day session with a prescribed protocol, which included an introduction to the nursing intervention audit tool, instruction in the operational definition of each nursing intervention item, and the opportunity to conduct a chart audit with feedback. The audit of a research team member was used as the standard against which the research assistants' chart audits were compared. This type of control aided the investigators' ability to draw conclusions, discuss the findings, and cite the need for further research in this area. For the consumer, constancy demonstrates a clear, consistent, and specific means of data collection.

When psychosocial interventions are implemented, researchers often describe the training of interventionists or data collectors that took place to ensure constancy. In a study by Kilty and Prentice (2010) on the outcomes of a school nurse referral to a family physician for adolescents identified with elevated cholesterol or blood pressure risk factors, interviews were conducted by research assistants. Training was done to ensure that the data collection, recording, and management methods were consistent and that completed forms were reviewed for quality assurance.

Manipulation of the Independent Variable

A third means of control is manipulation of the independent variable. *Manipulation* refers to the administration of a program, treatment, or inter-

vention to only one group within the study but not to the other participants in the study. The first group is known as the **experimental group,** and the other group is known as the **control group,** or comparison group. In a control group, the variables under study are held at a constant or comparison level. For example, Sinclair and Ferguson (2009) examined whether combining classroom learning with simulated learning activities would increase self-efficacy in nursing practice. The experimental group received the intervention, whereas the control group received the standard 2 hours of lectures per week.

Experimental and quasiexperimental designs involve manipulation, whereas in nonexperimental designs, the independent variable is not manipulated. This lack of manipulation does not decrease the usefulness of a nonexperimental design, but the use of a control group in an experimental or quasiexperimental design is related to the research question and, again, its theoretical framework.

Blinding is a technique used in experimental and quasiexperimental research in which the participants are not aware of whether they are receiving the intervention. Double blinding is a technique in which both the researchers and the participants are not aware of who is receiving the intervention and who is in the control group. For example, Newby and colleagues (2009) tested the feasibility of using topical tetracaine, in comparison with a placebo, to reduce the pain of intramuscular immunization injections in infants. The administration was video-recorded, and a paediatric nurse assessed the level of pain by watching the videos. This nurse was "blind" as to which infant received the tetracaine or placebo.

Helpful Hint

Be aware that the lack of manipulation of the independent variable does not mean that the study is weaker. The level of the problem, the amount of theoretical work, and the research that has preceded the project affect the researcher's choice of the design. If the problem is amenable to a design in which the independent variable can be manipulated, the power of a researcher to draw conclusions will increase, provided that all of the considerations of control are equally addressed.

Randomization

Researchers may also choose other forms of control, such as randomization. **Randomization** is a sampling selection procedure in which each participant in a population has an equal chance of being assigned to either the experimental group or the control group. Randomization eliminates bias, aids in the attainment of a representative sample, and can be used in various designs. Johnston and associates (2010) examined whether the use of iPod technology in medical-surgical nursing courses would have an effect on grades. Some students had their own iPod. Students without their own iPod were randomly assigned to one of three experimental groups or to the control group.

Randomization can also be accomplished with paper-and-pencil-type instruments. By randomly ordering items on the instruments, the investigator can assess whether a difference in responses is correlated with the order of the items. Randomization may be especially important in longitudinal studies, in which bias from giving the same instrument to the same participants on a number of occasions can be a problem (see Chapter 12).

QUANTITATIVE CONTROL AND FLEXIBILITY

The same level of control cannot be exercised in all types of designs. At times, when a researcher wants to explore an area in which little or no literature on the concept exists, the researcher will probably use an exploratory design. In this type of study, the researcher is interested in describing or categorizing a phenomenon in a group of individuals. Richard and colleagues (2010) engaged in survey research to identify areas that they considered priorities for change in cancer care. They obtained information on how

to improve care in the ambulatory care centre. In critiquing this type of study, the issue of control should be applied in a highly flexible manner because of the preliminary nature of the work.

If from a review of a study you determine that the researcher intended to conduct a correlational study (an examination of the relationship between or among the variables), then the issue of control takes on more importance. Control must be exercised as strictly as possible. At this intermediate level of design, it should be clear to the reviewer that the researcher considered the extraneous variables that may affect the outcomes.

All aspects of control are strictly applied to studies that use an experimental design. The reader should be able to locate in the research report how the researcher met these criteria: whether the conditions of the research were constant throughout the study, the assignment of participants was random, and experimental and control groups were used. Because of the control exercised in the study, the reader can determine that all issues related to control were considered and the extraneous variables were addressed.

Evidence-Informed Practice Tip ____

Remember that establishing evidence for practice is determined by assessing the validity of each step of the study, assessing whether the evidence assists in planning patient care, and assessing whether patients respond to the evidence-informed care.

INTERNAL AND EXTERNAL VALIDITY

Consumers of research must believe that the results of a study are valid, based on precision, and faithful to what the researcher wanted to measure. To form the basis of further research, practice, and theory development, a study must be credible and dependable. The two important criteria for evaluating the credibility and dependability of the results are internal validity and external validity. Threats to validity are listed in Box 9-1, and a discussion of each threat follows.

Internal Validity

Internal validity is the degree to which the experimental treatment, not an uncontrolled condition, resulted in the observed effects. To establish internal validity, the researcher rules out other factors or threats as rival explanations of the relationship between the variables. Threats to internal validity may be numerous and are considered by researchers in planning a study and by consumers before implementing the results in practice (Campbell & Stanley, 1996). Research consumers should note that the threats to internal validity are most clearly applicable to experimental designs, but attention to factors that can compromise outcomes should be considered to some degree in all quantitative designs. If these threats are not considered, they could negate the results of the research by affecting the design. Threats to internal validity include history threats, maturation effects, testing effects, instrumentation threats, **attrition,** and selection bias. Table 9-2 provides examples of these threats.

History Threats

Not only the independent variable but also another specific event may affect the dependent variable, either inside or outside the experimental setting. This threat to internal validity is referred to as the **history threat.** In a study of the effects of a breast-feeding education program on the length of time of breast-feeding, government-sponsored breast-feeding promotions on television and in newspapers could affect the length of time of breast-feeding and would be considered a threat of history. A published example of history affecting research findings is Bull and associates' (2000) study (see Table 9-2).

Maturation Effects

Maturation refers to the developmental, biological, or psychological processes that operate within an individual as a function of time; these processes are external to the events of the investigation. For example, suppose that a researcher wished to evaluate the effect of a specific teaching method on the achievements of baccalaureate students on a skills test. The investigator would record the students' abilities before and after the teaching method. Between the pretest and the posttest, the students would have grown older and wiser. The growth or change is unrelated to the investigation, and the differences between the two testing periods may be explained by such maturation rather than by the experimental treatment.

Maturation effects could also occur in a study of the relationship between two methods of teaching about children's knowledge of self-care measures. Posttests of student learning must be conducted relatively soon after the teaching sessions are completed. Such a short interval allows the investigator to conclude that the results were the outcome of the design of the study and not maturation in a population of children who are learning new skills rapidly. Maturation is more than change that results from an age-related developmental process; maturation can also be related to physical changes (see Table 9-2).

Testing Effects

Taking the same test repeatedly could influence participants' responses the next time the test is completed. For example, the effect on the

TABLE 9-2	
EXAMPLES OF INTERNAL VALIDITY THREATS	
THREAT	**EXAMPLE**
History threat	Bull, Hansen, and Gross (2000) tested a teaching intervention in one hospital and compared the outcomes with those at another hospital in which the usual care was given. During the final months of data collection, the control hospital implemented a critical care pathway for congestive heart failure; as a result, data from the control hospital (cohort 4) were not included in the analysis.
Maturation effect	Koniak-Griffin, Verzemnieks, Anderson, Brecht, Lesser, Kim, et al. (2003) evaluated the 2-year postbirth infant health and maternal outcomes of an early intervention program by public health nurses and noted that the lack of change in some of the variables may have been attributable to the general maturation changes experienced by new mothers rather than to the intervention.
Testing effect	A researcher wishes to measure acute pain with a repeated-measures design during a lengthy procedure. The researcher must consider the results in view of the possible bias of repeating the pain measurements over a short period of time. The measurements may prime the patients' responses, and the practice of reporting pain repeatedly on the same instrument during a procedure may influence the results. Bennett, Lyons, Winters-Stone, and Hanson (2007) evaluated the effect of a motivational intervention on increasing physical activity in long-term cancer survivors. Several established instruments were used to measure variables. The measure of physical activity was obtained through self-report, which the researchers noted to be a possible limitation. The repeated self-measurements may have primed the patients' responses and primed the results.
Instrumentation threat	Inoue, Kakehashi, Oomori, and Koizumi (2004) studied biochemical hypoglycemia in female nurses during shift work in Japan. The nurses determined their own blood glucose levels 12 times, at four points during each of three shifts. The researchers noted that the study depended on self-testing and self-reporting of blood glucose levels; thus, documenting the validity of the data was difficult. Even though the study was well developed and participants were ensured confidentiality, the researchers still were concerned with this threat to the study's validity. Holditch-Davis, Brandon, and Schwartz (2003) examined the development of eight behaviours in preterm infants. Data collectors were trained and assessed for interrater reliability, which thus precluded the threat of instrumentation.
Mortality (attrition)	Stewart, Reutter, Letourneau, and Makwarimba (2009) tested a support intervention for homeless youth to optimize peer influence. A total of 70 youths were recruited to the study; 56 completed some part of the intervention. Attrition over time was a major challenge, resulting in a small sample and affecting the power of the study.
Selection bias	Smith, Corso, Brown, and Cameron (2011) controlled for selection bias by establishing selection criteria and having two groups: one receiving an intensive brief smoking cessation intervention (like an experimental group), the other receiving a brief smoking cessation intervention, which was used as the comparator.

participant's posttest score as the result of having taken a pretest is known as a **testing effect.** The effect of taking a pretest may sensitize an individual and improve the score on the posttest. Individuals generally score higher when they take a test a second time, regardless of the treatment. The differences between posttest and pretest scores may be a result not of the independent variable but rather of the experience gained through the testing. For example, in a study of the effect of integrating simulated teaching/learning strategies in undergraduate nursing education,

Sinclair and Ferguson's (2009) pretests and posttests consisted of the same self-efficacy questionnaire. Whether the significant increase in self-efficacy resulted from the teaching/learning strategies or was the effect of taking the test more than once was difficult to determine. Table 9-2 provides another example of a testing effect.

Instrumentation Threats

Instrumentation threats are changes in the variables or observational techniques that may account for changes in the obtained measurement.

For example, a researcher may wish to study various types of thermometers (e.g., tympanic, digital, electronic, chemical indicator, plastic strip, and mercury) to compare the accuracy of the mercury thermometer with the other temperature-taking methods. To prevent instrumentation threats, the researcher must check the calibration of the thermometers according to the manufacturer's specifications before and after data collection.

Another example concerns techniques of observation or data collection. If a researcher has several raters collecting observational data, all must be trained in a similar manner. If they are not similarly trained, or even if they are similarly trained but unable to conduct the study as planned, a lack of consistency may occur in their ratings; therefore, a threat to internal validity will occur.

Boechler and colleagues (2003) examined whether the amount of caregiving is related to the behaviour of a father and his child during a structured teaching interaction. The father was observed teaching his child to use a standardized teaching item, such as grabbing a ring or taking the lid off a container. Two trained female observers watched the father and scored the interaction on the Nursing Child Assessment Teaching Scale; only consensus scores from both observers were used in the data analysis. (For another example, see Table 9-2.) Although the researcher takes steps to prevent problems of instrumentation, the threat of instrumentation may still occur. When a critiquer finds such a threat, it must be evaluated within the total context of the study.

Mortality

Mortality or attrition is the loss of study participants from the first data-collection point (pretest) to the second data-collection point (posttest). If the participants who remain in the study are not similar to those who dropped out, the results could be affected. The loss of participants may be from the sample as a whole, or, in a study that has both an experimental group and a control group, more of the participants may drop out from one group than from the other group; this effect is known as *differential loss of participants*. In a study of the ways in which a media campaign affects the incidence of breast-feeding, if most dropouts were non–breast-feeding women, the perception given could be that exposure to the media campaign increased the number of breast-feeding women, whereas the effect of experimental attrition led to the observed results. See Table 9-2 for an example of a study in which mortality (attrition) may have influenced the results.

Selection Bias

If precautions are not used to gain a representative sample, **selection bias**—the threat to internal validity that arises when pretreatment differences exist between the experimental group and the control group—could result from the way the participants were chosen. Selection effects are a problem in studies in which the individuals themselves decide whether to participate in a study. Suppose an investigator wishes to assess whether a new smoking cessation program contributes to smoking cessation. If the new program is offered to all smokers, chances are that only individuals who are more motivated to stop smoking will take part in the program. Assessment of the effectiveness of the program is problematic because the investigator cannot know for certain whether the new program encouraged smoking cessation behaviours or whether only highly motivated individuals joined the program. To avoid selection bias, the researcher could randomly assign participants to either the new teaching method group or a control group that receives a different type of instruction. Table 9-2 provides another example of selection bias.

Helpful Hint

The list of threats to internal validity is not exhaustive. More than one threat can be found in a study, depending on the type of study design. Finding a threat to internal validity in a study does not invalidate the results and is usually acknowledged by the investigator in the "Results" or "Discussion" section of the study.

Evidence-Informed Practice Tip

Avoiding threats to internal validity in clinical research can be difficult. However, this reality does not render studies that have threats useless. Take the threats into consideration, and weigh the total evidence of a study for not only its statistical meaningfulness but also its clinical meaningfulness.

External Validity

External validity concerns the generalizability of an investigation's findings to additional populations and to other environmental conditions. To achieve external validity, variation in the conditions and the types of participants should lead to the same results. The goal of the researcher is to select a design that maximizes both internal and external validity, but attaining this goal is not always possible. If it is not possible, the researcher must attain the minimum criterion of external validity.

The factors that may affect external validity are related to the selection of participants, study conditions, and type of observations. These factors are termed *selection effects, reactive effects,* and *testing effects.* You may notice the similarity in the names of the factors of selection and testing and those of the threats to internal validity. When considering factors as internal threats, the reader assesses them as they relate to the *independent* and *dependent* variables within the study; when assessing them as external threats, the reader considers them in terms of the generalizability, or use outside the study with other populations and settings.

The Critical Thinking Decision Path displays the ways in which threats to internal and external validity can interact. This path is not, however, exhaustive with regard to the type of threats and their interaction. In comparison with problems of internal validity, generalizability issues are typically more difficult to deal with because they mean that the researcher is assuming that other populations are similar to the one being tested.

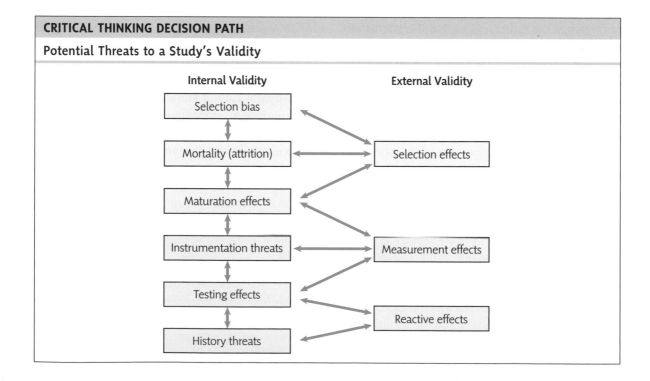

CRITICAL THINKING DECISION PATH

Potential Threats to a Study's Validity

Selection Effects

Selection concerns the generalizability of the results to other populations. An example of **selection effects** is when the researcher cannot attain the ideal sample population. At times, the number of available participants may be low, or they may not be accessible to the researcher. The researcher may then need to choose a nonprobability method of sampling, not a probability method. Therefore, the type of sampling method used and how participants are assigned to research conditions will affect the generalizability of findings to other groups, or the external validity. In the following quotations, the authors have noted selection effects:

- "The results of this study are limited by the small sample size." (Newby, Faschoway, & Souroroff, 2009, p. 531)
- "The relatively small sample size of Chinese youth and low variability of peer risky behaviours may account for the nonsignificant findings." (Wilgerodt, 2008, p. 404)
- "Study limitations include the possibility of selection bias. Our sample was chosen from two professional organizations whose members may have been more likely to be concerned about safety, skewing the results . . . which limits the generalizability of our findings." (Wagner, Capezuti, & Rice, 2009, p. 190)
- "One primary limitation of our study is that we only surveyed street youth in Toronto who accessed preventive health services. Therefore, the demographic and behavioural characteristics of street youth in our study may not be generalized to street youth elsewhere. Street youth of Toronto tend to come from a variety of racial and ethnic backgrounds, but in our study, categories of ethnicity were limited to three levels [Caucasian, Blacks and Other]; therefore, we cannot quantify the scope of diversity. Also,

street youth in Toronto come from various locations in Ontario and Canada." (Linton, Singh, Turbow, & Legg, 2009, p. 389)

These remarks are cautionary, but also they also point out the usefulness of the findings for practice and future research aimed at building the data in these areas.

Reactive Effects

Reactivity is defined as the participants' responses to being studied. Participants may behave in a certain way with the investigator not because of the study procedures but merely as an independent response to being studied. This response is also known as the **Hawthorne effect,** named after Western Electric Corporation's Hawthorne plant, where a study of working conditions was conducted in the 1930s. The researchers developed several different working conditions, such as turning up the lights, piping in music loudly or softly, and changing work hours. They found that no matter what was done, the workers' productivity increased. They concluded that production increased as a result of the workers' knowing that they were being studied rather than because of the experimental conditions.

For example, in a randomized controlled study, Bennett and colleagues (2007) tested the effect of telephone-based motivational interviewing on increasing physical activity and improving physical fitness, thus improving health self-efficacy in adults living in rural areas. The researchers noted that the physical activity counsellors knew to which group (control or experimental) the participants were assigned, which may have allowed the control group to become aware of components of the experimental treatment. The researchers also noted that each participant also participated in a 6-minute walk test in which a strict protocol was used, but it was also possible that conversation before the test might have influenced performance rate. The researchers made recommendations about how to avoid such threats in future studies.

Thomas and colleagues (2010), who assessed anaemia and red blood cell transfusion practices, noted that physicians in the intensive care unit were aware that phlebotomy and transfusion practices were being recorded. This could have led to temporary modifications in behaviour during the study, thereby affecting the outcomes.

Measurement Effects

Administration of a pretest in a study affects the generalizability of the findings to other populations; the resulting changes are known as **measurement effects.** Just as pretesting affects the posttest results within a study, pretesting affects the posttest results and generalizability outside the study. For example, suppose a researcher wants to conduct a study with the aim of changing attitudes toward acquired immune deficiency syndrome (AIDS). To accomplish this task, an education program on the risk factors for AIDS is incorporated. To test whether the education program changes attitudes toward AIDS, tests are given before and after the teaching intervention. The pretest on attitudes allows the participants to examine their attitudes regarding AIDS. The participants' responses on follow-up testing may differ from those of individuals who were given the education program and did not see the pretest. Therefore, when a study is conducted and a pretest is given, it may prime the participants and affect their subsequent answers, which in turn can affect the generalizability of the findings.

Helpful Hint

When you review a study, be aware of the internal and external threats to validity. These threats do not render a study useless; instead, they make it more useful to you. Recognition of the threats allows researchers to build on data and allows consumers to think through what part of the study can be applied to practice. Specific threats to validity depend on the type of design and generalizations that the researcher hopes to make.

Other threats to external validity depend on the type of design and methods of sampling used by the researcher but are beyond the scope of this text. Campbell and Stanley (1996) offered detailed coverage of the issues related to internal and external validity.

APPRAISING THE EVIDENCE

Quantitative Research

Critiquing the design of a study requires knowledge of the overall implications of a particular design for the study as a whole (see Critiquing Criteria box). Researchers want to consider the level of evidence provided by the design and how the study can be used to improve or change practice. Minimizing threats to internal and external validity enhances the strength of evidence for any quantitative design. The concept of the research design is all-inclusive and parallels the concept of the theoretical framework. The research design is similar to the theoretical framework in that it deals with a piece of the research study that affects the whole. This chapter has introduced the meaning, purpose, and important factors of design choice, as well as the vocabulary that accompanies these factors. Several criteria for evaluating the design can be drawn from this chapter. Remember that the criteria are applied differently with various designs. Differences in application do not mean that the consumer will find a haphazard approach to design but rather that each design has particular criteria that allow the consumer to classify the design by type (e.g., experimental or nonexperimental). These criteria must be met and addressed in conducting an experiment. The particulars of specific designs are addressed in Chapters 10 and 11. The following discussion primarily pertains to the overall evaluation of a quantitative research design.

The research outcome should demonstrate that an objective review of the literature and the establishment of a theoretical framework guided the choice of the design. No explicit statement regarding these areas is

APPRAISING THE EVIDENCE

Quantitative Research—cont'd

made in a research article. A consumer can evaluate the design by critiquing the theoretical framework (see Chapter 2) and literature review (see Chapter 5). Is the question new and not extensively researched? Has a great deal of research been conducted on the question, or is the question a new or different way of looking at an old question? Depending on the level of the question, the investigators make certain choices. These choices enable researchers to look for differences in a controlled, comparative manner.

The consumer should be alert for the methods that investigators use to maintain control (e.g., homogeneity in the sample, consistent data-collection procedures, manipulation of the independent variable, and randomization). As discussed in Chapter 10, all of these criteria must be met for an experimental design. As you begin to understand the types of designs (i.e., experimental, quasiexperimental, and nonexperimental designs such as survey and relationship designs), you will find that control is applied in varying degrees or—as in the case of a survey study—the independent variable is not manipulated (see Chapter 11). The level of control and its applications presented in Chapters 10 and 11 provide the remaining knowledge for fully critiquing the aspects of a study's design.

Once you have established whether the necessary control or uniformity of conditions has been maintained, you must determine whether the study is believable or valid. You should ask whether the findings are the result of the variables tested—and thus internally valid—or whether another explanation is possible. To assess this aspect, you should review the threats to internal validity. If the investigator's study was systematic, was well grounded in theory, and followed the criteria for each of the processes, you will probably conclude that the study is internally valid.

In addition, you must know whether a study has external validity or generalizability to other populations or environmental conditions. External validity can be claimed only after internal validity has been established. If the credibility of a study (internal validity) has not been established, a study has no generalizability to other populations (external validity). Determination of external validity is related directly to the sampling method (see Chapter 12). If the study is not representative of any one group or phenomena of interest, external validity may be limited or not present. The establishment of internal and external validity requires not only knowledge of the threats to internal and external validity but also knowledge of the phenomena being studied, which allows critical judgements to be made about the linkage of theories and variables for testing. You should find that the design follows from the theoretical framework, literature review, research question, and hypotheses. You should believe, on the basis of clinical knowledge and knowledge of the research process, that the investigators are not, as the expression goes, comparing apples with oranges.

CRITIQUING CRITERIA

1. Is the type of study design employed appropriate?
2. Does the researcher use the various concepts of control that are consistent with the type of design chosen?
3. Does the design seem to reflect feasibility?
4. Does the design flow from the proposed research question, theoretical framework, literature review, and hypothesis?
5. What are the threats to internal validity?
6. What are the controls for the threats to internal validity?
7. What are the threats to external validity?
8. What are the controls for the threats to external validity?
9. Is the design appropriately linked to the levels of evidence hierarchy?

CRITICAL THINKING CHALLENGES

- Consider the following statement: "All research attempts to solve problems." How would you support or refute this statement?
- As a consumer of research, you recognize that control is an important concept in the issue of research design. You are critiquing an assigned experimental study as part of your "open-book" midterm examination. From what is written, you cannot determine how the researchers kept the conditions of the study constant. How does this characteristic affect the study's use in an evidence-informed practice model?
- Box 9-1 lists six major threats to the internal validity of an experimental study. Prioritize them, and defend the one that you deem the essential, or number one, threat to address in a study.
- You are critiquing the research design of an assigned study as a consumer of research. How does the research design influence the findings of evidence in the study?
- How do threats to external validity contribute to the strength and quality of evidence provided by the findings of a research study?

KEY POINTS

- The purpose of the design is to provide the format of masterful and accurate research.
- Many types of designs exist. No matter which type of design the researcher uses, the purpose remains the same.
- The research consumer should be able to locate within the study a sense of the question that the researcher wished to answer. The question should be proposed with a plan or scheme for the accomplishment of the investigation. Depending on the question, the consumer should be able to recognize the steps taken by the investigator to ensure control.
- The choice of the specific design depends on the nature of the question. To specify the nature of the research question, the design must reflect the investigator's attempts to maintain objectivity, accuracy, pragmatic considerations, and, most important, control.

- Control affects not only the outcome of a study but also its future use. The design should also reflect how the investigator attempted to control threats to both internal and external validity.
- Internal validity must be established before external validity can be established. Both are considered within the sampling structure.
- No matter which design the researcher chooses, it should be evident to the reader that the choice was based on a thorough examination of the research question within a theoretical framework.
- The design, research question, literature review, theoretical framework, and hypothesis should all be interrelated.
- The choice of the design is affected by pragmatic issues. At times, two different designs may be equally valid for the same question.
- The choice of design affects the study's level of evidence.

REFERENCES

Bennett, J. A., Lyons, K. S., Winters-Stone K., & Hanson, G. (2007). Motivational interviewing to increase physical activity in long-term cancer survivors: A randomized controlled trial. *Nursing Research, 56*(1), 18-27.

Boechler, V., Harrison, M. J., & Magill-Evans, J. (2003). Father-child teaching interventions: The relationship to father involvement in caregiving. *Journal of Pediatric Nursing, 18*, 46-51.

Bull, M. J., Hansen, H. E., & Gross, C. R. (2000). A professional-patient partnership model of discharge planning with elders hospitalized with heart failure. *Applied Nursing Research, 13*, 19-28.

Campbell, D., & Stanley, J. (1996). *Experimental and quasi-experimental designs for research*. Chicago: Rand-McNally.

Doran, D., Harrison, M. B., Laschinger, H., Hirdes, J., Rukholm, E., Sidani, S., et al. (2006). Relationship between nursing interventions and outcome achievement in acute care settings. *Research in Nursing & Health, 29*, 61-70.

Hayward, K., Campbell-Yco, M., Price, S., Morrison, D., Whyte, R., Cake, H., & Vine, J. (2007). Co-bedding twins: How pilot study findings guided improvements in planning a larger multicenter trial. *Nursing Research, 56*, 137-143.

Holditch-Davis, D., Brandon, D. H., & Schwartz, T. (2003). Development of behaviors in preterm infants: Relation to sleeping and waking. *Nursing Research, 52*, 307-317.

Inoue, K., Kakehashi, Y., Oomori, S., & Koizumi, A. (2004). Endemic hypoglycemia among female nurses. *Research in Nursing and Health, 27*, 87-96.

Ireland, S. E., Arthur, H. M., Gunn, E. A., & Oczkowski, W. (2010). Stroke prevention care delivery: Predictors of risk factor management outcomes. *International Journal of Nursing Studies, 48*, 156-164.

Johnston, R., Hepworth, J., Goldsmith, M., & Lacasse, C. (2010). Use of iPod(tm) technology in medical-surgical nursing courses: Effect on grades. *International Journal of Nursing Education Scholarship, 7*(1), 1-17.

Kilty, H. L., & Prentice, D. (2010). Adolescent cardiovascular risk factors: A follow-up study. *Clinical Nursing Research, 19*(1), 6-20.

Koniak-Griffin, D., Verzemnieks, I. L., Anderson, N. L. R., Brecht, M., Lesser, J., Kim, S., et al. (2003). Nurse visitation for adolescent mothers: Two-year infant health and maternal outcomes. *Nursing Research, 52*, 127-136.

Linton, A., Singh, M., Turbow, D., & Legg, T. J. (2009). Street youth in Toronto: An investigation of demographic predictors of high risk behaviors and HIV status. *Journal of HIV/AIDS & Social Services, 8*, 375-396.

McGilton, K., Sorin-Peters, R., Sidani, S., Rochon, E., Boscart, V., & Fox, M. (2011). Focus on communication: Increasing the opportunity for successful staff-patient interactions. *International Journal of Older People, 6*(1), 13-24.

Newby, B. D., Faschoway, G. D., & Souroroff, C. I. (2009). Tetracaine (Ametop) compared to placebo for reducing pain associated with intramuscular injection of palivizumab (Synagis). *Journal of Pediatric Nursing, 24*(6), 529-533.

Ploeg, J., Brazil, K., Hutchison, B., Kaczorowski, J., Dalby, D. M., Goldsmith, C. H., & Furlong, W. (2010). Effect of preventive primary care outreach on health related quality of life among older adults at risk of functional decline: Randomised controlled trial. *British Medical Journal, 340*, c1480. doi:101136.bmj.c1480

Richard, M. L., Parmar, M. P., Calestagne, P. P., & McVey, L. (2010). Seeking patient feedback: An important dimension of quality in cancer care. *Journal of Nursing Care Quality, 25*(4), 344-351.

Sinclair, B., & Ferguson, K. (2009). Integrating simulated teaching/learning strategies in undergraduate nursing education. *International Journal of Nursing Education and Scholarship, 6*(1), Article 7.

Smith, P. M., Corso, L., Brown, K. S., & Cameron, R. (2011). Nurse case-managed tobacco cessation interventions for general hospital patients: Results of a randomized clinical trial. *Canadian Journal of Nursing Research, 43*(1), 98-117.

Sobieraj, G., Bhatt, M., LeMay, S., Rennick, J., & Johnston, C. (2009). The effect of music on parental participation during pediatric laceration repair. *Canadian Journal of Nursing Research, 41*(4), 68-82.

Steenbeek, A., Edgecombe, N., Durling, J., LeBlanc, A., Anderson, R., & Bainbridge, R. (2009). Using an interactive journal club to enhance nursing knowledge acquisition, appraisal, and application. *International Journal of Nursing Education Scholarship, 6*(1), 1-8.

Stewart, M., Reutter, L., Letourneau, N., & Makwarimba, E. (2009). A support intervention to promote health and coping among homeless youths. *Canadian Journal of Nursing Research, 41*(2), 54-77.

Thomas, J., Jensen, L., Nahirniak, S., & Gibney, R. T. N. (2010). Anemia and blood transfusion practices in the critically ill: A prospective cohort review. *Heart & Lung, 39*(3), 217-225.

Wagner, L. M., Capezuti, E., & Rice, J. C. (2009). Nurses' perceptions of safety culture in long-term care settings. *Journal of Nursing Scholarship, 41*(2), 184-192.

Wilgerodt, M. A. (2008). Family and peer influences on adjustment among Chinese, Filipino and white youth. *Nursing Research, 57*(6), 395-405.

FOR FURTHER STUDY

ⓔvolve Go to Evolve at http://evolve.elsevier.com/ Canada/LoBiondo/Research for Audio Glossary, how-to instructions for Writing Proposals for Funding, and additional research articles for practice in reviewing and critiquing.

CHAPTER 10

Experimental and Quasiexperimental Designs

Susan Sullivan-Bolyai | Carol Bova | Mina D. Singh

LEARNING OUTCOMES

After reading this chapter, you will be able to do the following:

- List the criteria necessary for inferring cause-and-effect relationships.
- Distinguish the differences between experimental and quasiexperimental designs.
- Define problems with internal validity that are associated with experimental and quasiexperimental designs.
- Describe the use of experimental and quasiexperimental designs for evaluation research.
- Critically evaluate the findings of selected studies in which cause-and-effect relationships were tested.
- Apply levels of evidence to experimental and quasiexperimental designs.

KEY TERMS

a priori
after-only design
after-only nonequivalent
  control group design
antecedent variable
attrition
control
dependent variable
evaluation research
experiment

experimental design
formative evaluation
independent variable
intervening variable
manipulation
mortality
nonequivalent control group
  design
one-group pretest–posttest
  design

posttest–only control group
  design
quasiexperiment
quasiexperimental design
randomization
Solomon four-group design
summative evaluation
testing effects
time series design
true experiment

STUDY RESOURCES

Go to Evolve at http://evolve.elsevier.com/Canada/LoBiondo/Research for Audio Glossary, how-to instructions for Writing Proposals for Funding, and additional research articles for practice in reviewing and critiquing.

CHAPTER 10 PROVIDED AN OVERVIEW OF the meaning, purpose, and issues related to quantitative research design. This chapter provides a discussion of specific types of quantitative designs, inasmuch as choosing the correct design is crucial for hypothesis testing or answering research questions. The design involves a *plan,* a *structure,* and a *strategy,* which guide a researcher in writing the hypothesis or research questions, conducting the project, and analyzing and evaluating the data.

Each design has specific characteristics to maintain control: for example, homogeneity in the sample, consistent data-collection procedures, manipulation of the independent variable, and randomization.

One of the fundamental purposes of scientific research in any profession is to determine cause-and-effect relationships. Nurses, for example, are concerned with developing effective approaches to maintaining and restoring wellness. Testing such nursing interventions to determine how well they actually work—that is, evaluating the outcomes in terms of efficacy and cost effectiveness—is accomplished with the use of experimental and quasiexperimental designs. These designs differ from nonexperimental designs in one important way: The researcher actively seeks to bring about the desired effect and does not passively observe behaviours or actions. In other words, the researcher is interested not merely in observing customary patient care but in making something happen. Experimental and quasiexperimental studies are also important to consider in relation to evidence-informed practice because they provide level II and level III evidence. The findings of such studies provide the validation of clinical practice and the rationale for changing specific aspects of practice (see Chapter 20).

Experimental designs are particularly suitable for testing cause-and-effect relationships because they help eliminate potential alternative explanations (threats to validity) for the findings. Inferring causality requires that the following three criteria be met.

1. The causal variable and effect variable must be associated with each other.
2. The cause must precede the effect.
3. The relationship must not be explainable by another variable.

When you critique studies in which experimental and quasiexperimental designs were used, the primary focus is on the validity of the conclusion that the experimental treatment, or the **independent variable,** caused the desired effect on the outcome, or **dependent variable.** The validity of the conclusion depends on how well the researcher controlled the other variables that may explain the relationship studied. Thus, the focus of this chapter is to explain how various types of experimental and quasiexperimental designs control extraneous variables.

The purpose of this chapter is to acquaint you with the issues involved in interpreting studies that involved the use of **experimental design** (characterized by three properties: randomization, control, and manipulation) and **quasiexperimental design** (in which random assignment is not used, but the independent variable is manipulated, and certain mechanisms of control are used). Examples of these designs are listed in Box 10-1. The Critical Thinking Decision Path shows an algorithm that influences a researcher's choice of experimental or quasiexperimental design.

BOX **10-1**

SUMMARY OF EXPERIMENTAL AND QUASIEXPERIMENTAL RESEARCH DESIGNS

EXPERIMENTAL DESIGNS
1. True experimental (pretest–posttest control group) design
2. Solomon four-group design
3. After-only design

QUASIEXPERIMENTAL DESIGNS
1. Nonequivalent control group design
2. After-only nonequivalent control group design
3. One group (pretest–posttest) design
4. Time series design

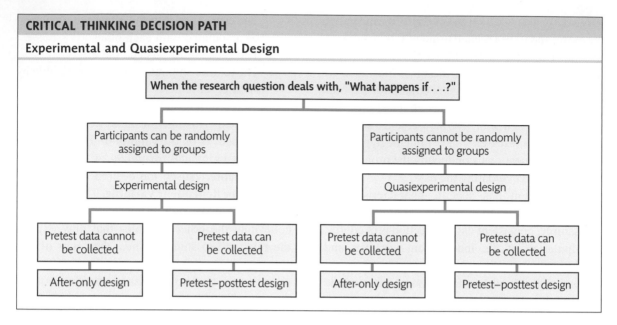

CRITICAL THINKING DECISION PATH

Experimental and Quasiexperimental Design

TRUE EXPERIMENTAL DESIGN

An **experiment** is a scientific investigation that makes observations and collects data according to explicit criteria. A **true experiment**—also known as a *pretest–posttest control group design* or *classic experiment*—has three identifying properties: randomization, control, and manipulation. These properties allow for other explanations of the phenomenon to be ruled out and thereby provide the strength of the design for testing cause-and-effect relationships.

A research study in which an experimental design is used is commonly called a *randomized clinical trial* (RCT). An RCT or experimental design is considered to be the best research design, "the gold standard," for providing information about cause-and-effect relationships. An individual RCT generates level II evidence because only minimal bias is introduced by this design. The higher level of evidence that a design produces, the more likely the results are to offer an unbiased estimate of the effect of an intervention and the more confident you are that the intervention will be effective and produce the same results over and over again.

An example of an RCT was the study by Ploeg and colleagues (2010), who compared the effect of a provider-initiated primary care outreach intervention with that of usual care among adults at risk for functional decline. They used a 1:1 allocation ratio to assign participants to the intervention or control group. The sequence of allocation was generated in blocks of 8 or 16, so that the allocation was balanced in blocks. A table of random digits was used to assign block size and allocation.

Randomization

Randomization, or random assignment to a group, is required for a study to be considered a true experimental design. It involves the assignment of participants to either the experimental or the control group on a purely random basis. In other words, each participant has an equal and known probability of being assigned to any group. Random assignment may be performed individually or by groups (LeMay, Johnston, Choiniére, Fortin, Huber, Fréchette, et al., 2010; Sobieraj, Bhatt, LeMay, Rennick, & Johnston, 2009 [see Appendix C]). Random assignment to experimental or control groups allows for the elimination of any systematic bias that may affect the dependent variable being studied. In randomization, it is assumed that any important intervening variable (a condition that occurs during the study that affects the dependent variable) will occur in an equal distribution between the groups (as discussed in Chapter 9). Randomization minimizes variance (as discussed in Chapter 12) and decreases selection bias. Participants are randomly assigned to groups through several procedures, such as a table of random numbers or computer-generated number sequences. Whatever method is used, it is important that the process be truly random, that it be tamper-proof, and that the group assignment is concealed. Note that random assignment to groups is different from the random sampling discussed in Chapter 12.

Control

Control refers to the introduction of one or more constants into the experimental situation. Control is acquired by manipulating the causal or independent variable, randomly assigning participants to a group, carefully preparing experimental protocols, and using comparison groups. In experimental research, the comparison group is the control group, or the group that receives the usual treatment rather than the innovative, experimental treatment.

Manipulation

As discussed previously, experimental designs are characterized by the researcher "doing something" to at least some of the participants. The experimental treatment is administered to some participants in the study but not to others, or different amounts of it are administered to different groups. This difference in how the treatment is provided is the **manipulation** of the independent variable. The independent variable might be a treatment, a teaching plan, or a medication. The effect of this manipulation is measured to determine the result of the experimental treatment.

The concepts of control, randomization, and manipulation and their application to experimental design are sometimes confusing for students. These concepts allow researchers to have confidence in the causal inferences they make by allowing them to rule out other potential explanations. Consider the use of control, randomization, and manipulation in the following example. Moore and colleagues (2009) used a cross-sectional RCT to examine whether catheter washouts would prevent or reduce catheter blockage in long-term indwelling urethral catheters. Participants were recruited from long-term care units and homecare agencies.

A computer-generated process was used for randomization to the control and experimental groups. The patients were randomly assigned to one of three groups: control (usual care, no washout), saline washout, or commercially available acidic (Contisol) washout solution. The use of random assignment meant that all patients who met the study criteria had an equal and known chance of being assigned to the control group or one of the experimental groups. The use of random assignment to groups helps ensure that the three study groups are comparable with regard to preexisting factors that might affect the outcome of interest, such as gender, age, length of stay in the hospital, and stage of cancer. Also, the researchers in this example checked statistically whether the procedure of random assignment did, in fact, produce groups that were similar at baseline.

Evidence-Informed Practice Tip

In health care research, the term *randomized clinical trial* (RCT) often refers to a true experimental design. These designs are being used more frequently in nursing research, which is critical to evidence-informed practice initiatives.

The degree of control exerted over the experimental conditions in Moore and colleagues' (2009) study is illustrated by its detailed descriptions of how to perform the washouts, with visual aids on how to properly irrigate the catheter. This control helped ensure that all members of the experimental group received similar treatment, and it assists the reader in understanding the nature of the experimental treatment. The control group provided a comparison against which the experimental group could be judged.

In Moore and colleagues' (2009) study, receiving the saline or Contisol wash were the manipulated treatments. Patient outcomes were measured for all participants, including mean urinary pH, incidence of microscopic hematuria and pyuria and incidence of urinary tract infections. The primary outcome variable was mean length of time until first catheter change. By controlling the experimental intervention with the use of standard protocol, Moore and colleagues were able to assert that the evidence is insufficient to state whether catheter washout with saline or Contisol is more effective than usual care with no washout to prevent obstruction and clogging.

The use of the experimental design allows researchers to rule out many of the potential threats to internal validity of the findings, such as selection bias, history, and maturation effects (see Chapter 9). The strength of the true experimental design lies in its ability to help the researcher control the effects of any extraneous variables—alternative events that could explain the findings—that might constitute threats to internal validity. Such extraneous variables can be either *antecedent* or *intervening*.

The **antecedent variable** occurs before the study but may affect the dependent variable and confound the results. Factors such as age, gender, socioeconomic status, and health status might be important antecedent variables in nursing research because they may affect dependent variables, such as recovery time and ability to integrate health care behaviours. Antecedent variables that might have affected the dependent variables in the study by Moore and colleagues (2009) included age, gender, and length of time that a urinary catheter was used. Random assignment to groups helps ensure that the groups are similar with regard to these variables so that differences in the dependent variable may be attributed to the experimental treatment. However, the researcher should check, and report, how the groups actually compared with regard to such variables. An **intervening variable** is a condition that occurs during the course of the study and is not part of the study; however, the intervening variable affects the dependent variable and can affect the study outcomes. An example of an intervening variable that might have affected the outcomes of Moore and colleagues' (2009) study is a change in health care status in any of the participants, such as a newly diagnosed medical condition or an infection. Thus, if the care provided to patients changed in any major way while the study was being implemented, the results of the study also would be affected.

Types of Experimental Designs

Several different experimental designs exist (Campbell & Stanley, 1966). Each is based on the classic design called the *true experiment,* diagrammed in Figure 10-1. Above the description diagram, symbolic notations are routinely used:

- *R* represents random assignment (for both the experimental group and the control group).
- *O* signifies observation through data collection on the dependent variable.
- O_1 signifies pretest data collection.
- O_2 represents posttest data collection.
- *X* represents exposure to the intervention.

Therefore, in Figure 10-1, note that the participants were assigned randomly *(R)* to the experimental or the control group. The experimental treatment *(X)* was given only to participants in the experimental group, and the pretests *(O_1)* and posttests *(O_2)* are the measurements of the dependent variables that were made before and after the experimental treatment was performed. In all true experimental designs, participants are randomly

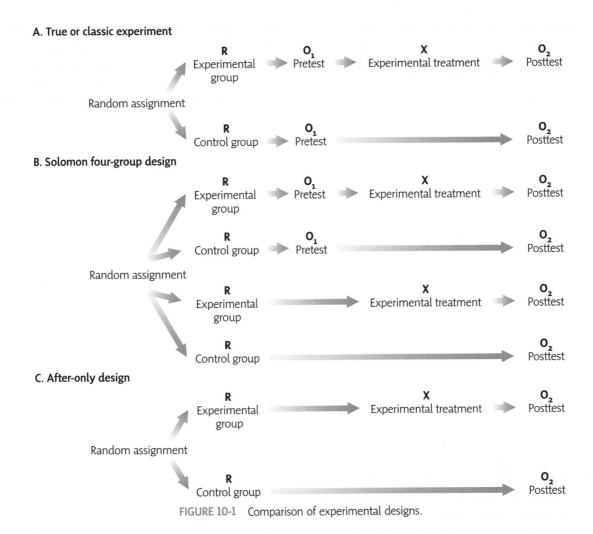

FIGURE 10-1 Comparison of experimental designs.

assigned to groups, an experimental treatment is introduced to some of the participants, and the effects of the treatment are observed. The variation in designs primarily concerns the number of observations that are made.

As shown in Figure 10-1, participants are randomly assigned to the two groups, experimental and control, so that antecedent variables are controlled. Next, pretest measurements or observations are made so that the researcher has a baseline for determining the effect of the independent

variable. The researcher then introduces the experimental variable to one of the groups and measures the dependent variable again to see whether it has changed. The control group receives no experimental treatment, but the dependent variable in that group is also measured later for comparison with the experimental group. The degree of difference between the two groups at the end of the study indicates the confidence the researcher has that a causal link exists between the independent and dependent variables. Because random assignment and the control inherent in this design minimize the effects of many threats to internal validity, the true experimental design is a strong design for testing cause-and-effect relationships.

However, the design is not perfect. Some threats cannot be controlled in true experimental studies (see Chapter 9). People tend to drop out of studies that require their participation over an extended period. The influence over the outcome of an experiment of people dropping out or dying is commonly known as **attrition** or **mortality.** If the number or type of people who drop out of the experimental group differs from that of the control group, a mortality effect might explain the findings. When you read such a work, examine the sample and the results carefully to see whether dropouts or deaths occurred.

Testing effects—the effects on the scores of a posttest as the result of having taken a pretest—also can be a problem in these studies because the researcher is usually administering the same test twice, and participants tend to score better the second time just by learning the test. Researchers can circumvent this problem in one of two ways: They might use different forms of the same test for the two measurements, or they might use a more complex experimental design called the Solomon four-group design.

The **Solomon four-group design,** shown in Figure 10-1, consists of two groups that are identical to those used in the classic experimental design plus two additional groups: an experimental after-group and a control after-group. As the diagram shows, all four groups have randomly assigned (R) participants, as in all experimental studies. However, the addition of these latter two groups helps rule out testing threats to internal validity that the before- and after-groups may experience. For example, suppose a researcher is interested in the effects of counselling on the self-esteem of patients with chronic illness. Just taking a test of self-esteem (O_1) may influence how the participants report themselves. The items might make the participants think more about how they view themselves so that the next time they fill out the questionnaire (O_2), their self-esteem might appear to have improved. In reality, however, their self-esteem may be the same as it was before; the scores are different only because the participants had previously taken the test. The use of this design with the two groups that do not receive the pretest allows for evaluating the effect of the pretest on the posttest in the first two groups. (See Practical Application box for another example of use of the Solomon four-group design.)

Although this design helps evaluate the effects of testing, the threat of mortality remains a problem, as in the classic experimental design.

Practical Application

Weinrich and colleagues (2007) used the Solomon four-group design to test an enhanced decision aid for prostate cancer screening versus standard education with middle-aged men. They hypothesized that participants who received the pretest would have higher posttest knowledge. The men were first randomly assigned to one of four groups: experimental and control groups that received both pretest and posttest and the other experimental and control groups that received only the posttest. They also tested and found no differences across the four groups in demographics, family history of prostate cancer, or previous history of screening prostate examinations, thus ensuring the success of the randomization process. The findings revealed that outcomes varied depending on group assignment (those who took both pretest and posttest had significantly higher scores than did the posttest–only intervention group) but also depending on whether the men had had previous digital rectal examinations.

A less frequently used experimental design is the **after-only design,** shown in Figure 10-1. This design, which is sometimes called the **posttest–only control group design,** is composed of two randomly assigned groups (R), but in contrast to the true experimental design, neither group is given a pretest or other measures. Again, the independent variable is introduced to the experimental group (X) and not to the control group. The process of randomly assigning the participants to groups is assumed to be sufficient to ensure a lack of bias so that the researcher can still determine whether the treatment (X) created significant differences between the two groups $(O_1$ and $O_2)$. This design is particularly useful when testing effects are expected to be a major problem and the number of available participants is too limited for a Solomon four-group design.

An example of this design would be a study of an intervention on postoperative pain management, inasmuch as pain cannot be measured before surgery and only an after-only design is required.

Helpful Hint

Remember that mortality is a problem in most experimental studies because data are usually collected more than once. The researcher should demonstrate that the groups are equivalent both when they enter the study and at the final analysis.

Field and Laboratory Experiments

Experiments also can be classified by setting. Field experiments and laboratory experiments share the properties of control, randomization, and manipulation and involve the same design characteristics but are conducted in different environments. Laboratory experiments take place in an artificial setting created specifically for the purpose of research. In the laboratory, the researcher has almost total control over the features of the environment, such as temperature, humidity, noise level, and participant conditions. Conversely, field experiments are exactly what the name implies: Experiments that take place in a real, preexisting social setting, such as a hospital or clinic, where the phenomenon of interest usually occurs.

Because most experiments in the nursing literature are field experiments and control is such an important element in the conduct of experiments, studies conducted in the field are subject to treatment contamination by factors specific to the setting that the researcher cannot control. However, studies conducted in the laboratory are by nature "artificial" because the setting is created for the purpose of research. Thus, laboratory experiments, although stronger with regard to internal validity questions than field studies, have more problems with external validity. For example, a participant's behaviour in the laboratory may be quite different from the person's behaviour in the real world; this dichotomy presents problems in generalizing findings from the laboratory to the real world. Therefore, when you read research reports, you need to consider the possible effect of the experiment's setting on the findings of the study.

Consider a hypothetical study on different types of wound treatment gels and creams for the management of pressure ulcers. This study could be performed in a laboratory with animals, which would have allowed complete control over the external environment of the study—a variable that might be important in studying wound healing. However, researchers cannot guarantee that the results found in a study in a laboratory would be applicable to human patients in hospital settings; thus, some external validity would be lost.

Advantages and Disadvantages of the Experimental Design

As previously discussed, experimental designs are the most appropriate for testing cause-and-effect relationships because the design enables the researcher to control the experimental situation. Therefore, experimental designs offer better corroboration than if the independent variable is manipulated in such a way that certain consequences can be expected. Such studies are important because one of nursing's major research priorities is documenting outcomes to provide a basis for changing or supporting current nursing practice.

Experimental designs are not commonly used in nursing research, for several reasons. First, experimentation is conducted under the assumption that all the relevant variables involved in a phenomenon have been identified. For many areas of nursing research, this is simply not the case, and descriptive studies need to be completed before experimental interventions can be applied. Second, these designs have some significant disadvantages. One problem with an experimental design is that many variables important in predicting outcomes of nursing care are not amenable to experimental manipulation. It is well known that health status varies with age and socioeconomic status. No matter how careful a researcher is, no one can assign participants randomly by age or a certain level of income. In addition, it may be technically possible to manipulate some variables, but their nature may preclude their actually manipulation.

For example, if a researcher tried to randomly assign groups to study the effects of cigarette smoking and asked the experimental group to smoke two packs of cigarettes a day, that researcher's ethics would be seriously questioned. It is also potentially true that such a study would not work because nonsmokers randomly assigned to the smoking group would be unlikely to comply with the research task. Thus, sometimes even when a researcher plans to conduct a true experiment, participants dropping out of the study or other factors may, in effect, make the study a quasiexperiment.

Quasiexperimental designs are considered when it is not possible to randomly assign participants or when a control group is lacking. For example, McGilton and associates (2003) found that health care professionals in long-term care facilities can be taught how to enhance their care without adding staff. To conduct the study, randomly assigning residents to nursing staff was not feasible; therefore, two separate units were used for the control condition and the intervention.

Another problem with experimental designs is that they may be difficult or impractical to perform in field settings. It may be quite difficult to randomly assign patients on a hospital floor to different groups when they might talk to each other about the different treatments. Experimental procedures also may be disruptive to the usual routine of the setting. If several nurses are involved in administering the experimental program, it may be impossible to ensure that the program is administered in the same way to each participant.

Because of these problems in carrying out true experiments, researchers frequently turn to another type of research design to evaluate cause-and-effect relationships. Such designs, because they seem experimental but lack some of the control of the true experimental design, are called *quasiexperiments*.

QUASIEXPERIMENTAL DESIGNS

Quasiexperimental designs are intended to test cause-and-effect relationships; however, in a quasiexperimental design, full experimental control is not possible. A **quasiexperiment** is a research design in which the researcher initiates an experimental treatment, but some characteristic of a true experiment is lacking. Control may not be possible because of the nature of the independent variable or the nature of the available participants. Quasiexperimental designs usually lack the element of randomization, as described earlier with McGilton and associates' (2003) study. In other cases, the control group may be missing. However, like experiments, quasiexperiments involve the introduction of an experimental treatment.

In comparison with the true experimental design, quasiexperimental designs are used similarly. Both types of designs are used when the researcher is interested in testing cause-and-effect relationships. However, the basic problem with the quasiexperimental approach is a weakened confidence in making causal assertions. Because of the lack of some controls in the research situation, quasiexperimental designs are subject to contamination by many, if not all, of the threats to internal validity discussed in Chapter 9.

Types of Quasiexperimental Designs

Many different quasiexperimental designs exist. Only the ones most commonly used in nursing research are discussed in this book. To illustrate, the symbols and notations introduced earlier in the chapter are used. Refer to the true experimental design shown in Figure 10-1 and compare it with the **nonequivalent control group design** shown in Figure 10-2. Note that the latter design looks exactly like that of the true experiment

except that participants are not randomly assigned to groups.

For example, suppose a researcher is interested in the effects of a new diabetes education program on the physical and psychosocial outcomes of patients with newly diagnosed diabetes. If the conditions were right, the researcher might be able to randomly assign participants to either the group receiving the new program or the group receiving the usual program, but for any number of reasons, that design might not be possible (e.g., nurses on the unit where patients are admitted might be so excited about the new program that they cannot help but include the new information for all patients). Thus, the researcher has two

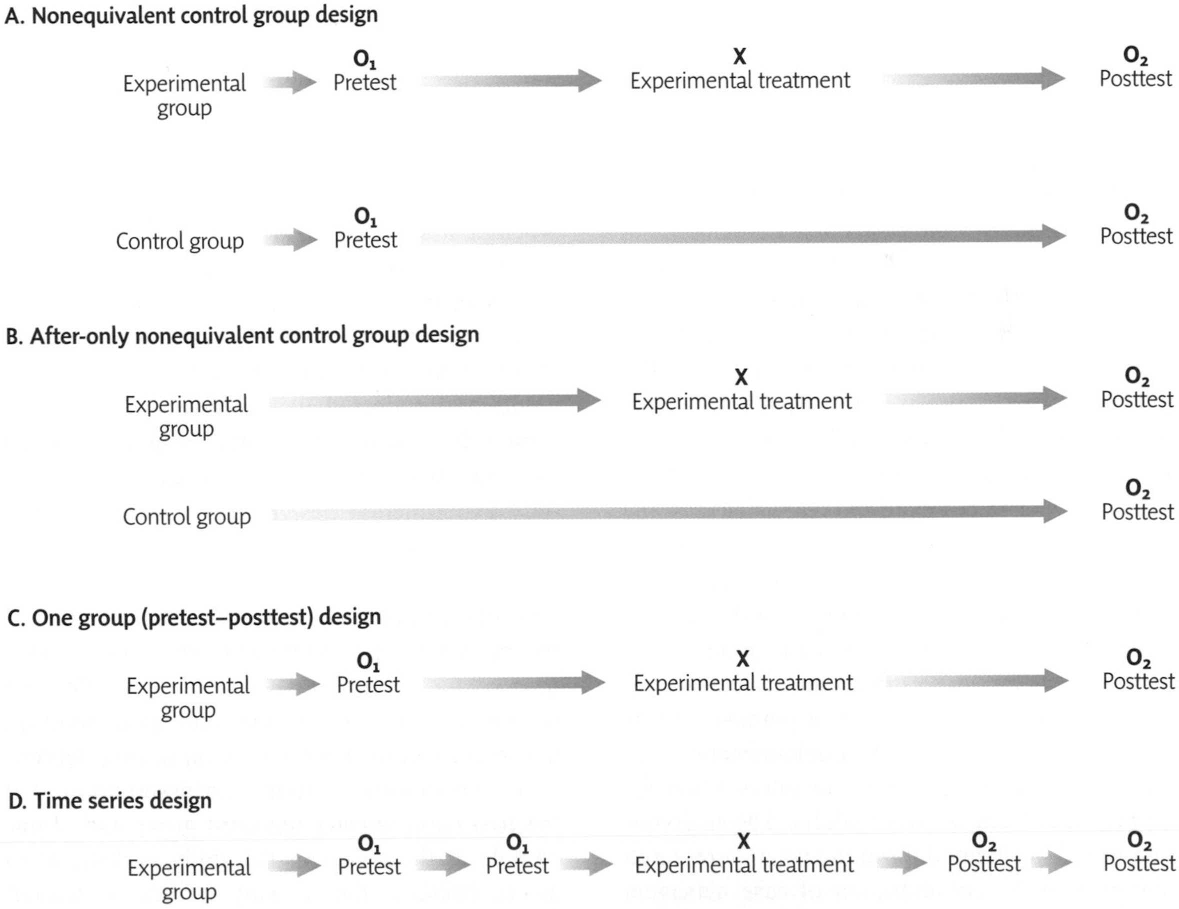

A. Nonequivalent control group design

Experimental group	O_1 Pretest		X Experimental treatment		O_2 Posttest

Control group	O_1 Pretest				O_2 Posttest

B. After-only nonequivalent control group design

Experimental group			X Experimental treatment		O_2 Posttest

Control group					O_2 Posttest

C. One group (pretest–posttest) design

Experimental group	O_1 Pretest		X Experimental treatment		O_2 Posttest

D. Time series design

Experimental group	O_1 Pretest	O_1 Pretest	X Experimental treatment	O_2 Posttest	O_2 Posttest

FIGURE 10-2 Comparison of quasiexperimental designs.

choices: to abandon the experiment or to conduct a quasiexperiment. To conduct a quasiexperiment, the researcher might find a similar unit that has not been introduced to the new program and study the patients with newly diagnosed diabetes who are admitted to that unit as a comparison group. The study would then involve the quasiexperimental type of design.

Studies in which both quantitative and qualitative methods are used are called *mixed-methods studies.*

Helpful Hint

Remember that researchers often make trade-offs and sometimes use a quasiexperimental design instead of an experimental design because it may be pragmatically impossible to randomly assign participants to groups. The fact that the design is not "pure" does not decrease the value of the study, although the utility of the findings may be decreased.

The nonequivalent control group design is commonly used in nursing research studies conducted in field settings. The basic problem with the design is the weakening of the researcher's confidence in assuming that the experimental and comparison groups are similar at the beginning of the study. Threats to internal validity, such as selection bias, maturation effects, testing effects, and mortality (attrition), are possible with this design. However, the design is relatively strong because the gathering of the data at the time of the pretest allows the researcher to compare the equivalence of the two groups on important antecedent variables before the independent variable is introduced.

In Ducharme and colleagues' (2006) study, the motivation of caregivers to learn about stress management might be important in determining the effect of this program. The purpose of this project was to evaluate the implementation and effects of a stress management intervention for family caregivers of older adults. The intervention was implemented through an action research design with the collaboration of case managers working in community health centers. A total of

81 caregivers participated in the study. The quasiexperimental design used to test the effects of the intervention showed significant effects on perceived challenge associated with caregiver role, control by self, use of social support, and use of problem solving. In the measures taken at the outset of the study, the researcher could include a measure of motivation to learn. The differences between the two groups on this variable could then be tested, and if significant differences existed, they could be controlled statistically in the analysis. Nonetheless, the strength of the causal assertions that can be made on the basis of such designs depends on the ability of the researcher to identify and measure or control possible threats to internal validity.

Suppose that the researcher did not measure the participants' responses before the introduction of the new treatment (or the researcher was hired after the new program began) but later decided that data demonstrating the effect of the program would be useful. Perhaps, for example, a third party asks for such data to determine whether it should pay the extra cost of the new teaching program. Sometimes the outcomes simply cannot be measured before the intervention, as with prenatal interventions that are expected to affect birth outcomes. The study that could be conducted would have an **after-only nonequivalent control group design,** illustrated in Figure 10-2. This design is similar to the after-only experimental design, but randomization is not used to assign participants to groups. In this design, the two groups are assumed to be equivalent and comparable before the introduction of the independent variable *(X).* Thus, the soundness of the design and the confidence that the researchers can have in the findings depend on the soundness of this assumption of preintervention comparability. Often, the assumption that the two nonrandomly assigned groups are comparable at the outset of the study is difficult to assert because the validity of the statement cannot be assessed.

In the example of the teaching program for patients with newly diagnosed diabetes, measuring the participants' motivation after the teaching program would not reveal whether their motivations differed before they received the program, and it is possible that the teaching program would motivate individuals to learn more about their health problem. Therefore, the researcher's conclusion that the teaching program improved physical status and psychosocial outcome would be subject to the alternative conclusion that the results were an effect of preexisting motivations (selection effect) in combination with greater learning by participants so motivated (selection-maturation interaction). Nonetheless, this design is frequently used in nursing research because opportunities for data collection are often limited and because this design is particularly useful when testing effects may be problematic.

Tranmer and Parry (2004) used an after-only design to test the effects of an advanced practice nursing intervention on health-related quality of life, symptom distress, and satisfaction with care among cardiac surgery patients. The intervention was telephone support for 4 weeks after hospital discharge.

Another quasiexperimental design is a **one-group pretest–posttest design** (Figure 10-2), which is used by researchers when only one group is available for study (see Practical Application box). Data are collected before and after an experimental treatment on this one group of participants. In this type of design, the participants act as their own controls, and no randomization occurs. Because controls and randomization are important characteristics that enhance the internal validity of the study, the evidence generated by the findings of this type of quasiexperimental design needs to be interpreted with careful consideration of the design limitations.

An approach used by researchers when only one group is available is to study that group over a longer period: that is, to test participants before an intervention and again afterwards. This

> ### Practical Application
>
> Martinez and associates (2007) conducted a one-group pretest–posttest design study to explore nurses' perceptions of the effect of the 15-minute family interview on the paediatric hospital admission process. The intervention consisted of two in-depth teaching sessions and hands-on coaching in the use of the 15-minute family interview. Each nurse acted as his or her own control by being interviewed twice, before receiving the intervention and after completing six family interviews. Findings revealed that the nurses perceived the genogram, therapeutic questions, and commendations as having a positive effect on their ability to conduct family assessment and family interventions.

quasiexperimental design is called a **time series design** and is illustrated in Figure 10-2. Time series designs are useful for determining trends, as in a study of the effect of adult day programs on family caregivers of elderly relatives (Warren, Ross-Kerr, Smith, & Godkin, 2003). The caregivers completed measures of burden, quality of life, perceived health, and opinion about institutionalization at four time points (just before patient admission and 2 weeks, 2 months, and 6 months after admission to the day program). Sometimes data are collected many times before the introduction of the treatment to establish a baseline point of reference on outcomes. The experimental treatment is then introduced, and data are collected multiple times afterward to determine a change from baseline. The broad range and number of data-collection points help rule out alternative explanations, such as history effects. However, a testing threat to internal validity is ever present because of multiple data-collection points, and without a control group, the threats of selection bias and maturation effects cannot be ruled out (see Chapter 9).

To rule out some alternative explanations for the findings of a one-group pretest–posttest design, researchers typically measure the phenomenon of interest over a longer period and introduce the experimental treatment sometime during the course of the data-collection period.

Even with the absence of a control group, the broader range of data-collection points helps rule out threats to validity such as history effects. Obviously, the earlier example of teaching patients with diabetes does not lend itself to this design because researchers do not have access to the patients before the diagnosis.

Helpful Hint

One of the reasons replication is so important in nursing research is that many problems cannot be subjected to experimental methods. Therefore, the consistency of findings across many patient populations helps support a cause-and-effect relationship even when an experiment cannot be conducted.

Advantages and Disadvantages of Quasiexperimental Designs

Because of the problems inherent in interpreting the results of studies with quasiexperimental designs, you may wonder why anyone would use them. Quasiexperimental designs are used frequently because they are practical and feasible, and the results are generalizable. These designs are more adaptable to the real-world practice setting than controlled experimental designs. In addition, for some hypotheses, these designs may be the only way to evaluate the effect of the independent variable of interest.

The weaknesses of the quasiexperimental approach involve mainly the inability to establish clear cause-and-effect relationships. However, if the researcher can rule out any plausible alternative explanations for the findings, such studies can lead to increased knowledge about causal relationships. Researchers have several options for ruling out these alternative explanations. They may control extraneous variables **a priori** (before initiating the intervention) by design.

Researchers can also use methods to control extraneous variables statistically. In some cases, common sense knowledge of the problem and

the population can suggest that a particular explanation is not plausible. Nonetheless, replicating such studies is important to support the causal assertions developed through the use of quasiexperimental designs.

The literature on cigarette smoking is an excellent example of how findings from many studies, experimental and quasiexperimental, can be linked to establish a causal relationship. A large number of well-controlled experiments with laboratory animals randomly assigned to smoking and nonsmoking conditions have documented that lung disease does develop in "smoking" animals. Although such evidence is suggestive of a link between smoking and lung disease in humans, it is not directly transferable because animals and humans are different. Because humans cannot be randomly assigned to smoking and nonsmoking groups for ethical and other reasons, researchers interested in this problem must use quasiexperimental data to test their hypotheses about smoking and lung disease.

Several different quasiexperimental designs have been used to study this problem, and all have yielded similar results: A causal relationship does exist between cigarette smoking and lung disease. Note that the combination of results from both experimental and quasiexperimental studies led to the conclusion that smoking causes lung disease because the studies together meet the causal criteria of relationship, timing, and lack of an alternative explanation.

The tobacco industry has argued that because the studies on humans are not true experiments, another explanation is possible for the relationships that have been found. For example, these relationships suggest that the tendency to smoke is linked to the tendency for lung disease to develop, and smoking is merely an unimportant intervening variable. The reader needs to review the evidence from studies to determine whether the cause-and-effect relationship postulated is believable.

Evidence-Informed Practice Tip ___

Findings from studies with experimental designs are considered level II evidence, and those from studies with quasiexperimental designs are considered level III evidence. Quasiexperimental designs are lower on the hierarchy of evidence because of a lack of a research control, which limits the ability to establish confident cause-and-effect statements that influence clinical decision making.

EVALUATION RESEARCH AND EXPERIMENTATION

As the science of nursing expands and the cost of health care rises, nurses and other health care professionals have become increasingly concerned with the ability to document the costs and the benefits of nursing care (see Chapter 1). This task is a complex process, but at its heart is the ability to evaluate or measure the outcomes of nursing care to inform health care decision making. Such studies usually are associated with quality assurance, quality improvement, and evaluation. Studies of evaluation or quality assurance do exactly what the name implies: They are concerned with the determination of the quality of nursing and health care and with the assurance that the public is receiving high-quality care.

Quality assurance and quality improvement in nursing are current and important topics for nursing care. Many early studies of quality assurance documented whether nursing care met predetermined standards. The goal of quality improvement studies is to evaluate the effectiveness of nursing interventions and to provide direction for further improvement in the achievement of quality clinical outcomes and cost effectiveness.

Evaluation research is the use of scientific research methods and procedures to evaluate a program, treatment, practice, or policy. In evaluation research, analytical means are used to document the worth of an activity such as an intervention, but such research is not a different

design. Both experimental and quasiexperimental designs (as well as nonexperimental designs) are used to determine the effect or outcomes of a program. When these designs are used in evaluating a program, the term *evaluation research* is used. Bigman (1961) listed the following purposes and uses of evaluation research:

1. To discover whether and how well the objectives are being fulfilled
2. To determine the reasons for specific successes and failures
3. To direct the course of the experiment with techniques for its effectiveness
4. To reveal principles that underlie a successful program
5. To base further research on the reasons for the relative success of alternative techniques
6. To redefine the means to be used for attaining objectives and to redefine subgoals in view of research findings

According to Clarke (2001), the following four levels of evaluation research are being highlighted in health care, especially nursing research: evaluation of the effectiveness of clinical interventions; evaluation of the effect of new ways of delivering health care; evaluation of structured programs aimed at specific patient groups; and evaluation of the quality of service. In many evaluation research studies, investigators use mixed methods, with both quantitative and qualitative information.

Evaluation studies may be either formative or summative. In **formative evaluation,** a program is assessed as it is being implemented; usually, the focus is on evaluation of the process of a program rather than the outcomes. In **summative evaluation,** the outcomes of a program are assessed after completion of the initial program.

Kuehn and colleagues (2011) used a summative evaluation to assess the effect of a North American nursing exchange program on student cultural awareness. In contrast, Jurasek and associates (2010) used formative evaluation to describe the collaborative development of an adolescent epilepsy transition clinic (i.e., for transition to adult care). They conducted a process evaluation (1) to gather information on whether the learning needs of the adolescents were met, (2) to demonstrate decreased fear associated with the transition, (3) to prepare parents for the expectations and differences of the adult program, and (4) to determine whether nurses were appropriate program leaders. Data were collected at the end of transition and 2 to 3 months into adult transition. Knowledge related to summative (outcomes) and formative (process) evaluation of programs is important in translating research into clinical practice.

The use of experimental and quasiexperimental designs in studies of quality improvement and

evaluation enables researchers to determine not only whether care is adequate but also which method of care is best under certain conditions. Furthermore, such studies can be used to determine whether a particular type of nursing care or intervention is cost effective: that is, that the care or intervention does what it is intended to do but at lower or equivalent cost. Cost studies are usually incorporated into the evaluation of an intervention. For example, Steel-O'Connor and associates (2003) evaluated the effects of programs of follow-up care by public health nurses in terms of infant health problems, breast-feeding rates, and the use of postpartum health services in Ontario. The authors compared the costs associated with routine home visiting by a public health nurse after early obstetrical discharge with the costs associated with a screening telephone

APPRAISING THE EVIDENCE

Experimental and Quasiexperimental Designs

As discussed earlier in the chapter, various designs for research studies differ in the amount of control the researcher has over the antecedent and intervening variables that may affect the results of the study. True experimental designs, which yield level II evidence, offer the most possibility for control, whereas nonexperimental designs, which yield level IV, V, or VI evidence, offer the least. Quasiexperimental designs, which yield level III evidence, offer somewhere in between. Research designs must balance the needs for internal validity and external validity in order to produce useful results. In addition, judicious use of design requires that the chosen design be appropriate to the problem, free of bias, and capable of answering the research question.

Questions that you should pose when reading studies that test cause-and-effect relationships are listed in the Critiquing Criteria box. All of these questions should help you judge, with confidence, whether a causal relationship exists.

For studies in which either experimental or quasiexperimental designs are used, first try to determine the type of design that was used. Often, a statement

describing the design of the study appears in the abstract and in the "Methods" section of the article. If such a statement is not present, the reader should examine the study for evidence of the following three characteristics: control, randomization, and manipulation. If all are discussed, the design is probably experimental. Conversely, if the study involves the administration of an experimental treatment but does not involve the random assignment of participants to groups, the design is quasiexperimental. Next, try to identify which of the variations within these two types of designs was used. Determining the answer to these questions gives you a head start because inherent in each design are particular threats to validity, and this step makes it easier to critically evaluate the study. The next question to ask is whether the researcher required a solution to a cause-and-effect problem. If so, the study is suited to these designs. Finally, think about the conduct of the study in the setting. Is it realistic to think that the study could be conducted in a clinical setting without some contamination?

The most important question to ask as you read experimental studies is "What else could have

APPRAISING THE EVIDENCE

Experimental and Quasiexperimental Designs—cont'd

happened to explain the findings?" Thus, the author must provide adequate accounts of how the procedures for randomization, control, and manipulation were carried out. The study should include a description of the procedures for random assignment to such a degree that the reader can determine the likelihood for any one participant to be assigned to a particular group. The description of the independent variable also should be detailed. The inclusion of this information helps the reader decide whether the treatment given to some participants in the experimental group might differ from what was given to others in the same group. In addition, threats to validity, such as testing effects and mortality (attrition), should be addressed. Otherwise, the conclusions of the study could potentially be erroneous and less believable to the reader.

This question of potential alternative explanations or threats to internal validity for the findings is even more important when you critically evaluate a quasiexperimental study because these study designs cannot possibly control for many plausible alternative explanations. A well-written report of a quasiexperimental study systematically reviews potential threats to the validity of the findings. Then your work as the reader is to decide whether the author's explanations make sense. When critiquing evaluation research, you should look for a careful description of the program, policy, procedure, or treatment being evaluated. In addition, you may need to determine the design used to evaluate the program and assess the appropriateness of the design for the evaluation. Once you have discerned the design, you assess threats to validity for the appropriate design in determining the appropriateness of the author's conclusions in relation to the outcomes. As with all research, the results of studies with these designs need to be generalizable to a larger population of people than was actually studied. Thus, researchers need to decide whether the experimental protocol eliminated some potential participants and whether this weakness affected not only internal validity but also external validity.

CRITIQUING CRITERIA

1. What design is used in the study?
2. Is the design experimental or quasiexperimental?
3. Is the problem one of a cause-and-effect relationship?
4. Is the method used appropriate to the problem?
5. Is the design suited to the setting of the study?

EXPERIMENTAL DESIGNS

1. What experimental design is used in the study, and is it appropriate?
2. How are randomization, control, and manipulation applied?
3. Are there reasons to believe that alternative explanations exist for the findings?

4. Are all threats to validity, including mortality (attrition), addressed in the report?
5. Whether the experiment was conducted in the laboratory or a clinical setting, are the findings generalizable to the larger population of interest?

QUASIEXPERIMENTAL DESIGNS

1. What quasiexperimental design is used in the study, and is it appropriate?
2. What are the most common threats to the validity of the findings of this design?
3. What are the plausible alternative explanations, and have they been addressed?
4. Are the author's explanations of threats to validity acceptable?
5. What does the author say about the limitations of the study?

6. Do other limitations related to the design exist that are not mentioned?

EVALUATION RESEARCH

1. Do the authors identify a specific problem, practice, policy, or treatment that they will evaluate?
2. Do the authors identify the outcomes to be evaluated?
3. Is the problem analyzed and described?
4. Is the program to be analyzed described and standardized?
5. Do the authors identify the measurement of the degree of change (outcome) that occurs?
6. Do the authors determine whether the observed outcome is related to the activity or to one or more other causes?

call. Steel-O'Connor and associates found that the direct, indirect, and total costs of health services per 100 infants were greater with home visits and concluded that a routine home visit is not always necessary to identify women who need that service. In an era of health care reform and cost containment for health expenditures, evaluating the relative costs and benefits of new programs of care is increasingly important. Relatively few studies in nursing and medicine have been dedicated to such evaluation, but in terms of outcomes, nursing costs and cost savings are important in future studies.

Helpful Hint

Think of quality assurance and quality improvement projects as research-related activities that enhance the ability of nurses to generate cost and quality outcome data. These outcome data contribute to documenting the effectiveness of nursing practice.

CRITICAL THINKING CHALLENGES

- Discuss the barriers to nurse researchers in meeting the three criteria of a true experimental design.
- How is it possible to have a research design that includes an experimental treatment intervention and a control group and yet is not considered a true experimental study? How does this affect the usefulness of the findings in an evidence-informed practice?
- Argue your case for supporting or not supporting the following claim: "The fact that true experimental design is not used does not decrease the value of the study, even though it may decrease the utility of the findings in practice." Include examples with your rationale.
- Respond to the following question: Why are experimental studies considered the best evidence for an evidence-informed practice model? Justify your answer.

KEY POINTS

- Experimental designs or randomized clinical trials provide the strongest evidence (level II) in terms of whether an intervention or treatment affects patient outcomes.
- Two types of design commonly used in nursing research to test hypotheses about cause-and-effect relationships are experimental and quasiexperimental designs. Both are useful for the development of nursing knowledge because they test the effects of nursing actions and lead to the development of prescriptive theory.
- True experiments are characterized by the ability of the researcher to control extraneous variation, manipulate the independent variable, and randomly assign participants to research groups.
- Experiments conducted in clinical settings or in the laboratory provide the best evidence in support of a causal relationship because the following three criteria can be met: (1) the independent and dependent variables are related to each other; (2) the independent variable chronologically precedes the dependent variable; and (3) the relationship cannot be explained by the presence of a third variable.
- Researchers frequently use quasiexperimental designs to test cause-and-effect relationships because experimental designs are often impractical or unethical.
- Quasiexperiments may lack either randomization or the comparison group, or both, which are characteristics of true experiments. Their usefulness in studying causal relationships depends on the ability of the researcher to rule out plausible threats to the validity of the findings, such as history, selection bias, and maturation and testing effects.
- The level of evidence (level III) provided by quasiexperimental designs weakens confidence that the findings were the result of the intervention rather than extraneous variables.
- The overall purpose of critiquing such studies is to assess the validity of the findings and to determine whether these findings are worth incorporating into the nurse's personal practice.

REFERENCES

Bigman, S. K. (1961). Evaluating the effectiveness of religious programs. *Review of Religious Research*, *2*, 99-110.

Campbell, D., & Stanley, J. (1966). *Experimental and quasiexperimental designs for research*. Chicago: Rand-McNally.

Clarke, A. (2001). Evaluation research in nursing and health care. *Nurse Researcher*, *8*(3), 4-14.

Ducharme, F., Lebel, P., Lachance, L., & Trudeau, D. (2006). Implementation and effects of an individual stress management intervention for family caregivers of an elderly relative living at home: A mixed research design. *Research in Nursing & Health*, *29*, 427-441.

Jurasek, L., Ray, L., & Quigley, D. (2010). Development and implementation of an adolescent epilepsy transition clinic. *Journal of Neuroscience Nursing*, *42*(4), 181-189.

Kuehn, A. F., Chircop, A., Downe-Wamboldt, B., Sheppard-LeMoine, D., Wittstock, L., Herbert, R., . . . Critchley, K. (2011). Evaluating the impact of a North American nursing exchange program on student cultural awareness. *International Journal of Nursing Education Scholarship*, *8*(1), Article 4.

LeMay, S., Johnston, C., Choinière, M., Fortin, C., Hubert, I., Fréchette, G., . . . Murray, L. (2010). Pain management interventions with parents in the emergency department: A randomized trial. *Journal of Advanced Nursing*, *66*, 2442-2449.

Martinez, A. M., D'Artois, D., & Rennick, J. E. (2007). Does the 15-minute (or less) family interview influence family nursing practice? *Journal of Family Nursing*, *13*(2), 157-178.

McGilton, K. S., O'Brien-Pallas, L. L., Darlington, G., Evans, M., Wynn, F., & Pringle, D. M. (2003). Effects of a relationship-enhancing program of care on outcomes. *Journal of Nursing Scholarship*, *35*, 151-156.

Moore, K. N., Hunter, K. F., McGinnis, R., Bacsu, C., Fader, M., Gray, M., . . . Voaklander, D. (2009). Do catheter washouts extend patency time in long-term indwelling urethral catheters? A randomized controlled trial of acidic washout solution, normal saline washout, or standard care. *Journal of Wound Ostomy Continence Nursing*, *39*(1), 82-90.

Ploeg, J., Brazil, K., Hutchison, B., Kaczorowski, J., Dalby, D. M., Goldsmith, C. H., & Furlong, C. (2010). Effect of preventive primary care outreach on health related quality of life among older adults at risk of functional decline: Randomised controlled trial. *British Medical Journal*, *340*, c1480. doi:101136.bmj.c1480

Sobieraj, G., Bhatt, M., LeMay, S., Rennick, J., & Johnston, C. (2009). The effect of music on parental participation during pediatric laceration repair. *Canadian Journal of Nursing Research*, *41*, 68-82.

Steel-O'Connor, K. O., Mowat, D. L., Scott, H. M., Carr, P. A., Dorland, J. L., & Young-Tai, K. F. (2003). A randomized trial of two public health nurse follow-up programs after early discharge. *Canadian Journal of Public Health*, *94*, 98-103.

Tranmer, J. E., & Parry, M. J. E. (2004). Enhancing postoperative recovery of cardiac surgery patients: A randomized clinical trial of an advanced practice nursing intervention. *Western Journal of Nursing Research*, *26*, 515-532.

Warren, S., Ross-Kerr, J., Smith, D., & Godkin, D. (2003). The impact of adult day programs on family caregivers of elderly relatives. *Journal of Community Health Nursing*, *20*(4), 209-221.

Weinrich, S. P., Seger, R., Curtsinger, T., Pumphrey, G., NeSmith, E. G., & Weinrich, M. (2007). Impact of pretest on posttest knowledge scores with a Solomon four research design. *Cancer Nursing*, *30*, E16-E28.

FOR FURTHER STUDY

⊖volve Go to Evolve at http://evolve.elsevier.com/Canada/LoBiondo/Research for Audio Glossary, how-to instructions for Writing Proposals for Funding, and additional research articles for practice in reviewing and critiquing.

CHAPTER 11

Nonexperimental Designs

Geri LoBiondo-Wood | Judith Haber | Mina D. Singh

LEARNING OUTCOMES

After reading this chapter, you will be able to do the following:

- Describe the overall purpose of nonexperimental designs.
- Describe the characteristics of survey and relationship/difference designs.
- Define the differences between survey and relationship/difference designs.
- List the advantages and disadvantages of surveys and each type of relationship/difference design.
- Identify methodological, secondary analysis, and meta-analysis research.
- Identify the purposes of methodological, secondary analysis, and meta-analysis research.
- Discuss relational inferences versus causal inferences as they relate to nonexperimental designs.
- Identify the criteria used to critique nonexperimental research designs.
- Apply the critiquing criteria to the evaluation of nonexperimental research designs as they appear in research reports.
- Apply levels of evidence to nonexperimental designs.

KEY TERMS

cohort
correlational study
cross-sectional study
descriptive/exploratory survey
developmental study
epidemiological study
ex post facto study
hierarchical linear modelling (HLM)

incidence
longitudinal study
meta-analysis
methodological research
nonexperimental research design
prediction study
prevalence

prospective study
psychometrics
relationship/difference study
retrospective data
retrospective study
secondary analysis
survey study

STUDY RESOURCES

Go to Evolve at http://evolve.elsevier.com/Canada/LoBiondo/Research for Audio Glossary, how-to instructions for Writing Proposals for Funding, and additional research articles for practice in reviewing and critiquing.

MANY PHENOMENA OF INTEREST AND RELEVANCE to nursing do not lend themselves to an experimental design. For example, nurses studying pain may be interested in knowing the amount of pain, variations in the amount of pain, and patients' responses to postoperative pain. The investigator would not design an experimental study that would potentially intensify a patient's pain just to study the pain experience; that would be unethical. Instead, the researcher would use a nonexperimental design to examine the factors that contribute to the variability in a patient's postoperative pain experience. Nonexperimental research designs are used in studies when the researcher wishes to construct a picture of a phenomenon; examine events, people, or situations as they naturally occur; or test relationships and differences among variables. Nonexperimental designs may enable the researcher to understand how a phenomenon occurs at one point or over a period of time.

In experimental research, the independent variable is manipulated; in a **nonexperimental research design,** the independent variable is not manipulated. In nonexperimental research, the independent variables have occurred naturally, and the investigator cannot directly control them by manipulation. In contrast, in an experimental design, the researcher actively manipulates one or more variables. The researcher in a nonexperimental design explores relationships or differences among the variables. Nonexperimental research requires a clear, concise research problem or hypothesis that is based on a theoretical framework. Even though the researcher does not actively manipulate the variables, the concepts of control (see Chapter 9) should be considered as much as possible.

Researchers do not agree on how to classify nonexperimental studies. A continuum of quantitative research designs is shown in Figure 11-1. This chapter divides nonexperimental designs into *survey studies* and *relationship/difference studies,* as illustrated in Box 11-1. These categories are flexible; nonexperimental studies may be classified in a different way in other sources. Some studies belong exclusively to one of these categories, whereas other studies have the characteristics of more than one category or more than one design label. As you read the research literature, you will often find that researchers who are conducting a nonexperimental study use several design classifications. This chapter introduces the various types of nonexperimental designs, their advantages and disadvantages, the use of nonexperimental research, the issues of causality, and the critiquing process as it relates to nonexperimental research. The Critical Thinking Decision Path outlines the path to the choice of a nonexperimental design.

Evidence-Informed Practice Tip

When you critically appraise nonexperimental studies, be aware of possible sources of bias that can be introduced at any point in the study.

BOX 11-1

SUMMARY OF NONEXPERIMENTAL RESEARCH DESIGNS

SURVEY STUDIES
- Descriptive
- Exploratory
- Comparative

RELATIONSHIP/DIFFERENCE STUDIES
- Correlational
- Developmental
  - Cross-sectional
  - Longitudinal or prospective
  - Retrospective or ex post facto

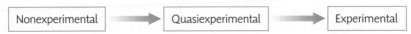

FIGURE 11-1 Continuum of quantitative research designs.

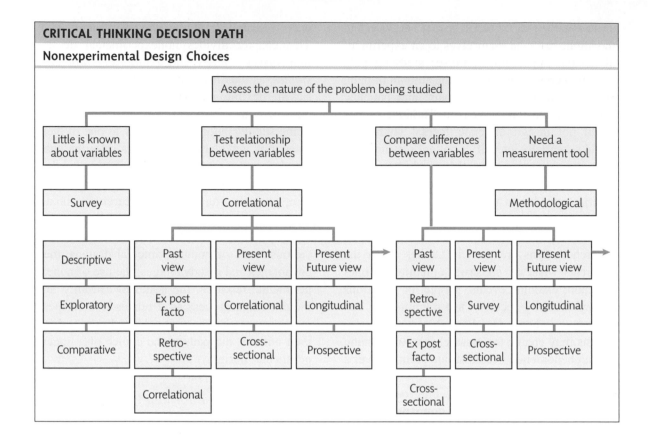

CRITICAL THINKING DECISION PATH

Nonexperimental Design Choices

SURVEY STUDIES

The broadest category of nonexperimental designs is the survey study. In a **survey study**—further classified as *descriptive, exploratory,* or *comparative*—detailed descriptions of existing variables are collected, and the data are used to justify and assess current conditions and practices or to make more plans for improving health care practices. When you read research, you will find that the terms *exploratory, descriptive, comparative,* and *survey* may be used either alone, inter-changeably, or together to describe the design of a study (see Table 11-1). For example, investigators may use a **descriptive/exploratory survey** to search for accurate information about the characteristics of particular participants, groups, institutions, or situations or about the frequency of a phenomenon's occurrence, particularly when

little is known about the phenomenon. The data are used to justify or assess current conditions or to make plans for improvement of conditions. Qualitative researchers also use the term *descriptive* in their reports, as in the study by Chojecki and colleagues (2010), who used a qualitative/descriptive design to explore the perceptions of a peer learning approach to paediatric clinical education. You will be able to determine the difference by checking in the analysis and findings sections, inasmuch as the qualitative descriptive study entails the use of the analyses outlined in Chapter 16, whereas the descriptive correlational or survey studies entail the use of descriptive and inferential statistical analyses.

In survey studies, the types of variables of interest can be classified as opinions, attitudes, or facts. For example, Sawhney and Sawyer (2008) conducted a cross-sectional study in which they used e-mailed surveys to explore and describe the role of nurses working in a specialty practice of pain management. The results of this study build on previous work in which the role of nurses in pain management was examined. Respondents to the survey reported several benefits and challenges to the role of these nurses. In another example, to explore nurses' perceptions of and level of satisfaction with the system of medication administration in long-term care, surveys were given to 301 licensed nurses (Kaasalainen, Agarwal, Dolovich, Papaioannou, Brazil, Akhtar-Danash, 2010).

Fact variables include attributes of individuals such as gender, income level, political and religious affiliations, ethnicity, occupation, and educational level. Koren and associates (2010) used the data from the annual tracking surveys of nurse practitioners in Ontario conducted by the Centre for Rural and Northern Health Research for the Ministry of Health and Long-term Care to describe current employment and practice.

Data in survey research can be collected through a questionnaire or an interview (see Chapter 13). For example, Yonge and colleagues (2010) administered a Web-based questionnaire to examine the willingness of nursing students to volunteer during a pandemic. Another example is the study by Hoe Harwood and associates (2010), who used an online national survey to describe nontraditional, "innovative" clinical placements within Canadian nursing education programs from the perspectives of clinical placement coordinators and nurse educators.

Survey researchers study either small or large samples of participants recruited from defined populations. The sample can be either broad or narrow and can be made up of people or institutions. For example, if a primary care rehabilitation unit based on a case-management model were to be established in a hospital, researcher might survey prospective applicants' attitudes with regard to case management before the unit staff members were selected. In a broader example, if a hospital were contemplating converting all patient care units to a case-management model, a survey might be conducted to determine the attitudes of a representative sample of nurses in the hospital toward case management. The data might provide the basis for projecting the in-service needs of nursing with regard to case management. The scope and depth of a survey are a function of the nature of the problem.

In surveys, investigators attempt only to relate one variable to another or to assess differences between variables; they do not attempt to determine causation. The two major advantages of surveys are the great deal of information that can be obtained from a large population in a more economical manner than face-to-face interviews and the surprising accuracy of survey research information. If a sample is representative of the population (see Chapter 12), a relatively small number of participants can accurately represent the views of the population.

However, survey studies have several disadvantages. First, the information obtained in a survey tends to be superficial. The breadth rather than the depth of the information is emphasized. Second, conducting a survey requires a great deal of expertise in various research areas. The survey

Helpful Hint
Research consumers should recognize that a well-constructed survey can provide a wealth of data about a particular phenomenon of interest, even though causation is not being examined.

Evidence-Informed Practice Tip
Evidence obtained from a survey population may be coupled with clinical expertise and applied to a similar population to develop an educational program to enhance knowledge and skills in a particular clinical area. For example, a survey designed to measure nursing staff's knowledge and attitudes about evidence-informed practice may yield data that are used to develop a staff development course in evidence-informed practice.

investigator must have skills in sampling techniques, questionnaire construction, interviewing, and data analysis to elicit reliable and valid data. Third, large-scale surveys can be time consuming and costly, although the use of on-site personnel can reduce costs.

RELATIONSHIP/DIFFERENCE STUDIES

Investigators endeavour to trace the relationships or differences between variables that can provide a deeper insight into a phenomenon. This type of study can be classified as a **relationship/difference study.** The following types of relationship/difference studies are discussed: *correlational studies* and *developmental studies.*

Correlational Studies

In a **correlational study,** an investigator examines the relationship between two or more variables. The researcher is not testing whether one variable causes another variable or how different one variable is from another variable. Instead, the researcher is testing whether the variables covary; in other words, as one variable changes, does a related change occur in the other variable? The researcher using this design is interested in quantifying the strength of the relationship between the variables or in testing a hypothesis about a specific relationship. The positive or negative direction of the relationship is also a central concern (see Chapter 16 for an explanation of the correlation between variables).

In their correlational study, Bailey and colleagues (2010) explored family member perception of informational support, anxiety, satisfaction with care, and their interrelationships to guide further refinement of a local informational support initiative. These researchers were not testing a cause-and-effect relationship.

Another example of correlational research was the study by Armstrong and associates (2009), who tested a theoretical model derived from Rosabeth Moss Kanter's theory of workplace empowerment. They found that total empowerment was most strongly related to management leadership ability and nurse participation in hospital affairs and least strongly to collaborative nurse-physician relationships.

Correlational studies offer researchers and research consumers the following advantages:

- An increased flexibility when investigating complex relationships among variables
- An efficient and effective method of collecting a large amount of data about a problem
- A potential for practical application in clinical settings
- A potential foundation for future experimental research studies
- A framework for exploring the relationship between variables that cannot be inherently manipulated

The correlational design has a quality of realism and is particularly appealing because it suggests the potential for practical solutions to clinical problems. The following, however, are the disadvantages of correlational studies:

- Inability to manipulate the variables of interest
- No randomization in the sampling procedures, because the study deals with preexisting groups; therefore, generalizability is decreased
- Inability to determine a causal relationship between the variables because of the lack of manipulation, control, and randomization

One of the most common misuses of a correlational design is the researcher's conclusion that a causal relationship exists between the variables. In their study, Bailey and colleagues (2010) appropriately concluded that informational support was positively correlated significantly with satisfaction with care. The report concluded with some very thoughtful recommendations for future studies in this area by stating that representativeness could be improved through probability sampling and sample size if a quasiexperimental study was to be conducted.

Correlational studies may be further labelled *descriptive correlational* or *predictive correlational*. A study by Plunkett and colleagues (2010) is an example of a predictive correlational study. The goal was to predict whether the intention of generic BScN students to further pursue graduate studies is influenced by their valuation of graduate studies and perceived self-efficacy for graduate studies. The researchers concluded that several of the variables were predictive of (did not cause) intention to pursue graduate studies.

The inability to draw causal statements should not lead you to conclude that a nonexperimental correlational study has a weak design. In terms of evidence for practice, researchers—on the basis of the literature review and their findings—frame the utility of the results in view of previous research and therefore help establish supportive evidence of the applicability of the results to a specific patient population. A correlational design is very useful for clinical research studies because many of the phenomena of clinical interest are beyond the researcher's ability to manipulate, control, and randomize.

Developmental Studies

Nonexperimental designs in which a time perspective is used can be further subclassified. A **developmental study** is concerned not only with the existing status and the relationship and differences among phenomena at one point in time but also with changes that occur as a function of time. The following three types of developmental study designs are discussed here: *cross-sectional*, *longitudinal* or *prospective*, and *retrospective* or *ex post facto*. Remember that in the literature, studies may be designated by more than one design name. This practice is accepted because many studies have elements of several nonexperimental designs. Table 11-1 provides examples of studies classified with more than one design label.

TABLE 11-1

EXAMPLES OF STUDIES WITH MORE THAN ONE DESIGN LABEL

DESIGN TYPE	STUDY'S PURPOSE
Descriptive with repeated measures	To determine whether there are psychosocial and physical benefits of a self-awareness intervention for adults with type 1 diabetes and hypoglycaemia (Hernandez, Hume, & Rodger, 2008)
Descriptive, correlational	To examine the associations between depression and work-related variables such as job strain, role overload, respect, social and employer supports, and nurses' perception of the quality of care they provide (Ohler, Kerr, & Forbes, 2010)
Cross-sectional, descriptive, correlational	To describe family member perception of informational support, anxiety, satisfaction with care, and their relationships, in order to guide further refinement of a local informational support initiative and its eventual evaluation (Bailey, Sabbagh, Loiselle, Boileau, & McVey, 2010)
Explanatory, correlational	To determine the stressors, academic performance, and learned resourcefulness in baccalaureate nursing students (Goff, 2011)
Retrospective, cross-sectional	To explore experiences of refugee and refugee claimant mothers with an ill preschooler on equitable access to health care (Wahoush, 2009)
Prospective, cohort	To assess for anemia and red blood cell transfusion practices in 100 consecutive adults admitted to a general systems intensive care unit (Thomas, Jensen, Nahirniak, & Gibney, 2010)

Cross-Sectional Studies

In a **cross-sectional study,** researchers examine data at one time; in other words, the data are collected on only one occasion with the same participants rather than with the same participants at several times.

An example of a cross-sectional study is provided by Richard and associates (2010), who explored patient satisfaction in ambulatory cancer care. Another cross-sectional study approach is to simultaneously collect data on the study's variables from different **cohort** (participants) groups. An example of a cross-sectional study with different cohort groups was conducted by Fox and colleagues (2010), who used a naturalistic cohort design to determine the relationship between bed rest and orthostatic intolerance of sitting in adults residing in chronic care facilities. Cohorts represented different amounts of bed rest that were occurring naturally: "no bed rest," "two to four days" of bed rest, and "five to seven days" of bed rest. In cross-sectional studies, researchers can investigate relationships and correlations, differences and comparisons, or both. For instance, Fox and colleagues (2010) posed research questions that allowed the researchers to investigate both differences and relationships among and between variables.

Evidence-Informed Practice Tip

Replication of significant findings in nonexperimental studies, with similar or different populations or both, increases your confidence in the conclusions offered by the researcher and the strength of evidence generated by consistent findings from more than one study.

Longitudinal or Prospective Studies

In contrast to the cross-sectional design, the **longitudinal study** or **prospective study** (also referred to as *repeated-measures* studies) collects data from the same group at different times. Researchers also use longitudinal studies to explore differences and relationships. For example, the investigator conducting a study with children with diabetes could use a longitudinal design. In that case, the investigator could collect yearly data or monitor the same children over a number of years to compare changes in the variables at different ages. By collecting data from each participant at yearly intervals, the investigator obtains a longitudinal perspective of the diabetic process.

In another example of a longitudinal study, Voyer and associates (2005) collected data from a sample of 138 older adults. The purpose of the study was to describe the mental health status of long-term users of benzodiazepines and to compare their status with the mental health of older adults who have either begun or stopped consuming benzodiazepines over a 1-year period.

Cross-sectional and longitudinal designs have many advantages and disadvantages. When assessing the appropriateness of a cross-sectional study versus a longitudinal study, the research consumer should first assess the researcher's goal in view of the theoretical framework. For example, in a hypothetical study of infant colic, the researchers are investigating a developmental process; therefore, a longitudinal design seems more appropriate. However, the disadvantages inherent in a longitudinal design also must be considered. The period of data collection may be long because of the time the participants take to progress to each data-collection point. In the infant colic study, it might take the researchers between 12 and 18 months to collect the data from the total sample. Threats to internal validity, such as testing and attrition also are ever present and unavoidable in a longitudinal study (see Chapter 16). As a result, longitudinal designs are costly in terms of time, effort, and money. Moreover, confounding variables could affect the interpretation of the results. Participants in these studies may respond in a socially desirable way that they believe is congruent with the investigators' expectations (see the discussion of the Hawthorne effect in Chapter 9).

Despite the pragmatic constraints imposed by a longitudinal study, the researcher should proceed with this design if the theoretical framework supports a longitudinal developmental perspective. The advantages of a longitudinal study are that participants are monitored separately and thereby serve as their own controls; an increased depth of responses can be obtained; and early trends in the data can be analyzed. The researcher can assess changes in the variables of interest over time and explore both relationships and differences between variables.

Cross-sectional studies, in comparison with longitudinal studies, are less time consuming and less expensive and are thus more manageable for the researcher. Because large amounts of data can be collected at one time, the results are more readily available. In addition, the confounding variable of maturation, which results from the passage of time, is not present. However, the investigator's ability to establish an in-depth developmental assessment of the interrelationships of the phenomena being studied is reduced. Thus, the researcher is unable to determine whether the change that occurred is related to the change that was predicted because the same participants were not monitored over a period of time. In other words, the participants are unable to serve as their own controls (see Chapter 10).

In summary, longitudinal studies begin in the present and end in the future, and cross-sectional studies encompass a broader perspective of a cross-section of the population at one specific time.

Evidence-Informed Practice Tip

The quality of evidence provided by a longitudinal cohort study is stronger than that from other nonexperimental designs because the researcher can determine the incidence of a problem and its possible causes.

Retrospective or Ex Post Facto Studies

A **retrospective study** is essentially the same as an **ex post facto study.** Epidemiologists primarily use the term *retrospective,* whereas social scientists prefer the term *ex post facto.* In either case, the dependent variable has already been

affected by the independent variable, and the investigator attempts to link current events to past events.

When scientists wish to explain causality or the factors that determine the occurrence of events or conditions, they prefer to use an experimental design. However, they cannot always manipulate the independent variable or use random assignments. In cases in which experimental designs cannot be employed, ex post facto studies may be used. *Ex post facto* literally means "from after the fact." These studies also are known as *causal-comparative* studies or *comparative* studies. As this design is discussed further, you will see that ex post facto research is similar to quasiexperimental research because in both, differences between variables are examined (Campbell & Stanley, 1963).

In retrospective studies, a researcher hypothesizes, for example, that variable X (cigarette smoking) is related to and a determinant of variable Y (lung cancer), but $X,$ the presumed cause, is not manipulated, and participants are not randomly assigned to groups. Instead, the researcher chooses a group of participants who have experienced X (cigarette smoking) in a normal situation and a control group of participants who have not experienced $X.$ The behaviours, performances, or conditions (lung tissue) of the two groups are compared in order to determine whether the exposure to X had the effect predicted by the hypothesis. Table 11-2 illustrates this example and reveals that although cigarette smoking

TABLE **11-2**

PARADIGM FOR THE EX POST FACTO DESIGN		
GROUPS (NOT RANDOMLY ASSIGNED)	**INDEPENDENT VARIABLE (NOT MANIPULATED BY INVESTIGATOR)**	**DEPENDENT VARIABLE**
Exposed group: cigarette smokers	X: cigarette smoking	Y_e: lung cancer
Control group: nonsmokers		Y_c: no lung cancer

appears to be a determinant of lung cancer, the researcher is still not able to conclude that a causal relationship exists between the variables because the independent variable has not been manipulated and the participants were not randomly assigned to groups.

Another example of a retrospective study is that of Tourangeau and associates (2006), who were interested in the effect of the structures and processes of hospital nursing care on the rate of 30-day mortality among patients with acute medical conditions. Tourangeau and associates collected **retrospective data** (data that have already been recorded, such as scores on a standard examination) from several clinical and administrative secondary databases, which included the Ontario Hospital Insurance Plan, the Ontario Registered Persons Database, and the Ontario Hospital Reporting System (file 2002–2003). In self-reports, collected through the Ontario Nurses Survey 2003, nurses described the type of clinical unit in which they worked, their evaluation of patient care quality, their career intentions, their feelings of burnout, and many other work-related variables. The study revealed that 30-day mortality rates were lower in association with hospitals that had a higher percentage of registered nurse staff, a higher percentage of nurses with bachelor's degrees, more extensive use of care maps or protocols to guide patient care, and higher rates of burnout among nurses.

The advantages of the retrospective design are similar to those of the correlational design. The additional benefit of the retrospective design is that it offers a higher level of control than a correlational study. For example, in a cigarette smoking study, the lung tissue samples from non-smokers and smokers could be compared. This comparison would enable the researcher to establish the existence of a differential effect of cigarette smoking on lung tissue. However, the researcher would remain unable to draw a causal link between the two variables. This inability is the major disadvantage of the retrospective design.

Another disadvantage of retrospective research is that an alternative hypothesis may be the reason for the documented relationship. If the researcher obtains data from two existing groups of participants, such as one that has been exposed to X and one that has not, and the data support the hypothesis that X is related to Y, the researcher cannot be sure whether X or an extraneous variable is the cause of the occurrence of Y. Finding naturally occurring groups of participants who are similar in all ways except for their exposure to the variable of interest is very difficult. The possibility always exists that the groups differ in another way (e.g., in exposure to another lung irritant, such as asbestos), which can affect the findings of the study and produce spurious results. Consequently, when you read about such a study, you need to cautiously evaluate the conclusions drawn by the investigator.

> **Helpful Hint**_____
> When you read research reports, you will note that, at times, researchers classify a study's design with more than one design label. This classification is correct because research studies often reflect aspects of more than one design.

Longitudinal or prospective (cohort) studies are less common than retrospective studies because it can take a long time for the phenomenon of interest to become evident in a prospective study. For example, if researchers were studying pregnant women who regularly consume alcohol, it would take 9 months for the effect of low birth weight in the participants' infants to become evident. The problems inherent in a prospective study are therefore similar to those of a longitudinal study. However, longitudinal or prospective studies are considered stronger than retrospective studies because of the degree of control that can be imposed on extraneous variables that might confound the data.

PREDICTION AND CAUSALITY IN NONEXPERIMENTAL RESEARCH

Researchers and research consumers are concerned with the issues of prediction and causality in explaining cause-and-effect relationships. Historically, researchers have said that only experimental research can support the concept of causality. For example, nurses are interested in discovering what causes anxiety in many settings. If nurses can uncover the causes, they can perhaps develop interventions that would prevent or decrease the anxiety. Causality makes it necessary to order events chronologically; therefore, if nurses find in a randomized experiment that event 1 (stress) occurs before event 2 (anxiety) and that participants who experienced stress were anxious, whereas those in the unstressed group were not, then the hypothesis that stress causes anxiety is supported. If these results occurred in a nonexperimental study in which some participants underwent the stress of surgery and were anxious, whereas others did not have surgery and were not anxious, an association or relationship would be said to exist between stress (surgery) and anxiety. The results of a nonexperimental study, however, do not imply that the stress of surgery caused the anxiety.

Many variables (e.g., anxiety) that nurse researchers wish to study to explore causation cannot be manipulated, nor would it be wise to try to manipulate the variables. However, studies that can assert a predictive or causal sequence are needed. In view of this need, many nurse researchers use several analytical techniques that can explain the relationships among variables to establish predictive or causal links. These techniques are called *causal modelling* (see the Practical Application box), *model testing,* and *associated*

causal analysis (Kaplan, 2008; Schumacker & Lomax, 2004).

Practical Application

Samuels-Dennis and colleagues (2010) used causal modelling to validate a theoretical model that highlights the process through which posttraumatic stress disorder (PTSD) develops among women. The results revealed that mothers' strains and personal resources played a significant mediating role in the relationship between cumulative trauma and posttraumatic stress disorder.

You will also find the terms *path analysis, LISREL, analysis of covariance structures, structural equation modelling* (SEM), and ***hierarchical linear modelling*** (HLM) (Raudenbush & Bryk, 2002) used to describe the statistical techniques (see Chapter 16) used in these studies. An HLM is a type of regression analysis that allows for analysis of hierarchically structured data simultaneously at all levels (see the Practical Application box for an example of the use of HLM).

Practical Application

An example of HLM appeared in a study by Letourneau and associates (2009), who examined the influences of fathers' characteristics on the behavioural development of children who were exposed to maternal postpartum depression. The findings indicated that fathers' workforce participation in the first 2 years of a child's life has a long-term effect on the behavioural outcomes of children in families affected by postpartum depression.

In a **prediction study,** a model may be tested to assess which independent variables can best explain the one or more dependent variables in order to make a forecast or prediction derived from particular phenomena. For example, Linton and colleagues (2009) investigated the demographic predictors of human immunodeficiency virus (HIV) seropositivity status among homeless youth. Results indicated that there are relationships between age and HIV status and between ethnicity and HIV status, although not of a predictive nature. Goff (2011) conducted an explanatory correlational study to explore learned resourcefulness, stressors, and academic performance in baccalaureate nursing students. Goff found that levels of personal and academic stressors were evident but were not significant predictors of academic performance. Age was a significant predictor of academic performance.

In another example, Singh and Cameron (2005) tested a model for predicting the psychosocial effect of caring for patients who had experienced a stroke. The variables of the model were developed from a previous systematic study and further tested in this study. Singh and Cameron explained the development of the model and the premise of the study. The explanation enables readers of the study to clearly understand the purpose and aim of the research and the test of the model with regression analyses. Although Singh and Cameron did not test a cause-and-effect relationship between the chosen independent predictor variables and the dependent criterion variable, the study did demonstrate a theoretically meaningful model of how variables work together in a group in a particular situation.

Helpful Hint

Nonexperimental clinical research studies have progressed to the point at which prediction models are used to explore or test relationships between independent variables and dependent variables.

As nurse researchers develop their programs of research in a specific area, more tests of models will be available. The statistics used in model-testing studies are advanced, but the beginning research consumer should be able to read the article, understand the purpose of the study, and determine whether the model generated was logical and developed with a solid basis from the literature and past research. This section cites several studies in which researchers conducted sound tests of theoretical models.

A full description of the techniques and principles of causal modelling is beyond the scope of this text.

Evidence-Informed Practice Tip

Research studies that entail the use of nonexperimental designs and provide level IV evidence can build the foundation for a program of research that leads to experimental designs in which the effectiveness of nursing interventions can be tested.

ADDITIONAL TYPES OF QUANTITATIVE STUDIES

Other types of quantitative studies complement the science of research. These additional designs provide a means of viewing and interpreting phenomena to provide further breadth and knowledge to nursing science and practice. These types of quantitative studies are methodological research, meta-analysis, secondary analysis, and epidemiological studies.

Methodological Research

Methodological research is the development and evaluation of data-collection instruments, scales, and techniques. As noted in Chapters 13 and 14, methodology has a strong influence on research. The most significant and important aspect of methodological research addressed in measurement development is **psychometrics:** the theory and development of measurement instruments (such as questionnaires) and measurement techniques (such as observational techniques) through the research process. Thus, psychometrics is concerned with the measurement of a concept, such as anxiety or interpersonal conflict, with reliable and valid tools. (See Chapter 14 for a discussion of reliability and validity.)

Nurse researchers have used the principles of psychometrics to develop and test measurement instruments that focus on nursing phenomena.

Nurse researchers also use instruments developed in other disciplines, such as psychology and sociology, in which tools have been psychometrically tested. Sound measurement tools are critical for the reliability and validity of a study. A study's purpose, problems, and procedures may be clear, and the data analysis may be correct and consistent, but if the measurement tool has inherent psychometric problems, the findings will be rendered questionable or of limited utility.

The main problem for nurse researchers is locating appropriate measurement tools. Many of the phenomena of interest in nursing practice and research are intangible, such as interpersonal conflict, caring, coping, and maternal-fetal attachment. The intangible nature of various phenomena, and yet the need to measure them, places methodological research in an important position in research. Methodological research differs from other designs of research. First, it does not include all of the research process steps discussed in Chapter 2. Second, to implement methical research techniques, the researcher must have a sound knowledge of psychometrics or must consult with a researcher knowledgeable in psychometric techniques. The methodological researcher is not interested in the relationship of the independent variable to a dependent variable or in the effect of an independent variable on a dependent variable. Instead, the methodological researcher is interested in identifying an intangible construct (concept) and making it tangible with a paper-and-pencil instrument or observation protocol.

A methodological study includes the following steps:

- Defining the construct, or concept, or behaviour to be measured
- Formulating the tool's items
- Developing instructions for users and respondents
- Testing the tool's reliability and validity

A sound, specific, and exhaustive literature review is necessary to identify the theories underlying the steps in this construct. The literature review provides the basis of item formulation. Once the

items have been developed, the researcher assesses the tool's reliability and validity (see Chapter 14). Various aspects of these procedures may differ according to the tool's use, purpose, and stage of development.

In an example of methodological research, Watson and associates (2008) documented the psychometric properties of the Nurses' Attitudes Toward Obesity and Obese Patients Scale (NATOOPS).

Common considerations that researchers incorporate into methodological research are outlined in Table 11-3. Many more examples of methodological research can be found in the nursing research literature (Akhtar-Danesh, Valaitis, Schofield, Underwood, Martin-Misener, Baumann, Kolotylo, 2010; Roberts & Ward-Smith, 2010; Sidani, Epstein, Bootzin, Moritz, & Miranda, 2009; Ward-Griffin, Keefe, Martin-Matthews, Kerr, Brown, Oudshoom, 2009). Psychometric or methodological studies are found primarily in journals that report research. The *Journal of Nursing Measurement* is devoted to the publication of information on instruments, tools, and approaches for measurement of variables.

The specific procedures of methodological research are beyond the scope of this book, but you are urged to look closely at the tools used in studies.

Meta-analysis

Meta-analysis is a statistical technique, not a research design. It is based on a strict scientific approach in systematic reviews, in which the results of many studies in a specific area are synthesized and statistically summarized to formulate an overall conclusion. Each study is a unit of analysis. The goal is to read all of the studies concerning a particular clinical question and, using rigorous inclusion and exclusion criteria, to determine which studies are similar and to analyze their results, in order to quantify the effectiveness of the intervention under study. This method is more powerful because it is a rigorous process of summarizing evidence rather than estimating the

TABLE 11-3

COMMON CONSIDERATIONS IN THE DEVELOPMENT OF MEASUREMENT TOOLS

CONSIDERATION	COMMENT
The well-constructed scale, test, interview schedule, or other form of index should consist of an objective, standardized measure of samples of a behaviour that has been clearly defined. Observations should be made on a small but carefully chosen sampling of the behaviour of interest, thus creating confidence that the samples are representative.	A new tool should be based on a thorough review of previous theoretical and research literature to ensure validity.
The tool should be standardized; that is, a set of uniform items and response possibilities are uniformly administered and scored.	Without specific criteria and rating procedures, the evaluations of the items would be based on the subjective impressions, which may have varied significantly between observers and conditions.
The items of a measurement tool should be unambiguous; they should be clear-cut, concise, exact statements with only one idea per item. Negative stems or items with negatively phrased response possibilities result in ambiguity in meaning and scoring.	For example, in constructing a tool to measure job satisfaction, a nurse scientist writes the following item: "I never feel that I don't have time to provide good nursing care." The response format consists of "Agree," "Undecided," and "Disagree." A response of "Disagree" will likely not reflect the respondent's true intention because of the confusion that is created by the double-negative phrasing "never . . . don't."
The type of items used in any one test or scale should be restricted to a limited number of variations. Participants who are expected to shift from one kind of item to another may fail to provide a true response as a result of the distraction of making such a change.	Mixing true-or-false items with questions that require a yes-or-no response and items that provide a response format of five possible answers can lead to a high level of measurement error.
Items should not provide irrelevant clues. Unless carefully constructed, an item may furnish an indication of the expected response or answer. Furthermore, the correct answer or expected response to one item should not be given by another item.	An item that provides a clue to the expected answer may contain value words that convey cultural expectations, such as "A good wife enjoys caring for her home and family."
The items of a measurement tool should not be made difficult by requiring unnecessarily complex or exact operations. Furthermore, the difficulty of an item should be appropriate to the level of the participants being assessed. Limiting each item to one concept or idea helps accomplish this objective.	A test constructed to evaluate learning in an introductory course in research methods may contain an item that is inappropriate for the designated group, such as "A nonlinear transformation of data to linear data is a useful procedure before a hypothesis of curvilinearity is tested."
The diagnostic, predictive, or measurement value of a tool depends on the degree to which it serves as an indicator of a relatively broad and significant area of behaviour, known as the *universe of content* for the behaviour. As already emphasized, a behaviour must be clearly defined before it can be measured. The definition is developed from the universe of content: that is, the information and research findings that are available for the behaviour of interest. The items should reflect that definition. The extent to which the test items appear to accomplish this objective is an indication of the validity of the instrument.	Two nurse researchers are studying the construct of quality of life. Each nurse has defined this construct in a different way. Consequently, the measurement tool that each nurse devises will include different questions. The questions on each tool will reflect the universe of content for quality of life as defined by each researcher.
The instrument also should adequately cover the defined behaviour. The primary consideration is whether the number and nature of items in the sample are adequate. If the sample has too few items, the accuracy or reliability of the measure must be questioned. In general, the sample should have a minimum of 10 items for each independent aspect of the behaviour of interest.	For example, few people would be satisfied with an assessment of intelligence if the scale were limited to three items.
The measure must prove its worth empirically through tests of reliability and validity.	The researcher should demonstrate to the reader that the scale is accurate and measures what it purports to measure (see Chapter 14).

effect of the results derived from single studies alone. Johnston (2005) noted that the meta-analysis of a number of randomized clinical trials (RCTs) gives due weight to the sample size of the studies included and provides an estimate of treatment effect; in other words, a meta-analysis helps determine whether the intervention makes a difference. A systematic review provides the most powerful and useful evidence available to guide practice: level I evidence (see Chapter 3).

When you critically appraise a systematic review, some of the questions to consider are the following:

- Does the systematic review address a focused research question?
- Does the meta-analysis include specific inclusion and exclusion criteria for judging the studies?
- Does a publication bias exist?
- Are the included studies homogeneous in terms of purpose, sample, research methods?
- Are the designs of the studies similar?
- Are the interventions similar?
- Are the outcome measures similar?

Think about the systematic review as progressively sifting and sorting data until the highest quality of evidence is used to establish the conclusions. First, the researcher combines the results of all of the studies that focus on a specific question. The studies considered of lowest quality are then excluded, and the quality of the remaining studies are reanalyzed. The researcher repeats this process sequentially, excluding studies until only the studies of highest quality available are included in the analysis. An alteration in the overall results as an outcome of this sifting and sorting process suggests the sensitivity of the conclusions to the quality of the studies included in the meta-analysis.

Such considerations determine whether it is reasonable to combine the studies for analysis. The consumer of research should note that a researcher who conducts a meta-analysis does not conduct the original analysis of data in the area but instead synthesizes the data from already published studies by following a set of controlled and systematic steps. Systematic reviews with a meta-analysis can be used to synthesize results of both nonexperimental and experimental research studies.

Finally, evidence-informed practice requires that you, the research consumer, determine—on the basis of the strength and quality of the evidence provided by the results of the meta-analysis, coupled with your clinical expertise and patients' values—whether you would consider a change in practice. For example, in their meta-analysis, Edwards and associates (2004) addressed the clinical question "Do psychological interventions (education, individual cognitive-behavioural or psychotherapeutic programs, or group support) improve survival and psychological outcomes in women with metastatic breast cancer?" The results of the systematic review were reported as follows:

A search was conducted of published and unpublished RCTs in any language that assessed the effectiveness of psychological or psychosocial interventions in women with breast cancer. Data sources included the following: Cochrane Breast Cancer Group Trials Register, Cochrane Central Register of Controlled Trials, Medline, CINAHL, PsychINFO, and SIGLE; references of relevant studies and reviews; hand searches of relevant journals; and known authors in the field. Two reviewers assessed the quality of individual RCTs using the Jadad scale and another method score that was more relevant for trials of psychological interventions.

The main results of the systematic review indicate that five studies ($N = 636$) met the selection criteria; in two studies, cognitive-behavioural group interventions were assessed, and in three studies, supportive-expressive group therapy was assessed. Meta-analysis conducted with a fixed-effects model showed that rates of survival at 1, 5, or 10 years did not differ between participants receiving group psychological interventions and those receiving usual care. Cognitive-behavioural therapy also did not differ from the usual care with regard to anxiety (one trial), self-esteem (one trial), or mood state (one trial) at 6 months. Supportive expressive group therapy improved scores on the Courtauld Emotional Control scale at 8 months (one trial) and reduced reported pain, assessed on a 10-point visual analogue scale (meta-analysis of two trials; weighted mean difference in reduction of 0.75; 95% confidence interval, 0.63 to 0.86) in comparison with the usual care. The groups did not differ in mood states at 10 to 12 months (two trials) or in quality of life at 1 year (one trial). Edwards and associates (2004) concluded that existing data did not provide evidence of a survival benefit for women with metastatic breast cancer who received group psychological interventions over those who received the usual care. Evidence on the effects on various aspects of psychological functioning is mixed.

Systematic reviews in which results from multiple RCTs are combined offer stronger evidence (level I) in estimating the magnitude of an effect for an intervention (see Chapter 3, Figure 3-1). The strength of evidence provided by systematic reviews has become the foundation of evidence-informed practice.

Evidence-Informed Practice Tip

Evidence-informed practice methods, such as systematic reviews, increase a nurse's ability to manage the ever-increasing volume of information produced to develop the best practices that are evidence based.

Secondary Analysis

Secondary analysis also is not a design but a form of research in which the previously collected and analyzed data from one study are reanalyzed for a secondary purpose. The original study may be either an experimental or a nonexperimental design. For example, Schneider and colleagues (2011) conducted a secondary analysis to examine the psychosocial outcomes of the meaning of caregiving, self-esteem, optimism, burden, depression, spirituality, and posttraumatic stress in parents caring for children with a life-limiting illness. The original study was a cross-sectional, descriptive study focusing on the theoretical construct of posttraumatic growth. In another study, Robinson and Molzahn (2007) conducted a secondary analysis of Canadian data from a larger international study designed to develop and test a new module for the measurement of quality of life of older adults. Data were available from a convenience sample of 426 older adults in British Columbia. The purpose of the study was to explore the relationships between sexual activity and intimacy and the quality of life of older adults.

Epidemiological Studies

In an **epidemiological study,** factors affecting the health and illness of populations are examined in relation to the environment. The purview of public health for many years, epidemiological studies are investigations of the distribution, determinants, and dynamics of health and disease. In these studies, investigators attempt to link effects with cause; however, a clear understanding of the causes is often not possible, especially when the illness or problem has already occurred and the method is to look retrospectively at the evidence.

Some of the questions that epidemiological researchers attempt to answer are "Did exposure to a certain environment affect health?" and "Does staff shortage or organizational issues affect burnout?" Research cannot answer such questions directly but can establish a statistically significant association between exposure to causative factors and disease or the effects of ill health.

Two frequently conducted types of epidemiological studies are studies of **prevalence** (the number of people affected by a disease or health problem) and studies of **incidence** (the number of cases occurring in a particular period).

APPRAISING THE EVIDENCE

Nonexperimental Designs

The criteria for critiquing nonexperimental designs are presented in the Critiquing Criteria box. When you critique nonexperimental research designs, keep in mind that such designs offer the researcher the least amount of control. The first step in critiquing nonexperimental research is to determine which type of design was used in the study. Often, a statement describing the design of the study appears in the abstract and in the "Methods" section of the report. If such a statement is not present, you should closely examine the report for evidence of which type of design was employed. You should be able to discern that either a survey or a relationship design was used, as well as the specific subtype. For example, you would expect an investigation of self-concept development in children from birth to 5 years of age to be a relationship study with a longitudinal design.

Next, you should evaluate the theoretical framework and underpinnings of the study to determine whether a nonexperimental design was the most appropriate approach to the problem. For example, in many of the studies on pain discussed throughout this text, the relationship between pain and any of the independent variables under consideration cannot be manipulated. For such studies, a nonexperimental correlational, longitudinal, or cross-sectional design is appropriate. Investigators use one of these designs to examine the relationship between the variables in naturally occurring groups. Sometimes, you may think that it would have been more appropriate for the investigators to use an experimental or a quasiexperimental design. However, you must recognize that pragmatic or ethical considerations also may have guided the researchers in their choice of design (see Chapters 6 and 10).

You should assess whether the problem is at a level of experimental manipulation. Often, researchers merely wish to examine whether relationships exist between variables. Therefore, when you critique such studies, you should be able to determine the purpose of the study. If the purpose of the study does not include the expectation of a cause-and-effect relationship, you need not look for one. However, be wary when the researcher in a nonexperimental study suggests a cause-and-effect relationship in the findings.

Finally, the factor or factors that influence changes in the dependent variable are often ambiguous in nonexperimental designs. As with all complex phenomena, multiple factors can contribute to variability in the participants' responses. When an experimental design is not used for controlling some of these extraneous variables that can influence results, the researcher must strive to provide as much control of these variables as possible within the context of a nonexperimental design.

When it has not been possible to randomly assign participants to treatment groups as an approach to controlling an independent variable, the researcher may use a strategy of matching participants for identified variables. For example, in a study of birth weight, pregnant women could be matched with regard to variables such as weight, height, smoking habits, drug use, and other factors that might influence the birth weights of their infants. The independent variable of interest, such as the type of prenatal care, would then be the major difference in the groups. You would then feel more confident that the only difference between the two groups was the differential effect of the independent variable because the other factors in the two groups were theoretically the same. However, you should also remember that other influential variables—such as income, education, and diet—might have been present but were not considered in matching. Threats to internal and external validity represent a major influence on the interpretation of a nonexperimental study because they impose limitations on the generalizability of the results.

If you are critiquing one of the additional types of research discussed, you must first identify the type of research used; then you must understand its specific purpose and format. The format and methods of secondary analysis, methodological research, and meta-analysis vary; knowing how they vary allows you to assess whether the process was applied appropriately. Some of the basic principles of these methods were presented in this chapter. The specific criteria for evaluating these designs are beyond the scope of this text, but the references provided can assist you in this process. Even though the format and methods vary, all research has a central goal: to answer questions scientifically.

CRITIQUING CRITERIA

1. Which nonexperimental design is used in the study?
2. In accordance with the theoretical framework, is the rationale for the type of design evident?
3. How is the design congruent with the purpose of the study?
4. Is the design appropriate for the research problem?
5. Is the design suited to the data-collection methods?
6. Does the researcher present the findings in a manner congruent with the design used?
7. Does the researcher theorize beyond the relational parameters of the findings and erroneously infer cause-and-
effect relationships between the variables?
8. Are alternative explanations for the findings possible?
9. How does the researcher discuss the threats to internal and external validity?
10. How does the researcher deal with the limitations of the study?

Helpful Hint

As you read the literature, you will find studies with labels such as *outcomes research, needs assessments, evaluation research,* and *quality assurance.* These studies are not designs per se; instead, these studies are conducted with either experimental or nonexperimental designs. Studies with these labels are designed to test the effectiveness of health care techniques, programs, or interventions. When reading such a research study, you should assess which design was used and whether the principles of the design, sampling strategy, and analysis are consistent with the study's purpose.

CRITICAL THINKING CHALLENGES

- Discuss which type of nonexperimental design might help validate the defining characteristics of a particular nursing diagnosis you use in practice. Do you think it is possible for nurses and patients to serve as the participants in this type of study?
- The midterm group (five-student) assignment for your research class is to critique an assigned quantitative study. To proceed, you must first decide the study's overall type. You think it is an ex post facto nonexperimental design, whereas the other students think it is an experimental design because the study has several explicit hypotheses. How would you convince the other students that you are correct?
- You are completing your senior practicum on a surgical step-down unit. The nurses completed an evidence-informed practice protocol for patient-controlled analgesics. Some of the nurses

want to implement it immediately, whereas others want to implement it with only some patients. You think that it should be implemented as a research study. Could either of the ways the nurses want to implement the protocol be considered in a research study?
- You are part of a journal club at your hospital. Your group has been examining a phenomenon specific to your patient population and noticed that 20 correlational studies on the topic have been published. Your group decides to perform a meta-analysis of the data. What steps need to be considered in performing the meta-analysis? What level of evidence would you expect to obtain with this method? Explain your answer.

KEY POINTS

- Nonexperimental research designs are used in studies that make an account of events as they naturally occur. The major difference between nonexperimental and experimental research is that in nonexperimental designs, the independent variable is not actively manipulated by the investigator.
- Nonexperimental designs can be classified either as survey studies or as relationship/difference studies.
- Survey studies and relationship/difference studies are both descriptive and exploratory in nature.
- In survey research, the investigator collects detailed descriptions of existing phenomena and uses the data either to justify current conditions and practices or to make more intelligent plans for improving them.

- In relationship/difference studies, researchers endeavour to explore the relationships or differences between variables in order to provide deeper insight into the phenomena of interest.
- In correlational studies, researchers examine relationships.
- Developmental studies are further divided into categories of cross-sectional, longitudinal (prospective), and retrospective (ex post facto) studies.
- Methodological research, secondary analysis, and meta-analysis are examples of other means of adding to the body of nursing research. Both the researcher and the reader must consider the advantages and disadvantages of each design.
- Nonexperimental research designs do not enable the investigator to establish cause-and-effect relationships between the variables. You must be wary of nonexperimental studies in which researchers make causal claims about the findings, unless a causal modelling technique is used.
- Nonexperimental designs offer the researcher the least amount of control. Threats to validity represent a major influence on the interpretation of a nonexperimental study because they impose limitations on the generalizability of the results and, as such, should be fully assessed by the critical reader.
- The critiquing process is directed toward evaluating the appropriateness of the selected nonexperimental design in relation to factors such as the research problem, the theoretical framework, the hypothesis, the methodology, and the data analysis and interpretation.
- Although nonexperimental designs do not provide the highest level of evidence (level I), they do provide a wealth of data that become useful for formulating both level I and level II studies that are aimed at developing and testing nursing interventions.

REFERENCES

Akhtar-Danesh, N., Valaitis, R. K., Schofield, R., Underwood, J., Martin-Misener, R., Baumann, A., & Kolotylo, C. (2010). A questionnaire for assessing community health nurses' learning needs. *Western Journal of Nursing Research, 32*(8), 1055-1072.

Armstrong, K., Laschinger, H., & Wong, C. (2009). Workplace empowerment and magnet hospital characteristics as predictors of patient safety climate. *Journal of Nursing Care Quality, 24*(1), 55-62.

Bailey, J. J., Sabbagh, M., Loiselle, C. G., Boileau, J., & McVey, L. (2010). Supporting families in the ICU: A descriptive correlational study of informational support, anxiety, and satisfaction with care. *Intensive and Critical Care Nursing, 26,* 114-122.

Campbell, D. T., & Stanley, J. C. (1963). *Experimental and quasi-experimental designs for research.* Chicago: Rand-McNally.

Chojecki, P., Lamarre, J., Buck, M., St-Sauveur, I., Eldaoud, N., & Purden, M. (2010). Perceptions of a peer learning approach to pediatric clinical education. *International Journal of Nursing Education Scholarship, 7*(1), Article 39. Epub 2010 Oct 29.

Edwards, A. G., Hailey, S., Maxwell, M. (2004). Psychological interventions for women with metastatic breast cancer. *Cochrane Database System Review, 2004*(2), CD004253.

Fox, M. T., Sidani, S., & Brooks, D. (2010). The relationship between bed rest and sitting orthostatic intolerance in adults residing in chronic care facilities. *Journal of Nursing and Healthcare of Chronic Illness, 2*(3), 187-196. doi:10.1111/j/1752-9824.2010.01058.x

Goff, A.-M. (2011). Stressors, academic performance, and learned resourcefulness in baccalaureate nursing students. *International Journal of Nursing Education Scholarship, 8*(1), Article 1.

Hernandez, C. A., Hume, M. R., & Rodger, N. W. (2008). Evaluation of a self-awareness intervention for adults with type 1 diabetes and hypoglycemia awareness. *Canadian Journal of Nursing Research, 40*(3), 38-56.

Hoe Harwood, C., Reimer-Kirkham, S., Sawatzky, R., Terblanche, T., & Van Hofwegen, L. (2010). Innovation of community clinical placements: A Canadian survey. *International Journal of Nursing Education Scholarship, 6*(1), Article 28.

Johnston, L. (2005). Critically appraising quantitative evidence. In B. M. Melnyk & E. Fineout-Overholt (Eds.), *Evidence-based practice in nursing and healthcare* (pp. 79-126). Philadelphia: Lippincott Williams & Wilkins.

Kaasalainen, S., Agarwal G., Dolovich, L., Papaioannou, A., Brazil, K., & Akhtar-Danesh, N. (2010). Nurses' perceptions of and satisfaction with the medication administration system in long-term-care homes. *Canadian Journal of Nursing Research, 42*(4), 58-79.

Kaplan, D. (2008). *Structure equation modeling: Foundations and extensions.* Thousand Oaks, CA: Sage.

Koren, I., Mian, O., & Rukholm, E. (2010). Integration of nurse practitioners into Ontario's primary health care system: Variations across practice settings.

Canadian Journal of Nursing Research, 42(2), 48-69.

Letourneau, N., Duffett-Leger, L., & Salmani, M. (2009). The role of paternal support in the behavioural development of children exposed to postpartum depression. *Canadian Journal of Nursing Research, 41*(3), 86-106.

Linton, A., Singh, M., Turbow, D., & Legg, T. J. (2009). Street youth in Toronto: An investigation of demographic predictors of high risk behaviors and HIV status. *Journal of HIV/AIDS & Social Services, 8*, 375-396.

Ohler, M., Kerr, M. S., & Forbes, D. A. (2010). Depression in nurses. *Canadian Journal of Nursing Research, 42*(3), 66-82.

Plunkett, R. D., Iwasiw, C. L., & Kerr, M. (2010). The intention to pursue graduate studies in nursing: A look at BScN students' self-efficacy and value influences. *International Journal of Nursing Education Scholarship, 7*(1), Article 23.

Raudenbush, S., & Bryk, A. (2002). *Hierarchical linear models: Applications and data analysis methods* (2nd ed.). Newbury Park, CA: Sage.

Richard, M. L., Parmar, M. P., Calestagne, P. P., & McVey, L. (2010). Seeking patient feedback: An important dimension of quality in cancer care. *Journal of Nursing Care Quality, 25*(4), 344-351.

Roberts, C. A., & Ward-Smith, P. (2010). Choosing a career in nursing: Development of a career search instrument. *International Journal of Nursing Education Scholarship, 7*(1), Article 2.

Robinson, J. G., & Molzahn, A. E. (2007, March). Sexuality and quality of life. *Journal of Gerontological Nursing, 33*(3), 19-27.

Samuels-Dennis, J., Ford-Gilboe, M., Wilk, P., Avison, W. R., & Ray, S. (2010). Cumulative trauma, personal and social resources, and post-traumatic stress symptoms among income-assisted single mothers. *Journal of Family Violence, 25*(6), 603-617. doi:10.1007/s10896-010-9323-7

Sawhney, M., & Sawyer, J. (2008). A cross-sectional study of the role of Canadian nurses with a specialty practice in pain management. *Acute Pain, 10*, 151-156.

Schneider, M., Steele, R., Cadell, S., & Hemsworth, D. (2011). Differences on psychosocial outcomes between male and female caregivers of children with life-limiting illnesses. *Journal of Pediatric Nursing, 26*(3), 186-199. doi:10.1016/j.pedn.2010.01.007

Schumacker, R. E., & Lomax, R. C. (2004). *A beginner's guide to structural equation modeling.* Hillsdale, NJ: Erlbaum.

Sidani, S., Epstein, D. R., Bootzin, R. R., Moritz, P., & Miranda, J. (2009). Assessment of preferences for treatment: Validation of a measure. *Research in Nursing and Health, 32*, 419-438.

Singh, M., & Cameron, J. (2005). The psychosocial aspects of caregiving to stroke patients. *AXON, 27*(1), 18-24.

Thomas, J., Jensen, L., Nahirniak, S., & Gibney, R. T. (2010). Anemia and blood transfusion practices in the critically ill: A prospective cohort review. *Heart & Lung, 39*(3), 217-225.

Tourangeau, A. E., Doran, D. M., McGillis-Hall, L., O'Brien-Pallas, L., Pringle, D., Tu, J. V. (2006). Impact of hospital nursing care on 30-day mortality for acute medical patients. *Journal of Advanced Nursing, 57*, 32-44.

Voyer, P., Cappeliez, P., Pérodeau, G., & Préville, M. (2005). Mental health for older adults and benzodiazepine use. *Journal of Community Health Nursing, 22*, 213-229.

Wahoush, E. O. (2009). Equitable health-care access: The experiences of refugee and refugee claimant mothers with an ill preschooler. *Canadian Journal of Nursing Research, 41*(3), 186-206.

Ward-Griffin, C., Keefe, J., Martin-Matthews, A., Kerr, M., Brown, J-B., & Oudshoom, A. (2009). Development and validation of the Double Duty Caregiving Scale. *Canadian Journal of Nursing Research, 41*(3), 108-128.

Watson, L., Oberle, K., & Deutscher, D. (2008). Development and psychometric testing of the Nurses' Attitudes Toward Obesity and Obese Patients (NATOOPS) scale. *Research in Nursing and Health, 31*, 586-593.

Yonge, O., Rosychuk, R. J., Bailey, T. M., Lake, R., Marrie, T. J. (2010). Willingness of university nursing students to volunteer during a pandemic. *Public Health Nursing, 27*(2), 174-180.

FOR FURTHER STUDY

evolve   Go to Evolve at http://evolve.elsevier.com/ Canada/LoBiondo/Research for Audio Glossary, how-to instructions for Writing Proposals for Funding, and additional research articles for practice in reviewing and critiquing.

PART FOUR

Processes Related to Research

RESEARCH **VIGNETTE**

Developing and Implementing a Framework for Interprofessional Education in Health Sciences Education: Can Nursing Contribute?

Julie Gaudet, RN, MN (Admin.)
Professor
School of Nursing
Centre for Health Sciences
George Brown College
Toronto, Ontario

As a teacher at George Brown College since 2002, I have always been interested in educational research. When I was asked to participate in the creation of interprofessional education (IPE) curricula in health sciences at the college, I was eager to get involved because of my belief that interdisciplinary collaboration is key to achieving high-quality patient care.

Through my work on a variety of IPE projects, I discovered that although the concept of "learning in an interdisciplinary context" as a preparatory step for "real world" practice intuitively makes sense to everyone, students generally lack the understanding of each member's role on a health care team and have limited opportunities to interact with students from other health care professions while in their respective programs. Moreover, at times, professional boundary issues are misinterpreted as barriers to learning collaboratively. Although a growing body of evidence exists on the short-term student outcomes of IPE focused on knowledge and skills related to collaboration, less is known about the long-term effect of IPE on student behaviour, postregistration collaborative practice, and patient care (Hammick, Freeth, Koppel, Reeves, & Barr, 2007).

In my former role as a mental health clinical nurse, it was natural for me to work collaboratively with multidisciplinary staff, including nurses, psychiatrists, psychologists, dietitians, physiotherapists, occupational therapists, and a myriad of other clinical consultants. From the outside looking in this type of collaborative working scenario does not appear unique to the mental health setting but is true of all specialties. Conversely, professionals who work or spend a considerable amount of time in psychiatric settings would argue that clinical discussions, and those related to the therapeutic milieu, decision making, and team dynamics have, at times, a different "feel" than within more traditional clinical settings.

Although reality in this context is highly subjective to the interpretation of the individuals involved, my curiosity related to the following research questions was, of course, expected and grounded in my past experience within a psychiatric interdisciplinary context:

- Does IPE, "when two or more professions learn with, from and about each other to improve collaboration and the quality of care" (Centre for the Advancement of Interprofessional Education,* 2002), result in the formation of a more collaborative nursing practitioner?
- Does IPE lead to entry-to-practice nurses' adoption of an inclusive view of a health care professional?

The answers to these questions have since preoccupied my thoughts and those of many of my colleagues. As a beginning step to meeting the identified need for IPE, a team of committed leaders and faculty members embarked on a developmental journey that involved the creation of an early curriculum framework for IPE and four key IPE learning outcomes (George Brown College, 2004) for all students attending programs in the Centre for Health Sciences. The IPE learning outcomes that follow were designed to enable students to accomplish the following objectives:

- Appraise the relationship between their own profession and the background, scope, and roles of other health care professionals
- Evaluate their ability to work in a team

---

*In the Centre for Health Sciences at George Brown College, the term *interprofessional education* is used to include all such learning in academic and work-based settings before and after qualification; an inclusive view of a professional is thereby adopted.

- Participate collaboratively as a health team member to support patients' achievement of their expected health outcomes
- Assess the effect of the broader legislative and ethical framework on interprofessional practice

In 2004, our team recognized that specific learning outcomes were paramount for the increased IPE focus and that appropriate interprofessional learning spaces were needed for this type of education to be sustained. Significant renovations were undertaken to create interdisciplinary learning spaces, which included a clinical simulation practice environment. According to the Society for Simulation in Healthcare (2010), health care simulation education is a form of learning that mimics real world health care scenarios in "safe" environments:

> Simulation is the imitation or representation of one act or system by another. Healthcare simulations can be said to have four main purposes—*education, assessment, research,* and *health system integration* in facilitating patient safety.
>
> Each of these purposes may be met by some combination of role play, low and high tech tools, and a variety of settings from tabletop sessions to a realistic full mission environment. Simulations may also add to our understanding of human behavior and true-to-life settings in which professionals operate. The link that ties together all these activities is the act of imitating or representing some situation or process from the simple to the very complex.

Interprofessional learning activities such as simulation education allows learners to gain a better understanding of interprofessional teamwork and to reflect on their attitudes toward working in an interprofessional team (Reeves, Lewin, Espin, & Zwarenstein, 2010). These spaces have enabled a variety of opportunities for interprofessional learning among students of the different disciplines, who previously used learning spaces in more insular ways.

A series of IPE programs and pilot projects have been designed to expose both faculty and students to this form of learning. For example, in one project, nursing and dental health students actively learned blood pressure monitoring skills and oral cleaning techniques from each other. In another, nursing students collaborated with students from the dental hygiene, fitness and lifestyle management, health information management, and health informatics programs to develop a common patient assessment tool. A more recent project involved health sciences students and interprofessional health care providers (from Revera Inc., a long-term and residential care service provider in Toronto) jointly involved in an interprofessional ethical decision-making workshop. This workshop, structured in a way that fostered open discussions among the participants in diverse health care roles, enabled both students and health care professionals to apply the framework to ethical issues and dilemmas relevant in the resident population of older adults.

These pilot projects provided several opportunities over a span of 7 years to gather insight into the perspectives of student participants and from faculty who facilitated those IPE/simulation learning activities. Evaluation data from these projects highlighted students' overall positive attitudes toward IPE, toward people from other professions, and toward one another, and teaching faculty gained considerable experience with this type of facilitation; however, additional research is needed to determine whether learning in interprofessional simulated contexts, real-life contexts, or both will result in nursing students' ability to practise in more collaborative ways as they enter the practice setting and whether it will ultimately lead to safer patient outcomes or to more holistic care. Because nurses make up the bulk of practitioners on a health care team in acute and chronic care settings, researchers must determine whether the health outcomes and well-being of patients can be improved as a result of training in this interdisciplinary team-based approach.

In order to move the interprofessional and simulation education and research agendas forward in the Centre for Health Sciences at George Brown College, and building on the initial learning outcomes work (George Brown College, 2004), my colleagues and I have further developed a framework by which to formally integrate IPE into our curriculum.

This framework involves six major foundations of interprofessional care and their associated levels of competencies: (1) health care systems and professions, (2) biomedical and social models of health, (3) communications, (4) collaboration, (5) conflict management, and (6) critical thinking.

The specific competencies are organized into steps or levels. For example, in relation to health care systems and professions, we have defined two main levels that encompass three competencies:

- Understanding the scopes of practice and the legislation (related to one's own profession and those of others)
- Social and political histories of professions (understanding power relationships and imbalances that produce barriers to effective interprofessional practice)

The competency ladder is as follows:

1. Demonstrates an understanding of *one's own* profession, history, legislation, regulation, and scope of practice
2. Appraises the relationship *between* one's own profession and the background/ history, scope, and roles of other health care professions
3. Critically assesses the impact of social history, and broader political, legislative, and ethical frameworks on one's own profession and on interprofessional practice

In the Centre for Health Sciences at George Brown College, the successful application of the framework and the competency levels on the competency ladder to be achieved by a specific program will, to a large extent, need to align with the professional entry to practice competencies (where relevant), and to the breadth, depth, and complexity of knowledge and vocational outcomes identified in the Ministry of Training, Colleges, and Universities' "Framework for Programs of Instruction." In addition, the planning for this program will need to account for other challenges, such as individual program structure and length, and for broader expectations about the health care system in order to ensure the success of the framework implementation.

In terms of next steps, we plan to identify the appropriate level of competency for each of our programs. For example, students in a 1-year dental assisting program will not be expected to achieve the same competencies as those in a 4-year BScN program. We also plan to develop and integrate curriculum into the programs to achieve these competencies. We will establish Centre-wide "IPE Days" to expose all students in the Centre for Health Sciences to IPE content and experiential learning. Last, but perhaps most important, we will begin to study and answer challenging but important operational and process questions, such as these: How do we get students from different programs/years together to practise interprofessionally? How will we overcome operational and logistical challenges in designating specific days each semester for IPE initiatives? How relevant and adequate are the foundations of interprofessional care and their associated levels of competencies? Are the competencies adequately grounded in learning theory (e.g., adult learning theory, experiential learning, problem-based learning, behavioural approaches, hybrid approaches)?

Pilot implementation projects began September 2011 and involve the BScN and Practical Nursing (PN) students (and possibly students from the Gerontology/Activation program). In 2012, we plan on expanding the number of programs involved until all our students are receiving the IPE curriculum and participating in the centre-wide interprofessional activities.

Engaging in IPE curriculum development and research has been tremendously rewarding. I have witnessed first-hand how willing and eager various students and faculty colleagues are to collaborate toward a common goal. Although learning what is unique to nursing is paramount for developing professional competence, optimal patient-centred holistic care cannot be achieved independently of the contributions of other health care professionals. The pursuit of excellence in team-based collaborative practice will take time, but nursing is a driving force toward achieving this goal!

REFERENCES

Centre for the Advancement of Interprofessional Education. (2002). *Defining IPE*. Retrieved from http://www.caipe.org.uk.

George Brown College. (2004, December 7). *The future of health science education: Framework for inter-professional education*. Toronto: Author.

Hammick, M., Freeth, D., Koppel, I., Reeves, S., & Barr, H. (2007). A best evidence systematic review of interprofessional education. *Medical Teacher, 22*, 461–467.

Johnston, C., & Toni, G. (2010, January). *A framework for IPE in non-degree health professions.* Paper presented at IPE Ontario 2010, Toronto.

Reeves, S., Lewin, S., Espin, S., & Zwarenstein, M. (2010). *Interprofessional teamwork for health and social care.* Oxford, UK: Wiley-Blackwell.

Society for Simulation in Healthcare. (2010). *What is health care simulation?* Retrieved from http://www.ssih.org/about-simulation.

CHAPTER 12

Sampling

Judith Haber | Mina D. Singh

LEARNING OUTCOMES

After reading this chapter, you will be able to do the following:

- Identify the purpose of sampling.
- Define population, sample, and sampling.
- Compare a population and a sample.
- Discuss the eligibility criteria for sample selection.
- Define nonprobability sampling and probability sampling.
- Identify the types of strategies for both nonprobability and probability sampling.
- Identify the types of qualitative sampling.
- Compare the advantages and disadvantages of specific nonprobability and probability sampling strategies.
- Discuss the contribution of nonprobability and probability sampling strategies to the strength of evidence provided by study findings.
- Discuss the factors that influence determination of sample size.
- Discuss the procedure for drawing a sample.
- Identify the criteria for critiquing a sampling plan.
- Use the critiquing criteria to evaluate the "Sample" section of a research report.

KEY TERMS

accessible population
cluster sampling
convenience sampling
data saturation
delimitations
effect size
element
eligibility criteria
heterogeneity
homogeneous
matching

multistage sampling
network sampling
nonprobability sampling
pilot study
population
probability sampling
purposive sampling
quota sampling
random selection
representative sample
sample

sampling
sampling frame
sampling interval
sampling unit
simple random sampling
snowball effect sampling
stratified random sampling
systematic sampling
target population
theoretical sampling

STUDY RESOURCES

Go to Evolve at http://evolve.elsevier.com/Canada/LoBiondo/Research for Audio Glossary, how-to instructions for Writing Proposals for Funding, and additional research articles for practice in reviewing and critiquing.

SAMPLING IS THE PROCESS OF SELECTING representative units of a population for study in a research investigation. Although sampling is a complex process, it is a familiar one. In their daily lives, people gather knowledge, make decisions, and formulate predictions on the basis of sampling procedures. For example, nursing students may make generalizations about the overall quality of nursing professors as a result of their exposure to a sample of nursing professors during their undergraduate programs. Patients may make generalizations about a hospital's food or quality of nursing care during a 1-week hospital stay. Limited exposure to a limited portion of these phenomena forms the basis of people's conclusions, so much of their knowledge and many of their decisions are based on their experience with samples.

Researchers also derive knowledge from samples. Many questions in scientific and naturalistic research cannot be answered without the use of sampling procedures. For example, when the effectiveness of a new education intervention for diabetic patients is tested, the intervention is administered to a sample of the population. The researcher must come to some conclusions without giving the intervention to the entire population of diabetic patients. To obtain the experiences or outcomes of engaging in this education, the researcher needs to select the appropriate sampling strategy in accordance with the research design and question. This is done to avoid erroneous conclusions or making generalizations from a nonrepresentative sample. Thus, research methodologists have expended considerable effort to develop sampling theories and procedures that produce accurate and meaningful information.

Essentially, researchers sample representative segments of the population because sampling the entire population of interest to obtain relevant information is rarely feasible or necessary.

This chapter will familiarize you with the basic concepts of sampling as they pertain to the principles of quantitative and qualitative research designs, nonprobability and probability sampling, sample size, and the related critiquing process.

SAMPLING CONCEPTS

Population

A **population** is a well-defined set that has certain specified properties or characteristics from which data can be gathered and analyzed. A population can be composed of people, animals, objects, or events. For example, if a researcher is studying undergraduate nursing students, the type of educational preparation of the population must be specified. In this example, the population consists of undergraduate students enrolled in a generic baccalaureate nursing program. Examples of other possible populations might be all female patients admitted to a certain hospital for lumpectomies for treatment of breast cancer during 2008, all children with asthma in the province of Alberta, or all men and women with a diagnosis of schizophrenia in North America. These examples illustrate that a population may be broadly defined and potentially involve millions of people, or it may be narrowly specified to include only a few people.

When you read a research report, you should consider whether the researcher has identified the population descriptors that form the basis for the inclusion (eligibility) or exclusion criteria (delimitations) that are used to select the sample from the array of all possible units, whether people, objects, or events. Consider the population previously defined as undergraduate nursing students enrolled in a generic baccalaureate program. Would this population include both part-time and full-time students? Would it include students who had previously attended another nursing program? What about international students? At which level (first year through senior year) would students qualify? As much as possible, the researcher must specifically delineate the exact criteria used to decide whether an individual would be classified as a member of a given population. The population descriptors that provide the basis for inclusion (eligibility) criteria should be evident in the sample; in other words, the characteristics of the population and the sample should be congruent. The degree of congruence is evaluated to assess the representativeness of the sample. For example, if a population is defined as full-time, Canadian-born, senior-level nursing students enrolled in a generic baccalaureate nursing program, the sample would be expected to reflect these characteristics.

Think about the concept of inclusion criteria, or **eligibility criteria** (characteristics of a population that meet requirements for inclusion in a study), applied to a research study in which the participants are patients. For example, in an investigation of the effects of music on dyspnea during exercise in individuals with chronic obstructive pulmonary disease (COPD), the participants had to meet all of the following inclusion (eligibility) criteria:

1. A confirmed medical diagnosis of COPD (i.e., chronic bronchitis, emphysema, or both)
2. Ability to speak and read English
3. Ability to ambulate independently
4. Experiencing dyspnea at least once a week
5. An increase in the level of dyspnea of at least two points on the Borg scale after a 6-minute walk

Examples of exclusion criteria, or **delimitations** (characteristics that restrict the population to a homogeneous group of participants), include gender, age, marital status, socioeconomic status, religion, ethnicity, level of education, age of children, health status, and diagnosis. In a study of the differences in sleep complaints in adults with varying levels of bed rest residing in extended-care facilities for chronic disease management, Fox and colleagues (2010) established the following exclusion criteria: ability to ambulate out of bed without physical assistance, receiving palliative care, admission for short-term rehabilitation, and being in the acute illness phase. These exclusion criteria, or delimitations, were selected because of their potential effect on the accurate evaluation of the varying levels of bed rest among patients in extended care.

In a randomized clinical trial, Smith and associates (2011) tested the efficacy of two smoking cessation interventions: one intensive and one brief. The inclusion criteria were as follows: age of 18 years or older, tobacco use in the past 30 days, minimum 36-hour stay, telephone access, and willingness to be randomly assigned to a group and to quit smoking. Exclusion criteria were as follows: enrollment in another smoking cessation trial, being pregnant, the presence of medical complications (e.g., receiving palliative care, unstable condition, or institutionalization), inability to speak English, communication difficulties, substance abuse, and a psychiatric history.

The **heterogeneity,** or dissimilarities, of a sample group inhibits the researchers' ability to interpret the findings meaningfully and to make generalizations. It is much wiser to study only one **homogeneous** group—that is, a group with limited variation in attributes or characteristics, as in the aforementioned study—or to include specific groups as distinct subsets of the sample and study the groups comparatively, as was the case in Ostry and colleagues' (2010) study. These researchers sought to determine mental health outcomes in sawmill workers in British Columbia. They compared rural workers with urban workers and, after controlling for socioeconomic variables, concluded that rural sawmill workers had better outcomes.

Remember that exclusion criteria or delimitations are not established in a casual or meaningless way but are established to control for extraneous variability or bias. Each exclusion criterion should have a rationale, presumably related to a potential contaminating effect on the dependent variable. Carefully established sample exclusion criteria, or delimitations, increase the precision of the study and contribute to accuracy while constraining the generalizability or transferability of the findings (see Chapter 9).

The population criteria establish the **target population:** that is, the entire set of cases about which the researcher would like to make generalizations. A target population might include all undergraduate nursing students enrolled in generic baccalaureate programs in Canada. Because of time, money, and personnel, however, using a target population is often not feasible. An **accessible population**—one that meets the population criteria and is available—is used instead. For example, an accessible population might include all full-time generic baccalaureate students attending school in Manitoba. Pragmatic factors must also be considered in identifying a potential population of interest.

Helpful Hint

Often, researchers do not clearly identify the population under study, or the population is not clarified until the "Discussion" section, when an effort is made to discuss the group (population) to which the study findings can be generalized.

A population is not restricted to human participants. The population may consist of hospital records; blood, urine, or other specimens taken from patients at a clinic; historical documents; or laboratory animals. For example, a population might consist of all urine specimens collected from patients in the Mount Sinai Hospital antepartum clinic or all patient charts on file at a day surgery centre. A population can be defined in a variety of ways. Of importance is that the basic unit of the population must be clearly defined because the generalizability of the findings is a function of the population criteria.

Evidence-Informed Practice Tip

Consider whether the sample selection was biased, thereby influencing the validity of the evidence provided by the outcomes of the study.

Samples and Sampling

Sampling is a process of selecting a portion or subset of the designated population to represent the entire population. A **sample** is a set of elements that make up the population; an **element** is the most basic unit about which information is collected. The most common element in nursing research is individuals, but other elements (e.g., places or objects) can form the basis of a sample or population. For example, a researcher plans a study to compare the effectiveness of different nursing interventions on reducing falls in older adults in long-term care facilities. Four facilities, in each of which a different treatment protocol is used, are identified as the sampling units—not the nurses themselves or the treatment alone. A sampling unit can be an organization, a group, or an individual person.

The purpose of sampling is to increase the efficiency of a research study. Examining every element or unit in the population would not be feasible. When sampling is done properly, the researcher can draw inferences and make generalizations about the population without examining each unit in the population.

In qualitative research, the results can have good generalizability to the population under study. Sampling procedures that entail the formulation of specific criteria for selection ensure that the characteristics of the phenomena of interest will be, or are likely to be, present in all of the elements being studied. The researcher's efforts to ensure that the sample is representative of the target population provide a stronger position from which to draw conclusions from the sample findings that are generalizable to the population (see Chapter 9).

After reviewing a number of research studies, you will recognize that samples and sampling procedures vary in terms of merit. The foremost criterion in evaluating a sample is its representativeness. A **representative sample** has key characteristics that closely approximate those of the population. If 70% of the population in a study of childrearing practices consisted of women and 40% were full-time employees, a representative sample should reflect these characteristics in the same proportions.

The representativeness of a sample cannot be guaranteed without access to a database about the entire population. Because it is difficult and inefficient to assess an entire population, the researcher must employ sampling strategies that minimize or control for sample bias. If an appropriate sampling strategy is used, the sample data will almost always enable a reasonably accurate understanding of the phenomena under investigation.

Evidence-Informed Practice Tip

Determining whether the sample is representative of the population being studied in journal articles will influence both your interpretation of the evidence provided by the findings and your decision making about the findings' relevance to the your patient population and practice setting.

TYPES OF SAMPLES

Sampling strategies are generally grouped into two categories: *nonprobability sampling* and *probability sampling*. In **nonprobability sampling,** elements are chosen through nonrandom methods. The drawback of this strategy is that each element's probability of being included in

the samples cannot be estimated. In other words, ensuring that every element has a chance for inclusion in the nonprobability sample is not possible. In **probability sampling,** some form of random selection is used when the sample units are chosen. This type of sample enables the researcher to estimate the probability that each element of the population will be included in the sample. Probability sampling is the more rigorous sampling strategy used in quantitative research and is more likely to result in a representative sample.

The remainder of this section is devoted to a discussion of different types of nonprobability and probability sampling strategies. A summary of sampling strategies appears in Table 12-1. You may refer to this table as the various nonprobability and probability strategies are discussed in the following sections. Note that if there is bias in sampling, it will distort the analysis and the findings of the study.

Helpful Hint

Research articles are not always explicit about the type of sampling strategy that was used. If the sampling strategy is not specified, assume that in a quantitative study, a convenience sample was used and that in a qualitative study, a purposive sample was used.

Nonprobability Sampling

Because of a lack of random selection, the nonprobability sampling strategy is less generalizable than probability sampling because it tends to produce less representative samples. Such samples are more feasible for the researcher to obtain, however, and most samples—in nursing research and the research of other disciplines—are nonprobability samples. When a nonprobability sample reflects the target population through the careful use of inclusion and exclusion criteria, you can have more confidence in the representativeness of the sample and the external validity of the findings. The major types of nonprobability sampling are *convenience, quota, network,* and

TABLE 12-1

SUMMARY OF SAMPLING STRATEGIES

SAMPLING STRATEGY	EASE OF DRAWING A REPRESENTATIVE SAMPLE	RISK OF BIAS	REPRESENTATIVENESS OF THE SAMPLE
NONPROBABILITY			
Convenience	Very easy	Greater than in any other sampling strategy	Because samples tend to be self-selecting; representativeness is questionable
Quota	Relatively easy	Contains an unknown source of bias that affects external validity	Builds in some representativeness by using knowledge about the population of interest
Purposive	Relatively easy	Bias increases with greater heterogeneity of the population; conscious bias is also a danger but is offset with maximal variation	Very limited ability to generalize because the sample is handpicked from a quantitative view, but this approach is necessary for the qualitative researcher to choose participants on the basis of the phenomenon under study
Network	Can be easy if the network is accessible	Minimal if a thorough sampling plan is developed	Represents the event, incident, or experience being studied
Theoretical	Requires a two-stage process; can be prolonged	Minimal if a thorough sampling plan is developed	Typically begins with another type of sampling, such as convenience or criterion sampling aimed at variation in the phenomenon, and thus represents aspects of the theory being constructed
PROBABILITY			
Simple random	Laborious	Low	Maximized; the probability of nonrepresentativeness decreases with increased sample size
Stratified random	Time-consuming	Low	Enhanced
Cluster	Less time consuming than simple or stratified sampling	Subject to more sampling errors than is simple or stratified sampling	Less representative than simple or stratified sampling
Systematic	More convenient and efficient than is simple, stratified, or cluster sampling	Bias in the form of nonrandomness can be inadvertently introduced	Less representative if bias occurs as a result of coincidental nonrandomness

purposive sampling strategies. Convenience and quota sampling can be used in both quantitative and qualitative research, whereas network and purposive sampling are used mostly in qualitative research and are discussed later in this chapter.

Convenience Sampling

Convenience sampling is the use of the most readily accessible persons or objects as participants in a study. The participants may include volunteers, the first 25 patients admitted to a certain hospital with a particular diagnosis, all of the people who enrolled in a certain program during the month of September, or all of the students enrolled in a certain course at a particular university during 2005. The participants are convenient and accessible to the researcher; hence the term *convenience sample.*

In studying the association between parental anxiety and compliance with preoperative requirements for pediatric outpatient surgery, Chahal and colleagues (2009) used convenience sampling to obtain a sample size of 203. Sinclair and Ferguson (2009) used a convenience sample of 250 collaborative baccalaureate nursing students to study the effect of integrating simulated teaching and learning strategies in undergraduate nursing education. The advantage of a convenience sample is that it is easy for the researcher to obtain participants. The researcher may need to be concerned only with obtaining a sufficient number of participants who meet the same criteria.

Linton and associates (2009) also obtained a convenience sample from health and social service agencies servicing homeless youth. Chiovitti (2006) used convenience sampling as a first stage of sampling in a qualitative, grounded theory study in order to explore nurses' meaning of caring with patients in acute psychiatric hospital settings.

The major disadvantage of a convenience sample is that the risk of bias is greater than in any other type of sample (see Table 12-1). Because convenience samples entail voluntary participation, the probability that researchers will recruit people who feel strongly about the issue being studied is increased, which may favour certain outcomes of the study. The problem of bias is related to the tendency of convenience samples to be self-selecting; in other words, the researcher obtains information only from the people who volunteer to participate. In this case, the following questions must be raised:

- What motivated some of the people to participate and others not to participate?
- What kind of data would have been obtained if nonparticipants had also responded?
- How representative of the population are the people who did participate?

For example, a researcher may stop people on a street corner to ask their opinion on an issue; place advertisements in the newspaper; or put signs in local churches, community centres, or supermarkets to recruit volunteers for a particular study. To study the prevention or treatment of osteoporosis in postmenopausal women who had completed treatment (except for tamoxifen) for breast cancer, and for whom hormone replacement therapy was contraindicated, Waltman and colleagues (2003) recruited participants from breast cancer support groups and through physician referrals and local television and radio announcements. To assess the degree to which a convenience sample approximates a random sample, a researcher can compare the convenience sample data with the known demographic information and by examining variability around the mean. In this manner, the researcher checks for the representativeness of the convenience sample and the extent to which bias is or is not evident (Cochran, 1977; Sousa, Zauszniewski, & Musil, 2004).

Because recruiting research participants is a problem that confronts many nurse researchers, innovative recruitment strategies are sometimes used. For example, a researcher may offer to pay the participants for their time. A relatively new method of accessing and recruiting participants is through online computer networks (e.g., disease-specific chat rooms and bulletin boards).

In evaluating a research report, you should recognize that the convenience sample strategy, although the most common, is the weakest form of sampling strategy in quantitative research in terms of generalizability. When a convenience sample is used, researchers should analyze and interpret the data cautiously. When you critique a research study in which this sampling strategy was used, you should be skeptical about the external validity of the findings (see Chapter 9).

Quota Sampling

Quota sampling refers to a form of nonprobability sampling in which knowledge about the population of interest is used to ensure some representativeness about the sample (see Table 12-1). Through quota sampling, the researcher identifies a particular strata of the population, and the quota sample proportionally represents the

TABLE **12-2**

NUMBERS AND PERCENTAGES OF STUDENTS IN STRATA OF A QUOTA SAMPLE OF 5000 GRADUATES OF NURSING PROGRAMS IN A PARTICULAR CITY			
CATEGORIES	**DIPLOMA GRADUATES**	**ASSOCIATE DEGREE GRADUATES**	**BACCALAUREATE GRADUATES**
Strata	1000 (20%)	2000 (40%)	2000 (40%)
Quota sample	100	200	200

strata. For example, the data in Table 12-2 reveal that of the 5000 nurses in a particular city, 20% are diploma graduates, 40% are post–RN degree graduates, and 40% are baccalaureate graduates. Each of these strata should be proportionately represented in the sample. In this case, the researcher used a proportional quota sampling strategy and decided to include 10% of a population of 5000 (i.e., 500 nurses). On the basis of the proportion of each stratum in the population, 100 diploma graduates, 200 post-RN graduates, and 200 baccalaureate graduates were the quotas established for the three strata. The researcher recruited participants who met the eligibility criteria of the study until the quota for each stratum was filled. In other words, once the researcher obtained the necessary 100 diploma graduates, 200 post-RN graduates, and 200 baccalaureate graduates, the sample was complete with regard to both the research design and other pragmatic matters, such as economy.

The researcher systematically ensures that proportional segments of the population are included in the sample. An example is the study by Kaasalainen and Crook (2004), who evaluated the ability of older adult residents of a long-term care facility to report their pain. The researchers stratified a sample of 130 residents according to their level of cognitive impairment: cognitively intact, mildly impaired, moderately impaired, and extremely impaired. The quota sample is not randomly selected (i.e., once the proportional strata have been identified, the researcher obtains participants until the quota for each stratum has been filled), but it does increase the representativeness of the sample. This sampling strategy addresses the problem of overrepresentation or underrepresentation of certain segments of a population in a sample.

An example of nonproportional quota sampling is the study by Fox and colleagues (2010), who examined differences in sleep complaints among adults with varying amounts of bed rest who were residing in extended-care facilities for chronic disease management. The three cohorts (comparative, moderate, and high) reflected different amounts of bed rest that were naturally occurring. To ensure equal representation of the different amounts of bed rest, nonproportional quota sampling was used.

The characteristics chosen to form the strata are selected according to a researcher's judgement on the basis of knowledge of the population and the literature review. The criterion for selection should be a variable that reflects important differences in the independent variables under investigation. Age, gender, religion, ethnicity, medical diagnosis, socioeconomic status, level of completed education, and occupation are among the variables that are likely to be important in stratifying samples in nursing research investigations.

In critiquing a research strategy, you seek to determine whether the sample strata appropriately reflect the population under consideration and whether the variables used are homogeneous enough to ensure a meaningful comparison. Even when the researcher has addressed these factors, you must remember that a quota strategy is a nonprobability sample and thus includes an unknown source of bias that affects the external validity. The people who choose to participate may not be typical of the population in terms of the variables being measured, and assessing the possible biases that may be operating is not possible. When the phenomena being investigated are relatively similar within the population, the risk of bias may be minimal; however, in heterogeneous populations, the risk of bias is greater.

Evidence-Informed Practice Tip ____

When you think about applying study findings to your clinical practice, consider whether the participants in the sample are similar to your own patients.

Probability Sampling

The primary characteristic of probability sampling is the random selection of elements from the population. In **random selection,** each element of the population has an equal and independent chance of being included in the sample. In the hierarchy of evidence, probability sampling represents the strongest type of sampling strategy. That means there is greater confidence that the sample is representative rather than biased and that it more closely reflects the characteristics of the population of interest. Four commonly used probability sampling strategies are *simple random sampling, stratified random sampling, cluster sampling,* and *systematic sampling.*

Random selection of sample participants should not be confused with random assignment of participants. As discussed in Chapter 10, *randomization* refers to the assignment of participants to either an experimental or a control group on a purely random basis.

Simple Random Sampling

Simple random sampling is a laborious and carefully controlled process. Because the principles of simple random sampling are incorporated in the more complex probability designs, the principles of this strategy are presented.

In **simple random sampling,** the researcher defines the population (a set), lists all units of the population (a **sampling frame**), and selects a sample of units (a subset) from which the sample will be chosen. For example, if Canadian hospitals specializing in the treatment of cancer were the sampling unit, a list of all such hospitals would be the sampling frame. If certified adult nurse practitioners constituted the accessible population, a list of those nurses would be the sampling frame.

Once a list of the population elements has been developed, the best method of selecting a sample is to employ a table of random numbers containing columns of digits, as shown in Figure 12-1. Such tables can be generated by computer programs. After assigning consecutive numbers to units of the population, the researcher starts at any point on the table of random numbers and reads consecutive numbers in any direction (i.e., horizontally, vertically, or diagonally). When a number is read that corresponds with the written unit on a card, that unit is chosen for the sample. The investigator continues to read until a sample of the desired size is drawn. The advantages of simple random sampling are as follows:

- The sample selection is not subject to the conscious biases of the researcher.
- The representativeness of the sample is maximized in relation to the population characteristics.
- The differences in the characteristics of the sample and the population are purely a function of chance.
- The probability of choosing a nonrepresentative sample decreases as the size of the sample increases.

Boscart (2009) used simple random sampling to select 30 patients from three different units to evaluate the effect of a brief, focused educational interaction on the quality of verbal interactions between nursing staff and patients in a chronic care facility. You must remember that although a researcher may use a carefully controlled

1000 random integers between 0 and 99

40	23	0	29	10	94	17	58	12	85	13	25	80	84	72	74	54	63	55	31
32	98	59	23	74	97	51	42	21	87	48	64	54	38	84	68	14	17	35	48
84	34	84	14	53	65	67	37	2	45	84	21	71	34	10	80	72	27	11	13
86	37	24	89	23	4	44	40	72	81	44	69	25	44	34	34	34	75	50	50
50	58	85	8	22	24	73	20	63	35	60	87	91	92	96	80	19	22	87	24
1	87	43	82	9	31	40	88	33	28	82	73	18	6	48	64	59	45	34	3
21	19	42	76	84	67	29	68	8	66	93	89	96	28	12	14	38	47	52	65
32	66	33	21	81	97	39	76	67	27	97	22	76	89	41	11	91	29	6	66
16	82	42	75	35	42	92	90	77	24	21	8	36	16	5	54	89	51	57	85
74	32	63	65	93	96	18	36	82	72	39	69	37	97	51	17	36	71	38	30
50	94	4	66	17	37	10	53	8	29	67	74	88	38	11	59	60	91	56	17
71	47	81	18	53	98	7	87	29	37	22	93	13	6	95	7	95	71	14	6
71	93	48	16	33	19	46	21	60	44	52	91	52	58	10	9	41	31	35	18
20	94	13	99	45	6	53	54	1	25	79	28	1	48	36	26	68	37	59	7
75	22	69	56	62	40	64	45	40	99	94	14	98	84	22	38	24	87	43	71
16	87	41	0	88	83	11	37	71	78	22	39	43	37	75	84	84	11	55	58
92	90	80	2	30	37	84	55	56	50	3	71	24	13	62	74	82	44	90	32
96	89	31	32	37	45	70	67	80	55	58	9	55	60	61	55	86	44	27	77
38	29	36	94	65	39	56	29	29	65	88	13	71	38	71	8	81	66	31	44
20	6	61	66	90	13	70	60	92	53	87	49	34	42	14	47	75	33	26	9
63	44	94	21	14	13	41	80	39	72	29	3	25	89	44	88	13	49	18	58
13	32	93	90	31	75	86	95	18	51	61	59	84	95	67	54	40	30	29	63
26	35	48	81	19	24	36	36	76	16	46	5	93	41	97	46	79	54	95	49
89	74	96	95	94	69	31	60	16	69	76	42	28	71	69	34	46	55	20	42
50	39	28	64	20	68	60	33	92	82	61	70	5	68	95	88	12	85	18	94
55	86	5	96	87	69	75	93	54	79	0	57	45	8	86	59	25	21	9	29
75	35	1	2	86	62	70	83	85	13	97	37	13	73	16	38	36	23	54	11
74	50	1	77	87	92	68	87	57	36	17	47	0	97	78	72	72	45	54	51
34	24	35	13	26	42	22	75	47	2	34	87	15	50	65	27	5	72	28	68
73	33	42	65	91	24	44	84	71	55	70	1	27	30	8	61	65	61	18	92
7	55	12	6	61	17	23	95	91	58	60	30	35	61	34	27	75	44	35	64
10	94	18	4	3	19	21	37	28	55	76	25	10	29	80	64	8	81	20	32
20	48	92	87	95	58	57	73	42	1	12	81	94	85	63	97	24	19	93	51
81	10	92	49	70	15	76	4	36	92	62	99	78	32	86	74	43	22	98	46
66	67	82	94	67	75	16	88	84	98	0	52	37	0	43	9	0	51	2	62
84	92	36	11	3	52	44	65	45	67	97	86	92	2	50	5	93	66	73	40
36	29	98	46	88	23	28	44	8	71	69	43	53	16	87	21	56	23	37	24
15	11	82	30	59	94	23	30	40	25	87	26	24	30	44	53	33	65	72	55
89	57	49	79	83	88	42	45	41	93	38	24	15	80	97	18	61	12	13	42
23	36	65	9	64	26	93	37	26	44	42	17	45	68	27	77	74	56	49	34
9	93	90	61	45	40	75	85	64	66	36	89	72	43	99	90	92	10	10	85
53	94	30	31	62	92	82	30	94	56	40	4	50	53	9	74	87	2	36	36
18	69	77	38	89	78	30	68	71	92	22	93	91	74	52	1	97	69	71	42
50	20	76	36	6	20	75	56	36	5	14	70	9	78	23	33	91	33	25	72
30	46	1	10	16	72	69	26	94	39	80	36	36	68	92	74	22	74	41	42
59	47	7	92	77	55	2	12	5	24	0	30	25	62	83	36	92	96	36	75
93	22	3	20	82	44	16	69	98	72	30	57	77	15	90	29	32	38	3	48
9	55	27	41	40	94	77	14	54	10	25	75	1	74	72	15	69	80	33	58
70	8	3	5	46	89	28	86	40	6	25	40	81	26	63	97	87	48	26	41
19	6	89	31	80	60	13	89	17	69	38	93	58	55	54	69	74	33	8	55

FIGURE 12-1   A table of random numbers.

sampling procedure that minimizes error, no guarantee exists that the sample will be representative. Factors such as sample heterogeneity and participant dropout may jeopardize the representativeness of the sample despite the most stringent random sampling procedure. In examining single mothers' adverse and traumatic experiences and posttraumatic stress symptoms, Samuels-Dennis and associates (2010) used simple random sampling to recruit 2400 single mothers from the active caseload of the provincial social assistance program. No simple answer exists as to an acceptable response rate of surveys, but researchers consider the accuracy of their results, whether the population is heterogeneous, and the sorts of biases introduced by the number of responses received. In Samuels-Dennis and associates' study, 247 single mothers completed the survey, which reflects a response rate of 11.3%. The author states that "this extremely low response rate diminishes our ability to generalize these findings to the wider population of income-assisted single mothers" (p. 20).

An assessment of the differences between responders and nonresponders can also provide valuable information, such as length of survey, degree of responder fatigue, and relevance of questions (Berk, 2003).

The major disadvantage of simple random sampling is that it is a time-consuming and inefficient method of obtaining a random sample. (Consider the task of listing all baccalaureate nursing students in Canada.) With random sampling, it may also be impossible to obtain an accurate or complete listing of every element in the population. Imagine trying to obtain a list of all completed suicides in Toronto for 2001. Although suicide may have been the cause of death, another cause (e.g., cardiac failure) often appears on the death certificate. It would be difficult to estimate how many elements of the target population would be eliminated from consideration. Bias would definitely be an issue, despite the researcher's best efforts. Thus, the evaluator

of a research article must exercise caution in generalizing from reported findings, even when random sampling is the stated strategy, if the target population has been difficult or impossible to list completely.

Stratified Random Sampling

Stratified random sampling requires that the population be divided into strata or subgroups. The subgroups or subsets that the population is divided into are homogeneous. An appropriate number of elements from each subset is randomly selected on the basis of the proportion in the population. The goal of this strategy is to achieve a greater degree of representativeness. Stratified random sampling is similar to the proportional stratified quota sampling strategy discussed earlier in this chapter. The major difference is that stratified random sampling involves a random selection procedure for obtaining sample participants. Figure 12-2 illustrates the use of stratified random sampling.

The population is stratified according to any number of attributes, such as age, gender, ethnicity, religion, socioeconomic status, or level of education completed. The variables selected to make up the strata lead to subgroups that share one or more of the attributes being studied (see Practical Application box). The following questions can be asked in the selection of a stratified sample:

- Does a critical variable or attribute exist that provides a logical basis for stratifying the sample?
- Does the population list contain sufficient information about the attributes that will be used to divide the sample into subsets?
- Is it appropriate for each subset to be equal in size, or is it more appropriate for each subset to be proportionally stratified on the basis of the proportion of each subset in the population?
- If proportional sampling is being used, is the number of participants in each subset

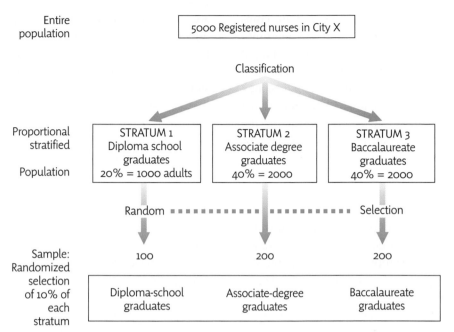

Entire population

5000 Registered nurses in City X

Classification

Proportional stratified

Population

| STRATUM 1 Diploma school graduates 20% = 1000 adults | STRATUM 2 Associate degree graduates 40% = 2000 | STRATUM 3 Baccalaureate graduates 40% = 2000 |

Random ▪▪▪▪▪▪▪▪▪▪▪▪▪▪▪ Selection

Sample: Randomized selection of 10% of each stratum

100   200   200

| Diploma-school graduates | Associate-degree graduates | Baccalaureate graduates |

FIGURE 12-2   Participant selection through the use of a proportional stratified random sampling strategy.

sufficient as a base for meaningful comparisons?

- Once the subset comparison has been determined, are random procedures used for selection of the sample?

Practical Application

A stratified random sampling plan was used by Ulrich and colleagues (2006) to identify ethical concerns and conflicts of nurse practitioners and physician assistants in relation to managed care and the factors that influence ethical conflict. A self-administered questionnaire was mailed to a stratified sample of 3900 nurse practitioners and physician assistants in the United States. Ulrich and colleagues calculated the sample size for each stratum to detect a correlation of 0.2, allowing for 75% eligibility, 40% response rate, and three different state practice environments (excellent or favourable, acceptable, and limiting or restricting) and allowing for a 10% difference in proportions among strata with 95% confidence and 80% power.

In one study (Akhtar-Danesh et al., 2010), a proportional random sampling was based on one strata—location of practice—in assessing community nurses' learning needs. The authors sampled 500 community health nurses: 350 from Ontario and 150 from Nova Scotia, representing equal proportions from each province.

As illustrated in Table 12-1, a stratified random sampling strategy has the following advantages: (1) The representativeness of the sample is enhanced; and (2) the risk of bias is low (i.e., the researcher has a valid basis for making comparisons among subsets if information about the critical variables has been available). A third advantage is that the researcher is able to oversample a disproportionately small stratum to adjust for the researchers' underrepresentation, statistically weigh the data accordingly, and continue to make legitimate comparisons.

The obstacles encountered by a researcher in using this strategy include (1) the difficulty of obtaining a population list containing complete critical variable information; (2) the time-consuming effort of obtaining multiple enumerated lists; (3) the challenge of enrolling proportional strata; and (4) the time and money involved in carrying out a large-scale study with a stratified sampling strategy. In critiquing the study, you must question the appropriateness of this sampling strategy for the problem under investigation.

To examine the effect of biographical factors (i.e., gender, age, nursing education, current position at work, and length of time in current workplace) on job satisfaction, Curtis (2008) recruited a stratified random sample from all eligible registrants with the Irish Nursing Board on the basis of these factors. It is appropriate for the researcher to strive to represent all strata proportionately in the study sample.

Multistage Sampling (Cluster Sampling)

Multistage sampling, or **cluster sampling,** involves a successive random sampling of units (clusters) that meet sample eligibility criteria; this sampling progresses from large to small. A **sampling unit** is an element or set of elements used for selecting the sample. The first-stage sampling unit consists of large units or clusters. The second-stage sampling unit consists of smaller units or clusters. Third-stage sampling units are even smaller.

Consider an example in which a sample of nurse practitioners is desired. The first sampling unit is a random sample of hospitals, obtained from a provincial nurses' association list, that meet the eligibility criteria (e.g., size, type). The second-stage sampling unit consists of a list of acute care nurse practitioners (ACNPs) practising at each hospital selected in the first stage (i.e., the list obtained from the vice president for nursing at each hospital). The criteria for inclusion in the list of ACNPs are as follows: (1) Participants must be certified ACNPs with at least 2 years' experience as an ACNP; (2) at least 75% of the

ACNPs' time must be spent in providing care directly to patients in acute or critical care practices; and (3) the participants must be in full-time employment at the hospital. The second-stage sampling strategy calls for random selection of two ACNPs from each hospital who meet the eligibility criteria.

When multistage sampling is used in relation to large national surveys, provinces are used as the first-stage sampling unit, followed by successively smaller units (such as counties, cities, districts, and blocks) as the second-stage sampling unit and then households as the third-stage sampling unit.

Sampling units or clusters can be selected by simple random or stratified random sampling methods (see Practical Application box). Suppose that the hospitals described in the preceding example are grouped into four strata according to size (i.e., number of beds) as follows: (1) 200 to 299; (2) 300 to 399; (3) 400 to 499; and (4) 500 or more. Stratum 1 comprises 25% of the population; stratum 2 comprises 30% of the population; stratum 3 comprises 20% of the population; and stratum 4 comprises 25% of the population. Thus, either a simple random or a proportional stratified sampling strategy can be used to randomly select hospitals that would proportionately represent the population of hospitals in the provincial nurses' association list.

The main advantage of cluster sampling, as illustrated in Table 12-1, is that it is considerably more economical in terms of time and money than other types of probability sampling, particularly when the population is large and geographically dispersed or when a sampling frame of the elements is not available. However, cluster sampling has two major disadvantages: (1) More sampling errors tend to occur than with simple random or stratified random sampling, and (2) the appropriate handling of the statistical data from cluster samples is very complex.

In critiquing a research report, you need to consider whether the use of cluster sampling is justified in light of the research design, as well as other pragmatic matters, such as economy.

> ## Practical Application
>
> Vlack and colleagues (2007) obtained survey estimates of immunization coverage for indigenous 2-year-old Australian children in Queensland and compared these estimates with those from the national Immunization Register. To select a survey sample, they first stratified 153 geographical areas in Queensland according to their accessibility, creating four strata (from "highly accessible" to "very remote"), and then randomly selected 30 of them for a total target sample of 210 children: 7 eligible children from each area. This sample represented 6% of the estimated population.

Systematic Sampling

Systematic sampling is a sampling strategy that involves the selection of every "kth" case drawn from a population list at fixed intervals, such as every tenth member listed in the directory of the College and Association of Registered Nurses of Alberta (CARNA). Systematic sampling might be used to recruit every "kth" person who enters a hospital lobby or who is hospitalized with a diagnosis of acquired immune deficiency syndrome (AIDS) in 2005. When systematic sampling is used, the population must be narrowly defined (e.g., as consisting of all people entering or leaving the hospital lobby) for the sample to be considered a probability sample. If older adults were sampled systematically on entering a hospital lobby, the resulting sample would not be a probability sample because not every older adult would have a chance of being selected. As such, systematic sampling can sometimes represent a nonprobability sampling strategy.

Systematic sampling strategies can be designed, however, to fulfill the requirements of a probability sample. First, the listing of the population (sampling frame) must be random in relation to the variable of interest. For example, suppose that participants were being selected from every tenth hospital room for a study on patient satisfaction with nursing care. In the hospital where the study was being conducted, every tenth room happened to be a private room. Patients in private rooms might respond differently regarding their satisfaction than patients in semiprivate rooms. Because of the nonrandom arrangement of the rooms, bias may be introduced.

Second, the first element or member of the sample must be selected randomly. In this case, the researcher—who has a population list, or sampling frame—first divides the population *(N)* by the size of the desired sample *(n)* to obtain the sampling interval width *(k)*. The **sampling interval** is the standard distance between the elements chosen for the sample. For example, to select a sample of 50 family nurse practitioners from a population of 500 family nurse practitioners, the sampling interval would be as follows:

$$k = \frac{500}{50} = 10$$

Essentially, every tenth case on the family nurse practitioner list would be sampled. Thus, if the starting point was participant 5, then next person chosen would be 15th, then 25th, etc.

Once the sampling interval has been determined, the researcher uses a table of random numbers (see Figure 12-1) to obtain a starting point for the selection of the 50 participants. If the population size is 500 and a sample size of 50 is desired, a number between 1 and 500 is randomly selected as the starting point. In this instance, if the first number is 51, the family nurse practitioners corresponding to numbers 51, 61, 71, and so forth would be included in the sample of 50.

Another procedure recommended in many texts is to randomly select the first element from within the first sampling interval. If the sampling interval is 5, a number between 1 and 5 is selected as the random starting point. For example, the number 3 is randomly chosen.

Keeping in mind the sampling interval of 5, the next elements selected would correspond to the numbers 8, 13, 18, and so on, until the sample was obtained. Although this procedure is technically correct, choosing a random starting point from across the total population of elements is more attractive because every element has a chance to be chosen for the sample during the first selection step.

Systematic sampling and simple random sampling are essentially the same type of procedure. The advantage of systematic sampling is that the results are obtained in a more convenient and efficient manner (see Table 12-1). The disadvantage of systematic sampling is that bias in the form of nonrandomness can be inadvertently introduced into the procedure. This problem may occur if the population list is arranged so that a certain type of element is listed at intervals that coincide with the sampling interval. For example, if every tenth nursing student on a population list of all types of nursing students in Ontario was a baccalaureate student and the sampling interval was 10, baccalaureate students would be overrepresented in the sample.

Cyclical fluctuations are also a factor in systematic sampling. For example, if a list is kept of nursing students using the college library each day to do computer literature searches, a biased sample would probably be obtained if every seventh day, such as Sunday, is chosen as the sampling interval: in the case of Sunday, because probably fewer and perhaps different nursing students use the library on Sundays than on weekdays. Therefore, caution must be exercised about departures from randomness because they affect the representativeness of the sample and, as a result, the external validity of the study.

You should note whether a satisfactory random selection procedure was performed. If randomization was not used, the systematic sampling may have become a nonprobability quota sample. You need to be cognizant of this issue because the implications related to interpretation and generalizability are drastically altered when a nonprobability sample is involved.

For example, in their study, Cho and associates (2003) sought to determine the effects of nurse staffing (that is, ratio of number of Registered Nurses to Registered Practical Nurses) on adverse events, including morbidity, mortality, and medical costs. The study used two existing databases: California Hospital Financial Data and 1997 data for the state of California released by the Agency for Healthcare Research and Quality (AHRQ). In the selection of hospitals and patients, the researchers strived to create a sample that included homogeneous hospital and patient groups while representing the majority of the target population. Hospitals were stratified by ownership, hospital size, teaching affiliation, and location; nurse staffing was stratified by type of care unit (e.g., medical-surgical acute care, medical-surgical intensive care, and coronary care). Patient characteristics were stratified by "diagnostic related group" and selected demographic variables. Because randomization was not used at any phase of this multilevel sampling procedure, you would consider this study to be a nonprobability stratified sample with the external validity limitations of that sampling strategy (see Chapter 9).

Evidence-Informed Practice Tip

The sampling strategy, whether probability or nonprobability, must be appropriate for the study design and evaluated in relation to the level of evidence provided by the design.

Special Sampling Strategies

Several special sampling strategies are used in nonprobability sampling. **Matching** is a special strategy used to construct an equivalent comparison sample group by filling it with participants who are similar to each participant in another sample group in terms of preestablished variables, such as age, gender, level of education, medical diagnosis, or socioeconomic status. Theoretically, any variable other than the independent variable that could affect the dependent variable should be matched. In reality, the more variables matched, the more difficult it is to obtain an adequate sample size.

Matching was used in a study that sought to determine whether unmarried adolescent mothers and married adult mothers differ in terms of satisfaction with inpatient postpartum nursing care. In this sample, adolescent and adult postpartum mothers were matched in terms of parity, mode of delivery, infant health status, and infant feeding method (Peterson & DiCenso, 2002). When an organization or institution composes the sampling unit, matching may also be an important consideration. For example, in a study of the effect of an ankle-strengthening and walking exercise program on improving fall-related outcomes in older adults, Schoenfelder and Rubenstein (2004) recruited participants from 10 private, urban nursing homes in eastern Iowa. Participants were matched in pairs by scores on the Risk Assessment for Falls Scale II and then the members of each pair were randomly assigned to opposite groups (the intervention or control condition).

Nonprobability Sampling Strategies Used in Qualitative Research

Because nonprobability sampling is the best method of obtaining individuals who are key informants of a phenomenon, these sampling methods are widely used in qualitative research. As described in Chapter 7, qualitative research methods are conducted to gain both insights into and in-depth meaning about experiences, incidents, or events. In qualitative research, the sampling procedure is governed by the methodology used. Many sampling strategies are used in qualitative sampling, but the most common approaches are *network sampling, purposive sampling,* and *theoretical sampling.*

Network Sampling

Network sampling, sometimes referred to as **snowball effect sampling** or *snowballing,* is a

strategy used for locating samples that are difficult or impossible to locate in other ways. This sampling strategy takes advantage of social networks and the tendency of friends to share characteristics. When a few participants with the necessary eligibility criteria are found, the researcher asks for their assistance in getting in touch with other people with similar characteristics that meet these criteria.

Chen (2010) recruited participants from purposive sampling and then, in her second round of recruitment, used network sampling by asking participants whether they knew any other interested women who would be part of the study. The study was about understanding the cultural context of Chinese mothers' perceptions of breast-feeding and infant health in Canada.

Today, online computer networks, as described in the following section on purposive sampling, can be used to assist researchers in recruiting participants who are otherwise difficult to locate, thereby taking advantage of the networking or snowball effect. The Critical Thinking Decision Path illustrates the relationship between the type of sampling strategy and the appropriate generalizability.

Purposive Sampling

Purposive sampling is an increasingly common strategy in which the researcher's knowledge of the population and its elements is used to handpick the cases to be included in the sample. The researcher usually selects participants who are considered typical of the population.

For example, in a qualitative study (see Appendix A), Seneviratne and associates (2009) used a subset of purposive sampling, maximum variation purposive sampling, to locate health care professionals in their ethnographic study. Maximum variation purposive sampling is the "process of deliberately selecting a heterogeneous sample and observing commonalities in their experiences" (Morse, 1994, p. 229).

CRITICAL THINKING DECISION PATH

Assessing the Relationship between the Type of Sampling Strategy and the Appropriate Generalizability

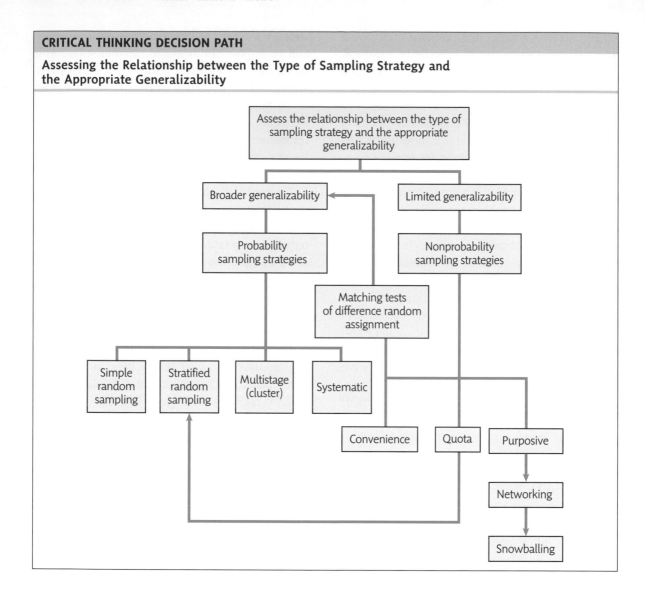

A purposive sample is also used when a highly unusual group is being studied, such as a population with a rare genetic disease (e.g., Tay-Sachs disease). In this case, the researcher would describe the sample characteristics precisely to ensure that the reader will have an accurate picture of the participants in the sample. This type of sample can also be used to study the differential effect of risk factors in a specific population longitudinally. For example, in the longitudinal

Delaware Valley Twin Study, Meininger and associates (1998) examined the differential effect of cardiovascular risk factors that have the potential to respond to environmental and lifestyle modification. They recruited participant families from Mothers of Twins clubs and schools in the Philadelphia metropolitan area. Same-sex monozygotic and dizygotic twin pairs who met the eligibility criteria were recruited into this study.

In another situation, the researcher may wish to interview individuals who reflect a particular characteristic. For example, Martin-Misener and colleagues (2010) studied the role of primary health care nurse practitioners in rural Nova Scotia. Nine chairpersons, six women and three men, were selected through the use of purposive sampling to form a group representative of the health boards in each district health authority.

Today, computer networks (e.g., online services) can be of great value in helping researchers access and recruit participants for purposive samples. For instance, Valaitis and associates (2008) used an online method to invite 91 schools of nursing to participate in their study of the barriers and enablers influencing the integration of community health nursing content in baccalaureate education in Canada.

The researcher who uses a purposive sample assumes that errors of judgement in overrepresenting or underrepresenting elements of the population in the sample will tend to balance each other. The validity of this assumption, however, cannot be determined objectively. You must be aware that the more heterogeneous the population, the greater the chance that bias is introduced in the selection of a purposive sample. As indicated in Table 12-1, conscious bias in the selection of participants remains a constant concern. Therefore, the findings from a study involving a purposive sample should be regarded with caution. As with any nonprobability sample, the ability to generalize is very limited. The following are several instances when a purposive sample may be appropriate:

- The effective pretesting of newly developed instruments with a purposive sample of diverse types of people
- The validation of a scale or test with a known-groups technique
- The collection of exploratory data in relation to an unusual or highly specific population, particularly when the total target population remains unknown to the researcher

- The collection of descriptive data (e.g., as in qualitative studies) with which researchers seek to describe the lived experience of a particular phenomenon (e.g., postpartum depression, caring, hope, or surviving childhood sexual abuse)
- The focus of the study population when it is related to a specific diagnosis (e.g., type 1 diabetes, multiple sclerosis), a specific condition (e.g., legal blindness, terminal illness), or a specific demographic characteristic (e.g., same-sex twin pairs)

Many types of purposive sampling exist (Miles & Huberman, 1994; Patton, 2010), but the following three types of cases are the most often used:

1. Typical cases: cases that are "normal" or "average" among those being studied
2. Deviant or extreme cases: cases that represent unusual manifestations of the phenomenon of interest
3. Confirming or disconfirming cases: cases that are exceptions, that represent variation, or for which an initial elaborate analysis is necessary

In any type of purposive sampling, sampling is stopped when **data saturation** occurs: that is, when the information being shared with the researcher becomes repetitive.

Criterion sampling is also a form of purposive sampling. The researcher needs to have a set of criteria for a sample, and all cases that meet these criteria are selected. It is important that the criteria are established so that cases that are chosen will yield rich data relevant to the research problem being explored: for example, all patients who were in a smoking cessation program and have resumed smoking. This criterion would enable an understanding of what is needed to support individuals who wish to quit smoking.

Theoretical Sampling

Theoretical sampling is associated with grounded theory research. As you learned in Chapter 8, the goal of grounded research is theory generation;

thus, a theoretical sampling strategy is used to fully elaborate and validate variations in the data by finding examples of a theoretical construct (Sandelowski, 1995). In **theoretical sampling,** the researcher selects experiences that will help test ideas and gather complete information about developing concepts. Sampling is stopped when theory saturation or redundancy occurs.

Theoretical sampling was used by Young and associates (2007), who evaluated the relative effectiveness of telephone and videophone follow-up for children and families after a child's surgery for scoliosis. Young and associates used memo writing to guide the initial coding of concepts and the theoretical sampling process. The views, situations, and experiences of different family members were compared, and data from the same individuals were gathered at different times. Young and associates engaged in constant comparative analyses as new categories arose.

Helpful Hint_____

Look for a brief discussion of a study's sampling strategy in the "Methods" section of a research article. Some articles have a separate subsection with the heading "Sample," "Participants," or "Study Participants." A statistical description of the characteristics of the actual sample often does not appear until the "Results" section of a research article.

SAMPLE SIZE: QUANTITATIVE

No single rule can be applied to the determination of a sample's size. When researchers estimate sample size, they must consider many factors, such as the following:

- The type of design used
- The type of sampling procedure used
- The type of formula used for estimating the optimal sample size
- The degree of precision required
- The heterogeneity of the attributes under investigation
- The relative frequency at which the phenomenon of interest occurs in the popu-

lation (i.e., a common vs. a rare health problem)
- The projected cost of using a particular sampling strategy

The sample size should be determined before the study is conducted. A general rule is always to use the largest sample possible. The larger the sample, the more likely it is to be representative of the population; smaller samples produce less accurate results.

An exception to the rule about sample size is the **pilot study,** which is a small sample study conducted as a prelude to a larger scale (parent) study. The pilot study typically is conducted with similar methods and procedures that both yield preliminary data for determining the feasibility of conducting a larger scale study and establish that sufficient scientific evidence exists to justify subsequent, more extensive research.

Hertzog (2008) summarized methods for justifying sample sizes on the basis of the aim of the pilot study. This author suggests that a sample size as small as 10 to 15 participants per group may be sufficient for the decisions being made. For pilot studies involving group comparisons, 10 to 20 participants per group may be enough. On the other hand, if a researcher is developing or testing an instrument, it is suggested that each group comprise 35 to 40 participants.

For example, Hayward and colleagues (2007) conducted a pilot study, "Co-Bedding Twins: How Pilot Study Findings Guided Improvements in Planning a Larger Multicenter Trial," using a sample with 70 babies per group. The researchers analyzed preliminary data to estimate effect size, determine staff and bedside care organization, evaluate feasibility of data-collection measures, and identify issues related to recruitment and follow-up before conducting a multicentre study.

The principle of "larger is better" holds true for both probability and nonprobability samples. Results based on small samples (fewer than 10 participants) tend to be unstable; the values fluctuate from one sample to the next. Small samples tend to increase the probability of obtaining a markedly nonrepresentative sample. As the sample size increases, the mean more closely approximates the population values; thus, fewer sampling errors are introduced.

An example of this concept is illustrated by a study in which the average monthly consumption of sleeping pills was investigated for patients on a rehabilitation unit after a cerebrovascular accident. The data in Table 12-3 indicate that the population consisted of 20 patients whose average consumption of sleeping pills was 15.2 per month.

The population of 20 patients was divided into sets of two simple random samples with sizes of 2, 4, 6, and 10. Each sample average in the right column represents an estimate of the population average, which is known to be 15.15. In most cases, the population value was unknown to the researchers, but because the population is so small, it could be calculated. In Table 12-3, note that with a sample size of two, the estimate might have been wrong by as much as eight sleeping pills in sample 1B. As the sample size increases,

the averages get closer to the population value, and the differences in the estimates between samples A and B also get smaller. Large samples permit the principles of randomization to work effectively (i.e., to counterbalance atypical values in the long run).

The sample size can be estimated with the use of a statistical procedure known as *power analysis* (see Chapter 16). A simple example illustrates this concept. Suppose that a researcher wants to determine the effect of nurse preoperative teaching on patient postoperative anxiety. Patients are randomly assigned to an experimental group or a control group. How many patients should be used in the study? When using power analysis, the researcher must estimate how large a difference will be observed between the groups (i.e., the difference in the mean amount of postoperative anxiety after the experimental preoperative teaching program). This difference is called the **effect size.** If a small difference is expected, the sample must be large (in this case, 196 patients in each group) to ensure that the differences will be revealed in a statistical analysis. If a medium-size difference is expected, the total sample size would be 128 (64 in each group). When expected differences are large, a small sample size can ensure that differences will be revealed through statistical analysis.

An example is illustrated by the study of Fox and colleagues (2010), who examined differences in sleep complaints among patients with varying amounts of bed rest. Before data collection, they conducted a power analysis based on prior research. With an alpha value set at .05 and the power set at .80, the power analysis indicated that 21 participants were required in each of the three cohorts in order to detect a large effect. Alpha is the probability of making a Type I error (rejecting the null hypothesis when the null hypothesis is true).

Power analysis is an advanced statistical technique that is commonly used by researchers and is a requirement for external funding. When

TABLE **12-3**

COMPARISON OF POPULATION AND SAMPLE VALUES AND AVERAGES IN STUDY OF SLEEPING PILL CONSUMPTION

NUMBER IN GROUP	GROUP	NUMBER OF SLEEPING PILLS CONSUMED (VALUES EXPRESSED MONTHLY)	AVERAGE
20	Population	1, 3, 4, 5, 6, 7, 9, 11, 13, 15, 16, 17, 19, 21, 22, 23, 25, 27, 29, 30	15.2
2	Sample 1A	6, 9	7.5
2	Sample 1B	21, 25	23.0
4	Sample 2A	1, 7, 15, 25	12.0
4	Sample 2B	5, 13, 23, 29	17.5
6	Sample 3A	3, 4, 11, 15, 21, 25	13.3
6	Sample 3B	5, 7, 11, 19, 27, 30	16.5
10	Sample 4A	3, 4, 7, 9, 11, 13, 17, 21, 23, 30	13.8
10	Sample 4B	1, 4, 6, 11, 15, 17, 19, 23, 25, 27	13.8

power analysis is not used, research studies may be based on samples that are too small, which may lead to a lack of support for the researcher's hypotheses and to a type I error (rejecting a null hypothesis when it should have been accepted); in other words, the researcher finds significant results when none exist (see Chapter 16). A researcher may also commit a type II error (accepting a null hypothesis when it should have been rejected) if the sample is too small; in other words, the sample is too small to detect treatment effects (see Chapter 16).

Despite the principles related to determining sample size that have been identified in this chapter, you should be aware that large samples do not ensure representativeness or accuracy. A large sample cannot compensate for faulty research design. The proportion of the population that is sampled does not provide a guarantee of accurate results. Accurate results can be obtained from only a small fraction of a large population. For example, a 10% probability sample of a population containing 1500 elements will yield more precise results than will a nonprobability 0.01% sample of a population with 100,000 elements.

You should evaluate the sample size in terms of (1) how representative the sample is of the target population and (2) to which population the researcher wishes to generalize the results of the study. The goal of sampling is to gather a sample as representative as possible with as few sampling errors as possible.

SAMPLE SIZE: QUALITATIVE

In qualitative research, no power analyses are conducted a priori to determine sample size requirements. According to Sandelowski (1995), sample size is determined by the purpose and type of the sampling and the research method to be used. Morse (1994) recommended about six participants for phenomenological studies and about 30 to 50 cases for ethnographies and grounded theory studies. These suggestions do not constitute a hard-and-fast rule because a one-person

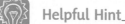

Helpful Hint

Remember to look for some rationale about the sample size and the strategies that the researcher has used (e.g., matching, test of differences on demographic variables) to ascertain or build in sample representativeness.

case study may be sufficient for a phenomenological study. When you critique a study, you must note how the researcher has explained the sampling plan and what limitations have been noted. Participants are added to the sample until data saturation is reached (i.e., new data no longer emerge during the data-collection process). The fittingness of the data is a more important concern than the representativeness of participants (see Chapter 14).

Evidence-Informed Practice Tip

Research designs and types of samples are often linked. You would expect to see experimental designs in which probability sampling strategies were used; if a nonprobability purposive sampling strategy is used to recruit participants to such a study, you would expect the participants to then be randomly assigned to intervention and control groups.

SAMPLING PROCEDURES

The criteria for selecting a sample vary according to the sampling strategy. Regardless of which strategy is used, the procedure must be systematically organized. Such organization will eliminate the bias that occurs when sample selection is carried out inconsistently. Bias in sample representativeness and generalizability of findings are important sampling issues that have generated national concern.

For example, many of the landmark adult health studies (e.g., the Framingham Heart Study and the Baltimore Longitudinal Study of Aging) historically excluded women as participants. The findings of these studies were generalized from men to all adults despite the lack of female representation in the samples. Similarly, the use of largely Euro-American participants in medication clinical trials limits the identification of variant responses to drugs in other ethnic or racially distinct groups (Campinha-Bacote, 1997). Findings based on Euro-American data cannot be generalized to Punjabis, Chinese, West Indians, or any other cultural group. Consequently, careful identification of the target population is a crucial step in the process.

In order to establish conclusions about psychosocial stressors related to all patients with a first-time myocardial infarction, both men and women must be included in the target population. To establish conclusions about the incidence of extrapyramidal side effects of haloperidol (Haldol) in a psychiatric ward among Chinese patients in comparison with Euro-Americans, the target population must be diverse. Sometimes, however, the target population must be gender specific, as when breast or prostate cancer or aspects of pregnancy or menopause are studied.

Several general steps (Figure 12-3) ensure the identification of a consistent approach by the researcher. Initially, the target population (i.e., the

entire group of people or objects about whom the researcher wants to establish conclusions or make generalizations) must be identified. The target population may consist, for example, of all female patients with a first-time diagnosis of breast cancer, all children with asthma, all pregnant teenagers, or all doctoral students in Canada.

Next, the accessible portion of the target population must be delineated. An accessible population might consist of all nurse practitioners in the province of New Brunswick, all male patients with AIDS admitted to a certain hospital during 2001, all pregnant teenagers in a specific prenatal clinic, or all children with rheumatoid arthritis under care at a specific hospital specializing in the treatment of autoimmune diseases.

Then a sampling plan or a protocol for actually selecting the sample from the accessible population is formulated. The researcher makes decisions about how participants will be approached, how the study will be explained, and who—the researcher or a research assistant—will select the sample. Regardless of who implements the sampling plan, consistency in how it is done is of paramount importance. In reading a research report, you want to find a description of the sample, as well as the sampling procedure, in the study. On the basis of the appropriateness of what has been reported, you can make judgements about the soundness of the sampling protocol, which, of course, will affect the interpretations of the findings.

Finally, once the accessible population and sampling plan have been established, permission is obtained from the institution's research board, which is commonly referred to as the *research ethics board*. This permission provides free access to the desired population.

When an appropriate sample size and sampling strategy have been used, the researcher can feel more confident that the sample is representative of the accessible population; however, it is more difficult to feel confident that the accessible population is representative of the target

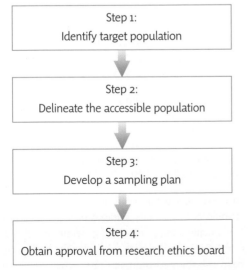

FIGURE 12-3 Summary of the general sampling procedures.

population. Are nurse practitioners in New Brunswick representative of all nurse practitioners in Canada? It is impossible to know for sure. Researchers must exercise judgement when assessing typicality. Unfortunately, no guidelines for making such judgements exist, and critiquers have even less basis to make such decisions. The best rule to use when evaluating the representativeness of a sample and its generalizability to the target population is to be realistic and con-

servative about making sweeping claims in relation to the findings.

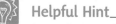 Helpful Hint_____

Remember to evaluate the appropriateness of the generalizations made about the findings of a quantitative study in view of the target population, the accessible population, the type of sampling strategy, and the sample size. In qualitative research, evaluate the transferability of the findings on the basis of the research design and its sampling strategy and size.

APPRAISING THE EVIDENCE

Sample

The criteria for critiquing the sampling technique of a study are presented in the Critiquing Criteria box. You (the reader) and the researcher approach the "Sample" section of a research report with different perspectives. You must raise the following two questions:

1. If this study were to be replicated, is enough information available about the nature of the population, the sample, the sampling strategy, and the sample size for another investigator to carry out the study?

2. Are the previously mentioned factors appropriate for the particular research design, and, if not, which factors require modification, especially if the study is to be replicated?

Sampling is considered to be one important aspect of the methodology of a research study. Thus, data pertaining to the sample usually appear in the "Methodology" section of the research report. The sampling content presented should reflect the outcome of a series of decisions based on sampling criteria appropriate to the design of the study, as well as the options and limitations inherent in the context of the investigation. The following discussion highlights several sampling criteria that you should consider when you evaluate the merit of a sampling strategy in relation to a specific research study.

Initially, the parameters or attributes of the study population should clearly specify to what population the findings may be generalized. In general, the target population of the study is not specifically identified by the researcher, but the nature of it is implied in the

description of the accessible population, the sample, or both. For example, if a researcher states that 100 participants were randomly selected from a population of men and women older than 65 and with a diagnosis of COPD who were treated in a respiratory rehabilitation program at a particular hospital during 2001, you can specifically evaluate the parameters of the population. The demographic characteristics of the sample (e.g., age, gender, diagnosis, ethnicity, religion, and marital status) should also be presented in either a tabular or a narrative summary because they provide further explication about the nature of the sample and enable you to evaluate the sampling procedure more accurately. For example, in their study on Canadian nurses' reports of workplace violence, Lemelin and associates (2009) presented detailed data summarizing demographic variables of importance. These data are reproduced as follows:

> Analysis of the sociodemographic variables showed that the average age of respondents was 32.63 years 65.0% of respondents had less than 10 years of nursing experience, and 68.5% of respondents had college-level nursing education. (Lemelin, Bonin, & Duquette, 2009, p. 158)

This example illustrates how a detailed description of the sample both provides a frame of reference for the study population and sample and generates questions to be raised. For example, note the variability in the range of mean risk-adjusted mortality rate. When this demographic sample information is available, you are able to

APPRAISING THE EVIDENCE

Sample—cont'd

question a sampling strategy that does not also account for the differential effect of the size or type of hospital on the mortality rate, which are factors that might affect the difference in the mortality rate. Also helpful is the researcher's rationale for having elected to study one type of population versus another. For example, why did Lemelin and associates (2009) use only nurses in Quebec in their study?

In a research study in which a nonprobability sampling strategy is used, it is particularly important to fully describe the population and the sample in terms of who the study participants were, how they were chosen, and the reason they were chosen. If these criteria are adhered to, the degree of heterogeneity or homogeneity of the sample can be determined. The use of a homogeneous sample minimizes the amount of sampling error introduced, a problem particularly common in nonprobability sampling.

Next, the defined representativeness of the population should be examined. Probability sampling is clearly the ideal sampling procedure for ensuring the representativeness of a study population. Use of random selection procedures (e.g., simple random, stratified random, cluster, or systematic sampling strategies) minimizes the occurrence of conscious and unconscious biases that affect the researcher's ability to generalize about the findings from the sample to the population. You should be able to identify the type of probability strategy used and determine whether the researcher adhered to the criteria for a particular sampling plan. In experimental and quasiexperimental studies, you must also know whether or how the participants were assigned to groups. If the criteria have not been followed, you have a valid reason for being skeptical about the proposed conclusions of the study.

Random selection is the ideal in establishing the representativeness of a study population; more often, however, realistic barriers (e.g., institutional policy, inaccessibility of participants, lack of time or money, and current state of knowledge in the field) necessitate the use of nonprobability sampling strategies. Many important research problems that are of interest to nurses do not lend themselves to experimental design and probability sampling, particularly qualitative research designs.

A well-designed, carefully controlled study with a nonprobability sampling strategy can yield accurate and meaningful findings that make a significant contribution to nursing's scientific body of knowledge. As the critiquer, you must ask a philosophical question: "If it is not possible or appropriate to conduct an experimental or quasiexperimental investigation with the use of probability sampling, should the study be abandoned?" The answer usually suggests that it is better to perform the investigation and be fully aware of the limitations of the methodology than not to acquire the potential knowledge. The researcher is always able to move on to subsequent studies that either replicate the initial study or entail the use of more stringent design and sampling strategies to refine the knowledge derived from a nonexperimental study.

The greatest difficulty in nonprobability sampling stems from the fact that not every element in the population has an equal chance of being represented in the sample. Therefore, some segment of the population will probably be systematically underrepresented. If the population is homogeneous with regard to critical characteristics, systematic bias will not be an important problem. Few of the attributes that researchers are interested in, however, are sufficiently homogeneous to render sampling bias an irrelevant consideration.

Next, the sampling plan's suitability to the research design should be evaluated. In experimental and quasiexperimental designs, some form of random selection or random assignment of participants to groups is used (see Chapter 10). In critiquing the report, you evaluate whether the researcher adhered to the principles of random selection and assignment. Lack of adherence to such principles compromises the representativeness of the sample and the external validity of the study. The following are questions that you might pose in relation to this issue:

- Has a random selection procedure (e.g., a table of random numbers) been identified?
- Has the appropriate random sampling plan been selected? In other words, has a proportional stratified sampling plan been selected instead of a simple random sampling plan in a study in which

Continued

APPRAISING THE EVIDENCE

Sample—cont'd

three distinct occupational levels appear to be critical variables for stratification?

- Has the particular random sampling plan been carried out appropriately? In other words, if a cluster sampling strategy was used, did the sampling units logically progress from the largest to the smallest?

Random sampling should not be regarded as a perfect method of obtaining a representative sample. Sometimes, bias is inadvertently introduced even when random selection is used. In many nonexperimental designs, nonprobability sampling strategies are used. For such studies, you can ask whether a nonexperimental design and a related nonprobability sampling plan were most appropriate. Sometimes, if the researchers had used another type of design or sampling plan, they could have constructed a stronger study that would have produced findings that were more generalizable and more reliable. In critiquing, however, you are rarely in a position to know what factors entered into the decision to plan one type of study rather than another.

You should then determine whether the sample size is appropriate and its size is justifiable. The researcher usually indicates in a research article how the sample size was determined; a similar indication is also seen commonly in doctoral dissertations. The method of arriving at the sample size and the rationale should be briefly mentioned. For example, a researcher may state the following:

A power analysis for the multiple regression with 2 independent variables ($p = .05$ and power = .80) determined that a sample of 76 was required to detect a moderate effect size of 0.15. A sample size of 300 was surveyed to offset the possibility of a low response rate typically found with mailed surveys, movement of nurses from employers, and any errors in the registry list. (Armstrong, Laschinger, & Wong, 2009, p. 57)

In Lemelin and associates' (2009) study on workplace violence reported by Canadian nurses, a power analysis was conducted, and

it was determined that 252 respondents were needed for a medium effect size (.25; alpha = .05; power = .95). (p. 158)

The importance of such examples lies in understanding that this type of statement meets the criteria stated at the beginning of the paragraph and should be evident in the research report. Other considerations with regard to sample size, especially when the sample size appears to be small or inadequate and no rationale is stated for the size, are as follows:

- How will the sample size affect the accuracy of the results?
- Are any subsets or cells of the sample overrepresented or underrepresented?
- Are any of the subsets so small as to limit meaningful comparisons?
- Has the researcher examined the effect of attrition on the results?
- Has the researcher recognized and identified any limitations posed by the size of the sample?

Essentially, these criteria necessitate that you carefully scrutinize several important elements pertaining to sample size that have implications for the generalizability of the findings. Keep in mind that in reports of qualitative studies, neither the predetermining nor the method of determining the sample size will be discussed. Rather, the sample size depends on the methodology used and is a function of data saturation (see Chapter 8).

With qualitative research designs, you apply criteria related to sampling strategies that are relevant for a particular type of qualitative study. In general, sampling strategies are purposive because the study of specific phenomena in their natural setting is emphasized; any participant belonging to a specified group is considered to represent that group. For example, in the qualitative study by Seneviratne and associates (2009; see Appendix A), the specified group was nurses on an acute stroke unit. The researchers' goal was to understand the nature of nursing on this type of unit—that is, the typicality or atypicality of the observed events and behaviours—and to reveal nurses' perceptions of the contexts of caring for survivors of acute stroke.

Finally, the "Sample" section of the research report should provide evidence that the rights of human participants have been protected. You will evaluate whether permission was obtained from an institutional research

APPRAISING THE EVIDENCE

Sample—cont'd

ethics board that reviewed the study with regard to maintaining ethical research standards (see Chapter 6). For example, the research ethics board examines the research proposal to determine whether the introduction of an experimental procedure may be potentially harmful and therefore undesirable. You also examine the report for evidence of the participants' informed consent, as well as protection of their confidentiality or anonymity. Research studies that do not demonstrate evidence of having met these criteria are highly unusual. Nevertheless, you will want to be certain that ethical standards that protect sample participants have been maintained.

Many factors must be considered when you critique the "Sample" section of a research report. The type and appropriateness of the sampling strategy become crucial elements in the analysis and interpretation of data, in the conclusions derived from the findings, and in the generalizability of the findings from the sample to the population. As stated earlier in this chapter, the major purpose of sampling is to increase the efficacy of a research study by representing the particular population so that not every element need be studied, while producing the findings that can be generalized from the sample to the population. You must demonstrate that the sampling strategy used provided a valid basis for the findings and their generalizability.

CRITIQUING CRITERIA

1. Have the sample characteristics been completely described?
2. Can the parameters of the study population be inferred from the description of the sample?
3. To what extent is the sample representative of the population as defined?
4. Are criteria for eligibility in the sample specifically identified?
5. Have sample delimitations been established?
6. Would it be possible to replicate the study population?
7. How was the sample selected? Is the method of sample selection appropriate?
8. What kind of bias, if any, is introduced by this method?
9. Is the sample size appropriate? How is it substantiated?
10. Does the researcher indicate that the rights of participants have been ensured?
11. Does the researcher identify the limitations in generalizability of the findings from the sample to the population? Are those limitations appropriate?
12. Is the sampling strategy appropriate for the design of the study and level of evidence provided by the design?
13. Does the researcher indicate how replication of the study with other samples would provide increased support for the findings?

CRITICAL THINKING CHALLENGES

- A research classmate asks the instructor the following question: "Why isn't it better to study an entire population of patients with lung cancer instead of using the research technique of sampling?" How would you answer this question? Include examples that will help the student see your point of view.
- In the report of a quasiexperimental study, the researchers indicated that they used a convenience sample with random assignment.

How is this possible? Would they have used a nonprobability or a probability sample? If you agree that this is a legitimate sampling technique, present both the advantages and the disadvantages; if you disagree, indicate your rationale.

- Your research class is having a debate on probability sampling versus nonprobability sampling with regard to desirability and feasibility. You are assigned to present the advantages of nonprobability sampling in nursing research. What arguments would you use?

- Discuss the principle of "larger is better" and its relationship to network sampling and the sample size of qualitative studies. Include in your discussion the concept of data saturation and the use of computer technology.
- Your research classmate is arguing that a random sample is always better, even if it is small and represents only one site. Another student is arguing that a very large convenience sample representing multiple sites can be very significant. Which classmate would you defend, and why?

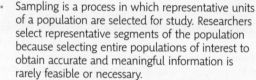

KEY POINTS

- Sampling is a process in which representative units of a population are selected for study. Researchers select representative segments of the population because selecting entire populations of interest to obtain accurate and meaningful information is rarely feasible or necessary.
- Researchers establish eligibility criteria; these are descriptors of the population and provide the basis for inclusion into a sample. Eligibility criteria can include age, gender, socioeconomic status, level of education, religion, and ethnicity.
- The researcher must identify the target population (i.e., the entire set of cases about which the researcher would like to make generalizations). Because of pragmatic constraints, however, the researcher usually uses an accessible population (i.e., one that meets the population criteria and is available).
- A sample is a set of elements that make up the population.
- A sampling unit is the element or set of elements used for selecting the sample. The foremost criterion in evaluating a sample is the representativeness or congruence of characteristics with the population.
- Sampling strategies consist of nonprobability and probability sampling.
- In nonprobability sampling, the elements are chosen by nonrandom methods. Types of nonprobability sampling include convenience, quota, and purposive sampling.
- Probability sampling is characterized by the random selection of elements from the population. In random selection, each element in the population has an equal and independent chance of being included in the sample. Types of

probability sampling include simple random, stratified random, cluster, and systematic sampling.
- Sample size is a function of the type of sampling procedure being used, the degree of precision required, the type of sample estimation formula being used, the heterogeneity of the study attributes, the relative frequency of occurrence of the phenomena under consideration, and the cost.
- Criteria for selecting a sample vary according to the sampling strategy. Systematic organization of the sampling procedure minimizes bias. The target population is identified, the accessible portion of the target population is delineated, permission to conduct the research study is obtained, and a sampling plan is formulated.
- In critiquing a research report, you evaluate the sampling plan for its appropriateness in relation to the particular research design.
- The completeness of the sampling plan is examined with regard to the potential replicability of the study. In critiquing, you evaluate whether the sampling strategy is the strongest plan for the particular study under consideration.
- An appropriate systematic sampling plan will maximize the efficiency of a research study. It will increase the accuracy and meaningfulness of the findings and enhance the generalizability of the findings from the sample to the population.

REFERENCES

Akhtar-Danesh, N., Valaitis, R. K., Schofield, R., Underwood, J., Martin-Misener, R., Baumann, A., & Kolotylo, C. (2010). A questionnaire for assessing community health nurses' learning needs. *Western Journal of Nursing Research, 32*(8), 1055-1072.

Armstrong, K., Laschinger, H., & Wong, C. (2009). Workplace empowerment and magnet hospital characteristics as predictors of patient safety climate. *Journal of Nursing Care Quality, 24*(1), 55-62.

Berk, R. (2003). *Regression analysis: A constructive critique.* Thousand Oaks, CA: Sage.

Boscart, V. M. (2009). A communication intervention for nursing staff in chronic care. *Journal of Advanced Nursing, 65*(9), 1823-1832.

Campinha-Bacote, J. (1997). Understanding the influence of culture. In J. Haber, B. Krainovich-Miller, & A. L. McMahon, & P. Price-Hoskins, (Eds.), *Comprehensive psychiatric nursing* (5th ed., pp. 70-95). St. Louis: Mosby.

Chahal, N., Manlhiot, C., Colapinto, K., Van Alphen, J., McCrindle, B. W., & Rush, J. (2009). Association between parental anxiety and compliance with preoperative requirements for pediatric outpatient surgery. *Journal of Pediatric Health Care, 23*(6), 372-377.

Chen, W. (2010). Understanding the cultural context of Chinese mothers' perceptions of breastfeeding and infant health in Canada. *Journal of Clinical Nursing, 19*, 1021-1029.

Chiovitti, R. F. (2006). Nurses' meaning of caring with patients in acute psychiatric hospital settings: A grounded theory study. *International Journal of Nursing Studies, 45*(2), 203-223.

Cho, S. H., Ketefian, S., Barkauskas, V. H., & Smith, D. G. (2003). The effects of nurse staffing on adverse events, morbidity, mortality, and medical costs. *Nursing Research, 52*, 71-79.

Cochran, W. G. (1977). *Sampling technique* (3rd ed.). New York: Wiley.

Curtis, E. A. (2008). The effects of biographical variables on job satisfaction among nurses. *British Journal of Nursing, 17*(3), 174-180.

Fox, M. T., Sidani, S., & Brooks, D. (2010). Differences in sleep complaints in adults with varying levels of bed days residing in extended care facilities for chronic disease management. *Clinical Nursing Research, 19*(2), 181-202.

Hayward, K., Campbell-Yeo, M., Price, S., Morrison, D., Whyte, R., Cake, H., & Vine, J. (2007). Co-bedding twins: How pilot study findings guided improvements in planning a larger multicenter trial. *Nursing Research, 56*, 137-143.

Hertzog, M. A. (2008). Consideration in determining sample sizes for pilot studies. *Research in Nursing & Health, 32*, 180-191.

Kaasalainen, S., & Crook, J. (2004). An exploration of seniors' ability to report pain. *Clinical Nursing Research, 13*, 199-215.

Lemelin, L., Bonin, J.-P., & Duquette, A. (2009). Workplace violence reported by Canadian nurses. *Canadian Journal of Nursing Research, 41*(3), 152-167.

Linton, A., Singh, M., Turbow, D., & Legg, T. J. (2009). Street youth in Toronto: An investigation of demographic predictors of high risk behaviors and HIV status. *Journal of HIV/AIDS & Social Services, 8*, 375-396.

Martin-Misener, R., Reilly, S. M., & Vollman, A. R. (2010). Defining the role of primary health care nurse practitioners in rural Nova Scotia. *Canadian Journal of Nursing Research, 42*(2), 30-47.

Meininger, J. C., Hayman, L. L., Coates, P. M., & Gallagher, P. R. (1998). Genetic and environmental influences on cardiovascular disease risk factors in adolescents. *Nursing Research, 47*, 11-18.

Miles, M. B., & Huberman, A. M. (1994). *Qualitative data analysis: An expanded sourcebook* (2nd ed.). Thousand Oaks, CA: Sage.

Morse, J. M. (1994). Designing funded qualitative research. In Denzin, N. K., & Lincoln, Y. S. (Eds.), *Handbook of qualitative research* (pp. 220-235). Thousand Oaks, CA: Sage.

Ostry, A., Maggi, S., Hershler, R., Chen, L., & Hertzman, C. (2010). Mental health differences among middle-aged sawmill workers in rural compared to urban British Columbia. *Canadian Journal of Nursing Research, 42*(3), 84-100.

Patton, M. Q. (2010). Evaluation checklists. Retrieved from http://www.wmich.edu/evalctr/checklists/ checklist_topics.

Peterson, W., & DiCenso, A. (2002). A comparison of adolescent and adult mothers' satisfaction with their postpartum nursing care. *Canadian Journal of Nursing Research, 34*, 117-127.

Samuels-Dennis, J., Ford-Gilboe, M., & Ray, S. (2010). Single mother's adverse and traumatic experiences and post-traumatic stress symptoms. *Journal of Family Violence, 26*(1), 9-20.

Sandelowski, M. (1995). Sample size in qualitative research. *Research in Nursing & Health, 18*, 179-183.

Schoenfelder, D. P., & Rubenstein, L. M. (2004). An exercise program to improve fall-related outcomes in elderly nursing home residents. *Applied Nursing Research, 17*(1), 21-31.

Seneviratne, C. C., Mather, C. M., & Then, K. L. (2009). Understanding nursing on an acute stroke unit: Perceptions of space, time and interprofessional practice. *Journal of Advanced Nursing, 65*(9), 1872-1881. doi: 10.1111/j.1365-2648.2009.05053.x

Sinclair, B., & Ferguson, K. (2009). Integrating simulated teaching/learning strategies in undergraduate nursing education. *International Journal of Nursing Education and Scholarship, 6*(1), Article 7.

Smith, P. M., Corso, L., Brown, K. S., & Cameron, R. (2011). Nurse case-managed tobacco cessation interventions for general hospital patients: Results of a randomized clinical trial. *Canadian Journal of Nursing Research, 43*(1), 98-117.

Sousa, V. D., Zauszniewski, J. A., Musil, C. M. (2004). How to determine whether a convenience sample represents the population. *Applied Nursing Research, 17*(2), 130-133.

Ulrich, C. M., Danis, M., Ratcliffe, S. J., Garrett-Mayer, E., Koziol, D., Soeken, K. L., & Grady, C. (2006) Ethical conflict in nurse practitioners and physician assistants in managed care. *Nursing Research*, 55(6), 391-401.

Valaitis, R. V., Rajsic, C. J., Cohen, B., Stamler, L. L., Meagher-Stewart, D., & Froude, S. A. (2008). Preparing the community health nursing workforce: Internal and external enablers and challenges influencing undergraduate nursing programs in Canada. *International Journal of Nursing Education Scholarship*, 5(1), Article 22.

Vlack, S., Foster, R., Menzies, R., Williams, G., Shannon, D., & Riley, I. (2007). Immunisation coverage of Queensland indigenous two-year-old children by cluster sampling and by register. *Australian & New Zealand Journal of Public Health*, 31(1), 67-72.

Waltman, N. L., Twiss, J. J., Ott, C. D., Gross, G. J., Lindsey, A. M., Moore, T. E., & Berg, K. (2003). Testing an intervention for preventing osteoporosis in postmenopausal breast cancer survivors. *Journal of Nursing Scholarship*, 35, 333-338.

Young, L., Siden, H., & Tredwell, S. (2007). Post-surgical telehealth support for children and family care-givers. *Journal of Telemedicine and Telecare*, 13, 15-19.

FOR FURTHER STUDY

Θvolve   Go to Evolve at http://evolve.elsevier.com/Canada/LoBiondo/Research for Audio Glossary, how-to instructions for Writing Proposals for Funding, and additional research articles for practice in reviewing and critiquing.

CHAPTER 13

Data-Collection Methods

Susan Sullivan-Bolyai | Carol Bova | Mina D. Singh

LEARNING OUTCOMES

After reading this chapter, you will be able to do the following:

- Define the types of data-collection methods used in nursing research.
- List the advantages and disadvantages of each of these methods.
- Compare how specific data-collection methods contribute to the strength of evidence in a research study.
- Critically evaluate the data-collection methods used in published nursing research studies.

KEY TERMS

biological measurement
closed-ended item
concealment
consistency
content analysis
debriefing
external criticism
internal criticism
interrater reliability

intervention
intervention fidelity
interview
Likert-type scale
measurement
objective
open-ended item
operational definition
operationalization

physiological measurement
questionnaire
reactivity
records or available data
scale
scientific observation
social desirability
systematic

STUDY RESOURCES

Go to Evolve at http://evolve.elsevier.com/Canada/LoBiondo/Research for Audio Glossary, how-to instructions for Writing Proposals for Funding, and additional research articles for practice in reviewing and critiquing.

NURSES USE ALL OF THEIR SENSES when collecting data from the patients to whom they provide care. Nurse researchers also have many ways to collect information about their research participants. Both the data collected when they perform patient care and the data collected for the purpose of research are objective and systematic. **Objective** means that the data must not be influenced by the person who collects the information, and **systematic** means that the data must be collected in the same methodical way by each person involved in the collection procedure. The methods that researchers use to collect information about participants are the identifiable and repeatable operations that define the major variables being studied.

Operationalization is the process of translating the concepts of interest to a researcher into observable and measurable phenomena. The same information may be collected in a number of ways. For example, Horgas and colleagues (2008) defined *disability* as having both physical and social functional limitations, and they operationally measured this variable by using the Sickness Impact Profile.

This purpose of this chapter is to familiarize you with the various ways in which researchers collect information from and about participants. The chapter provides nurse readers with the tools for evaluating the selection, use, and practicality of the various ways to collect data.

MEASURING VARIABLES OF INTEREST

To a large extent, the success of a study depends on the quality of the data-collection methods chosen and employed. Researchers have many types of methods available for collecting information from participants in research studies. **Measurement** is the assignment of numbers to objects or events according to rules; determining which measurement to use in a particular investigation may be the most difficult and time-consuming step in the study design. In addition, nurse researchers have an array of quality instruments with adequate reliability and validity (see Chapter

14). This aspect of the research process necessitates painstaking effort from the researcher. Thus, the process of evaluating and selecting the available tools to measure variables of interest is crucial for the potential success of the study. In this section, the selection of measures and the implementation of the data collection process are discussed. An algorithm that influences a researcher's choice of data collection methods is diagrammed in the Critical Thinking Decision Path.

Information about phenomena of interest to nurses can be collected in many different ways. Nurses are interested in the biological and physical indicators of health (e.g., blood pressure and heart rate), but they are also interested in complex psychosocial questions presented by patients. Psychosocial variables, such as anxiety, hope, social support, and self-concept, may be measured by several different techniques, such as observation of behaviour, self-reports of feelings, or self-reports about attitudes in interviews or questionnaires. To study variables of interest, researchers also may use data that have already been collected for another purpose, such as records, diaries, or other media.

The data-collection method must be appropriate to the problem, the hypothesis, the setting, and the population. For example, Van Cleve and associates (2004) were interested in studying the pain experiences of children across multiple age groups. Because they were studying children aged 4 to 17 years, the same type of instrument could not be used for all the children. To deal with the reading and development levels of the children, they used tested age-appropriate instruments. For example, the children who were 4 to 13 years of age used the poker chip tool, in which the child chooses from one to four red chips to represent "a little bit" to "the most pain" the child can experience. The older children, however, used the adolescent paediatric pain tool, in which words and graphics are used to rate the pain experience.

Selection of the data collection method begins during the literature review. As noted in Chapter 5,

CRITICAL THINKING DECISION PATH

Data Collection Methods

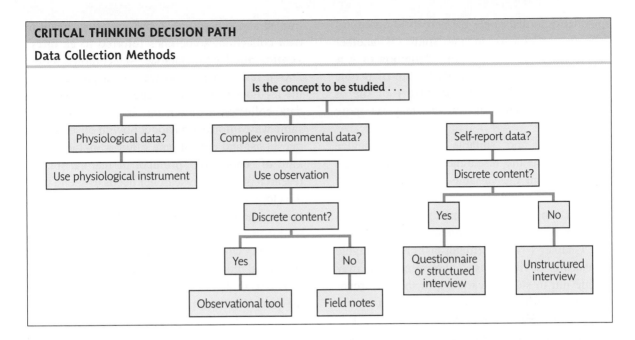

one purpose of the literature review is to provide clues about instrumentation. As the literature review is conducted, the researcher begins to explore how previous investigators defined and operationalized variables similar to those of interest in the current study. The researcher uses this information to define conceptually the variables to be studied. Once a variable has been defined conceptually, the researcher returns to the literature to define the variable operationally: that is, describe how a concept is measured and what instruments are used to capture the essence of the variable. This **operational definition** translates the conceptual definition into behaviours or verbalizations that can be measured for the study. In this second literature review, the researcher searches for measurement instruments that might be used "as is" or adapted for use in the study. If instruments are available, the researcher must obtain the author's permission for their use.

The following examples illustrate the relationship of conceptual and operational definitions. Stress research is of interest to researchers from many disciplines, including nursing. Definitions of stressors may be psychological, social, or physiological. If researchers are interested in studying stressors, they must first define what they mean by the concept of "stressor," both conceptually and operationally. Quality-of-life research is popular with researchers from many disciplines, including nursing. Definitions of quality of life may be related to health functioning, life satisfaction, or well-being.

Quality of life may also be interpreted in a general way (well-being) or be related specifically to a type of illness. Therefore, if researchers are interested in studying quality of life, they need first to define what they mean by the concept of "quality of life." For example, Molzahn (2007) was interested in quality of life as it relates to spirituality in later life. Molzahn wrote that this concept has many definitions but chose the World Health Organization's definition: "Quality of life is the individuals' perception of their position in life in the context of the culture and value systems in which they live and in relation to their goals, expectations, standards and concerns" (as cited in Molzahn, 2007, p. 35). According to this conceptual definition, the researcher would use a quality-of-life instrument specifically about spirituality to determine the perceived quality of life of participants in the study. If another researcher disagreed with this definition or was more interested in the quality of life of people with a specific illness or the quality of life of children, a different instrument may be more appropriate.

Sometimes no suitable measuring device exists, and so the researcher must then decide how important the variable is to the study and whether a new device should be constructed. The construction of new instruments for data collection that have reasonable reliability and validity (see Chapter 14) is a difficult task. If no suitable measuring device exists, the researcher may decide not to study a variable, or the researcher may decide to invest time and energy in instrument development. Either decision is acceptable, depending on the goals of the study and the goals of the researcher.

Helpful Hint_____

Remember that the researcher may not always present complete information about the way the data were collected, especially when established tools were used. To learn about the tool that was used, the reader may need to consult the original article that described the use or development of the tool.

Whether the researcher uses available methods or creates new ones, once the variables have been operationally defined in a manner consistent with the aims of the study, the population to be studied, and the setting, the researcher decides how the data-collection phase of the study will be implemented. This decision concerns how the instruments for data collection will be given to the participants. Consistency is the most important issue in this phase.

Consistency in data collection means that the method used to collect data from each participant in the study is exactly the same or as close to the same as possible. Consistency can minimize the bias introduced when more than one person collects the data. Data collectors must be carefully

trained and supervised. To ensure consistency in data collection, sometimes referred to as **intervention fidelity** (Santacroce, Maccarelli, & Grey, 2004), researchers must train data collectors in the methods to be used in the study so that each data collector acquires the information in the same way. Information about how to observe, ask questions, and collect data often is included in a kind of "cookbook" protocol or manual for the research project. A researcher needs to spend time developing the protocol and training data collectors to gather data systematically and reliably. Comments about their training and the consistency with which they collected data for the study should be provided by the researcher.

An example of intervention fidelity is given in the study by Ratner and colleagues (2004), who examined the efficacy of a smoking cessation intervention for patients about to undergo elective surgery. The researchers used several ways to ensure fidelity: (1) structured and rigorous training of research staff; (2) role playing to evaluate the competence of the study's registered nurses; (3) checks every 3 to 6 months to assess the extent of drift in role playing; (4) regular staff meetings to review the protocol and to address complex situations; (5) checklists for every timed intervention to ensure that all components of the intervention were covered; and (6) a video recording of an enactment of the intervention protocol for review by the registered nurses.

Another example of the importance of training data collectors appears in the study by Doran and associates (2006) on data collection of nursing-sensitive outcomes in acute care and long-term care settings. Doran and associates needed to assess nursing-sensitive outcomes accurately. Staff nurses were trained using didactic content and case studies on how to collect data on patient outcomes by research assistants. To assess inter-rater reliability, the research assistants (raters) conducted an independent assessment of three to five patients for each nurse over the 6-month period of data collection, and agreement between raters was calculated with the kappa statistic. The index of agreement in this study ranged from .64 to .93, and on average, the degree of agreement between rates was 86%; thus, the level of inter-rater agreement between the two observers, nurses and research assistants, was high. **Inter-rater reliability** (see Chapter 14) is the consistency of observations between two or more observers. It is often expressed as a percentage of agreement among raters or observers or as a coefficient of agreement that considers the element of chance (coefficient kappa).

 ### Evidence-Informed Practice Tip ____

It is difficult to place confidence in a study's findings if the data-collection methods are not consistent.

TYPES OF DATA-COLLECTION METHODS

In general, data-collection methods can be divided into the following five types: *physiological measurements, observational methods, interviews, questionnaires,* and *records or available data.* Each method has a specific purpose, as well as certain advantages and disadvantages inherent in its use. In the following sections, these data-collection methods are discussed, along with their respective uses and problems.

Physiological or Biological Measurements

In everyday practice, nurses collect physiological data about patients, such as their temperature, pulse rate, blood pressure, blood glucose level, urine specific gravity, and pH of bodily fluids. Such data are frequently useful to nurse researchers. For example, Bryanton and colleagues (2004) compared the effects of tub bathing versus traditional sponge bathing for healthy, full-term newborns and their mothers' ratings of pleasure and confidence. The physiological variable of newborn temperature was one of the outcome variables and was measured by one route, the axillary route, for standardization. Because physiological variables, such as cardiac output and blood pressure, can be measured in several

different ways, researchers need to measure these outcomes at similar intervals and in similar ways for all participants of the study.

Physiological measurement and **biological measurement** involve the use of specialized equipment to determine the physical and biological status of participants. Frequently, such measurements also require specialized training. These measurements can be *physical,* such as weight or temperature; *chemical,* such as blood glucose level; *microbiological,* as with cultures; or *anatomical,* as in radiological examinations. What distinguishes these measurements from others used in research is that special equipment is needed to make the observation. A researcher can say, "This participant feels warm," but to determine how warm the participant is requires the use of a sensitive instrument: a thermometer.

Physiological or biological measurement is particularly suited to the study of several types of nursing problems. Bryanton and colleagues' (2004) example is typical of studies dealing with ways to improve the performance of certain nursing actions, such as the measuring and recording of patients' physiological data. Physiological measures may yield important criteria for determining the effectiveness of certain nursing interventions. In the study of the effect of types of bathing and newborns' temperatures, Bryanton and colleagues (2004) reported that tub-bathed infants had significantly less temperature loss than did sponge-bathed infants.

The advantages of using physiological data-collection methods include their objectivity, precision, and sensitivity. Such methods are generally considered to yield objective findings because unless a technical malfunction occurs, two readings of the same instrument taken at the same time by two different nurses are likely to yield the same result. Because such instruments are intended to measure the variable being studied, they offer the advantage of being precise and sensitive enough to pick up subtle variations in the variable of interest. Also, the deliberate distortion of physiological information by a participant in a study is highly unlikely to occur.

Physiological measurements are not without inherent disadvantages, however. Some instruments, if not available through a hospital, may be quite expensive to obtain and use. In addition, the accurate use of such instruments often necessitates specialized knowledge and training. Another problem with physiological measurements is that simply by using them, the variable of interest may be changed. Although some researchers think of these instruments as being nonintrusive, the presence of some types of devices might change the measurement. For example, the presence of a heart rate monitoring device might make some patients anxious and thereby increase their heart rate. In addition, nearly all types of measuring devices are affected in some way by the environment. Even a simple thermometer can be affected by the participant's drinking something hot or cold immediately before the temperature is taken. Thus, you need to consider whether the researcher controlled such environmental variables in the study. Finally, a physiological way to measure the variable of interest may not exist. On occasion, researchers try to force a physiological parameter into a study in an effort to increase the precision of measurement. If the device does not measure the variable of interest, however, the validity of the device's use is suspect.

Observational Methods

Sometimes nurse researchers are interested in determining how participants behave under specific conditions. For example, the researcher might be interested in how children respond to painful situations. We might ask children how painful an experience was, but they may not be able to answer the question or to quantify the amount of pain, or they may distort their responses to please the researcher. Therefore, sometimes observing the participant may yield a more accurate description of the behaviour in question than does asking the patient.

Although observing the environment is a normal part of living, scientific observation places a great deal of emphasis on the objective and systematic nature of the observation. The researcher is not merely watching what is happening but is watching with a trained eye for certain specific events. **Scientific observation** fulfills the following four conditions:

1. The observations undertaken are consistent with the study's specific objectives.
2. A standardized and systematic plan exists for the observation and the recording of data.
3. All of the observations are checked and controlled.
4. The observations are related to scientific concepts and theories.

Observation is particularly suitable as a data-collection method in complex research situations that are best viewed as total entities and that are difficult to measure in parts, such as studies dealing with the nursing process, parent-child interactions, or group processes (see the Practical Application box for an example). In addition, observational methods can be the best way to operationalize some variables of interest in nursing research studies, particularly individual characteristics and conditions, such as traits and

---

Practical Application

Seneviratne and associates (2009; see Appendix A) conducted an ethnographic study to understand nursing on an acute stroke unit in regard to perceptions of space, time, and interprofessional practice. They made observations of 2 to 3 hours on 3 days of the week. The field worker made observations during every type of shift. The field work began with 3 months of general observation on the unit, in which the field worker watched at the charting desk and nursing station and while walking in the hall. Notes from observations were transcribed by means of computer. The field worker clarified gaps in field notes by returning to the field site and making more focused observations driven by the key informants.

symptoms; verbal and nonverbal communication behaviours, activities, and skill attainment; and environmental characteristics.

Observational methods can also be distinguished by the role of the observer. This role is determined by the amount of interaction between the observer and the people being observed. Each of the following four basic types of observational roles is distinguishable by the amount of concealment or intervention implemented by the observer:

1. Concealment without intervention
2. Concealment with intervention
3. No concealment without intervention
4. No concealment with intervention

These methods are illustrated in Figure 13-1; examples are given later. **Concealment** refers to is a study method in which participants do not know that they are being observed and in **intervention,** the observer provokes actions from those who are being observed.

In the study by Seneviratne and associates (2009), the field worker was not concealed while observing the nurses on the acute stroke unit.

When a researcher is concerned that the participants' behaviour will change as a result of being observed (reactivity), the type of observation most commonly employed is that of concealment without intervention. In this case, the researcher watches the participants without their knowledge of the observation and does not provoke them into action. Often, such concealed

observations involve the use of hidden television cameras, audio recordings, or one-way mirrors. Concealment without intervention is often used in observational studies of children. You may be familiar with rooms with one-way mirrors through which a researcher can observe the behaviour of the occupants of the room without being observed by them. Such studies allow the observation of children's natural behaviour and are often used in developmental research.

Observational studies commonly involve no concealment and no intervention. In this case, the researcher obtains informed consent from the participant to be observed and then simply observes the participant's behaviour.

Observing participants without their knowledge may violate assumptions of informed consent; therefore, researchers face ethical problems with this type of approach. However, researchers sometimes have no other way to collect such data, and the data collected are unlikely to have negative consequences for the participant. In these cases, the disadvantages of the study are outweighed by the advantages. Furthermore, the problem of consent is often handled by informing participants after the observation and allowing them the opportunity to refuse to have their data included in the study and to discuss any questions they might have. This process is called **debriefing.**

When the observer is neither concealed nor intervening, the ethical question is not a problem.

		Concealment	
		Yes	No
Intervention	Yes	Researcher hidden An intervention	Researcher open An intervention
	No	Researcher hidden No intervention	Researcher open No intervention

FIGURE 13-1   Types of observational roles in research.

Here, the observer makes no attempt to change the participants' behaviour and informs them that they are to be observed. Because the observer is present, this type of observation allows a greater depth of material to be studied than if the observer is separated from the participants by an artificial barrier, such as a one-way mirror. In a commonly used observational technique, the researcher functions as part of a social group to observe the participants. The problem with this type of observation is **reactivity** (also referred to as the Hawthorne effect; see Chapter 9), or the distortion created when the participants change behaviour because they know they are being observed.

In their study, Seneviratne and associates (2009) used unconcealed observation because the nurses and patients had given full consent for participation in the study. No concealment with intervention is used when the researcher is observing the effects of an intervention introduced for scientific purposes. Because the participants know they are participating in a research study, few problems with ethical concerns occur, but reactivity is a problem with this type of study.

Concealed observation with intervention involves staging a situation and observing the behaviours that are evoked in the participants as a result of the intervention. Because the participants are unaware of their participation in a research study, this type of observation has fallen into disfavour and is rarely used in nursing research.

Observational methods may be structured or unstructured. Unstructured observational methods are not characterized by a total absence of structure but usually involve collecting descriptive information about the topic of interest. In unstructured observations, the observer keeps field notes that record the activities, as well as the observer's interpretations of these activities. Field notes are usually not restricted to any particular type of action or behaviour; rather, they are intended to depict a social situation in a more general sense.

Another type of unstructured observation is the use of anecdotes. Despite popular usage of this term, anecdotes are not necessarily funny but usually focus on the behaviours of interest and frequently add to the richness of research reports by illustrating a particular point. In the study by Smith and associates (2006), interviews were conducted, and field notes were made and incorporated into the data set of this very innovative exploration of the topic.

In contrast, structured observations, such as the standardized tools used to evaluate mother-infant interaction in Koniak-Griffin and colleagues' (2003) study, require formal training and the competence of the evaluators. The use of structured observations without a standardized tool involves specifying in advance what behaviours or events are to be observed and preparing forms for record keeping, such as categorization systems, checklists, and rating scales. Whichever system is employed, the observer watches the participant and then marks on the recording form what was seen. In both cases, the observations must be similar among the observers (see the earlier discussion and Chapter 14 for an explanation of interrater reliability). Thus, observers need to be trained to be consistent in their observations and ratings of behaviour.

Evidence-Informed Practice Tip

When you read a research report that uses observation as a data-collection method, you will want to note evidence of consistency across data collectors through use of internal consistency reliability data in quantitative research and credibility in qualitative research. When that evidence is present, you can have greater confidence in the results.

Scientific observation has several advantages as a data-collection method. The main advantage is that observation may be the only way for the researcher to study the variable of interest. For example, what people say they do is often not what they really do. Therefore, if the study is designed to obtain substantive findings about human behaviour, observation may be the only way to ensure the validity of the findings. In addition, no other data-collection method can match the depth and variety of information that can be collected with the techniques of scientific observation. Such techniques are also flexible in that they may be used in both experimental and non-experimental designs and in laboratory and field studies.

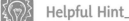 **Helpful Hint**_____

Sometimes researchers carefully train observers or data collectors, but the research report does not address this training. The limitations on length of research reports often prevent the inclusion of certain information. Readers can often assume that if reliability data are provided, then appropriate training occurred.

As with all data-collection methods, observation also has its disadvantages. Earlier in this chapter, the problems of reactivity and ethical concerns were mentioned with regard to concealment and intervention. In addition to these problems, data obtained by observational techniques are vulnerable to the bias of the observer. Emotions, prejudices, and values can influence the way that behaviours and events are observed. In general, the more the observer needs to make inferences and judgements about what is being observed, the more likely it is that distortion will occur. Thus, in judging the adequacy of observational methods, you will need to consider how observational tools were constructed and how observers were trained and evaluated.

Interviews and Questionnaires

Participants in a research study often have information that is important to the study and that can be obtained only by asking the participants. Such questions may be asked through the use of interviews and questionnaires. For both, the purpose is to ask participants to report data for themselves, but each method has unique advantages and disadvantages. The **interview** is a method of data collection in which a data collector questions a participant verbally. Interviews may be face to face or performed over the telephone, Skype, or other electronic means, and may consist of open-ended or closed-ended questions. In contrast, the **questionnaire** is an instrument designed to gather data from individuals about knowledge, attitudes, beliefs, and feelings. Survey research relies almost entirely on questioning participants with either interviews or questionnaires, but these methods of data collection can also be used in other types of research.

No matter what type of study is conducted, the purpose of questioning participants is to seek information. This information may be of either direct interest, such as the participant's age, or indirect interest, such as when the researcher uses a combination of items to estimate the degree to which the respondent has a particular trait or characteristic. An intelligence test is an example of how individual items are combined with several others to develop an overall scale of intelligence. When items of indirect interest on a survey or questionnaire are combined to obtain an overall score, the measurement tool is called a **scale.**

The investigator determines the content of an interview or questionnaire from the literature review (see Chapter 5). When evaluating interviews and questionnaires, you should consider the content of the scale, the individual items, and the order of the items. The basic standard for evaluating the individual items in an interview or questionnaire is that the item must be clearly written so that the intention of the question and the nature of the information sought are clear to the respondent. The only way to know whether the questions are understandable to the respondents is to pilot test them in a similar population. It is also critical not to rely on only the instrument developer's reports of reliability and validity (see Chapter 14). A pilot test allows researchers to test the reliability and validity for their unique sample rather than relying only on previously reported results.

Although each questionnaire item must consist of only one question or concept, be free of suggestions, and be worded with correct grammar, such items may be either open-ended or close-ended. An **open-ended item** is used when the researcher wants the participants to respond in their own words or when the researcher does not know all of the possible alternative responses. A **closed-ended item** is a question that the respondent may answer with only one of a fixed number of alternative responses. Many scales use a fixed-response format called a Likert-type scale. A **Likert-type scale** is a list of statements for which responses are varying degrees of agreement or opinion; for example, whether respondents "strongly agree," "agree," "disagree," or "strongly disagree." Sometimes finer distinctions are given, or a neutral category (e.g., "no opinion") may be provided. The use of the neutral category, however, sometimes creates problems because it is often the most frequent response and is difficult to interpret. Fixed-response items also can be used for questions requiring a "yes" or "no" response or when the interview or questionnaire has categories, as with income.

Structured, fixed-response items are best used when the question has a finite number of responses and the respondent is to choose the option closest to the right response. Fixed-response items have the advantage of simplifying the respondent's task and the researcher's analysis, but they may miss some important information about the participant. Sword and colleagues (2006) used self-reported fixed-response items via a structured telephone interview in their study of experiences of immigrant and Canadian-born women with regard to postpartum health, service needs, and access to care. Unstructured response formats allow such information to be included, but a special technique is needed to analyze the responses. This technique, called **content analysis,** is a method for the objective, systematic, and quantitative description of communications and documentary evidence.

Evidence-Informed Practice Tip

Scales used in nursing research should have evidence of adequate reliability and validity so that readers feel confident that the findings reflect what the researcher intended to measure (see Chapter 14).

Figure 13-2 shows a few items from a fictional survey of paediatric nurse practitioners. The first items are taken from a list of similar items, and they are both closed-ended and of a Likert-type format. Note that respondents are asked to choose how strongly they agree with each item. In using these questions in the survey, respondents are forced to choose from only these answers because it is thought that these will be the only responses. The only possible alternative response is to skip the item, leaving it blank.

Sometimes researchers have no idea or only a limited idea of what the respondent will say, or researchers want the answer in the respondent's own words, as with the second (open-ended) set of items. In this situation, respondents may also leave the item blank but are not forced to make a particular response.

Interviews and questionnaires are commonly used in nursing research. Both are strong approaches to gathering information for research because they enable the researcher to approach the task directly. In addition, both can elicit certain kinds of information, such as the participants' attitudes and beliefs, that would be difficult to obtain without asking the participant directly.

All methods that involve verbal reports, however, share a problem with accuracy. Often, it is impossible to know whether what the researcher is told is indeed true. For example, people are known to respond to questions in a way that makes a favourable impression. This response style is known as **social desirability,** which can be regarded as resulting from two factors: self-deception and other-deception.

Neyerhof (2006) discussed the two main modes of coping with social desirability bias. The

Close-Ended (Likert-Type Scale)
A. How satisfied are you with your current position?
     1. Very satisfied
     2. Moderately satisfied
     3. Undecided
     4. Moderately satisfied
     5. Very dissatisfied
B. To what extent do the following factors contribute to your current level of positive satisfaction?

	Not at all	Very little	Somewhat	Moderate amount	A great deal
1. % of time in patient care	1	2	3	4	5
2. Type of patients	1	2	3	4	5
3. % of time in educational activity	1	2	3	4	5
4. % of time in administration	1	2	3	4	5

Close-Ended
A. On average, how many patients do you see in one day?
     1. 1 to 3
     2. 4 to 6
     3. 7 to 9
     4. 10 to 12
     5. 13 to 15
     6. 16 to 18
     7. 19 to 20
     8. More than 20
B. How would you characterize your practice?
     1. Too slow
     2. Slow
     3. About right
     4. Busy
     5. Too busy

Open-Ended
A. Are there incentives that the National Association of Pediatric Nurse Associates and Practitioners ought to provide for members that are not currently being provided?

_____
_____
_____
_____
_____

FIGURE 13-2   Examples of close-ended and open-ended questions.

first mode is aimed at the detection and measurement of social desirability bias and is represented by two methods: the use of social desirability scales and the rating of item desirability. The second mode is aimed at preventing or reducing social desirability bias and is represented by the following methods: forced-choice items, the randomized response technique, the bogus pipeline, self-administration of the questionnaire, the selection of interviewers, and the use of proxy participants. Neyerhof found that no one method excelled completely and suggested that a combination of prevention and detection methods is the best strategy to reduce social desirability bias.

Questionnaires and interviews also have some specific purposes, advantages, and disadvantages. Questionnaires are useful tools when the purpose is to collect information. If questionnaires are too long, however, respondents are not likely to complete them. Questionnaires are most useful when the set of questions to be asked is finite and the researcher can be assured of the clarity and specificity of the items. Face-to-face techniques or interviews are most appropriate when the researcher may need to clarify the task for the respondent or is interested in obtaining more personal information from the respondent. Telephone interviews allow the researcher to reach more respondents than do face-to-face interviews and provide more clarity than do questionnaires.

Helpful Hint_____

Remember that sometimes researchers make trade-offs when determining the measures to be used. For example, if a researcher wants to learn about an individual's attitudes regarding practice, and practicalities preclude using an interview, a questionnaire may be used instead.

Seneviratne and associates (2009; see Appendix A) used both unconcealed observations and interviews to understand more about work practices. The participants were asked "grand tour" questions, such as "Can you walk me through your typical day?" and were asked for examples

of nursing practice. This use of multiple measures provides a more complete picture than the use of just one measure.

When determining whether to use interviews or questionnaires, researchers face difficult choices. The final decision is often based on the instruments available and their relative costs and benefits.

Both face-to-face and telephone interviews have some advantages over questionnaires. The rate of response to interviews is almost always better than that to questionnaires, which helps eliminate bias in the sample (see Chapter 12). Respondents seem to be less likely to hang up the telephone or to close the door in an interviewer's face than to throw away a questionnaire. Another advantage of the interview is that some people—such as young children, people with visual impairments, and people who are illiterate—cannot fill out a questionnaire but can participate in an interview. With an interview, the data collector knows who is giving the answers. When questionnaires are mailed, for example, anyone in the household could be the person who supplies the answers.

Interviews also allow for some safeguards to be built into the interview situation. Interviewers can clarify misunderstood questions and observe the level of the respondent's understanding and cooperativeness. In addition, the researcher has strict control over the order of the questions. With questionnaires, the respondent can answer questions in any order. Changing the order of the questions can sometimes change the response.

Finally, interviews allow for richer and more complex data to be collected, particularly when open-ended responses are sought. Richard and associates (2010) used open-ended questions in their individual interviews to investigate conceptualizations of disease prevention and health promotion among nurses from local public health organizations in Montreal. An example of such an approach is "To begin the interview, I'll ask you to describe a disease prevention or health promotion activity in which you have recently been involved within the context of your work" (p. 452).

Even when closed-ended response items are used, interviewers can probe to understand why a respondent answered in a particular way. Interviews can also be conducted in a group setting, called a *focus group interview,* which may include about 6 to 8 participants. Wagner and colleagues (2010) used a semistructured interview schedule to guide focus group discussions among nursing staff working in long-term care settings to explore patterns in communications about falls. These small-group interviews allow the participants to freely explain and share information individually and collectively. Agreement and disagreement among participants may be elicited, which allows the researchers to obtain specific information from a number of participants efficiently and simultaneously.

Questionnaires are much less expensive to administer than interviews because interviews may require the hiring and training of interviewers. Thus, if a researcher has a fixed amount of time and money, a larger and more diverse sample can be obtained with questionnaires. Questionnaires also provide complete anonymity, which may be important if the study deals with sensitive issues. Finally, the fact that no interviewer is present assures the researcher and the reader that no interviewer bias will occur. Interviewer bias occurs when the interviewer unwittingly leads the respondent to answer in a certain way. This problem is especially pronounced in studies with unstructured interview formats. A subtle nod of the head, for example, could lead a respondent to change an answer to correspond with what the researcher wants to hear.

Questionnaires were employed by Starzomski and Hilton (2000) to collect data on patient and family adjustment to kidney transplantation with and without an interim period of dialysis. To reach a large sample, save time, and reduce the labour costs of interviewing, questionnaires are mailed. Armstrong-Stassen and Cameron (2005) mailed questionnaires to 3000 community health nurses randomly selected from the College of Nurses of Ontario to investigate the work-related concerns, level of job satisfaction, and factors influencing the retention of community health nurses. The questionnaire packets contained a cover letter from the researchers, an informed consent form, a questionnaire booklet, and a reply envelope.

Records or Available Data

All of the data-collection methods discussed thus far concern the ways that nurse researchers gather new data to study phenomena of interest. Not all studies, however, require a researcher to acquire new information. Existing information can sometimes be examined in a new way to study a problem. The use of records and available data is sometimes considered to be primarily the concern of historical research, but hospital records, care plans, and existing data sources (e.g., the census) are frequently used for collecting information. What sets these studies apart from a literature review is that these available data are examined in a new way and not merely summarized; they also answer specific research questions.

Records or available data, then, are forms of information that are collected from existing materials, such as hospital records, historical documents, or audio or video recordings, and are used to answer research questions in a new manner. For example, the data analyzed in a study by Mammel and Kmet (2010) on the perioperative administration of antibiotics in orthopaedic trauma consisted of medical records to conduct the quality assurance review. The use of available data has certain advantages. Because the data-collection step of the research process is often the most difficult and time consuming, the use of available records often produces a significant saving of time. If the records have been kept in a similar manner over time, analysis of these records allows examination of trends over time.

In addition, the use of available data decreases problems of reactivity and response set bias. The researcher also does not have to ask individuals to participate in the study.

However, institutions are sometimes reluctant to allow researchers access to their records. If the records are kept so that an individual cannot be identified, access for research purposes is usually not a problem. Also, the Privacy Act, a federal law, protects the rights of individuals who may be identified in records, which would be a violation of anonymity.

One problem that affects the quality of available data concerns survival of records. If the records available are not representative of all of the possible records, the researcher may have a problem with bias. Often, because researchers have no way to tell whether the records have been saved in a biased manner, they need to make an intelligent guess as to their accuracy. For example, a researcher might be interested in studying socioeconomic factors associated with the suicide rate. These data frequently are underreported because of the stigma attached to suicide, and so the records would be biased. Recent interest in computerization of health records has led to an increase in the discussion about the desirability of access to such records for research. At this time, how much of such data will continue to be readily available for research without consent is unclear.

Another problem is related to the authenticity of the records. The distinction of primary and secondary sources is as relevant in this discussion as it was in the discussion of the literature review to determine the source of the work (see Chapter 5). A book, for example, may have been ghost-written, but all credit was accorded to the known author. The researcher may have a difficult time ferreting out these subtle types of biases.

Lastly, existing records may be missing a significant amount of data. For example, years of education may be recorded on only a portion of the sample records. Nonetheless, records and available data constitute a rich source of data for study.

ONLINE AND COMPUTERIZED METHODS OF DATA COLLECTION

With the fast-paced progression of the Internet and computer technology, many researchers are using online data collection. The information obtained can be quantitative or qualitative, closed-ended or open-ended. This method of data collection can take the form of Web-based surveys or data input directly into microcomputers.

Many online survey tools, such as Survey-Monkey or QuestionPro, are available; a survey can be downloaded quickly and the results obtained for a small fee. The advantages of this method are that it is anonymous and inexpensive; respondents can fill out the survey in their own time; a large number of participants can be accessed; respondent time is reduced; data-collection time is reduced; duplicate responses can be identified; and, for the researcher, implementation is time efficient. The disadvantages are that not everyone has access to a computer or is computer literate, the response rates may be low, and a large amount of data may be missing.

Computerized data collection can be accomplished through the use of personal digital assistants (PDAs). Researchers can input their data directly into these handheld microcomputers. The data can then be transferred to a larger computer for analysis.

Evidence-Informed Practice Tip
A critical evaluation of any data collection method includes evaluating the appropriateness, objectivity, consistency, and credibility of the method employed.

CONSTRUCTION OF NEW INSTRUMENTS

As already mentioned in this chapter, researchers sometimes cannot locate an existing instrument or method with acceptable reliability and validity to measure the variable of interest. This situation is often the case when part of a nursing theory is tested or when the effect of a clinical intervention is evaluated. For example, Gillis (1997) developed and tested an instrument to evaluate adolescent lifestyle. The instrument was used to assess lifestyle patterns for identification of health education and counselling priorities (see Chapter 14).

Instrument development is complex and time consuming, however. It consists of the following steps:

- Defining the construct to be measured
- Formulating the items (questions)
- Assessing the items for content validity
- Developing instructions for respondents and users
- Pretesting and pilot testing the items
- Estimating reliability and validity

Defining the construct (concepts at a higher level of abstraction) to be measured requires that the researcher develop an expertise in the construct, which necessitates an extensive review of the literature and of all tests and measurements that deal with related constructs. The researcher uses all this information to synthesize the available knowledge so that the construct can be defined.

Once the construct is defined, the individual items for measuring the construct can be developed. The researcher will develop many more items than are needed to address each aspect of the construct or subconstruct. A panel of experts in the field evaluates the items so that the researcher is assured that the items measure what they are intended to measure (content validity; see Chapter 14). Eventually, the number of items is decreased because some items will not elicit the intended information and will be dropped. In this phase, the researcher needs to ensure consistency both among the items and in testing and scoring procedures.

Finally, the researcher administers or pilot tests the new instrument by applying it to a group of people who are similar to those who will be studied in the larger investigation. The purpose of this analysis is to determine the quality of the instrument as a whole (reliability and validity) and the ability of each item to discriminate individual respondents (variance in item response). The researcher also may administer a related instrument to see whether the new instrument is sufficiently different from the older one.

It is important that researchers who invest significant time in tool development publish their results. For example, Goulet and associates (2003) were interested in understanding the attitudes of Quebec's adolescents toward breastfeeding and how other people influenced their opinions. From their literature review, Goulet and associates determined that no suitable instrument was available to measure this concept. They devised their own instrument on the basis of the theory of reasoned action (Fishbein & Ajzen, 1975). To ensure reliability and validity, they took the following steps: (1) A panel composed of lactation consultants and nurse researchers reviewed the items for content validity; (2) pilot testing was performed before the full study to ensure ease of administration, clarity, and precision of the instrument; (3) a factor analysis was performed to determine clusters of variables linked to form a construct; and (4) reliability analysis produced Cronbach's alpha between .71 and .70 for different parts of the instrument. This type of research serves not only to introduce other researchers to the tool but also to ultimately enhance the field, inasmuch as the ability to conduct meaningful research is limited only by the ability to measure important phenomena.

Helpful Hint

Determine whether a newly developed survey or questionnaire was pilot tested to obtain preliminary evidence of reliability and validity.

APPRAISING THE EVIDENCE

Data-Collection Methods

Evaluating the adequacy of data collection methods from written research reports is often problematic for new nursing research readers. Because the tool itself is not available for inspection, you may not feel comfortable judging the adequacy of the method without seeing it. However, you can ask questions to judge the method chosen by the researcher. These questions are listed in the Critiquing Criteria box.

In all studies, data collection methods should be clearly identified. The conceptual and operational definitions of each important variable should be present in the report. Sometimes it is useful for the researcher to explain why a particular method was chosen. For example, if the study dealt with young children, the researcher may explain that a questionnaire was deemed to be an unreasonable task, and so an interview was chosen.

Once you have identified the method chosen to measure each variable of interest, you should decide whether the method used was the best way to measure the variable. For example, if a questionnaire was used, you might wonder why the researcher decided not to use an interview. Also consider whether the method was appropriate to the clinical situation. Does it make sense to interview patients in the recovery room, for example?

Once you have decided whether all relevant variables are operationalized appropriately, you can begin to determine how well the method was carried out. For studies involving physiological measurement, determine whether the instrument was appropriate to the problem and not forced to fit it. The rationale for selecting a particular instrument should be given. For example, it may be important to know that the study was conducted under the auspices of a manufacturing firm that provided the measuring instrument. In addition, the researcher should have made provisions to evaluate the accuracy of the instrument and the skill level of the people who used it.

Several considerations are important when you read studies that involve observational methods. Who were the observers, and how were they trained? Is there any reason to believe that different observers perceived events or behaviours differently? Remember that the more inferences the observers are required to make, the more likely it is that observations will be biased. Also, consider the problem of reactivity: In any observational situation, it is possible that the mere presence of the observer will cause the participant to change the behaviour in question. Of importance is not that reactivity could occur but the extent to which reactivity could affect the data. Finally, consider whether the observational procedure was ethical. You need to consider whether the participants were informed that they were being observed, whether any intervention was performed, and whether the participants had agreed to be observed.

Interviews and questionnaires should be clearly described to allow the reader to decide whether the variables were adequately operationalized. Sometimes the researcher will reference the original report about the tool, and you may wish to read this study before deciding whether the method was appropriate for the current study. Also, the respondents' task should be clear. Thus, the researcher should have made provisions for the participants to understand both their overall responsibilities and the individual items of the interview or questionnaire. The following questions must be considered: Who were the interviewers in the interview situation? Does the researcher explain how they were trained to decrease any interviewer bias?

Available data, such as medical records, are subject to internal and external criticism. **Internal criticism** concerns the evaluation of the worth of the records and refers primarily to the accuracy of the data. The researcher should present evidence that the records are genuine. **External criticism** is concerned with the authenticity of the records. Are the records really written by the first author? The researcher may have a biased sample of all of the possible records in the problem area, which may have a profound effect on the validity of the results.

Once you have decided that the data collection method used was appropriate for the problem and the procedures were appropriate for the population studied, the reliability and validity of the instruments themselves need to be considered. These characteristics are discussed in Chapter 14.

CRITIQUING CRITERIA

1. Is the framework for research clearly identified?

DATA-COLLECTION METHODS

1. Are all of the data-collection instruments clearly identified and described?
2. Is the rationale for their selection given?
3. Is the method used appropriate for the problem being studied?
4. Were the methods used appropriate for the clinical situation?
5. Are the data-collection procedures similar for all participants?
6. Were efforts made to ensure intervention fidelity through the data-collection protocol?

PHYSIOLOGICAL MEASUREMENT

1. Is the instrument used appropriate for the research problem and not forced to fit it?
2. Is a rationale given for why a particular instrument was selected?
3. Is there a provision for evaluating the accuracy of the instrument

and the skill of the people who used it?

OBSERVATIONAL METHODS

1. Who conducted the observation?
2. Were the observers trained to minimize any bias?
3. Was an observational guide provided?
4. Were the observers required to make inferences about what they saw?
5. Is there any reason to believe that the presence of the observers affected the behaviour of the participants?
6. Were the observations performed according to the principles of informed consent?

INTERVIEWS

1. Is the interview schedule described adequately enough for you to know whether it covers the purpose of the study?
2. Is it clear that the participants understood the task and the questions?
3. Who were the interviewers, and how were they trained?

4. Is any interviewer bias evident?

QUESTIONNAIRES

1. Is the questionnaire described well enough for you to know whether it covers the purpose of the study? Is evidence provided that participants were able to perform the task?
3. Is it clear that the participants understood the questionnaire?
4. Are the majority of the items appropriately closed- or open-ended?

AVAILABLE DATA AND RECORDS

1. Are the records used appropriate for the problem being studied?
2. Are the data examined in such a way as to provide new information and not summarize the records?
3. Has the author addressed questions of internal and external criticism?
4. Is there any indication of selection bias in the available records?

CRITICAL THINKING CHALLENGES

- Physiological measurements are objective, precise, and sensitive. Discuss factors that might influence their validity and feasibility.
- A student in research class asks why nurses who participate in a clinical research study in the role of a data collector or who perform a "treatment intervention" need to be trained. What important factors or rationale would you

offer to support the establishment of interrater reliability?
- Observation is a data-collection method used frequently in nursing research. Discuss the factors that make nurses perfect potential candidates for this role and the disadvantages of using this method.
- Studies often use a survey to collect data. How can researchers increase their return rate for the survey, and how do they determine whether the survey return is adequate?

KEY POINTS

- Data-collection methods are described as being both objective and systematic. The data-collection methods of a study provide the operational definitions of the relevant variables.
- Types of data-collection methods include physiological measurements, observational methods, interviews, questionnaires, and records or available data. Each method has advantages and disadvantages.
- Physiological measurements are the methods in which technical instruments are used to collect data about patients' physical, chemical, microbiological, or anatomical status. These methods are suited to studying how to improve the effectiveness of nursing care. Physiological measurements are objective, precise, and sensitive, but they may be very expensive and may distort the variable of interest.
- Observational methods are used in nursing research when the variables of interest deal with events or behaviours. Scientific observation requires preplanning, systematic recording, controlling the observations, and determining the relationship to scientific theory. This method is best suited to research problems that are difficult to view as part of a whole. Observers may be required to perform or not perform interventions, and their activity may be concealed or obvious.
- Observational methods have several advantages: (1) they provide flexibility to measure many types of situations, and (2) they enable a great depth and breadth of information to be collected.
- Observation has disadvantages as well: (1) data may be distorted as a result of the observer's presence (reactivity), (2) concealment requires the consideration of ethical issues, and (3) data from observations may be biased by the person who is doing the observing.
- Interviews are data-collection methods commonly used in nursing research. Items on interview schedules may be of direct or indirect interest. Participants may be asked either open-ended or closed-ended questions. The form of the question should be clear to the respondent, free of suggestion, and grammatically correct.
- Questionnaires, or surveys, are useful when the number of questions to be asked is finite. The questions need to be clear and specific. Questionnaires are less costly and less time consuming to administer to large groups of participants, particularly if the participants are geographically widespread. Questionnaires also can be completely anonymous and prevent interviewer bias.
- Interviews are most appropriate when a large response rate and an unbiased sample are important because the refusal rate for interviews is much lower than that for questionnaires. Interviews enable the participation of people who cannot use a questionnaire, such as children and people who are illiterate. An interviewer can clarify and maintain the order of the questions for all participants.
- Records or available data are also an important source of research data. The use of available data may save the researcher considerable time and money in conducting a study. This method reduces problems with both reactivity and ethical concerns. However, records and available data are subject to problems of availability, authenticity, and accuracy.
- A critical evaluation of data-collection methods should emphasize the appropriateness, objectivity, and consistency of the method employed.

REFERENCES

Armstrong-Stassen, M., & Cameron, S. (2005). Concerns, satisfaction, and retention of Canadian community health nurses. *Journal of Community Health Nursing, 22*, 181-194.

Bryanton, J., Walsh, D., Barrett, M., & Gaudet, D. (2004). Tub bathing versus traditional sponge bathing for the newborn. *Journal of Obstetric, Gynecologic, and Neonatal Nursing, 33*, 704-712.

Doran, D. M., Harrison, M. B., Laschinger, H. S., Hirdes, J. P., Rukholm, E., Sidani, S., . . . Tourangeau, A. E. (2006). Nursing-sensitive outcomes data collection in acute care and long-term-care settings. *Nursing Research, 55*(2S), S75-S81.

Fishbein, M., & Ajzen, I. (1975). *Belief, attitude, intention, and behavior: An introduction to theory and research.* Reading, MA: Addison-Wesley

Gillis, A. J. (1997). The Adolescent Lifestyle Questionnaire: Development and psychometric testing. *Canadian Journal of Nursing Research, 29*, 29-46.

Goulet, C., Lampron, A., Marcil, I., & Ross, L. (2003). Attitudes and subjective norms of male and female adolescents toward breastfeeding. *Journal of Human Lactation, 19*, 402-410.

Horgas, A. L., Yoon, S. L., Nichols, A. L., & Marsiske, M. (2008). The relationship between pain and functional status in black and white older adults. *Research in Nursing and Health, 31*(94), 341-354.

Koniak-Griffin, D., Verzemnieks, I. L., Anderson, N. L. R., Brecht, M. L., Lesser, J., Kim, S., & Turner-Pluta, C. (2003). Nurse visitation for adolescent mothers: Two-year infant health and maternal outcomes. *Nursing Research, 52,* 127-136.

Mammel, J., & Kmet, L. (2010). Perioperative antibiotic administration in orthopaedic trauma. *Orthopaedic Nursing, 29*(2), 77-83.

Molzahn, A. E. (January 2007). Spirituality in later life: Effect on quality of life. *Journal of Gerontological Nursing, 15*(1), 32-39.

Neyerhof, A. J. (2006). Methods of coping with social desirability bias: A review. *European Journal of Psychology, 15,* 263-280.

Ratner, P. A., Johnson, J. L., Richardson, C. G., Bottorff, J. L., Moffatt, B., Mackay, M., . . . Budz, B. (2004). Efficacy of a smoking-cessation intervention for elective-surgical patients. *Research in Nursing & Health, 27,* 148-161.

Richard, L., Gendron, S., Beaudet, N., Boisvert, N., Sauvé, M. S., & Garceau-Brodeur, M. (2010). Health promotion and disease prevention among nurses working in local public health organizations in Montréal, Québec. *Public Health Nursing, 27*(5), 450-458.

Santacroce, S. J., Maccarelli, L. M., & Grey, M. (2004). Intervention fidelity. *Nursing Research, 53,* 63-66.

Seneviratne, C. C., Mather, C. M., & Then, K. L. (2009). Understanding nursing on an acute stroke unit: Perceptions of space, time and interprofessional practice. *Journal of Advanced Nursing, 65*(9), 1872-1881. doi: 10.1111/j.1365-2648.2009.05053.x

Smith, D., Edwards, N., Varcoe, C., Martens, P. J., & Davies, B. (2006). Bringing safety and responsiveness into the forefront of care for pregnant and parenting Aboriginal people. *Advances in Nursing Science, 29*(2), E27-E44.

Starzomski, R., & Hilton, A. (2000). Patient and family adjustment to kidney transplantation with and without an interim period of dialysis. *Nephrology Nursing Journal, 27*(1), 17-32.

Sword, W., Watt, S., & Kreuger, P. (2006). Postpartum health, service needs, and access to care experiences of immigrant and Canadian-born women. *Journal of Obstetric, Gynecologic, and Neonatal Nursing, 35*(6), 717-727.

Van Cleve, L., Bossert, E., Beecroft, P., Adlard, K., Alvarez, O., & Savedra, M. C. (2004). The pain experience of children with leukemia during the first year after diagnosis. *Nursing Research, 53,* 1-10.

Wagner, L. M., Damianakis, T., Mafrici, N., & Robinson-Holt, K. (2010). Falls communication patterns among nursing staff working in long-term care settings. *Clinical Nursing Research, 19*(3), 311-326.

FOR FURTHER STUDY

ℰvolve   Go to Evolve at http://evolve.elsevier.com/ Canada/LoBiondo/Research for Audio Glossary, how-to instructions for Writing Proposals for Funding, and additional research articles for practice in reviewing and critiquing.

CHAPTER 14

Rigour in Research

Geri LoBiondo-Wood | Judith Haber | Mina D. Singh

LEARNING OUTCOMES

After reading this chapter, you will be able to do the following:

- Discuss the purposes of reliability and validity.
- Define reliability.
- Discuss the concepts of stability, equivalence, and homogeneity as they relate to reliability.
- Compare the estimates of reliability.
- Define validity.
- Compare content validity, criterion-related validity, and construct validity.
- Discuss how measurement error can affect the outcomes of a research study.
- Discuss the purpose of credibility, auditability, and fittingness.
- Identify the criteria for critiquing the reliability and validity of measurement tools.
- Use the critiquing criteria to evaluate the reliability and validity of measurement tools.
- Discuss how evidence related to research rigour contributes to clinical decision making.

KEY TERMS

alpha coefficient
alternate-form reliability
auditability
chance error
Cohen's kappa
concurrent validity
constant error
construct validity
content validity
contrasted-groups approach
convergent validity
credibility
criterion-related validity
Cronbach's alpha
divergent validity

equivalence
error variance
face validity
factor analysis
fittingness
homogeneity
hypothesis-testing approach
internal consistency
interrater reliability
item-to-total correlation
known-groups approach
Kuder-Richardson (KR-20)
  coefficient
multitrait-multimethod
  approach

observed test score
parallel-form reliability
predictive validity
random error
reliability
reliability coefficient
rigour
split-half reliability
stability
systematic error
test-retest reliability
validation sample
validity

STUDY RESOURCES

Go to Evolve at http://evolve.elsevier.com/Canada/LoBiondo/Research for Audio Glossary, how-to instructions for Writing Proposals for Funding, and additional research articles for practice in reviewing and critiquing.

IN BOTH QUANTITATIVE AND QUALITATIVE RESEARCH, the purpose is to collect trustworthy data that can be used for analyses to make generalizations about the population and that are transferable to other groups. Because findings need to be generalizable and transferable, measurement of nursing phenomena is a major concern of nursing researchers, and rigour is strived for. **Rigour** refers to the strictness with which a study is conducted to enhance the quality, believability, or trustworthiness of the study findings. Rigour in quantitative research is determined by measurement instruments that validly and reliably reflect the concepts of the theory being tested, so that conclusions drawn from a study will be valid and will advance the development of nursing theory and evidence-informed practice. Thus, psychometric assessments are designed to obtain evidence of the quality of these instruments: that is, their reliability and validity.

Issues of reliability and validity are of central concern to the researcher, as well as to you as the critiquer of research. From either perspective, the measurement instruments that are used in a research study must be evaluated. Many new constructs are relevant to nursing theory, and a growing number of established measurement instruments are available to researchers. However, researchers often face the challenge of developing new instruments and, as part of that process, establishing the reliability and validity of those tools.

In qualitative research, rigour is ascertained by credibility, auditability, and fittingness. The growing importance of measurement issues, tool development, and related issues (e.g., reliability and validity, qualitative rigour) is evident in issues of the *Journal of Nursing Measurement,*

Canadian Journal of Nursing Research, International Journal of Qualitative Methods, and other nursing research journals. In this chapter, concepts related to quantitative rigour are discussed first, followed by factors that contribute to the trustworthiness of qualitative research.

When you read quantitative research studies and reports, you must assess the reliability and validity of the instruments used in each study to determine the soundness of the selection of these instruments in relation to the concepts or variables under investigation. The appropriateness of the instruments and the extent to which reliability and validity are demonstrated have a profound influence on the findings and on the internal and external validity of the study. Invalid measures produce invalid estimates of the relationships between variables, thus affecting internal validity. The use of invalid measures also leads to inaccurate generalizations to the populations being studied, thus affecting external validity and the ability to apply or not apply research findings in clinical practice. Thus, the assessment of reliability and validity is an extremely important skill to develop for critiquing nursing research.

Regardless of whether a new or already developed measurement tool is used in a research study, evidence of reliability and validity is crucial. Box 14-1 identifies several Internet resources that you can use to access and evaluate the reliability and validity of the measurement instruments used in research studies.

RELIABILITY

People are considered reliable when their behaviour is consistent and predictable. Likewise, the **reliability** of a research instrument is the extent to which the instrument yields the same results on repeated measures. Reliability, then, is concerned with consistency, accuracy, precision, stability, equivalence, and homogeneity. Concurrent with questions of validity, or after these questions are answered, the researcher and you, as the critiquer, ask how reliable the instrument is.

A reliable measure can produce the same results if the behaviour is measured again by the same scale. Reliability, then, refers to the propor-

tion of accuracy to inaccuracy in measurement. In other words, if researchers use the same or comparable instruments on more than one occasion to measure behaviours that ordinarily remain relatively constant, the researchers would expect similar results if the tools are reliable.

The three main attributes of a reliable scale are stability, homogeneity, and equivalence. The **stability** of an instrument refers to the instrument's ability to produce the same results with repeated testing. The **homogeneity,** or **internal consistency,** of an instrument means that all of the items in a tool measure the same concept or characteristic. An instrument is said to exhibit **equivalence** if the tool produces the same results when equivalent or parallel instruments or procedures are used. Each of these attributes and the means to estimate them are discussed here. Before these are discussed, however, an understanding of how to interpret reliability is essential.

Interpretation of the Reliability Coefficient

Because all of the attributes of reliability are concerned with the degree of consistency between scores that is obtained at two or more independent times of testing, these attributes often are expressed in terms of a correlation coefficient. The **reliability coefficient,** or **alpha coefficient,** expresses the relationship between the error variance, true variance, and the observed score, and it ranges from 0 to 1. A correlation of 0 indicates no relationship, and thus the error variance is high. When the error variance in a measurement instrument is low, the reliability coefficient is closer to 1. The closer to 1 the coefficient is, the more reliable the tool is. For example, suppose that a reliability coefficient of a tool is reported to be .89. This number indicates that the error variance is small and the tool has little measurement error. But if the reliability coefficient of a measure is reported to be .49, the error variance is high, and the tool has a problem with measurement error. For a tool to be considered reliable, a level of .70 or higher should be reported, although the intended purpose of the instrument needs to be considered if lower levels are accepted.

The interpretation of the reliability coefficient depends on the proposed purpose of the measure. Seven major tests of reliability can be used to calculate a reliability coefficient, depending on the nature of the tool: *test-retest reliability, parallel-* or *alternate-form reliability, item-to-total correlation, split-half reliability, Kuder-Richardson coefficient, Cronbach's alpha,* and *interrater reliability.* These tests are discussed as they relate to the attributes of stability, homogeneity, and equivalence (Box 14-2). In critiquing research reports, you should be aware that no single best way exists to assess reliability in relation to these attributes and that the researcher's method should be consistent with the aim of the research.

Stability

An instrument is thought to be stable or to exhibit stability when repeated administration of the instrument yields the same results. Researchers are concerned with an instrument's stability because they expect the instrument to measure a concept consistently over a period of time. Measurement over time is important in a longitudinal study because in that type of research, an

instrument is used on several occasions. Stability is also a consideration when a researcher is conducting an intervention study that is designed to effect a change in a specific variable. In this case, the instrument is administered once and then again after the alteration or change intervention has been completed. The tests that are used to estimate stability are test-retest reliability and parallel- or alternate-form reliability.

Test-Retest Reliability

Test-retest reliability is the stability of the scores of an instrument when it is administered more than once to the same participants under similar conditions. Scores from repeated testing are compared. This comparison is expressed by a correlation coefficient, usually a Pearson r (see Chapter 16). The interval between repeated administrations varies and depends on the concept or variable being measured. For example, if the variable that the test measures is related to developmental stages in children, the interval between test administrations should be short. The amount of time over which the variable was measured should also be recorded in the report.

An example of an instrument that was assessed for test-retest reliability is Akhtar-Danesh and associates' (2010) learning needs assessment questionnaire for community health nurses. Test-retest reliability was assessed at approximately a 2-week interval, and a high test-retest reliability coefficient ($r = .89$, $p < .01$) was obtained. The interval was adequate (2 weeks between testing), and coefficients exceeded .80 and were thus very good (Nunnally & Bernstein, 1994).

Parallel- or Alternate-Form Reliability

Parallel-form reliability is applicable and can be tested only if two comparable forms of the same instrument exist. **Parallel-form reliability,** or **alternate-form reliability,** is like test-retest reliability in that the same individuals are tested more than once within a specific interval, but in the assessment of parallel-form reliability, a

---

BOX 14-2

MEASURES USED TO TEST RELIABILITY

STABILITY
  Test-retest reliability
  Parallel- or alternate-form reliability

HOMOGENEITY
  Item-to-total correlation
  Split-half reliability
  Kuder-Richardson (KR-20) coefficient
  Cronbach's alpha

EQUIVALENCE
  Parallel- or alternate-form reliability
  Interrater reliability

different form of the same test is given to the participants on the second testing. Parallel forms or tests contain the same types of items that are based on the same domain or concept, but the wording of the items is different. The development of parallel forms is desired if the instrument is intended to measure a variable for which a researcher believes that "testwiseness" will be a problem, that is, respondents might recognize the test items and try to answer them in the same way as previously, instead of spontaneously.

For example, in their randomized controlled trial, Budin and colleagues (2008) compared the differential effect of a phase-specific standardized educational video intervention with that of a telephone counselling intervention on physical, emotional, and social adjustment in women with breast cancer and their partners. Because repeated measures over the four data-collection points—coping with the diagnosis, recovering from surgery, understanding adjuvant therapy, and ongoing recovery—were used, it was appropriate to use two alternative forms of the Partner Relationship Inventory (Hoskins, 1988) to measure emotional adjustment in partners. Each item on one scale (e.g., "I am able to tell my partner how I feel") is paired with one item on the second form (e.g., "My partner tries to understand my feelings"), and the responses should therefore be consistent.

Practically speaking, developing alternative forms of an instrument is difficult because of the many issues of reliability and validity. If alternative forms of a test exist, they should be highly correlated if they are to be considered reliable.

Helpful Hint

When a longitudinal design with multiple data-collection points is being conducted, look for evidence of test-retest reliability or parallel-form reliability.

Homogeneity, or Internal Consistency

Another attribute related to reliability of an instrument is the homogeneity with which the items within the scale reflect or measure the same concept. In other words, the items within the scale are correlated with, or complementary to, each other, and the scale is *unidimensional*. A unidimensional scale measures one concept, such as exercise self-efficacy. A total score is then used in the analysis of data.

When Akhtar-Danesh and associates' (2010) learning needs assessment questionnaire was tested for homogeneity, the reliability (alpha) coefficient was .99. In exceeding .70, the reliability coefficient provided sufficient evidence of the internal consistency of the instrument. Homogeneity can be assessed with one of four methods: item-to-total correlations, split-half reliability, Kuder-Richardson coefficient, or Cronbach's alpha.

Helpful Hint

When the characteristics of a study sample differ significantly from those of the sample in the original study, check to see whether the researcher has reestablished the reliability of the instrument with the current sample.

Item-to-Total Correlation

The **item-to-total correlation** is a measure of the relationship between each scale item and the total scale. When item-to-total correlations are calculated, a correlation for each item on the scale is generated (Table 14-1). Items that do not achieve a high correlation may be deleted from the

TABLE 14-1	
EXAMPLES OF ITEM-TO-TOTAL CORRELATIONS FROM COMPUTER-GENERATED DATA	
ITEM	**ITEM-TO-TOTAL CORRELATION**
1	.5069
2	.4355
3	.4479
4	.4369
5	.4213
6	.4216

instrument. In a research study, the lowest and highest item-to-total correlations are typically reported; the other correlations are usually not reported unless the study is a methodological investigation. An example of an item-to-total correlation report is illustrated in the study by Sidani and associates (2009), who evaluated the psychometric properties of the treatment and preferences measure. In that study, the item-to-total correlations ranged between .47 and .82, According to Nunnally and Bernstein (1994), these results are acceptable because the minimal mandatory correlation should be greater than .30.

Heaman and Gupton (2009) conducted a study to refine a new instrument, the Perception of Pregnancy Risk Questionnaire (PPRQ). A correlation matrix was constructed to summarize the interrelationships among the 11 items in the scale. The matrix was examined to identify any items to be dropped if they were either too highly correlated ($r \geq .80$) or not correlated sufficiently ($r < .30$) with one another. The results indicated that all items were adequately correlated ($r \geq .30$) with at least seven other items in the matrix. There were concerns about redundancy of items, inasmuch as no correlations exceeded .74.

Split-Half Reliability

Split-half reliability involves dividing a scale into halves and making a comparison. The halves may be, for example, odd-numbered and even-numbered items or a simple division of the first from the second half, or items may be randomly grouped into halves that will be analyzed opposite one another. Split-half reliability provides a measure of consistency in terms of sampling the content. The two halves of the test or the contents in both halves are assumed to be comparable, and a reliability coefficient is calculated. If the scores for the two halves are approximately equal, the test may be considered reliable.

The Spearman-Brown formula is one method of calculating the reliability coefficient. In a test of the Worry Interference Scale, a seven-item self-report measure was developed to assess the degree to which respondents believe that thoughts about breast cancer are interfering with daily functioning. The measure is embedded within a larger questionnaire that is also used to assess perceived risk, intention to undergo genetic testing, and frequency of worry about getting breast cancer. The Worry Interference Scale items concern disruptions in sleep, work, concentration, relationships, having fun, feeling sexually attractive, meeting family needs, and reproductive decisions. Ibrahim (2002) computed a Spearman-Brown split-half reliability and found a reliability coefficient that ranged from .83 to .92 for the first four items and from .75 to .83 for the other items. Split-half reliabilities of at least .75 are considered internally consistent.

Kuder-Richardson Coefficient

The **Kuder-Richardson (KR-20) coefficient** is the estimate of homogeneity used for instruments that have a dichotomous response format. A *dichotomous response format* is one in which the answer to a question should be either "yes" or "no" or either "true" or "false." The technique yields a correlation that is based on the consistency of responses to all items of a single form of a test that is administered once.

For example, in an investigation of the effectiveness of a randomized support group intervention for women with breast cancer, breast cancer knowledge was assessed with a 25-item true/false questionnaire developed for the study. Items were obtained from the American Cancer Society's publication *Cancer Facts and Figures* and were categorized as follows: knowledge of risk factors for developing breast cancer (10 items; e.g., "Most women diagnosed with breast cancer have at least one known risk factor for the disease"); symptoms of breast cancer (5 items; e.g., "Women who have breast cancer never experience any symptoms of the disease"); side effects of treatment (3 items; e.g., "A common side effect of radiation is sunburn-like symptoms"); treatment efficacy (4 items; e.g., "For women with small tumors that may not have spread outside the breast, having either a mastectomy or lumpectomy with axillary lymph node dissection results in the same overall life expectancy"); and methods of treatment (3 items; e.g., "Hormone treatment is used only for premenopausal women"). Because the scale was a binary format (true/false), the Kuder-Richardson reliability for the entire scale was calculated at .75, which is acceptable, having exceeded the minimum acceptable score of .70; however, the magnitude of the correlation is not robust.

Cronbach's Alpha

The fourth and most commonly used test of internal consistency is Cronbach's alpha. **Cronbach's alpha** is a test of internal consistency in which each item in the scale is simultaneously compared with the others, and a total score is then used to analyze the data. Many tools used to measure psychosocial variables and attitudes have a Likert-type scale response format, which is very suitable for testing internal consistency. In a Likert-type scale format, the participant responds to a question on a scale of varying degrees of intensity between two extremes. The two extremes are anchored by responses ranging from, for example, "strongly agree" to "strongly disagree" or from "most like me" to "least like me." The points between the two extremes may range from 1 to 5 or 1 to 7. Participants are asked to circle the response that most closely represents what they believe.

Figure 14-1 displays examples of items from a tool in which a Likert-type scale format was used to develop a career search instrument (Roberts & Ward-Smith, 2010). The psychometric properties of Sidani and colleagues' (2009) Treatment and Preferences measure were tested for internal consistency and construct validity. The testing revealed that there were four separate treatment options: sleep education and hygiene, stimulus control instructions, sleep restriction therapy, and, lastly, a multicomponent option involving the other three options, as illustrated in

Table 14-2. Cronbach's alpha exceeded .70 for each option, thereby providing sufficient evidence of the internal consistency of the instrument. Examples of reported Cronbach's alpha are shown in Box 14-3.

Helpful Hint

If a research article provides information about the reliability of a measurement instrument but does not specify the type of reliability, it is probably safe to assume that internal consistency reliability was assessed with Cronbach's alpha.

TABLE **14-2**

CRONBACH'S ALPHASCORES FOR THE FOUR OPTIONS OF THE TREATMENT AND PREFERENCES MEASURE

OPTIONS	CRONBACH'S ALPHA
Sleep education and hygiene	.86
Stimulus control instructions	.80
Sleep restriction therapy	.84
Multicomponent	.87

Adapted from Sidani, S., Epstein, D. R., Bootzin, R. R., Moritz, P., & Miranda, J. (2009). Assessment of preferences for treatment: Validation of a measure. *Research in Nursing and Health, 32*, 419–438.

BOX **14-3**

EXAMPLES OF REPORTED CRONBACH'S ALPHA

- "Interitem correlation for the learning needs subscales ranged from $r = .53$ to $r = .72$, which was in the acceptable range." (Akhtar-Danesh, Valaitis, Schofield, Underwood, Martin-Misener, Baumann, Kolotylo, 2010, p. 1061)
- "The total 9-item scale had a Cronbach's alpha of .87, the 5-item scale had an alpha of .84, and the 4-item Risk For Self-subscale had an alpha of .81." (Heaman & Gupton, 2009, p. 500)
- "For this study, the Cronbach α reliabilities for the subscales ranged from .72 to .85 and a total PES [Practice Environment Scale] reliability was found to be .92." (Armstrong, Laschinger, & Wong, 2009, p. 58)
- "Reliability, determined using Cronbach's alpha, was 0.87 for the CSQ [Career Search Questionnaire]. Subscale reliability for the 23 items purported to measure career interest was 0.77. Reliability for the 25 items which aimed to determine self-efficacy was 0.82." (Roberts & Ward-Smith, 2010, p. 8)

Career Search Questionnaire

	No interest	Little interest	Neutral	Some interest	Much interest
2. I am interested in learning new words and terminology to perform a job.					
3. I am interested in fine arts activities such as design or performance.					
5. I enjoy working with other people to find the best possible solutions to their problems.					
7. I enjoy thinking about things I have done and figuring out ways to do them better.					
8. I am interested in people who express opinions very different from my own.					
9. I would like to advance my career by being a lifelong learner, even if it requires additional classes.					
22. I am interested in a job where I can empower other people.					
23. I am interested in a job where I make my own decisions.					
	No confidence at all	Very little confidence	Moderate confidence	Much confidence	Complete confidence
2. I believe I could write speeches for people.					
6. I am able to be compassionate with ill people.					
7. I am able to use algebra to solve technical problems.					
8. I am capable of communicating well even in stressful situations.					
10. I believe that I can demonstrate concern for other people's privacy and dignity.					
11. I am able to keep a healthy boundary between my work and my own life.					
12. I am capable of keeping my workplace safe for myself and others.					
22. I believe I can get people to do things my way.					

FIGURE 14-1   Examples of portions of Likert-type scales.
Adapted from Roberts, C. A., & Ward-Smith, P. (2010). Choosing a career in nursing: Development of a career search instrument. *International Journal of Nursing Education Scholarship, 7*(1), Article 2.

Equivalence

Equivalence is either the consistency or agreement among observers who use the same measurement tool or the consistency or agreement between alternative forms of a tool. An instrument is thought to demonstrate equivalence when two or more observers have a high percentage of agreement about a certain behaviour or when alternative forms of a test yield a high correlation. Two methods to test equivalence are interrater reliability and alternate- or parallel-form reliability.

Interrater Reliability

Some measurement instruments are not self-administered questionnaires but instead are direct measurements of observed behaviour that must be systematically recorded. Such instruments must be tested for **interrater reliability** (the consistency of observations between two or more observers with the same tool). To accomplish interrater reliability, either two or more individuals should make an observation or one observer should observe the same behaviour on several occasions. The observers should score their observations with regard to the definition and operationalization of the behaviour to be observed.

When the research method of direct observation of a behaviour is required, consistency (or reliability) of the observations among all observers is extremely important. Interrater reliability concerns the reliability (or consistency) of the observer, not the reliability of the instrument. Interrater reliability is expressed either as a percentage of agreement between scorers or as a correlation coefficient of the scores assigned to the observed behaviours.

Resnick and colleagues (2001) established interrater reliability for the step activity monitor (SAM), a step counter developed for a wide variety of gait styles (ranging from a slow shuffle, such as a Parkinsonian-type gait, to a fast run) and used to measure activity in older adults.

Resnick and colleagues noted that other tools available to assess activity or exercise in older adults are generally self-report instruments that provide researchers or nurses with the individual's perception of the amount of activity performed. In contrast, the SAM provides objective information about step activity (the total number of steps taken over a period of time).

Participants in the study ($N = 30$) were recruited from the outpatient office in a continuing care retirement community. They were asked to walk at their own speed on a carpeted level surface for 1 minute, rest for 2 minutes, and then ambulate over the same path for another minute. Two observers, observing at the same time, counted steps during both episodes of ambulation. The two observers, both advanced practice nurses, had prior experience in observational gait assessment of older adults and step counting.

Interrater reliability was based on intraclass correlations of the two separate 1-minute observations of the SAM performed 2 minutes apart. Statistically significant correlations of .80 or greater between the means of the two observers and the results of the SAM at each testing interval (in which the average deviation between the SAM and the mean of the two observers was calculated) produced an interrater reliability estimate of .98, indicating a high level of agreement between observers. According to Santacroce and associates (2004), consistency in observation or intervention delivery is evidence that the study findings are valid and reliable.

Another type of interrater reliability is Cohen's kappa, a coefficient of agreement between two raters that is considered to be a more precise estimate of interrater reliability. **Cohen's kappa** expresses the level of agreement that is observed beyond the level that would be expected by chance alone. A Cohen's kappa of .80 or better is generally assumed to indicate good interrater reliability. A Cohen's kappa of .68 allows tentative conclusions to be drawn when lower levels of reliability are acceptable (McDowell & Newell,

1996). In her study on metacognitive factors that affect student nurses' use of point-of-care technology in clinical settings, Kuiper (2010) established interrater reliability (.70 to .90) to determine consistency in order to reflect self-regulated learning processes in journal prompts.

 Evidence-Informed Practice Tip _____

Interrater reliability is important for minimizing bias.

Parallel- or Alternate-Form Reliability

Parallel- or alternate-form reliability was described in the discussion of stability (see pp. 309–310). Use of parallel forms is thus a measure of stability and equivalence. The procedures for assessing equivalence through the use of parallel forms are the same.

VALIDITY

Validity refers to whether a measurement instrument accurately measures what it is intended to measure. To be valid, an instrument must first be reliable; without reliability, the instrument cannot have validity. However, reliability, although necessary, is not a sufficient condition for validity. Internal and external validity of a study are discussed in Chapter 9.

For example, a valid instrument that is intended to measure anxiety does so; it does not measure another construct, such as stress. A reliable measure can consistently rank participants on a given construct (e.g., anxiety), but a valid measure correctly measures the construct of interest. A measure can be reliable but not valid. Suppose that a researcher wanted to measure anxiety in patients by measuring their body temperatures. The researcher could obtain highly accurate, consistent, and precise temperature recordings, but such a measure would not be a valid indicator of anxiety. Thus, the high reliability of an instrument is not necessarily congruent with evidence of validity. A valid instrument, however, is reliable.

If an instrument is erratic, inconsistent, and inaccurate, it cannot validly measure the attribute of interest.

The three major kinds of validity—content, criterion-related, and construct validity—vary according to the kind of information provided and the investigator's purpose. In critiquing research articles, you will want to evaluate whether sufficient evidence of validity is present and whether the type of validity is appropriate to the design of the study and instruments used in the study. The sample that provides the initial data for determining the reliability and validity of a measurement tool is termed a **validation sample.**

 Evidence-Informed Practice Tip _____

Selecting measurement instruments that have strong evidence of validity increases the reader's confidence in the study findings: that the researchers actually measured what they intended to measure.

Content Validity

Content validity is the degree to which the content of the measure represents the universe of content: that is, the domain of a given construct. The universe of content provides the framework and basis for formulating the items that will adequately represent the content. When an investigator is developing a tool and issues of content validity arise, the concern is whether the measurement tool and the items it contains are representative of the universe of content that the researcher intends to measure. The researcher begins by defining the concept and identifying the dimensions that are the components of the concept. The items that reflect the concept and its dimensions are formulated (see Practical Application box for two examples).

When the researcher has completed this task, the items are submitted to a panel of judges considered to be experts on this concept. Researchers typically request that the judges indicate their level of agreement with the scope of the items and the extent to which the items reflect the concept under consideration.

> ### Practical Application
>
> Gélinas and colleagues (2008) reported on the item selection process and evaluation of the content validity of the Critical-Care Pain Observation Tool for nonverbal adults who were critically ill. A version of this tool was developed to include both behavioural and physiological indicators. Items were developed through the use of several sources: literature review, review of medical files, and consultation with critical care nurses and physicians. Content validity was measured with 13 critical care nurses and 4 physicians through the use of a content validity questionnaire. A content validity index was calculated to determine the relevance of each indicator and clinicians' agreement with the scales.
>
> Roberts and Ward-Smith (2010) sought content validity for the Career Search Questionnaire by including local nursing school advisers and counsellors for applicability and usability. Research support personnel were consulted for readability. Three educational psychologists reviewed the format of the instrument to ensure that it was consistent with that of established occupational inventories. Then, doctorally prepared nurse educators reviewed the instrument for content validity. There was consensus that the instrument was appropriate.

A subtype of content validity is **face validity,** which is a rudimentary type of validity in which the instrument intuitively gives the appearance of measuring the concept. To establish face validity, colleagues or participants are asked to read the instrument and evaluate the content in terms of whether it appears to reflect the concept that the researcher intends to measure. This procedure may be useful in the tool development process in terms of determining the readability and clarity of the content. Face validity, however, should in no way be considered a satisfactory alternative to other types of validity. In the development of the Adolescent Lifestyle Questionnaire (Gillis, 1997), the concept of healthy lifestyle was derived from qualitative interviews with adolescents. The scale comprised two subscales: health-promoting and health-protecting behaviours. To establish face validity, in addition to content validity, a panel of eight nurses reviewed the items for clarity and relevance.

> ### Evidence-Informed Practice Tip
>
> When face validity and content validity, the most basic types of validity, are the only types of validity reported in a research article, you, as a research consumer, cannot appraise the measurement tools as having strong psychometric properties; thus, you would lack confidence in the usefulness of the study findings.

Criterion-Related Validity

Criterion-related validity is the degree of relationship between the participant's performance on the measurement tool and the participant's actual behaviour. The criterion is usually the second measure, which is used to assess the same concept being studied.

Two types of criterion-related validity are concurrent and predictive. **Concurrent validity** is the degree of correlation of two measures of the same construct administered at the same time. A high correlation coefficient indicates agreement between the two measures. **Predictive validity** is the degree of correlation between the measure of the concept and a future measure of the same concept. Because of the passage of time, the correlation coefficients are likely to be lower for predictive validity studies.

McGilton and associates (2005) evaluated the concurrent validity of the newly developed Relational Care Scale (RCS) and the Relational Behaviour Scale (RBS) because both scales are based on the empathic and reliable behaviours of care providers and on Winnicott's (1965) relational theory. In addition, the RCS was assessed with the Relationship Visual Analogue Scale. The results indicated that the RCS was positively correlated with the Relationship Visual Analogue Scale ($r = .63$, $p < .0001$; $n = 50$), and the RBS was positively moderately correlated with the RCS ($r = .42$, $p < .001$; $n = 72$).

An example of predictive validity appears in the study of McCarter-Spaulding and Dennis (2010), who assessed the psychometric properties of the short form of the Breastfeeding Self-Efficacy Scale, a measure of the self-confidence of mothers in breast-feeding. The researcher assessed the predictive validity of this scale by checking the correlation of the mothers' scores with their method of infant feeding at 4 months post partum because infant feeding was determined to be a strong and objective comparison criterion.

Construct Validity

Construct validity is the extent to which a test measures a theoretical construct or trait. To establish this type of validity, the researcher attempts to validate a body of theory underlying the measurement and testing of the hypothesized relationships. Empirical testing confirms or fails to confirm the relationships that would be predicted among concepts and, as such, provides more or less support for the construct validity of the instruments measuring those concepts. Establishing construct validity is a complex process, often involving several studies and approaches. The following approaches are discussed in this section: hypothesis-testing, convergent and divergent, contrasted-groups, and factor-analytical.

McCarter-Spaulding and Dennis (2010) also assessed construct validity by analyzing the relationship between network support and breast-feeding self-efficacy. As hypothesized, network support for breast-feeding was significantly correlated with the scores on the short form of the Breastfeeding Self-Efficacy Scores.

Hypothesis-Testing Approach

When the **hypothesis-testing approach** is used, the investigator uses the theory or concept underlying the measurement instrument to validate the instrument. The investigator accomplishes this task first by developing hypotheses about the behaviour of individuals with varying scores on

the measure; then by gathering data to test the hypotheses; and finally, on the basis of the findings, by making inferences about whether the rationale underlying the instrument's construction is adequate to explain the findings.

For example, Barnason and colleagues (2002) used a hypothesis-testing approach to establish the construct validity of the Barnason Efficacy Expectation Scale (BEES). Construct validity was tested on the basis of the empirically supported hypothesis that individuals with better health status and functioning also would have higher levels of self-efficacy. To explore this hypothesis, correlations were made between the BEES total score and physiological behaviours of interest in a population of patients who had received a coronary artery bypass graft. Measures of physiological functioning used in this psychometric study were subscales of the Medical Outcomes Study Short-Form 36, which has been used extensively in the literature as a measure of health status and functioning with established reliability and validity. This instrument is a multidimensional scale on which health concepts are measured. However, in this study, the physiological functioning subscales of physical functioning, role-physical functioning (role limitations caused by physical problems), and general health were used specifically because those aspects of functioning were more closely related to the behaviours measured with the BEES.

The BEES mean score was correlated with aspects of physiological functioning (physical, role-physical, and general health), with significant weak to moderate correlations ranging from .25 to .41. These findings provide support for the hypothesis and therefore preliminary support for the theoretical basis, conceptual accuracy, and construct validity of the BEES in the patient population: Individuals with better health status have higher levels of self-efficacy. Because of the homogeneous nature of the sample and the use of a convenience sampling strategy, however, further testing of the BEES is necessary with adults from various age, gender, socioeconomic, and cultural groups.

Convergent and Divergent Approaches

Two strategies for assessing construct validity are convergent and divergent approaches.

Convergent validity exists when two or more tools that are intended to measure the same construct are administered to participants and are found to be positively correlated. A correlational analysis (i.e., a test of relationship; see Chapters 11 and 16) determines whether the measures are positively correlated, in which case convergent validity is said to be supported.

Powers and colleagues (2004) evaluated the convergent validity of one of the most widely used tools for predicting the risk for pressure sores: the mobility subscale of the Braden Scale (Braden & Bergstrom, 1994). Patient immobility had been identified as an important risk factor in the development of pressure sores, and the mobility subscale of the Braden Scale was designed to quantify levels of mobility, on the basis of individual clinical observations.

To assess convergent validity, actigraphy (a noninvasive method of monitoring rest and activity cycles) was used to measure participants' frequency of movement. Powers and colleagues (2004) hypothesized that a lower mean frequency of movement would be recorded by actigraphy for participants scoring low (i.e., a score of 1) on the mobility subscale than for participants with higher scores. Powers and colleagues further hypothesized that as the mobility subscale scores increased, the mean frequency of the movements recorded by actigraphy would also increase.

Two consecutive data-collection periods, from 6 A.M. to 6 P.M. in a 48-hour interval, were chosen for analysis. Powers and colleagues (2004) found that only spontaneous patient movement was noted in the data analysis of the actigraph recordings. The statistically significant difference in the mean activity by subscale groups—$F(3, 15) =$ 31.69, $p = .001$—supported the hypothesis that as the mean activity in each group increased, the mean frequency of the movements recorded by actigraphy would also increase, and the greatest amount of activity occurred in the group with the highest scores. The researchers also found that the mean activity of participants whose mobility subscale level was 4 (no mobility limitations) was significantly greater than the activity of participants in the other three levels, which supported the convergent validity of the mobility subscale of the Braden Scale.

More recently, causal modelling has been used to develop and test a hypothesized explanation of causes of a phenomenon, and to establish convergent validity, as in the development of the Caregiver Reciprocity Scale by Carruth (1996). As illustrated in Table 14-3, several indicators have been recommended to assess convergent validity: standardized item loadings, item/composite reliability, examination of standard error, and estimated average variance, as extracted by each construct. For the data in Table 14-3, these indicators were calculated by the Linear Structural Relationships (LISREL) computer program.

The item loadings indicate the extent to which a single variable is related to the cluster of variables; for example, in Table 14-3, under the cluster of variables for *warmth and regard,* item 30 has a loading of .82, which is closer to the composite reliability of .89 and thus is more related to the cluster than item 2, which has a loading of .52. Item reliability is the reliability of that item within that subscale; for example, in Table 14-3, the reliability for item 4 on the subscale *love and affection* is .60, whereas the reliability for the subscale of *love and affection* with the four items is .88. Average variance is the amount of variance explained by a cluster of variables in that construct; for example, of the four subscales, *love and affection* has the highest estimate, .64. Standard error is the standard deviation divided by the sample size. Table 14-3 presents

TABLE 14-3

ESTIMATED LISREL PARAMETERS OF CONSTRUCT VALIDITY

CONSTRUCT	STANDARDIZED LOADINGS	ITEM/COMPOSITE RELIABILITY	2 × SE	VARIANCE EXTRACTED ESTIMATE
WARMTH AND REGARD				
		.89*		.48
Item 2	.52	.27	—†	
Item 10	.70	.48	.40	
Item 12	.76	.58	.42	
Item 21	.60	.35	.37	
Item 22	.71	.51	.40	
Item 25	.67	.45	.39	
Item 28	.70	.49	.40	
Item 30	.82	.66	.43	
Item 33	.74	.54	.41	
INTRINSIC REWARDS OF GIVING				
		.83*		.49
Item 1	.62	.38	—†	
Item 13	.64	.40	.29	
Item 17	.74	.55	.30	
Item 29	.76	.60	.30	
Item 32	.74	.55	.30	
LOVE AND AFFECTION				
		.88*		.64
Item 4	.77	.60	—†	
Item 5	.73	.53	.18	
Item 8	.90	.80	.18	
Item 15	.81	.65	.18	
BALANCE WITHIN FAMILY CAREGIVING				
		.77*		.47
Item 6	.72	.51	—†	
Item 19	.69	.48	.24	
Item 20	.75	.56	.24	
Item 34	.56	.31	.23	

From Carruth, A. K. (1996). Development and testing of the Caregiver Reciprocity Scale. *Nursing Research, 45,* 92–97.
LISREL, Linear Structural Relationships (computer program); *SE,* standard error.
*Denotes composite reliabilities.
†Denotes that the value was not estimated (parameter constrained at 1.0 in LISREL).

data indicating significant findings between the factor structure of the Caregiver Reciprocity Scale and the relevant causal modelling indicators, thereby offering support for the convergent validity of the items in each factor of the Caregiver Reciprocity Scale.

In contrast to convergent validity, the calculation of **divergent validity** requires measurement approaches that differentiate one construct from others that may be similar. Sometimes research-

ers search for instruments that measure the opposite of the construct. If the divergent measure is negatively related to other measures, the measure's validity is strengthened.

McGilton and associates (2003) assessed the divergent validity of the RBS, which consisted of three subscales related to the empathic and reliable relational behaviours of people who provided care to older adults. More positive behaviour of care providers was illustrated by higher scores on the RBS. The researchers hypothesized that the RBS would be negatively correlated with a negative affect scale. This hypothesis was supported through the use of the Philadelphia Center Affect Rating Scale, on which the RBS was found to be negatively correlated with anxiety ($r = .59$, $p < .005$), sadness ($r = -.59$, $p < .005$), and agitation ($r = -.39$, $p < .05$); thus, the construct validity of the RBS in measuring empathy and reliable relational behaviours was verified. More recently, the data from a factor analysis being conducted for other validity purposes has been used to determine divergent (sometimes called *discriminant*) validity. Carruth (1996) assessed the divergent validity of the four factors (subscales) of the Caregiver Reciprocity Scale by examining the correlations between each factor or subscale that appears in Table 14-3.

A specific method of assessing convergent and divergent validity is the **multitrait-multimethod approach.** Similar to the divergent validity approach just described, this method, proposed by Campbell and Fiske (1959), also involves examining the relationships between instruments that are intended to measure the same construct and between those that are intended to measure different constructs. A variety of measurement strategies, however, are used. In other words, this approach is a type of validation in which more than one method is used to assess the accuracy of an instrument. For example, anxiety could be measured by the following:

- Administering the State-Trait Anxiety Inventory
- Recording blood pressure readings
- Asking the participant about anxious feelings
- Observing the participant's behaviour

The results of one of these measures should then be correlated with the results of each of the others in a multitrait-multimethod matrix (Waltz, Strickland, & Lenz, 1991).

In their classic study designed to develop, validate, and normalize a measure of dimensions of interpersonal relationships (including social support, reciprocity, and conflict), Tilden and associates (1990) used the multitrait-multimethod approach to validity assessment. The two traits of social support and conflict listed in the Interpersonal Relationship Inventory were each measured with two different methods: a participant self-report tool and an investigator-observation visual analogue rating. Reciprocity was not included because of its high correlation with social support.

The use of multiple measures of a concept decreases systematic error. The use of a variety of data-collection methods (e.g., self-report, observation, interview, and collection of physiological data) also diminishes the effect of systematic error.

Contrasted-Groups Approach

In the **contrasted-groups approach** (sometimes called the **known-groups approach**) to the development of construct validity, the researcher identifies two groups of individuals expected to score extremely high or extremely low in the characteristic being measured by the instrument. The instrument is administered to both groups, and the differences in scores are examined. If the instrument is sensitive to individual differences in the trait being measured, the mean performance of these two groups should differ significantly, and evidence of construct validity would be supported. A *t* test or analysis of variance is used to statistically measure the difference between the two groups.

Secco (2002) sought to develop and assess the psychometric properties of the Infant Care Questionnaire, a self-report scale designed to measure a mother's perception of her abilities and competence in providing care to her infant. The researcher used the contrasted-groups approach to provide evidence of construct validity for the "Mom and Baby" dimension of the Infant Care Questionnaire.

The known groups were healthy mothers of different parity (low-risk primiparous and multiparous mothers [$n = 164$] of full-term infants) and mothers with different amounts of past infant care experience. Multiparous mothers, mothers with higher ratings of past infant care experience, and mothers with greater time in the mothering role were expected to have significantly higher "Mom and Baby" scores than were primiparous mothers with lower ratings of infant care experience.

As illustrated in Table 14-4, repeated-measures analysis of variance demonstrated significantly higher "Mom and Baby" scores for the multiparous mothers than for primiparous mothers by time [$F(2, 134) = 21.78, p = .000$] and parity [$F(1, 134) = 10.78, p = .001$]. Over time, certain trends were observed: lower scores for primiparous mothers at all three measurement times and diminished mean differences between parity groups. Secco (2002) proposed that these findings are associated with the maternal role attainment theory, which is that knowledge, skill, and competence perceptions are acquired during the postnatal period and that experience is a key factor in attainment of competence. The significantly higher scores on the "Mom and Baby" dimension for the multiparous mothers suggest that the Infant Care Questionnaire was sensitive enough to capture the differences between primiparous and multiparous mothers, thereby providing evidence of construct validity with the contrasted-groups approach.

Factor-Analytical Approach

A final approach to assessing construct validity is **factor analysis.** This procedure gives the researcher information about the extent to which a set of items measures the same underlying construct or the same dimension of a construct. In factor analysis, the researcher assesses the degree to which the individual items on a scale truly cluster around one or more dimensions. Items designed to measure the same dimension should load on the same factor; those designed to measure differing dimensions should load on different factors (Anastasi, 1988; Nunnally & Bernstein, 1994).

A factor analysis also indicates whether the items in the instrument reflect a single construct or several constructs. Several factors may be identified in a set of data. The study must have a large sample size in order to conduct a factor analysis. Nunnally and Bernstein (1994) recommended 10 observations for each variable. Thus, to develop the factor structure and reliability of the Brain Impairment Behavior Scale, Cameron and associates (2008) used data from several small studies in which this scale was used to obtain a sample size of 300. Table 14-5 gives an example of how factor analysis can be used, as it was in causal modelling.

Roberts and Ward-Smith (2010) conducted a factor analysis in the development of the Career Search Questionnaire. By performing exploratory factor analysis and using principal component analysis with a varimax rotation, they obtained five factors that accounted for 57.4% of the total variance. The findings from the factor analysis are presented in Table 14-5.

TABLE 14-4
RESULTS OF REPEATED-MEASURES ANALYSIS OF VARIANCE FOR MEAN "MOM AND BABY" DIMENSION SCORES BY TIME* AND PARITY†

POSTPARTUM WEEK	PRIMIPAROUS ($n = 97$)	MULTIPAROUS ($n = 43$)	ALL MOTHERS ($n = 140$)
1	3.74	4.09	3.85
2	4.00	4.23	4.10
3	4.07	4.18	4.10

*$F(2, n = 140) = 21.78, p < .001$.
†$F(1, n = 140) = 10.78, p < .001$.

Helpful Hint_____

When validity data about a study's measurement instruments are not included in a research article, you cannot determine whether the intended concept is being captured by the measurement tool. Before you use the results, check the instrument's validity by reviewing the original source.

TABLE 14-5

CAREER SEARCH QUESTIONNAIRE FACTORS AND HIGHEST FACTOR LOADINGS ON NURSING ITEMS: POPULATIONS BEFORE NURSING STUDY

FACTOR/ITEM	LOADING
FACTOR 1: ASSESSMENT AND SAFETY	
Safety for self, others	.713
Flexibility to changes	.706
Healthy boundaries	.704
Concerns for privacy, dignity	.688
Gather information	.660
Protect others, ethical treatment	.588
Understand physiology	.482
Health teaching	.471
FACTOR 2: ACTIVE PROBLEM SOLVING	
Learn technical skills	.752
Assign duties to others	.735
Plan goals for others	.690
Communicating during stress	.576
Empowering others	.545
Work with blood, human waste	.533
FACTOR 3: WORKING WITH PEOPLE	
Enjoy working with people	.797
Find solutions to problems	.742
Working with different people	.694
FACTOR 4: SCIENTIFIC LEARNING	
Lifelong learner	.739
New terminology	.659
Read research	.655
Ways to do things better	.447
FACTOR 5: COMPASSION	
Emotional and physical support	.724
Help people at end of life	.708
Compassion with ill people	.567

Adapted from Roberts, C. A., & Ward-Smith, P. (2010). Choosing a career in nursing: Development of a career search instrument. *International Journal of Nursing Education Scholarship, 7*(1), Article 2.

Evidence-Informed Practice Tip _____

When the tools used in a study are presented, note whether the sample used to develop the measurement instruments is similar to your patient population.

The Critical Thinking Decision Path will help you assess the appropriateness of the type of validity and reliability selected for use in a particular research study.

Researchers may be concerned about whether the scores that were obtained for a sample of participants were consistent, true measures of the behaviours, and thus an accurate reflection of the differences between individuals. The extent of variability in test scores that is attributable to error rather than a true measure of the behaviours is the **error variance.**

An **observed test score** that is derived from a set of items consists of the true score plus error (Figure 14-2). The error may be either chance (random) error or systematic error.

A **chance error** or a **random error** is an error that is difficult to control (e.g., a respondent's anxiety at the time of testing). These errors are unsystematic and are not predictable; thus, they cannot be corrected. However, awareness of the sources of these errors may help the researcher minimize their effect on measurement accuracy. These sources are as follows:

1. Transient human conditions, such as hunger, fatigue, health, lack of motivation, and anxiety, which are often beyond the awareness and control of the examiner.
2. Variations in the measurement procedure, such as misplacement of the blood pressure cuff, not waiting for a specific time period before taking the blood pressure, or placing the arm randomly in relation to the heart while measuring blood pressure; changing the wording of interview questions between administrations; or environmental factors, such as the presence of others while data are being obtained, a cold room, or discomfort with the researcher (who is part of the environment).
3. Errors in data processing, such as coding errors and incorrect inputting into the computer.

Chance errors affect an individual's observed score, so that the person's observed score may be higher than his or her true score, whereas another person's observed score may be lower than his or her true score. Instruments that are free

CRITICAL THINKING DECISION PATH

Determining the Appropriate Type of Validity and Reliability Selected for a Study

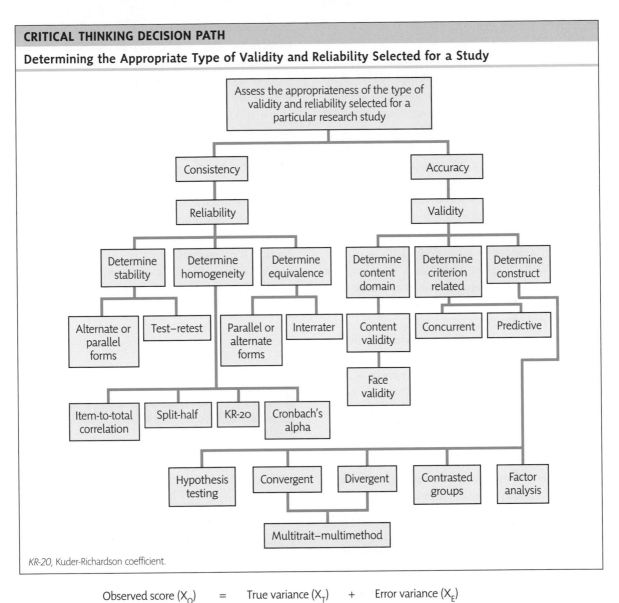

KR-20, Kuder-Richardson coefficient.

Observed score (X_O) = True variance (X_T) + Error variance (X_E)

Actual score
obtained

Consistent,
hypothetical,
stable, or
true score

Chance/Random Error
• Transient participant
  factors
• Instrumentation variations
• Transient environmental
  factors

Systematic Error
• Consistent instrument,
  participant, or environmental
  factors

FIGURE 14-2 Components of observed scores.

of chance errors are considered reliable (Nunnally, 1978).

A **systematic error** or a **constant error** is a measurement error that is attributable to relatively stable characteristics of the study population that may bias their behaviour, cause incorrect instrument calibration, or both. Such error has a systematic biasing influence on the participants' responses and thereby influences the validity of the instruments. Level of education, socioeconomic status, social desirability, response pattern, or other characteristics may influence the validity of the instrument by altering the measurement of the "true" responses in a systematic way. For example, a participant who wants to please the investigator may constantly answer items in a socially desirable way, thus making the estimate of validity inaccurate.

Systematic error also occurs when an instrument is improperly calibrated. Consider a scale that consistently gives a person's weight at 1 kg less than the actual body weight. The scale could be quite reliable (i.e., capable of reproducing the precise measurement), but the result is consistently invalid. Systematic error is considered part of the true score. The multimethod-multitrait approach is one method of decreasing systematic error. The validity of an instrument is the extent to which it is free of both chance errors and systematic errors (Nunnally, 1978).

The amount of detail about reliability and validity varies considerably among research articles. When the focus of a study is tool development, psychometric evaluation—including extensive reliability and validity data—is carefully documented and appears throughout the article rather than briefly in the "Instruments" section, as in other research studies.

RIGOUR IN QUALITATIVE RESEARCH: CREDIBILITY, AUDITABILITY, AND FITTINGNESS

As in quantitative research, the basic approach to ensure rigour in qualitative research is methodical research design, data collection, interpretation, and communication. Qualitative researchers seek to achieve two goals: (1) to account for the method and the data, which must be independent so that another researcher can analyze the same data in the same way and make the same conclusions, and (2) to produce a credible and reasoned explanation of the phenomenon under study. Thus, this rigour in qualitative methodology is judged by unique criteria appropriate for the research approach. Credibility, auditability, and fittingness are the scientific criteria proposed for qualitative research studies by Guba (1981). Although these criteria are not new, they still capture the rigorous spirit of qualitative inquiry and are reasonable for evaluation. The meanings of credibility, auditability, and fittingness are briefly explained in Table 14-6.

TABLE **14-6**

CRITERIA FOR JUDGING SCIENTIFIC RIGOUR: CREDIBILITY, AUDITABILITY, FITTINGNESS

CRITERIA	CHARACTERISTICS
Credibility	Truth of findings as judged by participants and others within the discipline. For example, you may find the researcher returning to the participants to share interpretation of findings and query accuracy from the perspective of the persons living the experience.
Auditability	Accountability as judged by the adequacy of information leading the reader from the research question and raw data through various steps of analysis to the interpretation of findings. For example, you should be able to follow the reasoning of the researcher step by step through explicit examples of data, interpretations, and syntheses.
Fittingness	Faithfulness to the everyday reality of the participants, described in enough detail so that others in the discipline can evaluate importance for their own practice, research, and theory development. For example, you will know enough about the human experience being reported that you can decide whether it "rings true" and is useful for guiding your practice.

Credibility

Credibility is a characteristic of qualitative research that refers to the accuracy, validity, and soundness of data. It is similar to internal validity in qualitative research. The methods to ensure credibility are prolonged engagement, persistent observation, peer debriefing, and member checks (Lincoln, 1995). In prolonged engagement and persistent observation, the researchers spend sufficient time with the study's participants to check for discrepancies in responses. Peer debriefing is conducted with experts in the field, whose probing questions and review about the research can assist the researchers in improving trustworthiness in the data. Member checking verifies the accuracy of participants' responses by asking the study participants to review the themes and narratives to determine whether the researchers accurately described their experiences (Lincoln & Guba, 1985).

Triangulation, crystallization, and searching for disconfirming evidence through negative case analyses are also used to ensure credibility and confirmability. In Chapter 7, triangulation—the cross-checking and verification of data through the use of different information sources, such as a variety of data sources, investigators, theoretical models, and research methods—and crystallization in both qualitative and mixed method research are discussed. Triangulation is viewed as offering completeness to naturalistic inquiry (Tobin & Begley, 2004).

Auditability and Fittingness

Engaging in an inquiry audit establishes both the auditability and the fittingness of the data. **Auditability** is the characteristic of a qualitative study, developed by the investigator's research process, that allows another researcher or a reader to follow the thinking or conclusions of the investigator. **Fittingness** is the degree to which study findings are applicable outside the study situation and the degree to which the results are meaningful to individuals not involved in the research. The audit trail was proposed by Guba (1981) to allow external auditors to follow the trail of qualitative data gathering and has been described by Lincoln and Guba (1985) as "the most important trustworthiness technique available to the naturalistic" (p. 285). The audit trail involves reviewing all documents relating to the study, such as research protocol, memos and correspondences, research tools, and field notes. See the Practical Application box for an example of establishing rigour through use of an audit trail.

> ### Practical Application
>
> In an illustration of how rigour is ascertained, Tourangeau and associates (2009) conducted a qualitative study to identify nurse-reported determinants of intention to remain employed and to develop a model explaining determinants of hospital nurses' intention to remain employed. Tourangeau and associates established trustworthiness in the data by engaging in a variety of methods: for credibility, they used verbatim quotations to illustrate findings, member checking, presenting their preliminary findings to some participants, and requesting participants' views on the accuracy of interpretation. "Transferability of findings was supported through descriptions of the time and context in which these data were found. These allow readers to make decisions about transferability. Both dependability and confirmability were strengthened through an audit trail (e.g., transcripts, history of theme development)" (p. 26).

As noted by Seneviratne and associates (2009) (see Appendix A), ethnographers keep track of changes in their ideas, beliefs, and values as they are engaged in the research. In this particular study, reflexive techniques were used to control for biases from having an insider (emic) perspective.

Luhanga and colleagues (2010) incorporated several strategies to ascertain rigour. They explored the preceptor role support and development within the context of a rural northern mid-sized Canadian community. Credibility was established when the participant preceptors validated recognition of the research findings as reflective of their own experiences in follow-up debriefing sessions. Excerpts from preceptor transcripts were presented in the findings to facilitate auditability of the data analysis and findings. A comprehensive audit trail and record of the theoretical memos maintained auditability. An independent reviewer read and commented on the fittingness of the results. Because the four criteria of credibility, fittingness, and auditability were met, confirmability was then achieved.

Emden and Sandelowski (1999) inferred that one set of criteria cannot "fit the bill" for every research study. Thus, Chiovitti and Piran (2003, p. 427) developed a framework of rigour that consisted of the following eight methods of research practice to enhance rigour during the research process and for critiquing published reports on research in grounded theory:

1. Let participants guide the inquiry process.
2. Check the theoretical construction generated against participants' meanings of the phenomenon.
3. Use participants' actual words in the theory.
4. Articulate the researcher's personal views and insights about the phenomenon explored.
5. Specify the criteria built into the researcher's thinking.
6. Specify how and why participants in the study were selected.
7. Delineate the scope of the research
8. Describe how the literature relates to each category that emerged in the theory.

Streubert and Carpenter (2007) commented that these criteria can provide a guide for critiquing grounded theory research.

Another concept to increase rigour that has not received much attention is goodness, represented as a "means of locating situatedness, trustworthiness and authenticity" (Tobin & Begley, 2004, p. 391). Tobin and Begley recommended that goodness be reflected by the entire study and discussed Arminio and Hultgren's (2002) six elements of goodness:

1. Foundation (epistemology and theory)
2. Approach (methodology)
3. Collection of data (method)
4. Representation of voice
5. The art of meaning making
6. Implication for professional practice

These six elements of goodness will help you as a research consumer when you critique a study for research utilization.

APPRAISING THE EVIDENCE

Reliability and Validity

Reliability and validity are two crucial aspects in the critical appraisal of a measurement instrument. The reviewer evaluates an instrument's level of reliability and validity, as well as how they were established. In a research report, the reliability and validity for each measure should be presented. If these data have not been presented, the reviewer must seriously question the merit and use of the tool and the study's results. Criteria for critiquing reliability and validity are presented in the Critiquing Criteria box.

If reliable and valid questionnaires are not used in a study, the results cannot be credible. As a critiquer, you have an ethical responsibility to question the reliability and validity of instruments used in research studies and to examine the findings in view of the quality of the instruments used and the data presented. The following discussion highlights key areas related to reliability and validity that should be evident in a research article.

Appropriate reliability tests should have been performed by the developer of the measurement tool and should then have been included by the current user in the research report. If the initial standardization sample and the current sample have different characteristics, the reader would find either (1) that a pilot study for the

APPRAISING THE EVIDENCE

Reliability and Validity—cont'd

present sample would have been conducted to determine whether the reliability was maintained or (2) that a reliability estimate was calculated for the current sample. For example, if the standardization sample for a tool that measures "satisfaction in an intimate heterosexual relationship" comprises undergraduate college students and if an investigator plans to use the tool with married couples, the reliability of the tool should be established with the latter group.

The investigator determines which type of reliability procedure is used in the study, depending on the nature of the measurement tool and how it will be used. For example, if the instrument is to be administered twice, you might determine that test-retest reliability should have been used to establish the stability of the tool. If an alternate form of the instrument has been developed for use in a repeated-measures design, evidence of alternate-form reliability should be presented to determine the equivalence of the parallel forms.

If the degree of internal consistency among the items is relevant, an appropriate test of internal consistency should be presented. In some instances, more than one type of reliability is presented, but you should determine whether all are appropriate. For example, the Kuder-Richardson formula implies that a single right or wrong answer exists, which makes use of the coefficient inappropriate with scales that provide a format of three or more possible responses. In such cases, another formula is applied, such as Cronbach's alpha.

Another important consideration is the acceptable level of reliability, which varies according to the type of test. Coefficients with reliability of .70 or higher are desirable. The validity of an instrument is limited by its reliability; in other words, less confidence can be placed in scores from tests with low-reliability coefficients.

Satisfactory evidence of validity is probably the most difficult determination for you as reviewer. This aspect of measurement is most likely to fall short of meeting the required criteria. Validity studies are time consuming and complex, and researchers sometimes settle for presenting minimal validity data.

Therefore, you should closely examine the item content of a tool when you evaluate its strengths and weaknesses and try to find conclusive evidence of content validity. In the body of a research article, however, it is unusual to have more than a few sample items available for review. Thus, you should determine whether the appropriate assessment of content validity was used to meet the researcher's goal.

Such procedures provide assurance that the tool is psychometrically sound and that the content of the items is consistent with the conceptual framework and the construct definitions. Construct validity and criterion-related validity are two of the more precise statistical tests of whether the tool measures what it is intended to measure. Ideally, an instrument should provide evidence of content validity, as well as criterion-related or construct validity, before a reviewer invests a high level of confidence in the tool.

You should also expect to see the strengths and weaknesses of instrument reliability and validity presented in the "Discussion," "Limitations," or "Recommendations" section, or in all of these sections, of a research article. In this context, the reliability and validity might be discussed in relation to other tools devised to measure the same variable. The relationship of the study's findings to the strengths and weaknesses in instrument reliability and validity is another important discussion point.

Finally, the researcher should propose recommendations for improving future studies in relation to instrument reliability and validity. For example, in the "Discussion" section of a report about developing and validating the Double Duty Caregiving Scale, Ward-Griffin and associates (2009) noted that nine factors were extracted with five subscales. Additional analyses were required to establish the psychometric properties of this Scale, including test-retest reliability to assess construct validity. The reliability coefficients for the five subscales ranged from .85 to .71. Reliability and validity in research reports can be evaluated to varying degrees. As a research consumer, you should not feel inhibited by the complexity of these topics but may use the guidelines presented in this chapter to systematically assess the reliability and validity of a research study.

Collegial dialogue is also an approach to evaluating the merits and shortcomings of an existing instrument,

Continued

APPRAISING THE EVIDENCE

Reliability and Validity—cont'd

as well as a newly developed one, that is reported in the nursing literature. Such an exchange promotes the understanding of methodologies and techniques of reliability and validity, stimulates the acquisition of a basic knowledge of psychometrics, and encourages the exploration of alternative methods of observation and the use of reliable and valid tools in clinical practice.

CRITIQUING CRITERIA

1. Was an appropriate method used to test the reliability of the tool?
2. Is the reliability of the tool adequate?
3. Was an appropriate method used to test the validity of the instrument?
4. Is the validity of the measurement tool adequate?
5. If the sample from the developmental stage of the tool was different from the current sample, were the reliability and validity recalculated to determine whether the tool is still adequate?
6. Have the strengths and weaknesses of the reliability and validity of each instrument been presented?
7. Did the researcher accurately depict the participant's reality?
8. Is evidence provided that the researcher's interpretation accurately represented the participant's meaning?
9. Have other professionals confirmed the researcher's interpretation?
10. Are the strengths and weaknesses of the research appropriately addressed in the "Discussion," "Limitations," or "Recommendations" sections of the report?

CRITICAL THINKING CHALLENGES

- Discuss the three types of validity that must be established before a reviewer invests a high level of confidence in the tool. Include examples of each type of validity.
- What are the major tests of reliability? Is it necessary to establish more than one measure of reliability for each instrument used in a study? Which do you think is the most essential measure of reliability? Include examples in your answer.
- Is it possible to have a valid instrument that is not reliable? Is the reverse possible? Support your answer with instruments you might use in the clinical setting with your patients.
- What are some ways in which credibility, auditability, and fittingness can be evaluated?
- How do you think the concept of evidence-informed practice has changed research utilization models? Is the review of the literature the same when a research proposal is developed as it is when the steps of research utilization or an evidence-informed practice protocol is implemented? Support your position.

KEY POINTS

- Reliability and validity are crucial aspects of conducting and critiquing research.
- Validity refers to whether an instrument measures what it is purported to measure. It is a crucial aspect of evaluating a tool.
- Three types of validity are content validity, criterion-related validity, and construct validity.
- The choice of a validation method is important and is made by the researcher on the basis of the characteristics of the measurement device in question and its use.
- Reliability refers to the ratio between accuracy and inaccuracy in a measurement device.
- The major tests of reliability are test-retest reliability, parallel- or alternate-form reliability, split-half reliability, item-to-total correlation, the Kuder-Richardson coefficient, Cronbach's alpha, and interrater reliability.
- The selection of a method for establishing reliability depends on the characteristics of the tool, the testing method that is used for collecting data from the standardization sample, and the kinds of data that are obtained.
- Credibility, auditability, and fittingness are criteria for judging the scientific rigour of a qualitative research study.

REFERENCES

Akhtar-Danesh, N., Valaitis, R. K., Schofield, R., Underwood, J., Martin-Misener, R., Baumann, A., & Kolotylo, C. (2010). A questionnaire for assessing community health nurses' learning needs. *Western Journal of Nursing Research, 32*(8), 1055-1072.

American Cancer Society. (2010). *Cancer facts and figures.* Atlanta: Author.

Anastasi, A. (1988). *Psychological testing* (6th ed.). New York: Macmillan.

Arminio, J. L., & Hultgren, F. H. (2002). Breaking out from the shadow: The question of criteria in qualitative research. *Journal of College Student Development, 43,* 446-456.

Armstrong, K., Laschinger, H., & Wong, C. (2009). Workplace empowerment and magnet hospital characteristics as predictors of patient safety climate. *Journal of Nursing Care Quality, 24*(1), 55-62.

Barnason, S., Zimmerman, L., Atwood, J., Nieveen, J., & Schmaderer, M. (2002). Development of a self-efficacy instrument for coronary artery bypass graft patients. *Journal of Nursing Measurement, 10,* 123-133.

Braden, B., & Bergstrom, N. (1994). Predictive validity of the Braden Scale for pressure sore risk in a nursing home population. *Research in Nursing and Health, 17,* 459-470.

Budin, W., Hoskins, C. N., Haber, J., Sherman, D. W., Maislin, G., Cater, J. R., . . . Shukla, S. (2008). Education, counselling, and adjustment among patient and partners: A randomized clinical trial. *Nursing Research, 57,* 199-213.

Cameron, J., Chung, A., Coyote, D., Streiner, D., Singh, M., & Stewart, D. (2008). Factor structure and reliability of the Brain Impairment Behavior Scale. *Journal of Neuroscience Nursing, 40*(1), 40-47.

Campbell, D., & Fiske, D. (1959). Convergent and discriminant validation by the matrix. *Psychological Bulletin, 53,* 273-302.

Carruth, A. K. (1996). Development and testing of the Caregiver Reciprocity Scale. *Nursing Research, 45,* 92-97.

Chiovitti, R. F., & Piran, N. (2003). Rigour and grounded theory research. *Journal of Advanced Nursing, 44*(4), 427-435.

Dennis, C. L. (2003). The Breastfeeding Self-Efficacy Scale: Psychometric assessment of the short form. *Journal of Obstetric, Gynecologic, & Neonatal Nursing, 32,* 734-744.

Doran, D. M., Harrison, M. B., Laschinger, H. S., Hirdes, J. P., Rukholm, E., Sidani, S., . . . Tourangeau, A. E. (2006). Nursing-sensitive outcomes data collection in acute care and long-term-care settings. *Nursing Research, 55*(2S), S75-S81.

Emden, C., & Sandelowski, M. (1999). The good, the bad and relative, part two: Goodness and the criterion problem in qualitative research. *International Journal of Professional Nursing Practice, 5*(1), 2-7.

Gélinas, C., Fillion, L., & Puntillo, K. A. (2008). Item selection and content validity of the Critical-Care Pain Observation Tool for non-verbal adults. *Journal of Advanced Nursing, 65*(1), 203-216.

Gillis, A. J. (1997). The Adolescent Lifestyle Questionnaire: Development and psychometric testing. *Canadian Journal of Nursing Research, 29,* 29-46.

Guba, E. G. (1981). Criteria for assessing the trustworthiness of naturalistic enquiries. *Educational Communication and Technology Journal, 29,* 75-91.

Heaman, M. I., & Gupton, A. L. (2009). Psychometric testing of the perception of pregnancy risk questionnaire. *Research in Nursing and Health, 32,* 493-503.

Hoskins, C. N. (1988). *The Partner Relationship Inventory.* Palo Alto, CA: Consulting Psychologists Press.

Ibrahim, S. E. R. (2002). Rates of adherence to pharmacological treatment among children and adolescents with attention deficit hyperactivity disorder. *Human Psychopharmacology, 17,* 225-231.

Jack, S. M., DiCenso, A., & Lohfeld, L. (2005). A theory of maternal engagement with public health nurses and family visitors. *Journal of Advanced Nursing, 49,* 182-190.

Kuiper, R.-A. (2010). Metacognitive factors that impact student nurse use of point of care technology in clinical settings. *International Journal of Nursing Education Scholarship, 7*(1), Article 5. doi: 10.2202/1548-923X.1866

Lincoln, Y. S. (1995). Emerging criteria for qualitative and interpretive research. *Qualitative Inquiry, 3,* 275-289.

Lincoln, Y., & Guba, E. (1985). *Naturalistic inquiry.* New York: Sage.

Luhanga, F. L., Dickeson, P., & Mossey, S. D. (2010). Preceptor preparation: An investment in the future generation of nurses. *International Journal of Nursing Education, 7*(1), Article 38, 1-15.

McCarter-Spaulding, D., & Dennis, C.-L. (2010). Psychometric testing of the Breastfeeding Self-efficacy Scale-Short Form in a sample of Black women in the United States. *Research in Nursing & Health, 33,* 111-119.

McDowell, I., & Newell, C. (1996). *Measuring health: A guide to rating scales and questionnaires.* New York: Oxford University Press.

McGilton, K. S., O'Brien-Pallas, L. L., Darlington, G., Evans, M., Wynn, F., & Pringle, D. M. (2003). Effects of relationship-enhancing program of care on outcomes. *Journal of Nursing Scholarship, 35,* 151-156.

McGilton, K. S., Pringle, D. M., O'Brien-Pallas, L. L., Wynn, F., & Streiner, D. (2005). Development and psychometric testing of the Relational Care Scale. *Journal of Nursing Measurement, 13,* 51-57.

Nunnally, J. C. (1978). *Psychometric theory* (2nd ed.). New York: McGraw-Hill.

Nunnally, J. C., & Bernstein, I. H. (1994). *Psychometric theory* (3rd ed.). New York: McGraw-Hill.

Powers, G. C., Zentner, T., Nelson, F., & Bergstrom, N. (2004). Validation of the mobility subscale of the Braden Scale for predicting pressure sore risk. *Nursing Research, 53,* 340-346.

Resnick, B., Nahm, E. S., Orwig, D., Zimmerman, S. S., & Magaziner, J. (2001). Measurement of activity in older adults: Reliability and validity of the step activity monitor. *Journal of Nursing Measurement, 9,* 275-290.

Roberts, C. A., & Ward-Smith, P. (2010). Choosing a career in nursing: Development of a career search instrument. *International Journal of Nursing Education Scholarship, 7*(1), Article 2.

Santacroce, S. J., Maccarelli, L. M., & Grey, M. (2004). Intervention fidelity. *Nursing Research, 53,* 63-66.

Secco, L. (2002). The Infant Care Questionnaire: Assessment of reliability and validity in a sample of healthy mothers. *Journal of Nursing Measurement, 10,* 97-109.

Seneviratne, C. C., Mather, C. M., & Then, K. L. (2009). Understanding nursing on an acute stroke unit: perceptions of space, time and interprofessional practice. *Journal of Advanced Nursing, 65*(9), 1872-1881, doi: 10.1111/j.1365-2648.2009.05053.x

Sidani, S., Epstein, D. R., Bootzin, R. R., Moritz, P., & Miranda, J. (2009). Assessment of preferences for treatment: Validation of a measure. *Research in Nursing and Health, 32,* 419-438.

Streubert, H. S., & Carpenter, D. (2007). *Qualitative research in nursing: Advancing the humanistic imperative.* Philadelphia: Lippincott, Williams, & Wilkins.

Tilden, V. P., Nelson, C. A., & May, B. A. (1990). The IPR inventory: Development and psychometric characteristics. *Nursing Research, 39,* 337-343.

Tobin, G. A., & Begley, C. M. (2004). Methodological rigour within a qualitative framework. *Journal of Advanced Nursing, 48,* 388-396.

Tourangeau, A. E., Cummings, B., Cranley, L. A., Ferron, E. M., & Harvey, S. (2009). Determinants of hospital nurse intention: Broadening our understanding. *Journal of Advanced Nursing, 66*(1), 22-32.

Waltz, C., Strickland, O., & Lenz, E. (1991). *Measurement in nursing research* (3rd ed.). Philadelphia: F. A. Davis.

Ward-Griffin, C., Keefe, J., Martin-Matthews, A., Kerr, M., Brown, J.-B., & Oudshoorn, A. (2009). Development and validation of the Double Duty Caregiving Scale. *Canadian Journal of Nursing Research, 41*(3), 108-128.

Winnicott, D. W. (1965). The maturational process and the facilitating environment. New York: International Universities Press.

FOR FURTHER STUDY

evolve Go to Evolve at http://evolve.elsevier.com/Canada/LoBiondo/Research for Audio Glossary, how-to instructions for Writing Proposals for Funding, and additional research articles for practice in reviewing and critiquing.

CHAPTER 15

Qualitative Data Analysis

Cherylyn Cameron

LEARNING OUTCOMES

After reading this chapter, you will be able to do the following:

- Describe the processes of qualitative data analysis.
- Outline the steps common to qualitative data analysis.
- Describe how data are reduced to meaningful units (themes).
- Describe the process of identifying themes and categories and the relationships between them.
- Assess the validity of a data analysis from a study.

KEY TERMS

codes	data display	thematic analysis
coding	data reduction	themes
constant comparative method	member checking	

STUDY RESOURCES

Go to Evolve at http://evolve.elsevier.com/Canada/LoBiondo/Research for Audio Glossary, how-to instructions for Writing Proposals for Funding, and additional research articles for practice in reviewing and critiquing.

AS DISCUSSED IN EARLIER CHAPTERS, qualitative analysis is not an analysis of the statistical tests used in the study but an analysis of the qualitative text. The text includes transcripts of interviews, narratives, documents, media such as newspapers and movies, and field notes. Qualitative researchers collect enormous amounts of data, which must be managed carefully: More than 150 pages of transcript can result from 25 interviews. To add to the complexity of qualitative data analysis, many researchers take different approaches to analysis. This chapter expands on the discussion in Chapter 8, in which the analysis of data was introduced in the context of several qualitative research traditions, such as phenomenology, grounded theory, ethnography, and case study.

AUDIO RECORDING INTERVIEWS

As discussed in Chapter 7, qualitative researchers gather data from a variety of sources, including interviews, observations, narrative, and focus groups (Streubert & Carpenter, 2011). Interviews are the most common source and serve as the primary source of data for many qualitative research projects. For example, Thorne and associates (2009) completed face-to-face interviews with each of the participants and followed up with bimonthly telephone interviews (see Appendix D). In addition to the field observations conducted in an ethnographic study, Seneviratne and associates (2009) conducted interviews to explore the participants' work practices (see Appendix A). Although some researchers believe that a recording device inhibits the free flow of discussion, Seidman (1998) and other authors have found that most participants and interviewers forget about the presence of the device. Consequently, most researchers record interviews and then transcribe them verbatim into written text. Some researchers may consider summarizing or paraphrasing the spoken words (Seidman, 1998), but this is not commonly practised. Most researchers wish to use the original words from the participants so that their own interpretations and personal biases are not juxtaposed with the participant's thoughts. The presence of the original words allows the reader to check the authenticity of the data. New researchers may transcribe the recording into text themselves; however, most researchers use a transcriptionist. It is recommended that the researcher spot-check interviews to ensure accuracy of the transcription (Streubert & Carpenter, 2011).

DATA MANAGEMENT

The open nature of qualitative inquiry typically results in the collection of more data than required. Glesne (2011) referred to the sheer volume of the data collected as "fat data." Consequently, researchers must be methodical in their organization and management of the data. Fortunately, computer software simplifies the storage and retrieval of data. In addition, researchers are also required to develop a decision or audit trail, which necessitates the tracking of the participants, the original audio recordings, and original and photocopied documents. Moreover, all of the data must be kept secure to maintain confidentiality.

Computer software to organize and retrieve data is referred to as computer-assisted qualitative data analysis software (CAQDAS). There are many computer programs to choose from, such as ATLAS.ti, Ethnograph, HyperRESEARCH, Inspiration, QSR NVivo, QSR XSight, and C-I-SAID. When choosing software, researchers have to understand what their needs are to determine the best fit. Meadows and Dodendorf (1999) categorized computer programs into the following three types:

1. Code-and-retrieve programs, which assist in organizing and grouping data (e.g., Data Collector)
2. Theory builders, which move to a different level of data organization by connecting themes and categories (e.g., QSR NVivo)
3. Conceptual network builders, which incorporate graphics with theory-building capabilities (e.g., Inspiration)

Unlike computer programs used with quantitative data, these programs do not analyze data. Data analysis and interpretation remain largely the task of the researcher. In other words, CAQDAS cannot "think for the researcher" (Glesne, 2011, p. 207). However, using computer programs for orderly organization and grouping of data facilitates the researcher's job of analysis and interpretation.

The researcher needs to test software to determine which program will be the most useful. Often, this process is one of trial and error before the most appropriate computer program is found. Most Web sites allow the downloading of a demonstration trial for a short time. Reviewing online tutorials (e.g., http://www.qsrinternational.com/solutions_multimedia.aspx) can also assist the researcher in selecting the most appropriate software. Although learning new software is very time consuming, the benefits of using computerized software outweigh the time spent researching and learning about it (Streubert & Carpenter, 2011). Qualitative discussion groups such as QUALR-L@LISTSERV.UGA.EDU, hosted at the University of Georgia, may also provide valuable insight and tips.

OVERVIEW OF DATA ANALYSIS

When does data collection end and data analysis begin? This is a controversial area of qualitative research because not all researchers agree on whether data collection should be completed before analysis begins or whether the two processes ought to take place concurrently. Therefore, the researcher needs to identify the process used.

As mentioned previously, many researchers begin a preliminary analysis as the material accumulates. Typically, the qualitative researcher transcribes all of the interviews, field notes, and observations as they are collected. As each piece of data is transcribed, researchers begin a preliminary analysis during which they determine what additional data need to be collected. Many researchers believe that the stages of data collection and data analysis should be integrated (Denzin & Lincoln, 2000; Miles & Huberman, 1994; Streubert & Carpenter, 2011), whereas others believe that these stages should be separate (Seidman, 1998).

The overall goal of qualitative data analysis is to make meaning out of massive amounts of text or data, and many methods for analysis are available. Patton (2002) encouraged researchers to do their "very best with . . . full intellectual capacity to fairly represent the data and communicate what the data reveal given the purpose of study" (p. 433). As described earlier, qualitative analysis is not a linear process; rather, it is cyclical, transformative, reciprocal, and iterative. Miles and Huberman (1994, p. 9) identified some common features among different approaches to qualitative data analysis:

- Affixing codes to a set of field notes taken during observations or interviews
- Noting reflections of other remarks in the margins
- Sorting and shifting though these materials to identify similar phrases, relationships between variables, patterns, themes, distinct differences between subgroups, and common sequences
- Isolating these patterns, processes, commonalities, and differences and taking them out to the field in the next wave of data collection
- Gradually elaborating a small set of generalizations that cover the consistencies discerned in the database
- Confronting those generalizations with a formalized body of knowledge in the form of constructs or theories

Guidelines such as these are useful, but they serve only as recommendations. Each qualitative study is unique and is reliant on the creativity, intellect, style, and experience of the researcher.

During the data analysis phase, all researchers fully immerse themselves in the data over a period of weeks to months. This process requires constant reading and rereading of the text until an understanding of what the data conveys is reached (Streubert & Carpenter, 2011). Many researchers also listen to the recorded interviews several times to increase their understanding and to remember the emotive component. Using an electronic player is helpful during this intense period of immersion. For example, during the interviews in Cameron's (2005) study, some participants were very emotional as they relived their experiences; the transcribed text did not reflect the emotions. Observations written by the researcher can capture these important elements. An important part of the data analysis is the interplay between data gathering or questioning and verifying what is heard and understood. Researchers continue to ask whether what they understood before is still relevant after subsequent interviews, observations, and reading of related documents. This "cyclic nature of questioning and verifying is an important aspect of data collection and analysis" (Streubert & Carpenter, 2011, p. 46).

Miles and Huberman (1994) referred to three discrete stages of data analysis: data reduction, data display, and conclusion drawing and verification (Figure 15-1). Many of the common methods used in nursing research fit into this general view of qualitative analysis.

Data Reduction

According to Miles and Huberman (1994), **data reduction** is "the process of selecting, focusing, simplifying, abstracting, and transforming the data that appear in written-up field notes or transcriptions" (p. 10). This process is ongoing as data are collected. Initially, the data can be organized into meaningful clusters of data by grouping related or similar data. Often, these clusters or groups of data are labelled as **themes,** or structured meaning units of data that occur frequently in the text. **Thematic analysis**—the process of recognizing and recovering the emergent themes—is an important aspect of organizing data. In the qualitative tradition, as van Manen (1997) stated, "grasping and formulating a thematic understanding is not a rulebound but a free act of 'seeing' meaning" (p. 79).

Glesne (2011) described several methods to help researchers discover the meanings embedded in data. The first method is to write memos or keep a reflective journal during the data-collection stage, which allows researchers to record thoughts about the data as these thoughts occur. Analytical files are developed to sort data into general categories, such as interview

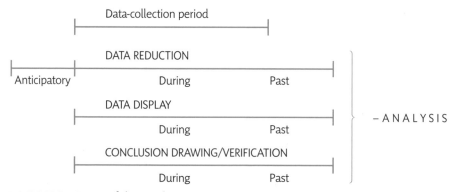

FIGURE 15-1   Stages of data analysis.
From Miles, M. B., & Huberman, A. M. (1994). Qualitative data analysis. Thousand Oaks, CA: Sage (Figure 1.3, p. 10). *Qualitative data analysis: An expanded sourcebook* by MILES, MATTHEW B.; HUBERMAN, A. MICHAEL. Copyright 1994 Reproduced with permission of SAGE PUBLICATIONS INC BOOKS in the format Other book via Copyright Clearance Center.

questions, people, and places, as well as useful quotations from the interviews and relevant quotations from the literature. These files help organize researchers' thoughts and those of others.

Next, Glesne (2011) recommended the development of rudimentary coding schemes. Coding, as Denzin and Lincoln (2000) described it, "is the heart and soul of whole-text analysis" (p. 780). **Coding** is a progressive marking, sorting, resorting, and defining and redefining of the collected data. Coding allows researchers to transform the "unstructured and messy data to ideas about what is going on in the data" (Richards & Morse, 2007, p. 133).

Last, Glesne (2011) recommended that researchers write themselves monthly field reports as a way of systematically reviewing the progress and determining the next steps. Aside from helping researchers keep track of their progress and communicate progress with other members of the research team, monthly summaries often result in new insights and new ways of approaching the research.

Denzin and Lincoln (2000) provided an overview of the fundamental steps in the coding of data: sampling, identifying themes, building codebooks, and marking texts. Richards and Morse (2007) described three types of coding: descriptive, topic, and analytic. Researchers use some or all of these steps when coding. *Descriptive coding* helps the researcher keep track of factual knowledge (e.g., gender). In *topic coding,* used most commonly, the data are grouped together by topic "to reflect on all the different ways people discuss particular topics, to seek patterns in their responses, or to develop dimensions of that experience" (Richards & Morse, 2007, p. 134). As the categories become more complicated, the topic coding becomes analytic. *Analytic coding* is more theoretical and leads to the development of themes. Although coding may sound complicated to you, remember that this process is evolutional, and it varies from project to project and from researcher to researcher. For

example, many researchers conducting narrative inquiry do not use coding, data reduction, and some of the other commonly used methods of data analysis. Moreover, remember that meanings are waiting to be discovered, not imposed on the data.

The next step, finding themes, is the most exciting step of the process, which occurs during and after data collection. These themes or basic units of analysis can be entire texts (e.g., interview transcripts, responses to surveys), grammatical segments (words, phrases, sentences, paragraphs), formatting units (rows, pages), or clusters of texts that reflect a single theme. Most researchers try to divide data into units of analysis that do not overlap with others. Researchers approach this step in a variety of ways; for example, experts in grounded theory recommend that the researcher read the text line by line.

The coding process itself is analysis (Miles & Huberman, 1994). Glesne (2006) stated that coding is as simple as identifying "what is important and giving it a name (code)" (p. 154). **Codes** are simply tags or labels that are assigned to the themes; often, the code itself is only one to four words long. Major codes may exist along with subcodes. Codes evolve during the analysis; more may be added, and others may be blended together. They mean something to the researcher and are not typically included in the research study. As the coding and themes are fine-tuned and finalized, much of the analysis is completed.

The next step is to build codebooks by organizing codes into lists, composed of either words or numbers that are used by the researcher. Then the text is marked, whereby the codes are assigned to the units of text. During this process, the researcher is immersed in the data, which results in new insights and interpretations.

Richards and Morse (2007) described two primary steps to data analysis: categorizing and conceptualizing: "Categorizing is how we understand and come to terms with the complexity of data in everyday life" (p. 157). Coding is one

TABLE 15-1

DOING ABSTRACTION IN THREE DIFFERENT METHODS

METHOD	WHEN DOES ABSTRACTION OCCUR?	WHERE DOES ABSTRACTION COME FROM?	HOW IS ABSTRACTION DONE?	WHAT ANALYTICAL OUTCOME IS BEING SOUGHT?
Phenomenology	Not until one has the data: Previous ideas and knowledge are bracketed	Themes and meanings in accounts, texts	Deep immersion, focus, thorough reading	To describe the essence of a phenomenon
Ethnography	Prior knowledge of site, situation; understanding develops during field research	Knowledge of social and economic setting; observation and learning from the setting	Rich description; combination of qualitative and quantitative patterning, coding, comparing, reviewing field notes	To identify themes and patterns; to explain and account for a social and cultural situation
Grounded theory	Abstraction is from the data, but can be informed by previously derived theories	Categories derived from data (observations or line-by-line analysis of texts); constant comparison with other situations or settings	Theoretical sensitivity; seeking concepts and their dimensions; open coding, dimensionalizing, memo writing, diagramming	To identify a core category and theory grounded in data

Reproduced with permission from Richards, L. & Morse, J. M. (2007). Readme first for a user's guide to qualitative methods (2nd ed). Thousand Oaks, CA: Sage (p. 159). *Readme first for a user's guide to qualitative methods* by MORSE, JANICE M.; RICHARDS, LYN Copyright 2007 Reproduced with permission of SAGE PUBLICATIONS INC BOOKS in the format Textbook via Copyright Clearance Center.

method for categorizing the data: however, other researchers in qualitative studies can think about data without coding. Many studies do not extend beyond categorizing if their research goal is to describe "what is going on" in a specific phenomenon. Conceptualizing moves up the ladder of abstraction (see Chapter 2) to build frameworks of concepts or theory. Phenomenology, ethnography, and grounded theory are all methods that necessitate conceptualization. In Table 15-1, the differences in the methods of abstraction are described by means of the following questions:

- When does abstraction occur?
- Where does abstraction come from?
- How is abstraction done?
- What analytical outcome is being sought?

Some researchers explicitly describe the process of data analysis. For example, Wuest and colleagues (2002) described the data analysis of grounded theory with an example of an earlier study by Wuest (2001) on women's caring. Wuest read each field note, transcript, or document line

TABLE 15-2

CODE ASSIGNMENTS AS DESCRIBED BY WUEST AND COLLEAGUES

CODE	TEXT EXAMPLE
Time for self	I steal an hour during the day.
Social interaction	I work not only for the money but to get out . . . for the social contacts.
Cultivating the marital relationship	So, after I get the kids to bed, I usually go downstairs and sit with him [partner] for an hour.

From Wuest, J., Merritt-Gray, M., Berman, H., & Ford-Gilboe, M. (2002). Illuminating social determinants of women's health using grounded theory. *Health Care International, 23*, 794-808.

by line while asking herself two questions: "What is this a conceptual indicator of?" and "What is going on here?" (Wuest, Merritt-Gray, Berman, & Ford-Gilboe, 2002). Codes were assigned to each grouping of data, from sentences to paragraphs to whole pages (Table 15-2). The codes (time for self, social interaction, and cultivating the marital relationship) were eventually grouped together into a single category: "replenishing."

In the study by Seneviratne and associates (2009; see Appendix A), data were gathered from field notes that were based on observations in the naturalistic setting and on interviews. The researchers analyzed the field notes and discovered three main themes. The researchers then kept returning to the field for further observations to cross-check their findings. Thorne and associates (2009) used a semistructured interview guide for the first face-to-face meeting to interview participants. The initial analysis identified themes to guide the subsequent bimonthly interviews that took place for up to 2 years. Through this constant comparative analysis process, the emerging themes were clarified with each interview.

Cameron (2003) analyzed the transcripts of interviews with 13 participants about their experiences transferring from a college to a university in a collaborative baccalaureate nursing program. She identified an initial set of themes at three points: as they emerged while she transcribed the interviews, after she relistened to the recorded interviews, and after a reading and a rereading of the transcripts. Differences, similarities, contradictions, and gaps in the data were noted as she returned to the original material to confirm the

TABLE **15-3**

CAMERON'S (2005) CODING SCHEME

MAJOR THEME	SUBTHEME	CODE
Academic shock	Workload	AS-Work
	Underprepared	AS-Uprep
	Curriculum	AS-C
	Unfulfilled promises	AS-prom
	Academic shock	AS
Professional transformation	Hospital to community	PT-H to C
	Practice to theory	PT-P to T
	Professionalization	PT-prof
Geographic relocation	Financial	GR-Fin
	Time and commuting	GR-T/C
	University structure	GR-US
	Campus size	GR-Size
	University culture	GR-Cul
	Guinea pigs	GR-GP
Transition stress	Self-doubt	TS-SD
	Going back	TS-GB
	Family and personal responsibility	TS-F
	Rumours	TS-R
	Emotions	TS-E
What social life?	Separation	S-sep
	Loneliness	S-L
	Bonding	S-B
Adaptation	Supports	A-Supp
	Personal attributes	A-P
	Learning the ropes	A-L
	Satisfaction	A-Sat
	Personal change	A-C
	Recommendations—college	A-RC
	Recommendations—university	A-RU

From Cameron, C. (2005). Experiences of transfer students in a collaborative baccalaureate nursing program. *Community College Review, 33*(2), 22-44. Reprinted by Permission of SAGE Publications.

findings. As a result of highlighting the students' stories, 29 subthemes emerged. From these, six major themes surfaced. Table 15-3 shows the coding scheme used to code the transcripts, and Table 15-4 shows how one small section of the text was coded to validate the themes after the data had been collected.

Data Display

The second major step in data analysis is the data display. Miles and Huberman (1994) defined **data display** as "an organized, compressed assembly of information that permits conclusion drawing and action" (p. 11). This display helps

the researcher understand the data and can be in the form of graphs, flowcharts, matrices, or any other visual representation. Like the rest of the analysis, the data display changes as more is known about the phenomenon under study. For example, Seneviratne and associates (2009) identified three themes (domains) and eight subthemes (theme components) resulting from their analysis of the nurses' perception of the contexts of caring for survivors of acute stroke (Table 15-5). The themes framed how nurses understand the challenges in organizing stroke care: (1) "space" concerned working in exceptionally close quarters; (2) "time" concerned how nurses had to find novel ways to provide care when there was not enough time; and (3) "interprofessional practice" referred to the importance that nurses ascribed to communications and collaboration among the interdisciplinary professionals. Ford-Gilboe and colleagues (2005) studied how women and their children promote their health after leaving abusive male partners. The researchers found that the families limit intrusion by the male partner through a process of strengthening capacity by means of four subprocesses: providing, regenerating family, renewing self, and rebuilding security. The structural components and how the

TABLE **15-4**

SAMPLE CODING

TEXT	CODE
"The first week of school?—Going out of my mind—coming home and crying. It was the expectations, they seem to be going on and on about these expectations that they were expecting of us. I don't think the information that was given to us was, I don't think was clarified properly or they didn't say it in a way to us that made us want to do it. It was . . . I felt very intimidated by the way they were talking to us by the expectations . . . you are going to do this and this and this . . . starting next week. I'm just in there—going out of my mind . . . . I don't know if I am going to be able to do this and it was again the self-doubt. It was . . . I don't think I'm going to be able to handle this. I want to go back to my college. And I remember me and my friends were just outside of our class and we were just like . . . this is unbearable and a couple of my friends wanted to call the college to see if they could get back in and . . . I knew if I could just last this week and last through a month . . . then I will see . . . Because I wasn't going to give up, just then. But it was definitely an eye opening experience. It wasn't at all what I expected. The professors were great but they just, it was too much information during that one week of the orientation."	TS-E AS-Work AS-Uprep TS-SD AS-Uprep TS-GB TS-E A-P AS-Uprep AS-Work

From Cameron, C. (2005). Experiences of transfer students in a collaborative baccalaureate nursing program. *Community College Review, 33*(2), 22-44.

TABLE **15-5**

THEMES AND SUBTHEMES IN RESULTS FROM APPENDIX A

THEMES	SUBTHEMES
Space	Nursing in a submarine Nursing too close Nursing under a state of "code burgundy"
Time	Lack of time Preserving time Time with and without space
Interprofessional practice	Relationships between stroke professionals Communication and collaboration

From Seneviratne, C. C., Mather, C. M., & Then, K. L. (2009). Understanding nursing on an acute stroke unit: Perceptions of space, time and interprofessional practice. *Journal of Advanced Nursing, 65*(9), 1872-1881. doi: 10.1111/j.1365-2648.2009.05053.x subprocesses relate to the theoretical structure are depicted in Figure 15-2.

Although many researchers use figures and charts as part of their data display, profiles or vignettes can also display what is to be learned from the participant's experience. Vignettes of the participant's experience can summarize what was learned from each participant and can then be shared with each participant for validation (Seidman, 1998). This narrative form transforms the text into a story—a compelling way of sharing meaning.

For example, Cameron (2003) studied the lived experience of transfer students in a collaborative nursing program and, as part of the mixed-methods design, interviewed 13 students. Vignettes were developed for each interview participant, who, in turn, selected a pseudonym that had personal meaning. The vignette was shared with each participant, who then had the opportunity to change or modify the description. An example of one vignette is as follows:

Zion, a young minority student, immigrated to Canada as a child. She attended college directly after graduating from high school. She chose the collaborative program because she was aware that the degree would be mandatory for nursing in the future and her mother felt that nursing, as a career choice, was perfect. During the college portion she struggled academically as she was commuting four hours per day. However, through perseverance, she managed to achieve a "B" average in her second year at college and was admitted to the university portion of the program. Zion rated her transition as fairly difficult. Her primary concern was financial and resulted in the delay of purchase of textbooks and course materials. The ensuing stress led to a breakdown in class. With the intervention of a professor, she stuck it out. Now in the final days of her first year at the university, Zion reflects that she settled in by February and at that point realized that she would not quit and could make it. Driving Zion is her determination and to be a good example for other minority students living below the poverty line. Her motto is "I don't let circumstances determine my outcome." Zion reports that this transition has made her stronger, more self-confident, and that overall she will be a better nurse. (Cameron, 2003, p. 120)

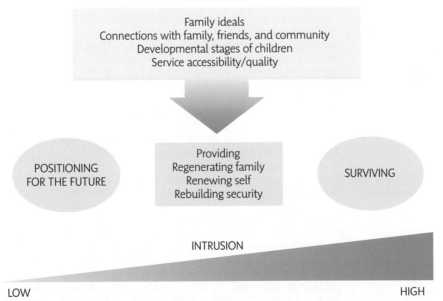

FIGURE 15-2 Subprocesses in strengthening capacity.
Ford-Gilboe, M., Wuest, J., & Merritt-Gray, M. (2005). Strengthening capacity to limit intrusion: Theorizing family health promotion in the aftermath of woman abuse. *Qualitative Health Research, 15*(4), 477–501. doi:10.1177/1049732305274590. Reprinted by Permission of SAGE Publications.

Rich descriptions, such as those found in vignettes or direct quotations, enliven the data and give meaning to people's experiences. Most qualitative research includes selected quotations to illustrate the themes and to provide readers with the opportunity to understand and validate the themes chosen by the researcher. For example, in studying patient-provider communications at the time of cancer diagnosis from the patients' perspective, Thorne and associates (2009) chose the following quotation to exemplify the shift in the intensity and recollection of the original account of cancer diagnosis:

> There's sort of a haziness of memory about the actual sequence of events but the feelings that I felt at the time are still pretty clear, you know. I felt concerned and worried. And you're so thirsty for as much information as I possibly could get, but also cognizant of the fact that I had a limited ability to take it in. (p. 1389)

Table 15-6 includes selected quotations from participants to support the themes emerging from Seneviratne and associates' (2009) study.

When the data are presented, the most important consideration for the research is to ensure that the presentation supports the findings and relays what needs to be known (Streubert & Carpenter, 2011). The purpose of the study determines how the story is told. If the method is descriptive phenomenology, the focus is on the description of the lived experiences, whereas in a grounded theory study, the focus is on a more careful description of how the narrative gives rise to the analysis and interpretation, which results in theory development.

TABLE **15-6**

EXAMPLES OF SELECTED QUOTATIONS TO SUPPORT THE THEMES FROM APPENDIX A

THEMES	EXAMPLE OF A QUOTATION
Space: Nursing in a submarine	"Our submarine . . . it's just a more condensed unit. But the thing that most bothers me is it's not centred. If you have patients in the last room . . . at the other end you are not in close proximity to anything—you're alone. That drives me crazy because the nursing station is so far away." "I'm too claustrophobic on this unit. It's like I am closed in . . . if you look down the hall from the nursing station you feel like the walls and curtains are closing in around you. It is so narrow. I feel constricted because I cannot work in a cramped space. I bump into other people all the time."
Time: Lack of time	"We are always injuring ourselves because we rush around. There is just not enough time for us to do things properly without patients. . . . So if things get missed, so be it." "It is easier to take over for patients, dressing them or brushing their teeth, rather than helping them do the tasks. It is a matter of accomplishing what is required for patients in a specific window of time."
Interprofessional practice: Relationships between stroke professionals	"We are not recognized for the mobility things we do or in any concerns we have about our patients. So, sometimes we don't work hard at it. The physios are only concerned that we get the patients ready for their rehab time at the gym. So we do that for them and then concentrate on our patient's medical needs." "It should be interprofessional, ideally. In general, stroke units are interdisciplinary. Only a small part of stroke unit care is the physician roles. So during most of stroke care, beyond the acute phase, when you have somebody settled, the physician's role is relatively minor. It's all about excellent nursing care and rehabilitation. So the team, by accident of history and hierarchy, is led by a physician but we have an NP, all the nurses, the physiotherapist, and social work . . . Everybody is involved in care including home planning, etc."

Based on Seneviratne, C. C., Mather, C. M., & Then, K. L. (2009). Understanding nursing on an acute stroke unit: Perceptions of space, time and interprofessional practice. *Journal of Advanced Nursing, 65*(9), 1872-1881. doi: 10.1111/j.1365-2648.2009.05053.x

Conclusion Drawing and Verification

Conclusion drawing starts at the beginning of data collection but is not finalized until the project is completed. Although qualitative research is inductive, it is tempting to draw conclusions prematurely. The challenge for the researcher is to remain amenable to new ideas, themes, and concepts as they appear.

Conclusion drawing is essentially the description of the relationship between the themes. Richards and Morse (2007) described this process as "doing abstraction" (p. 158), in which data are moved from categories (codes and themes) to concepts and constructs. As discussed earlier and shown in Table 15-1, the ways of abstracting vary with the type of method. Grounded theory formalizes this stage through the development of models, which lead to theory. Verification occurs as the data are collected; this process can vary from questioning one's own conclusion through the rechecking of the text to verification by colleagues and to finding new cases and applying the model to them. In grounded theory, researchers use the **constant comparative method,** in which new data are compared as they emerge with data previously analyzed.

Miles and Huberman (1994) stated that that this process of making sense of the data is a skill that all nurses have. People make sense of the world around them by organizing and interpreting it; this skill is applied to drawing and verifying conclusions. Miles and Huberman listed the following 13 tactics for generating meaning (pp. 245-246):

1. Noting patterns and themes (repetitive or recurring patterns among many separate pieces of data)
2. Seeing plausibility (realizing that the finding or conclusion sounds true or makes sense)
3. Clustering (grouping together things that seem to share characteristics)
4. Making metaphors (using a literary device in which different things are compared to make sense of the experience)
5. Counting (noting that something is happening a number of times)
6. Making contrasts or comparisons (comparing sets of things)
7. Partitioning variables (breaking down the themes into smaller units)
8. Subsuming particulars into the general (using a higher level of abstraction)
9. Factoring (generating words [factors] to express common findings)
10. Noting relationships between variables (depicting the relationships between the findings)
11. Finding intervening variables (discerning other variables that may link findings together)
12. Building a logical chain of evidence (validating each of the relationships identified)
13. Making conceptual or theoretical coherence (linking the findings into an overarching "how" and "why" of the phenomenon under study)

Refer to Miles and Huberman (1994) for more detail about these tactics. Richards and Morse's (2007) text on qualitative methods also describes the step-by-step process.

To verify the emergent themes and subthemes, Seneviratne and associates (2009) returned to the field to recheck their findings. Verbatim quotations provided a context for the themes (see Table 15-5). Thorne and associates (2009) used the themes to guide conversations in subsequent interviews to further develop the emerging analytic themes and to "clarify individual variations across accounts" (p. 1385).

Other researchers can use different methods to validate their themes. For example, Bottorff and colleagues (2004) used NVivo to search the data for content related to explanations of nicotine dependence, addiction, lack of control over smoking, and experiences associated with cessation. These data were then subjected to a thematic analysis in which the participants' explanations of addiction were compared. To verify the findings, the research team regularly discussed the analysis and interpretation. Once the initial analysis was complete, secondary analysis took place with a second set of interviews. As a final analysis, further interviews took place with eight selected participants to validate the findings.

No matter what method is used, researchers ask themselves, "What have I learned? How do I understand this, make sense of it and see the connections in it?" (Seidman, 1998). The conclusions drawn are simply to "describe, make contributions and contribute to greater understanding, or at least, more informed questioning" (Glesne, 2011, p. 210). As discussed in Chapter 7, through the processes of reflexivity and bracketing, researchers constantly compare their findings with their own personal beliefs and knowledge to ensure that the analysis reflects the participants' beliefs rather than their own.

SPECIFIC ANALYTIC PROCEDURES

The processes of data analysis vary according to the type of qualitative research. Table 15-7 summarizes the methods of analysis in qualitative methods, including phenomenology, ethnography, grounded theory, and case study. Excerpts from Canadian studies are included to exemplify the methods.

TRUSTWORTHINESS

As described in Chapter 14, rigour in qualitative research is determined by credibility, auditability, and fittingness as the criteria for evaluation. Trustworthiness is also important for determining the validity of the data interpretation or analysis. To ensure the trustworthiness of their findings, qualitative researchers must ask themselves the following questions (Hollway & Jefferson, 2000):

- What do you notice? The researcher has captured some impressions about the data; however, information may be missing.
- Why do you notice what you notice? Researchers must consider their own biases and predispositions as they interpret the data to produce trustworthy interpretations.
- How can you interpret what you notice? As discussed in Chapter 14, credibility stems from prolonged engagement and persistent observation. To be able to complete a full interpretation, the researcher must spend a sufficient amount of time in the field to build sound relationships with the participants.
- How can you know that your interpretation is the "right" one? The quickest way to know whether the interpretation is accurate is through sharing the findings with the participants. This sharing is an integral part of participatory action research, as outlined in Chapter 8, and is referred to in many studies as **member checking.** The researcher is also checking whether the connections between the categories or themes are logical. Inviting other experts to review the data analysis is another option for many researchers. In addition, some researchers analyze their data from several different frameworks (a form of triangulation) to increase the trustworthiness of the data analysis.

Finally, it is important to consider the limitations of the study. Many researchers describe the issues they faced so that readers will understand the research in the proper context (Glesne, 2006).

TABLE 15-7

METHODS OF ANALYSIS

TRADITION	METHOD OF ANALYSIS	EXAMPLE
Phenomenology: includes a variety of traditions	• Immersion in the data: listen to recordings, read and reread transcripts • Identify and extract significant statements • Determine relationships among the extracted statements (themes) • Prepare exhaustive description of the phenomena and the relationship among the themes • Synthesize the themes into a consistent description or statement of the phenomenon under study (essence)	Charlebois and Bouchard (2007): "'The Worst Experience': The Experience of Grandparents Who Have a Grandchild with Cancer" Eight grandparents were interviewed. Three central themes emerged: living the "worst experience"; giving support, a crucial role for grandparents; and feeling supported to carry on. The authors synthesized their findings in this way: "The essence of the phenomenon is described as follows: having a grandchild with cancer is, for all the grandparents in the study, the worst experience they can ever live, a vital duty to support members of the family, a duty that is closely related to the perception they have of their grandparental role, and a need to feel supported by calling upon several strategies to better carry on" (p. 27).
Ethnography	• Immersion in the data • Identify patterns and themes • Complete a cultural inventory • Interpret the findings • Compare the findings with those in the literature	Seneviratne, Mather, & Then (2009): "Understanding Nursing on an Acute Stroke Unit: Perceptions of Space, Time and Interprofessional Practice" The authors described their method as follows: "Analysis of field notes focused on identifying central domains, specific domain components and related work typologies. . . . Through an ongoing process of reading field notes, transcripts, and then returning to the field setting for further observations, we crosschecked our findings and were assured that our study domains, components and related subcategories were culturally salient" (p. 1874).
Grounded theory	• Examine data carefully line by line • Divide data into discrete parts • Compare data for similarities and differences • Compare data with other data continuously in a process: constant comparative method • Cluster codes to form categories • Expand and develop categories or collapse them into one another • Determine relationships between categories	Schreiber and MacDonald (2010): "Keeping Vigil over the Patient: A Grounded Theory of Nurse Anaesthesia Practice" The authors described their study as follows: "We used constant comparative method of grounded theory, which involves line-by-line coding to compare incident to incident and concept to concept. Second level or theoretical coding involves grouping concepts into higher level codes and exploring relationships among them. The emerging conceptualizations drive additional sampling and data collection . . . the resulting basic social process . . . presents how CRNA's enact their daily practice" (pp. 553-554).
Case study	• Identify unit of analysis (person, family, organization) • Code continuously as data are collected • Find commonalities and themes • Analyze field notes • Review description of themes to identify patterns and connections between them	Wittich and Southall (2008): "Coping with Extended Facedown Positioning After Macular Hole Surgery" In this study, all data were gathered from one patient's diary. The authors described their analysis as follows: "First each section was summarized to reveal the main themes. Each theme was designated with a meaningful name (i.e., sleep information). This data driven approach to thematic analysis resulted in a preliminary coding schema. The two investigators then together read line by line through the text, scrutinizing the content while adjusting the coding theme accordingly. . . . Using the ATLAS-ti query tool, meaningful patterns were sought in the text" (p. 438).

APPRAISING THE EVIDENCE

Qualitative Data Analysis

The general criteria for critiquing qualitative data analysis are proposed in the Critiquing Criteria box; however, remember that many different approaches to data analysis exist. The data analysis is consistent with the research philosophy, the question, and the design. For example, researchers using grounded theory build a case for substantive theory, explaining the phenomenon under study, whereas a researcher in phenomenological studies is interested in expressing the meaning of the phenomenon itself.

Regardless of the study's research method, several commonalities exist among methods used in qualitative data analysis. For example, analysis is conducted alongside the data collection, and in most cases the two processes are interrelated. Researchers become immersed in the data; they listen over and over to the interviews, read

and reread the transcripts, and spend substantial time in the field. Although the methods may differ, the text is coded to search for themes and categories through a process of data reduction. The emergent themes are then verified through member checking. As themes emerge, logical connections and relationships between the themes are identified to form a whole picture. The results are displayed in such a manner that the reader can understand and validate the conclusions that the researcher has drawn through the use of diagrams, tables, charts, direct quotations from the participants, and rich descriptions of the findings. In summary, qualitative data analysis involves much disparate data and transforms them into a coherent whole or story to provide meaning about the human experience.

CRITIQUING CRITERIA

1. The method of data analysis should be clearly stated.
2. The strategy of data analysis should be appropriate for the methodology of the study.
3. The steps of analysis should be listed for readers to follow.
4. The researcher should provide evidence that his or her interpretation captures the phenomenon under study.
5. The researcher should address the credibility, auditability, and fittingness of the data.

CRITICAL THINKING CHALLENGES

- How do researchers determine whether they have spent enough time with the data?
- Is it important for the researcher to personally transcribe the interviews?
- Why do some researchers reread the literature as themes emerge from the data?
- Often, data analysis takes place as data are collected. How can analysis of the data change the data collection?
- Researchers validate their interpretation of the data through a process of member checking. What happens if the participants indicate that the analysis does not reflect their experience?

KEY POINTS

- Qualitative data are text derived from transcripts of interviews, narratives, documents, media such as newspapers and movies, and field notes.
- Computer software can simplify the storage and retrieval of data.
- Qualitative research data can be managed through the use of computers, but the researcher must interpret the data.
- Data analysis and data collection are parallel processes.
- Qualitative analysis is not a linear process; rather, it is a cyclical and iterative process.
- The three discrete stages of data analysis are data reduction, data display, and conclusion drawing and verification.

- Data are organized into meaningful chunks of data through a clustering of related or similar data and are labelled as themes.
- Coding is the process of progressively marking, sorting, resorting, and defining and redefining the collected data.
- Data display involves the use of graphs, flowcharts, matrices, or any other visual representation to assemble data and to allow for conclusion drawing.
- Grounded theorists use the constant comparative method, in which new data are compared with data previously analyzed.
- Member checking is the process of sharing findings with the participants in order to check whether the interpretation of the findings is accurate

REFERENCES

Bottorff, J. L., Johnson, J. L., Moffat, B., Grewal, J., Ratner, P., & Kalaw, C. (2004). Adolescent constructions of nicotine addiction. *Canadian Journal of Nursing Research, 38*, 22-39.

Cameron, C. (2003). *The lived experience of transfer students in a collaborative baccalaureate nursing program*. Unpublished doctoral dissertation, University of Toronto.

Cameron, C. (2005). Experiences of transfer students in a collaborative baccalaureate nursing program. *Community College Review, 33*(2), 22-44.

Charlebois, S., & Bouchard, L. (2007). "The worst experience": The experience of grandparents who have a grandchild with cancer. *Canadian Oncological Nursing Journal, 17*(1), 26-36.

Denzin, N., & Lincoln, Y. (2000). *Handbook of qualitative research* (2nd ed.). Thousand Oaks, CA: Sage.

Ford-Gilboe, M., Wuest, J., & Merritt-Gray, M. (2005). Strengthening capacity to limit intrusion: Theorizing family health promotion in the aftermath of woman abuse. *Qualitative Health Research, 15*, 477-501.

Glesne, C. (2006). *Becoming qualitative researchers: An introduction* (3rd ed.). Don Mills, ON: Longman.

Glesne, C. (2011). *Becoming qualitative researchers: An introduction* (4th ed.). Toronto: Pearson.

Hollway, W., & Jefferson, T. (2000). *Doing qualitative research differently: Free association, narrative and the interview method*. Thousand Oaks, CA: Sage.

Meadows, L. M., & Dodendorf, D. M. (1999). Data management and interpretation using computers to assist. In B. Crabtree & W. L. Miller (Eds.), *Doing qualitative research* (2nd ed., pp. 195-220). Thousand Oaks, CA: Sage.

Miles, M. B., & Huberman, A. M. (1994). *Qualitative data analysis* (2nd ed.). Thousand Oaks, CA: Sage.

Patton, M. (2002). *Qualitative research & evaluation methods* (3rd ed.). Thousand Oaks, CA: Sage.

Richards, L., & Morse, J. M. (2007). *Read me first for a user's guide to qualitative methods* (2nd ed.). Thousand Oaks, CA: Sage.

Schreiber, R., & MacDonald, M. (2010). Keeping vigil over the patient: A grounded theory of nurse anaesthesia practice. *Journal of Advanced Nursing, 66*(3), 552-561. doi: 10.1111/j.1365-2648.2009.05207.x

Seidman, I. (1998). *Interviewing as qualitative research: A guide for researchers in education and social sciences* (2nd ed.). New York: Teachers College Press.

Seneviratne, C. C., Mather, C. M., & Then, K. L. (2009). Understanding nursing on an acute stroke unit: Perceptions of space, time and interprofessional practice. *Journal of Advanced Nursing, 65*(9), 1872-1881. doi: 10.1111/j.1365-2648.2009.05053.x

Streubert, H. J., & Carpenter, D. (2011). *Qualitative research in nursing: Advancing the humanistic imperative* (5th ed.). Philadelphia: Wolters Kluwer.

Thorne, S., Armstrong, E., Harris, S. R., Hislop, T. G., Kim-Sing, C., Oglov, V., et al. (2009). Patient real-time and 12 month-retrospective perceptions of difficult communications in the cancer diagnostic period. *Qualitative Health Research, 19*(10), 1383-1394. doi: 10.1177/1049732.309348382

van Manen, M. (1997). *Researching lived experience*. London, ON: Althouse Press.

Wittich, W., & Southall, K. (2008). Coping with extended facedown positioning after macular hole surgery: A qualitative diary analysis. *Nursing Research, 57*(6), 436-443.

Wuest, J. (2001). Precarious ordering: Towards a formal theory of women's caring. *Health Care for Women International: Special volume, Using Grounded Theory to Study Women's Health, 22*(1-2), 167-193.

Wuest, J., Merritt-Gray, M., Berman, H., & Ford-Gilboe, M. (2002). Illuminating social determinants of women's health using grounded theory. *Health Care International, 23*, 794-808.

FOR FURTHER STUDY

⊖volve   Go to Evolve at http://evolve.elsevier.com/Canada/LoBiondo/Research for Audio Glossary, how-to instructions for Writing Proposals for Funding, and additional research articles for practice in reviewing and critiquing.

CHAPTER 16

Quantitative Data Analysis

Susan Sullivan-Bolyai | Carol Bova | Mina D. Singh

LEARNING OUTCOMES

After reading this chapter, you will be able to do the following:

- Differentiate between descriptive and inferential statistics.
- State the purposes of descriptive statistics.
- Identify the levels of measurement in a research study.
- Describe a frequency distribution.
- List measures of central tendency and their use.
- List measures of variability and their use.
- Identify the purpose of inferential statistics.
- Distinguish between a parameter and a statistic.
- Explain the concept of probability as it applies to the analysis of sample data.
- Distinguish between type I and type II errors and their effects on a study's outcome.
- Distinguish between parametric and nonparametric tests.
- List the commonly used statistical tests and their purposes.
- Critically analyze the statistics used in published research studies.

KEY TERMS

alpha
analysis of covariance (ANCOVA)
analysis of variance (ANOVA)
chi-square (χ^2)
confidence interval
correlation
degree of freedom
descriptive statistics
factor analysis
Fisher's exact probability test
frequency distribution
inferential statistics
interval measurement
kurtosis

level of significance (alpha level)
levels of measurement
logistic regression (logit analysis)
mean *(M)*
measurement
measures of central tendency
measures of variability
median
modality
mode
multiple analysis of variance (MANOVA)
multiple regression

nominal measurement
nonparametric statistics
nonparametric tests of significance
normal curve
null hypothesis
odds ratio
ordinal measurement
P value
parameter
parametric statistics
Pearson correlation coefficient (Pearson *r*)
percentile
population

post hoc analysis	scientific hypothesis	statistic
power	semiquartile range (semi-	systematic review
probability	interquartile range)	*t* statistic
range	skew	type I error
ratio measurement	standard deviation	type II error
sampling error	standard error of the mean	Z score
scatter plots		

STUDY RESOURCES

Go to Evolve at http://evolve.elsevier.com/Canada/LoBiondo/Research for Audio Glossary, how-to instructions for Writing Proposals for Funding, and additional research articles for practice in reviewing and critiquing.

STATISTICS ARE USED EXTENSIVELY IN THE nursing and health care literature. Descriptive and inferential statistics are described in the "Methods" section, the "Results" section, or both sections of a research article. Before you become overwhelmed by the complexity of the information, bear in mind that you do not need to be familiar with or to be able to calculate a large number of complex statistical formulas to analyze data. An understanding of which tests are used with which kind of design and which type of data is sufficient. This basic understanding will help you to appraise evidence from a research study, which is essential for informing decisions you make in your practice.

As a reader, you do not analyze the data yourself, but it is important to understand the researcher's challenge in analyzing the data. After carefully collecting data, the researcher is faced with the task of organizing and analyzing the individual pieces of information so that the meaning of study results is clear. The researcher must choose methods of organizing and analyzing the raw data on the basis of the design, the type of data collected, and the hypothesis or question that was tested. Statistical procedures are used to organize and give meaning to the data.

The "Results" section of a research article contains the data generated from the testing of the hypothesis or research questions. These data are the result of analysis with both *descriptive* and *inferential statistics.* An example of what may be found is as follows: "A notable finding was the high average age of SNLs [senior nurse leaders] ... current SNLs were very experienced individuals [inasmuch] as over 80% ... had at least 15 years of management experience" (Wong, Laschinger, Cummings, Vincent, & O'Connor, 2010, p. 127; see Appendix B). The data in Table B-2 of Wong and colleagues' article are known as descriptive statistics, which are usually the first set of statistical results in a report or published article.

Descriptive statistics are obtained through descriptive statistical techniques that reduce data to manageable proportions by summarizing and organizing them. These techniques allow researchers to arrange data visually to display meaning and to help in understanding the sample characteristics and variables before the researchers engage in inferential data analyses. In some studies, descriptive statistics may be the only results sought from statistical analysis. Descriptive statistical techniques include **measures of central tendency,** which describe the average member of a sample, such as mode, median, and mean; measures of variability, such as range and standard deviation; and some correlation techniques, such as a **scatter plots,** which is a visual representation of the strength and magnitude of the relationship between two variables.

In contrast to descriptive statistics, inferential statistics allow researchers to estimate how reliably they can make predictions and generalize findings on the basis of the data. **Inferential statistics** are statistical details that combine mathematical processes and logic to test hypotheses about a population with the help of sample data. Through the use of inferential statistics, researchers can draw conclusions that extend beyond the immediate data of the study. An example of inferential statistics was provided by Sobieraj and colleagues (2009): "The greatest predictors of child distress were age ($\beta = -0.434$, $t = -4.017$, $P < 0.01$), with younger children being more distressed, and the presence of the father in the procedure room ($\beta = -0.419$, $t = -3.888$, $P < 0.01$)" (p. 75; see Appendix C).

The purpose of this chapter is to demonstrate how researchers use descriptive and inferential statistics in nursing research studies so that you, as a reader, will be better able to determine the appropriateness of the statistics used and to interpret the strength and quality of the reported findings, their clinical significance, and their applicability to practice. Basic concepts and terminology common in evidence-informed practice publications are presented in Chapter 20. The information in this chapter will help you begin to make sense of the statistics used in research papers.

DESCRIPTIVE STATISTICS

Levels of Measurement

Measurement is the assignment of numbers to variables or events according to rules. Every variable in a research study that is assigned a specific number must be similar to every other variable assigned that number. For example, male participants may be assigned the number 1 and female participants the number 2. The measurement level is determined by the nature of the object or event being measured. **Levels of measurement**—categorization of the precision with which an event can be measured—from low to high are nominal, ordinal, interval, and ratio. The levels of measurement help determine the type of statistics to be used in analyzing data. The higher the level of measurement, the greater the flexibility the researcher has in choosing statistical procedures. Every attempt should be made to use the highest level of measurement possible so that the maximum amount of information will be obtained from the data, as highlighted in Table 16-1. The Critical Thinking Decision Path on the facing page illustrates the relationship between levels of measurement and appropriate choice of specific descriptive statistics.

In **nominal measurement,** variables or events are classified into categories. The categories are mutually exclusive; a variable or an event either

TABLE 16-1

LEVEL OF MEASUREMENT SUMMARY TABLE

MEASUREMENT	DESCRIPTION	MEASURES OF CENTRAL TENDENCY	MEASURES OF VARIABILITY
Nominal	Classification	Mode	Modal percentage, range, frequency distribution
Ordinal	Relative rankings	Mode, median	Modal percentage, range, frequency, percentile, semiquartile range, frequency distribution
Interval	Rank ordering with equal intervals	Mode, median, mean	Modal percentage, range, percentile, semiquartile range, standard deviation
Ratio	Rank ordering with equal intervals and absolute zero	Mode, median, mean	All

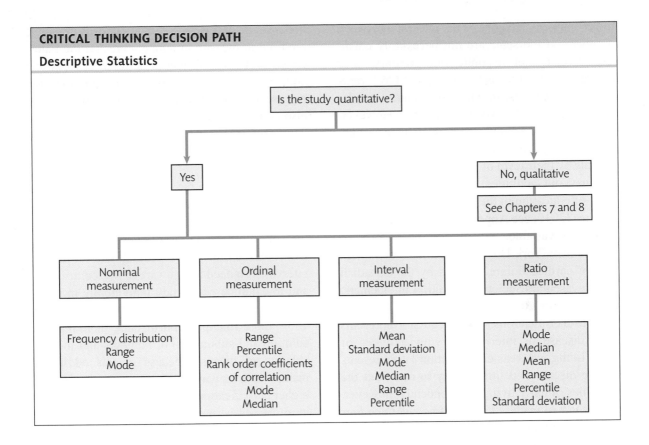

CRITICAL THINKING DECISION PATH

Descriptive Statistics

has or does not have the characteristic of a particular category. The numbers assigned to each category are nothing more than labels; such numbers do not indicate more or less of a characteristic. Nominal measurement can be used to categorize a sample with regard to such information as gender, hair colour, marital status, or religious affiliation.

Sobieraj and colleagues' (2009) study regarding the effect of music on parental participation during paediatric laceration repair included examples of nominal measurement, including location of laceration, type of tissue repair, and presence of a parent (see Appendix C). The nominal level of measurement allows the least amount of mathematical manipulation. Most commonly, the frequency of each event is counted, as is the percentage of the total that each category represents.

A variable at the nominal level can also be considered a *dichotomous* or a *categorical* variable. A dichotomous nominal variable has only two true values, such as true/false or gender (male/female). Nominal variables that are categorical still have mutually exclusive categories but have more than two true values, such as marital status (single, married, divorced, separated, or widowed). In both cases, the nominal variables are mutually exclusive. The gender of the patient in the article by Wong and colleagues (2010; see Appendix B) would be considered a dichotomous nominal variable (male/female).

Ordinal measurement reveals relative rankings of variables or events. The numbers assigned to each category can be compared, and the members of a higher ranked category can be said to have more of an attribute than members of a lower ranked category. The intervals between numbers on the scale are not necessarily equal, and zero is not absolute but arbitrary,. For example, ordinal measurement is used to formulate class rankings, in which one student can be ranked higher or lower than another. However, the actual grade-point averages of students may differ widely. Another example is ranking individuals by their level of wellness and their ability to carry out activities of daily living. Highest level of education in the article by Wong and colleagues (2010; see Appendix B) is an example of an ordinal variable.

The New York Heart Association's classification of cardiac failure adopted by the Canadian Cardiovascular Society (Arnold, Liu, Demers, Dorian, Giannetti, Haddad, et al, 2006) consists of four classifications. Classification I represents little disease or interference with activities of daily living, whereas classification IV represents severe disease and little ability to carry out the activities of daily living independently; however, an individual in class IV cannot be said to be four times sicker than an individual in class I. A similar scale based on an individual's current health status is used to classify an individual's risk for adverse effects from anaesthesia.

With ordinal-level data, the amount of mathematical manipulation possible is limited. In addition to what is possible with nominal-level data, medians, percentiles, and rank-order coefficients of correlation can be calculated. In most cases, ordinal variables in a scale are treated as interval measurements when converted to numerical codes. For example, when patients are asked to rate their level of satisfaction with life as "not satisfied," "satisfied," or "very satisfied," their responses are an ordinal measurement. When their ratings are treated numerically and coded as 1, 2, and 3, respectively, their responses are an interval measurement.

In **interval measurement,** events or variables are ranked on a scale with equal intervals between the numbers. The zero point remains arbitrary and not absolute. For example, interval measurements are used in measuring temperatures on the Fahrenheit scale. The distances between degrees are equal, but the zero point is arbitrary and does not represent the absence of temperature. Test scores also represent interval-level data. The differences between test scores represent equal intervals, but a score of zero does not represent the total absence of knowledge.

In many areas in the social sciences, including nursing, the classification of the level of measurement of intelligence, aptitude, and personality tests is controversial; some researchers regard these measurements as ordinal and others as interval. You need to be aware of this controversy and to examine each study individually in terms of how the data are analyzed. Interval-level data allow more manipulation of data, including the addition and subtraction of numbers and the calculation of means. Because of this additional manipulation, many authorities argue for the higher classification level. The Procedure Behaviour Check List used by Sobieraj and colleagues (2009) is an example of ordinal measurements but used as an interval measurement (see Appendix C).

In **ratio measurement,** events or variables are ranked on scales with equal intervals and absolute zeros. The number represents the actual amount of the property the object possesses. Ratio measurement is the highest level of measurement but is usually achieved only in the physical sciences. Examples of ratio-level data are height, weight, pulse, and blood pressure. All mathematical procedures can be performed with data from ratio scales. Therefore, the use of any statistical procedure is possible as long as it is appropriate for the design of the study.

Helpful Hint_____

Descriptive statistics assist in summarizing the data. The descriptive statistics calculated must be appropriate for both the purpose of the study and the level of measurement.

Frequency Distribution

One of the most basic ways of organizing data is in a frequency distribution. In a **frequency distribution,** the number of times each event occurs is counted, or the data are grouped and the frequency of each group is reported. For example, an instructor reporting the results of an examination could report the number of students receiving each individual grade or could group the grades in ranges and report the number of students who received each group of grades. When reviewing a frequency distribution, symmetry and kurtosis are noted. A distribution can be symmetrical (shaped like a bell) or asymmetrical, where most of the information is to one side, either to the left or the right. **Kurtosis** is the peakedness of the distribution. Table 16-2 shows the results of an examination given to a class of 51 students. The

results are reported in two ways. The columns on the left give the raw data tally and the frequency for each grade, whereas the columns on the right give the grouped data tally and grouped frequencies. In research studies, the results are grouped rather than reported individually for each participant (Sobieraj, Bhatt, LeMay, Rennick, & Johnston, 2009; see Appendix C).

When data are grouped, the researcher needs to define the size of the group or the interval width so that no score is categorized into two groups and all groups are mutually exclusive. The groupings of the data in Table 16-2 prevent overlap; each score is categorized into only one group. If the grouping had been 70 to 80 and 80 to 90, scores of 80 would have been categorized into two categories. The grouping should allow for a precise presentation of the data without serious loss of information. Very large interval

TABLE **16-2**

FREQUENCY DISTRIBUTION

	INDIVIDUAL			GROUP	
SCORE	TALLY	FREQUENCY	SCORE	TALLY	FREQUENCY
90	|	1	>89	|	1
88	|	1	80–89	卌 卌 卌	15
86	|	1			
84	卌 |	6			
82	||	2			
80	卌	5			
78	卌	5	70–79	卌 卌 卌 卌 |||	23
76	|	1			
74	卌 ||	7			
72	卌 ||||	9			
70	|	1			
68	|||	3	60–69	卌 卌	10
66	||	2			
64	||||	4			
62	|	1			
60		0			
58	|	1	<59	||	2
56		0			
54	|	1			
52		0			
50		0			
Total		51	Total		51

Mean, 74.51; standard deviation, +12.1; median, 74; mode, 72; range, 36 (54–90).

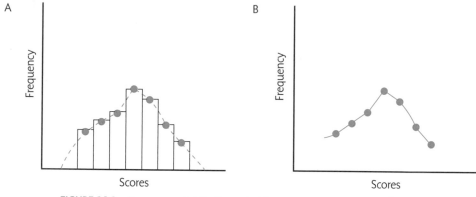

FIGURE 16-1   Frequency distributions. **A,** Histogram. **B,** Frequency polygon.

widths lead to loss of data information and may obscure patterns in the data. If the test scores in Table 16-2 had been grouped as 40 to 69 and 70 to 99, the pattern of the scores would have been obscured.

Information about frequency distributions may be presented in the form of a table, such as Table 16-2, or in the form of a graph. Figure 16-1 illustrates the most common graph forms: the histogram and the frequency polygon. These two methods are similar in that in both, scores or percentages of occurrence are plotted against frequency. The greater the number of points plotted, the smoother is the resulting graph. The shape of the resulting graph allows for observations that further describe the data. For example, in their study of parents' knowledge about the use of child safety systems, Snowdon and colleagues (2006) used histograms to illustrate the rate at which parents transitioned their infant from a rear-facing seat to a forward-facing seat and the timing of this transition (Figure 16-2).

Measures of Central Tendency

Measures of central tendency answer questions such as "What does the average nurse think?" and "What is the average temperature of patients on a unit?" These measures yield a single number that describes the middle of the group and summarizes the members of a sample. In statistics, the three measures of central tendency are the mode, the median, and the mean. Depending on the distribution, these measures may not all give the same answer to the question "What is the average?" Each measure of central tendency has a specific use and is most appropriate for specific kinds of measurement and types of distributions.

MODE. The **mode** is the most frequent score or result and can be obtained by inspection of the frequency distribution table or graph. Note that a sample distribution can have more than one mode. The number of modes, or peaks, contained in a distribution is called the **modality** of the distribution. The mode is the type of descriptive statistic most appropriately used with nominal-level data but can be used with all levels of measurement (see Table 16-1). The mode cannot be used for any subsequent calculations and is unstable; in other words, the mode can fluctuate widely from sample to sample from the same population. A change in just one score in Table 16-2 would change the mode from 72.

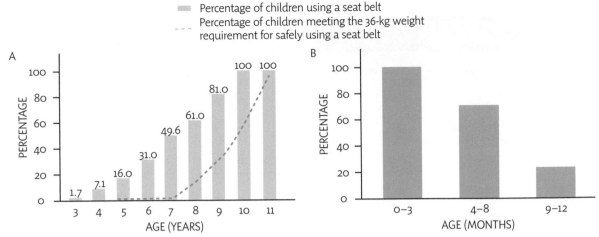

FIGURE 16-2 Histograms. **A,** Premature use of seat belts in children aged 3 to 11 years. **B,** Use of rear-facing safety seats in infants up to 12 months ($N = 296$). From Snowdon, A. W., Polgar, J., Patrick, L., & Stamler, L. (2006). Parents' knowledge about use of child safety systems. *Canadian Journal of Nursing Research, 38*(2), 107–108.

MEDIAN. The **median** is the middle score: of the other scores, 50% are higher and 50% are lower. The median is not sensitive to extremes in high and low scores; thus, it is a more accurate estimator of central tendency in non-normal distributions. In the series of scores in Table 16-2, the twenty-sixth score is always the median, regardless of how much the high and low scores change. The median is best used when the data are skewed (see the "Normal Distribution" section) and the researcher is interested in the "typical" score. For example, if age is a variable, and if a wide range with extreme scores may affect the mean, it would be appropriate to also report the median. The median is easy to find either by inspection or by calculation and can be used with ordinal or higher data, as shown in Table 16-1.

MEAN. The **mean** *(M)* is the arithmetical average of all scores and is used with interval- or ratio-level data (see Table 16-1). Most statistical tests of significance refer to the mean, the most widely used measure of central tendency, which is referred to in general conversations as the average.

Because the mean is affected by every score, it is affected by extreme scores; however, the larger the sample size, the less effect a single extreme score will have on the mean. For normally distributed populations, the mean is an appropriate measure of central tendency and is generally considered the single best point for summarizing data.

Helpful Hint_____
Of the three measures of central tendency, the mean is the most stable, the least affected by extremes, and the most useful for other calculations. The mean can be calculated only with interval- and ratio-level data.

Profetto-McGrath and associates (2010) used a table and narrative to describe the sample characteristics in their study examining the approaches used by clinical nurse specialists to select and use evidence in their daily practice.

The summary statistics in Table 16-3 may also be reported in narrative form.

TABLE 16-3

SUMMARY STATISTICS FOR STUDY BY PROFETTO AND ASSOCIATES

VARIABLE	CHARACTERISTIC	NUMBER OF PARTICIPANTS (%)
Sex	Male	2 (2.1)
	Female	2 (97.9)
Age	Mean/SD: 48.53 ± 7.643	
	Range: 30–66 years	
Highest level of nursing education	Certificate	1 (1.1)
	Diploma	22 (23.4)
	Bachelor's	37 (39.4)
	Master's	33 (35.0)
	Doctorate	1 (1.1)
Years as a registered nurse	Mean: 25.12 ± 8.521	
	Range: 2–45 years	

Adapted from Profetto-McGrath, J., Negrin, K., Hugo, K., & Bulmer Smith, K. (2010) Clinical nurse specialists' approaches in selecting and using evidence to improve practice. *Worldviews on Evidence-Based Nursing, 7*(1), 36-50, Table 1.

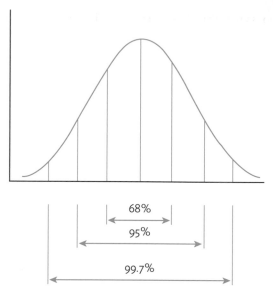

FIGURE 16-3 The normal distribution and associated standard deviations.

[The] sample was predominantly female (97.9%) with a mean age of 48.53 years (*SD* [standard deviation] = 7.643). and an average experience of 10.24 years (*SD* = 7.282) . . . On average, [clinical nurse specialists] reported 38.83% of their work responsibilities were devoted to clinical practice, 22.11% to education and training, 16.6% to consultation, and 6.32% to research. (Profetto-McGrath, Negrin, Hugo, & Bulmer Smith, 2010, pp. 39-40)

Of the measures of central tendency, the mean is the most stable and the median the most typical. If the distribution of a sample is symmetrical and unimodal, the mean, median, and mode coincide.

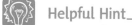 **Helpful Hint**_____

Measures of central tendency are descriptive statistics that describe the characteristics of a sample.

Normal Distribution

The theoretical concept of normal distribution is based on the observation that data from repeated interval or ratio measurements will gather at a midpoint in a distribution, approximating the normal curve illustrated in Figure 16-3. In addition, if the means of a large number of samples of the same interval- or ratio-level data are calculated and plotted on a graph, that curve also approximates the normal curve. This tendency of the means to approximate the normal curve is termed the *sampling distribution of the means*. The mean of the sampling distribution of the means is the mean of the population.

In visual representations of statistics, the **normal curve** is unimodal and symmetrical about the mean. The mean, median, and mode are equal. An additional characteristic of the normal curve is that a fixed percentage of the scores is located within a given distance of the mean. As shown in Figure 16-3, about 68% of the scores or means are within one standard deviation of the mean, 95% within two standard deviations of the mean, and 99.7% within three standard deviations of the mean.

SKEWNESS. **Skew** is a measure of the asymmetry of a set of scores. Not all samples of data approximate the normal curve. Some samples are nonsymmetrical, and the peak is off centre. For example, worldwide individual income has a positive skew: Most individuals have incomes in the low-to-moderate range and few in the upper range. In a positive skew, the peak of the distribution curve would be to the left of a normal curve, and the mean is to the right of the median. In contrast, age at death in Canada has a negative skew because most deaths occur at older ages. In a negative skew, the peak of the distribution curve would be to the right of a normal curve, and the mean is to the left of the median. Figure 16-4 illustrates positive and negative skew. In each diagram, the peak is off centre, and one "tail" of the curve is longer.

If the distribution is skewed, the mean will be pulled in the direction of the long tail of the distribution. With a skewed distribution, all three statistics should be reported. For example, national income in Canada is skewed. The mean wage differs from the median wage because the high salaries greatly outnumber the low salaries.

Evidence-Informed Practice Tip ———

The descriptive statistics for a sample indicate whether the sample data are skewed.

Interpreting Measures of Variability

Variability or dispersion is concerned with the spread of data. **Measures of variability**—statistical procedures that describe the level of dispersion in sample data—answer questions such as "Is the sample homogeneous or heterogeneous?" and "Is the sample similar or different?" If a researcher measures oral temperatures in two samples, one sample drawn from a healthy population and one sample from a hospitalized population, it is possible that the two samples will have the same mean. However, a wider range of temperatures is more likely to be found in the hospitalized sample than in the healthy sample. Measures of variability are used to describe these differences in the dispersion of data. As with measures of central tendency, the various measures of variability are appropriate to specific kinds of measurement and types of distributions.

Helpful Hint ———————

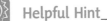

Descriptive statistics related to variability enable you to evaluate the homogeneity or heterogeneity of a sample.

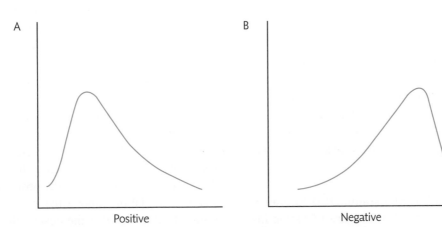

A   B

Positive   Negative

FIGURE 16-4   Positive and negative skew. **A,** Positive skew. **B,** Negative skew.

RANGE. The range is the simplest but most unstable measure of variability. **Range** is the distance between the highest and lowest scores. A change in either of these two scores would change the range. The range should always be reported with other measures of variability. For example, Schneider and colleagues (2011), who examined differences in psychosocial outcomes between male and female caregivers of children with life-limiting illnesses, found that the range of ages among female caregivers was 22.99 to 68.38 years, whereas the range of ages among the male caregivers was 26.98 to 57.02 years (Table 16-4). Thus, the age range was 45 years among the female caregivers and 30 years among the male caregivers. Range affects the standard deviation, as discussed later. The range in Table 16-4 could easily change with an increase or decrease in the high scores or the low scores with a different sample.

SEMIQUARTILE RANGE. The **semiquartile range (semi-interquartile range)** is the range of the middle 50% of the scores. It is more stable than the overall range because it is less likely to be changed by a single extreme score. The semiquartile range lies between the upper and lower quartiles; the upper quartile consists of the top 25% of scores, and the lower quartile consists of the lowest 25% of the scores. In Table 16-2, the middle 50% of the scores are between 68 and 78, and the semiquartile range is 10.

PERCENTILE. A **percentile** represents the percentage of scores that a given score exceeds. The median is the 50th percentile, and in Table 16-2, it is a score of 74. A score in the 90th percentile is exceeded by only 10% of the scores. The zero percentile and the 100th percentile are usually not used.

STANDARD DEVIATION. The **standard deviation** is the most frequently used measure of variability and is based on the concept of the normal curve

(see Figure 16-3). The standard deviation is a measure of average deviation of the scores from the mean and, as such, should always be reported with the mean. The standard deviation accounts for all scores and can be used to interpret individual scores. For the examination in Table 16-2, the mean was 73.1 and the standard deviation was 12.1; thus, a student should know that 68% of the grades were between 85.1 and 61. If the student received a grade of 88, he or she would know that this grade was better than those of most of the class, whereas a grade of 58 would indicate that the student did not do as well as most of the class. Table C-2 in Appendix C from the study by Sobieraj and colleagues (2009), reports the mean and standard deviation of the study variables' distress score for the both the control and intervention groups. As illustrated in this table, the mean score for the control group was 33.1 ($SD = 29$), whereas the mean score for the intervention group was 28.6 ($SD = 26$). This means that 68% of the control group scored between 2.1 and 62.1 on this measure and 68% of the intervention group scored between 2.6 and 54.6 on this measure. This table allows the reader to inspect the data and see the variation in the data.

The standard deviation is used in the calculation of many inferential statistics. One limitation of the standard deviation is that it is expressed in terms of the units used in the measurement and cannot be used to compare means that have different units. If researchers were interested in the relationship between height measured in centimetres and weight measured in kilograms, it would be necessary to convert the height and weight measurements to standard units, or Z scores. The **Z score** is used to compare measurements in standard units. Each of the scores is converted to a Z score, and then the Z scores are used to examine the relative distance of the scores from the mean. A Z score of 1.5 means that the observation is 1.5 standard deviations above the mean, whereas a score of -2 means that the observation is 2 standard deviations below the mean. By using Z

TABLE 16-4

DEMOGRAPHIC INFORMATION OF CAREGIVER BY GENDER

VARIABLE	TOTAL (N = 273)			WOMEN (N = 224)			MEN (N = 49)			TEST STATISTIC
	M	SD	RANGE	M	SD	RANGE	M	SD	RANGE	
AGE IN YEARS	41.74	7.61	22.99–68.38	41.19	7.62	22.99–68.38	44.29	7.08	26.98–57.02	t = – 2.61, P = .009
DIFFICULTY IN MANAGING COSTS	5.71	2.56	1–10	5.90	2.56	1–10	4.92	2.42	1–10	t = 2.42, P = .016
HOURS PER WEEK SPENT PROVIDING CARE	62.16	44.72	0–126	68.00	43.88	0–126	37.64	39.97	1.50–126	t = 4.29, P = .000
IMPORTANCE OF RELIGION*	3.04	1.03	1–4	3.10	1.01	1–4	2.76	1.09	1–4	t = 2.16, P = .002
MARITAL STATUS										$\chi^2 = 12.37, P = .015$
Married or lives as married	219	80.2		172	76.8		47	95.9		
Widowed	2	0.7		1	0.4		1	2.0		
Divorced/separated	34	12.5		33	14.7		1	2.0		
Never married	13	4.8		13	5.8		0	0		
Other	5	1.8		5	2.2		0	0		
HIGHEST EDUCATION LEVEL										$\chi^2 = 3.83, P = .429$
Elementary school completed	13	4.8		9	4.1		4	8.2		
High school completed	98	36.2		85	38.3		13	26.5		
College completed	39	14.4		30	13.3		9	18.4		
University degree completed	64	23.6		51	23.0		13	26.5		
Postgraduate degree completed	57	21.0		47	21.2		10	20.4		
SIZE OF COMMUNITY										$\chi^2 = 0.61, P = .737$
Metropolitan area/large city	120	44.0		97	43.3		23	46.9		
Medium city/small city	91	33.3		77	34.4		14	28.6		
Smaller communities	62	22.7		50	22.3		13	24.5		
CURRENT EMPLOYMENT STATUS										$\chi^2 = 59.95, P = .000$
Full-time	114	41.8		70	31.3		44	89.8		
Part-time	38	13.9		37	16.5		1	2.0		
Paid leave	5	1.8		5	2.2		0	0		
Unpaid leave	3	1.1		3	1.3		0	0		
Self-employed	16	5.9		13	5.8		3	6.1		
Not employed	78	28.6		78	34.8		0	0		
Other	19	7.0		18	8.0		1	2.0		

Continued

TABLE 16-4

DEMOGRAPHIC INFORMATION OF CAREGIVER BY GENDER—cont'd

VARIABLE	TOTAL (N = 273)			WOMEN (N = 224)			MEN (N = 49)			TEST STATISTIC
	M	SD	RANGE	M	SD	RANGE	M	SD	RANGE	
CHANGE IN EMPLOYMENT STATUS										$\chi^2 = 29.05, P = .000$
No	136	50.9		94	43.1		42	85.7		
Yes	131	49.1		124	56.9		7	14.3		
WORK ALLOWS TIME OFF										$\chi^2 = 13.11, P = .001$
No	10	5.2		5	3.4		5	10.0		
Yes completely	110	57.0		93	64.1		17	35.4		
Only partially	73	37.8		47	32.4		26	54.2		
INCOME CHANGED: CHILD'S ILLNESS										$\chi^2 = 5.52, P = 0.19$
No	96	35.3		72	32.1		24	50		
Yes	176	64.7		152	67.9		24	50		
AVERAGE HOUSEHOLD INCOME PER YEAR ($)										$U = 3,515.50, P = .001$
<19,999	21	8.0		20	9.2		1	22		
20,000–39,999	39	14.8		37	17.0		2	4.3		
40,000–59,999	39	14.8		33	15.1		6 031F,			
60,000–79,999	47	17.8		39	17.9		8 (|IA)			
80,000–99,999	32	12.1		27	12.4		5 COSI)			
100,000–119,999	38	14.4		27	12.4		11	219		
120,000–139,999	18	6.8		11	5.0		7	352		
140,000–199,999	22	8.3		16	7.3		6	03.0		
≤200,000	8	3.0		8	3.7		0	C		
CURRENT INCOME MEETS NEEDS										$U = 3,515.50, P = .004$
Totally inadequate	10	3.7		10	4.5		0	0		
Not very well	30	11.1		29	13.0		1	2.1		

Adapted from Schneider, M., Steele, R., Cadell, S., & Hemsworth, D. (2011). Differences on psychosocial outcomes between male and female caregivers of children with life-limiting illnesses. *Journal of Pediatric Nursing, 26*(3), 186–199. doi:10.1016/j.pedn.2010.01.007, p. 6, Copyright 2011, with permission from Elsevier.
SD, standard deviation.
*Range: 1 = *not important at all* to 4 = *very important.*

TABLE 16-5

TESTS OF DIFFERENCES BETWEEN MEANS

| LEVEL OF MEASUREMENT | ONE GROUP | TWO GROUPS | | MORE THAN TWO GROUPS |
		RELATED	INDEPENDENT	
NONPARAMETRIC				
Nominal	Chi-square	Chi-square Fisher's exact probability test	Chi-square	Chi-square
Ordinal	Kolmogorov-Smirnov test	Sign test Wilcoxon matched-pairs test	Chi-square	Chi-square
PARAMETRIC				
Interval or ratio	Correlated *t* test ANOVA (repeated measures)	Correlated *t* test	Independent *t* test ANOVA	ANOVA ANCOVA MANOVA

ANCOVA, Analysis of covariance; *ANOVA*, analysis of variance; *MANOVA*, multivariate analysis of variance.

scores, a researcher can compare results from scales that use different measurement units, such as height and weight.

Helpful Hint

Many measures of variability exist. The standard deviation is the most stable and useful because it provides a visual image of how the scores are dispersed around the mean.

INFERENTIAL STATISTICS

Inferential statistics combine mathematical processes with logic and allow researchers to test hypotheses about a population by using data obtained from probability samples. Statistical inference is generally used for two purposes: to estimate the probability that statistics found in the sample accurately reflect the population parameter and to test hypotheses about a population.

In the first purpose, a **parameter** is a characteristic of a **population**—a well-defined set that has certain specified properties—whereas a **statistic** is a characteristic of a *sample*. Statistics are used to estimate population parameters. Suppose that a researcher randomly selects 100 people with chronic lung disease and use an interval-level scale to study their knowledge of

TABLE 16-6

TESTS OF ASSOCIATION

LEVEL OF MEASUREMENT	TWO VARIABLES	MORE THAN TWO VARIABLES
NONPARAMETRIC		
Nominal	Phi coefficient Point-biserial correlation	Contingency coefficient
Ordinal	Kendall's tau Spearman's rho	Discriminant function analysis
PARAMETRIC		
Interval or ratio	Pearson *r*	Multiple regression Path analysis Canonical correlation

the disease. A mean score of 65 for these participants represents the sample statistic. If the researcher were able to study every participant with chronic lung disease, he or she also could calculate an average knowledge score, and that score would be the parameter for the population. Researchers are rarely able to study an entire population, but inferential statistics provide evidence that allow them to make statements about the larger population from studying the sample.

Both parametric and nonparametric inferential tests can be used in data analyses (see Tables 16-5 and 16-6). Parametric statistical models are based on assumptions about the distributions of sample values and parameters; thus, in these models, means and variances are used to test significance. Nonparametric tests are used when populations have non-normal distributions or when researchers wish to explore associations among variables. In these tests, no assumptions about the distribution of the data are made.

The example of the study of patients with lung disease alludes to two important qualifications of how a study must be conducted so that inferential statistics may be used. First, the sample was selected randomly: that is, through the use of probability methods (see Chapter 12). Because you are already familiar with the advantages of probability sampling, you know that in order to make generalizations about a population from a sample, that sample must be representative. All procedures for inferential statistics are based on

the assumption that the sample was drawn with a known probability. Second, the scale had to reflect the interval level of measurement. The mathematical operations involved in inferential statistics require this level of measurement. Note that researchers who use nonprobability methods of sampling also use inferential statistics. To compensate for the use of nonprobability sampling methods, researchers use techniques such as sample size estimation through power analysis. The following two Critical Thinking Decision Paths provide algorithms that reflect inferential statistics and that researchers use for statistical decision making.

Evidence-Informed Practice Tip ____

Try to determine whether the statistical test chosen was appropriate for the design, the type of data collected, and the level of measurement.

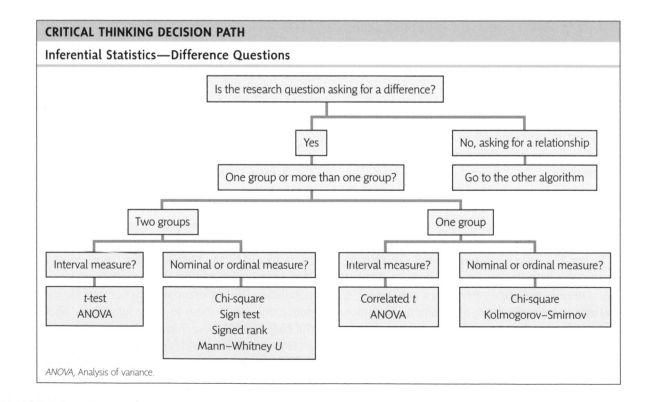

CRITICAL THINKING DECISION PATH

Inferential Statistics—Difference Questions

Is the research question asking for a difference?

- Yes
  - One group or more than one group?
    - Two groups
      - Interval measure? → t-test, ANOVA
      - Nominal or ordinal measure? → Chi-square, Sign test, Signed rank, Mann–Whitney U
    - One group
      - Interval measure? → Correlated t, ANOVA
      - Nominal or ordinal measure? → Chi-square, Kolmogorov–Smirnov
- No, asking for a relationship
  - Go to the other algorithm

ANOVA, Analysis of variance.

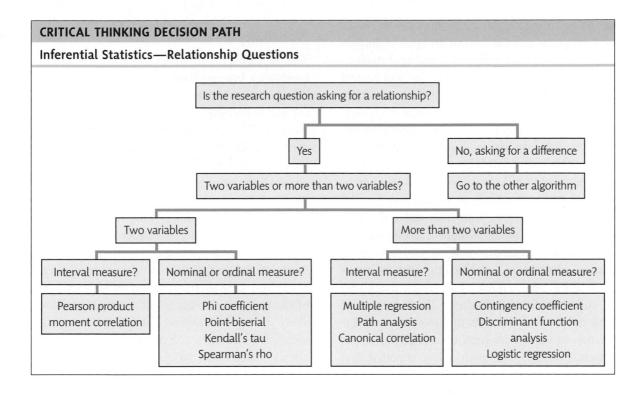

Hypothesis Testing

The second and most commonly used purpose of inferential statistics is hypothesis testing. Statistical hypothesis testing allows researchers to make objective decisions about the outcome of their study and to answer questions such as "How much of this effect is a result of chance?"; "How strongly are these two variables associated with each other?"; and "What is the effect of the intervention?"

The procedures used to make inferences are based on principles of negative inference. For example, to study the effect of a new educational program for patients with chronic lung disease, the researcher would actually have two hypotheses: the scientific hypothesis and the null hypothesis. The research or **scientific hypothesis** (H_1) is what the researcher believes the outcome of the study will be. In this example, the scientific hypothesis would be that the educational intervention would have a marked effect on the outcome in the experimental group in comparison with that in the control group. The **null hypothesis** (also called the *statistical hypothesis* or H_0), which is the hypothesis that actually can be tested by statistical methods, would be that no difference exists between the groups. In inferential statistics, the null hypothesis is used to test the validity of a scientific hypothesis in sample data. According to the null hypothesis, no relationship exists between the variables. and any observed relationship or difference is merely a function of chance fluctuations in sampling.

The concept of the null hypothesis is often confusing. An example may help clarify this concept. Sobieraj and colleagues (2009) used music during simple laceration repair to promote parent-led distraction; they were interested in determining whether this protocol would affect children's distress during the procedure (see Appendix C). On the basis of this hypothesis, Sobieraj and colleagues wanted to determine whether the differences found in the dependent variables differed significantly between the intervention group and the control group. The authors had to use the null hypothesis—that no difference would exist between the intervention and control groups—to test the scientific hypothesis. They found no difference in distress scores, regardless of parental participation. In other words, the differences between the control and intervention group scores were not large enough to conclude that they were unlikely to be caused by chance. Thus, the null hypothesis was not rejected.

On the other hand, Schneider and colleagues (2011) were examining psychosocial outcomes of meaning in caregiving, self-esteem, optimism, burden, depression, spirituality, and posttraumatic stress between male and female caregivers of children with life-limiting illnesses. One of their null hypotheses was that there was no difference in meaningfulness of caregiving scores between women and men. They reported that women had higher average scores than did men for meaningfulness in caregiving ($t = 2.66$, $df = 270$, $P = .008$). In other words, the null hypothesis was rejected, and the differences between the men and women were large enough to conclude that they were unlikely to be caused by chance. See information on the interpretation of P values in the later "Level of Significance" section.

All statistical hypothesis testing is a process of disproof or rejection. It is impossible to prove that a scientific hypothesis is true, but it is possible to demonstrate that the null hypothesis has a high probability of being incorrect. To reject the null hypothesis, therefore, is to show support for the scientific hypothesis, which is the desired outcome of most reports of inferential statistics.

Helpful Hint

Remember that most samples used in clinical research are samples of convenience, but most researchers use inferential statistics. Although such use violates one of the assumptions of such tests, the tests are robust enough to not seriously affect the results unless the data are skewed in unknown ways.

Probability

The researcher can never *prove* the scientific hypothesis but can show support for it by rejecting the null hypothesis: that is, by showing that the null hypothesis has a high probability of being incorrect. The theory underlying all of the procedures discussed in this chapter is probability theory. Probability is a concept that people talk about all the time, such as the chance of rain, but have a difficult time defining it. The **probability** of an event is the event's long-run relative frequency in repeated trials under similar conditions. In other words, the statistician does not think of the probability of obtaining a single result from a single study but rather of the chances of obtaining the same result from an idealized study that can be carried out many times under identical conditions. The notion of repeated trials allows researchers to use probability to test hypotheses.

Statistical probability is based on the concept of sampling error. The use of inferential statistics is based on random sampling. However, even when samples are randomly selected, the possibility of errors in sampling always exists. Therefore, the characteristics of any given sample may be different from those of the entire population.

Suppose that a large group of patients with decubitus ulcers is available for study and that researchers wish to learn the average length of time for such ulcers to heal with the usual nursing care. If the researchers studied the entire population, they might obtain an average healing time of 50 days, with a standard deviation of 10 days. Now, suppose that the researchers did not have the money necessary to study all the patients but wished to conduct several consecutive studies of this condition. For this study, the researchers first select a sample of 25 patients, calculate the mean and standard deviation, and then select the next sample. If this process is repeated many times in different samples, a different mean for each sample would probably result. For example, the researchers might find that one sample's mean might be 50.5 days, the next 47.5, and the next 62.5. The tendency for statistics to fluctuate from one sample to another is known as **sampling error.**

Sampling distributions are theoretical. In practice, researchers do not routinely draw consecutive samples from the same population; they usually compute statistics and make inferences on the basis of data from one sample. However, the knowledge of the properties of the sampling distribution—if these repeated samples are hypothetically obtained—enables the researcher to draw a conclusion on the basis of data from one sample. Such a conclusion is possible because the sampling distribution of the means has certain known properties.

The sampling distribution of the means is shaped like a normal curve, and the mean of the sampling distribution is the mean of the population. As discussed in the earlier "Normal Distribution" section, because the sampling distribution of the means is normal, several other important characteristics are revealed. When scores are normally distributed, 68% of them are between +1 standard deviation and −1 standard deviation, or the probability is 68 per 100 that any one randomly drawn sample mean is within the range of values between +1 standard deviation and −1 standard deviation (see Figure 16-3). In the example described earlier, if only one sample were selected, the chance of finding a sample mean between 40 and 60 would be 68%. The standard deviation of a theoretical distribution of sample means is called the **standard error of the mean.** The word *error* is used because the various means that make up the distribution contain an error in their estimates of the population mean. The error is considered to be standard because it implies the magnitude of the average error, just as a standard deviation implies the average variation from one mean. The *smaller* the standard error, the *less* variable are the sample means and

the *more accurate* are those means as estimates of the population value.

Although researchers rarely construct sampling distributions, standard error can be estimated because it bears a systematic relationship to the sample standard deviation and the size of the sample. Thus, increasing the size of the sample will increase the accuracy of estimates of population parameters. It is intuitive that an increase in the size of a sample will decrease the likelihood that one outlying score will dramatically affect the sample mean (see Chapter 12). The other reason that the sampling distribution is so important is that all statistics have sampling distributions. Researchers consult these distributions when making determinations about rejecting the null hypothesis.

Evidence-Informed Practice Tip

Remember that the strength and quality of evidence are enhanced by repeated trials that have consistent findings, thereby increasing the generalizability of the findings and applicability to clinical practice.

Type I and Type II Errors

The researcher's decision to accept or fail to accept (reject) the null hypothesis is based on a consideration of the probability that the observed differences are a result of chance alone. Because data on the entire population are not available, the researcher cannot flatly assert that the null hypothesis is or is not true. Thus, statistical inference is always based on incomplete information about a population, and errors can occur when such inferences are made. These errors are classified as type I and type II.

A **type I error** is the researcher's incorrect decision to reject the null hypothesis (Kline, 2005); that is, the researcher has found that results are statistically significant, but in fact they are not, and has accepted the alternate hypothesis. If, however, the researcher had found that the groups did not differ perhaps because only a few patients had been studied or the design of the study was poor for determining differences, a type II error might occur. In a **type II error**—also known as beta (β)—the results from the sample data lead to the failure to reject the null hypothesis when it is actually false; that is, no statistically significant differences between groups were found but there are indeed real differences. **Power** is the conditional prior probability that the researcher will decide correctly to reject the null hypothesis when it is actually false (Kline, 2005). A standard value of power of .8 is used to conduct power analyses in studies to determine sample size before the study begins. Power and beta are complementary and sum to 1.00. When power is increased, type II error is decreased, and vice versa.

In Schneider and colleagues' (2011) study of male and female caregivers, one null hypothesis of the study was that no differences in the psychological outcome of depression would exist between the genders. Schneider and colleagues reported a significant difference in rates of depression ($t = 3.27$, $df = 271$, $P = .001$). If the differences found were truly a function of chance (because this group of participants was unusual in some way) and if the number of participants was too small, a type I error would occur.

The relationship of the two types of errors is shown in Figure 16-5. When you critique a study to determine whether a type I error has occurred (rejecting the null hypothesis when it is actually true), you should consider the reliability and validity of the instruments used. For example, if the instruments did not accurately and precisely measure the intervention variables, the conclusion could be that the intervention made a difference, but, in reality, it did not. It is critical to consider the reliability and validity of all of the measurement instruments reported (see Chapter 14). In a practice discipline, type I errors usually are considered more serious because if a researcher declares that differences exist where none are present, then patient care can potentially be affected adversely. Type II errors (accepting the null hypothesis when it is false) may occur if the sample in the study is too small, thereby limiting the opportunity to measure the *treatment effect,* a true difference between two groups. A larger sample size improves the ability to *detect the treatment effect:* that is, the differences between two groups. If no significant difference is found between two groups with a large sample, this finding provides stronger evidence (than with a small sample) not to reject the null hypothesis.

Level of Significance

The researcher does not know when an error in statistical decision making has occurred. It is possible to know only that the null hypothesis is indeed true or false if data from the total population are available. However, the researcher can control the risk of making type I errors by setting the level of significance before the study begins (a priori). Slakter and colleagues (1991) explained

Conclusion of test of significance	REALITY	
	Null hypothesis is true	Null hypothesis is not true
Not statistically significant	Correct conclusion	Type II error
Statistically significant	Type I error	Correct conclusion

FIGURE 16-5 Outcome of statistical decision making.

in detail the importance of setting the level of significance before the study is conducted. The **level of significance (alpha level)** is the probability of making a type I error: in other words, the conditional probability of rejecting the null hypothesis when it is actually true. **Alpha,** or the level of significance, is considered an a priori probability because it is set before the data are collected, and it is a conditional probability because the null hypothesis is assumed to be true (Kline, 2005). The minimum level of significance acceptable for nursing research is .05. If the researcher sets alpha at .05, the researcher is willing to accept the fact that if the study were done 100 times, the decision to reject the null hypothesis would be wrong in 5 of those 100 trials, only if the null hypothesis is true.

Sometimes the researcher wants to have a smaller risk of rejecting a true null hypothesis; in that case, the level of significance may be set at .01. In this case, the researcher is willing to make the wrong decision only once in 100 trials. The decision as to how strictly the alpha level should be set depends on how important it is not to make an error. For example, if the results of a study are to be used to determine whether a great deal of money should be spent in an area of nursing care, the researcher may decide that the accuracy of the results is so important that an alpha level of .01 is chosen. In most studies, however, alpha is set at .05.

Another concept, the P value, is needed to interpret the alpha value. The ***P* value** is the conditional probability of obtaining, from the study data, a value of the test statistic that is at least as extreme as that obtained from the data that is like itself given that the null hypothesis is true (Kline, 2005). The P value is different from alpha because it is calculated from the sample data and is considered the *exact level of significance* (Gigerenzer, 1993). Thus, if this exact level of significance is less than the conditional a priori probability of making a type I error ($P <$ alpha), then the null hypothesis is rejected, and the result is considered

statistically significant at that alpha level. For example, if the alpha is set at .05 and the P value is found to be .04, then the results are considered statistically significant.

Whatever level of significance is set, the researcher either rejects or accepts the null hypothesis when comparing the statistical results with the preset alpha. For example, in Schneider and colleagues' (2011) study, the null hypothesis regarding participants' psychological outcomes was rejected because the variables of the hypothesis were significant at the .05 level or lower; in other words, the P values were less than alpha. Sobieraj and colleagues (2009), however, failed to reject the null hypothesis and found that the intervention group's distress scores were not significantly improved over those of the control group because the P values were greater than alpha (see Appendix C).

Perhaps you are thinking that researchers should always use the lowest alpha level possible because it makes sense that they would like to keep the risk of both types of errors at a minimum. Unfortunately, decreasing the risk of making a type I error increases the risk of making a type II error; that is, the stricter the researcher is in preventing the rejection of a true null hypothesis, the more likely the researcher is to accept a false null hypothesis. Therefore, researchers always have to accept more of a risk of one type of error when setting the alpha level.

Another method of determining the level of significance and whether to accept or reject the null hypothesis is called the *critical values method.* In this method, by calculating the estimates of population mean and standard deviation, a range of values is determined from which the researcher can compare the sample mean findings and decide whether to reject the null hypothesis.

Suppose researchers want to know the importance of support groups for caregivers of older adults. They ask 100 caregivers to rate the importance of support groups to them by using an instrument that ranges from 0 (not important at all) to 100 (very important). If Figure 16-3 represents the theoretical distribution for this study (a normal distribution with a mean of 50), 68% of the population would score between 40 and 60, and 95% would score between 30 and 70. Thus, the null hypothesis would be that the mean score for the population of caregivers would be 50, and the scientific hypothesis would be greater or less than 50. After measurements with this sample are completed, the researchers find that the sample mean score is 75. This mean is consistent with the scientific hypothesis, and the researchers can be 95% sure that, most of the time, the sample mean score would fall under this cut-off; thus, they would have confidence in rejecting the null hypothesis. In other words, only 5 of 100 times would they obtain this result by chance alone.

Helpful Hint

Decreasing the alpha level acceptable for a study increases the chance that a type II error will occur. When a researcher is conducting many statistical tests, the probability that some of the test results will be significant increases as the number of tests increases. Therefore, when a large number of tests are being conducted, many researchers decrease the alpha level to .01.

Practical and Statistical Significance

Statistical significance and practical significance are not the same. When a researcher finds a hypothesis statistically significant, this finding is unlikely to have happened by chance. In other words, if the level of significance has been set at .05, the odds are 95% that the researcher will make the correct conclusion on the basis of the results of the statistical test performed on sample data. The researcher would reach the wrong conclusion only 5 times in 100.

Suppose that a researcher is interested in the effect of loud rock music on the behaviour of laboratory mice. The researcher could design an experiment to study this question and find that loud music makes the mice act strangely. A statistical test suggests that this finding is not the result of chance. However, such a finding may or may not have practical significance, even though the finding has statistical significance. Whereas some authorities would argue that this study might have relevance to understanding the behaviour of teenagers, others would argue that the study has no practical value. Thus, the findings of a study may have statistical significance, but they may have no practical value or significance.

Although researchers should consider the practicality of a problem in the early stages of a research project (see Chapter 3), a distinction between the statistical and practical significance of the findings also should be made in the discussion of the results of a study. Some authorities believe that if the findings are not statistically significant, they have no practical value. In Sobieraj and colleagues' (2009) study, the research hypothesis was not statistically supported, but nonsupported hypotheses provide as much information about the intervention as do the supported hypotheses. The data allowed Sobieraj and colleagues to return to the previous literature in the area and discern from those findings both statistical and practical significance.

Evidence-Informed Practice Tip

You study the results to determine the effectiveness of the new treatment and the size and clinical importance of the effect.

Tests of Statistical Significance

Tests of statistical significance may be parametric or nonparametric. In most studies in nursing research literature, investigators use parametric tests that have the following three attributes:

1. The estimation of at least one population parameter
2. Measurement at the interval level or higher
3. Assumptions about the variables being studied

One assumption is usually that the variable is normally distributed in the overall population.

In contrast to parametric tests, **nonparametric tests of significance** are not based on the estimation of population parameters, so their assumptions about the underlying distribution are less restrictive. Nonparametric tests are usually applied when the variables have been measured on a nominal or ordinal scale.

Some debate surrounds the relative merits of the two types of statistical tests. The moderate position taken by most researchers and statisticians is that **nonparametric statistics**—also called *distribution-free tests*—are best used when the data cannot be assumed to be at the interval level of measurement or when the sample is small and the normality of the underlying distribution cannot be inferred. If these assumptions can be made, however, most researchers prefer to use **parametric statistics,** which are more powerful and more flexible than nonparametric statistics. Because stringent assumptions for parametric tests makes them more powerful than nonparametric tests, researchers are able to formulate simple sample statistics, such as the mean and the standard deviation, which enables them to accurately estimate population parameters with standard sampling distributions to obtain probabilities regarding the null hypotheses.

Researchers use many different statistical tests of significance to test hypotheses; however, the procedure and the rationale for their use are similar from test to test. Once the researcher has chosen a significance level and collected the data, the data are used to compute the appropriate test statistic. Each test has a related theoretical distribution that shows the probable and improbable values for that statistic. On the basis of the statistical result and the values in the distribution, the researcher either accepts or rejects the null hypothesis and then reports both the statistical result and its probability. Thus, a researcher may perform a *t* test, obtain a value of 8.98, and report that it is statistically significant at the $P <$ .05 level. This means that in 100 tests, the researcher had five chances to conclude wrongly that this result could not have been obtained by chance.

The likelihood of finding a statistic that is high enough to be statistically significant is increased as the sample size increases. This likelihood is indicated by the degrees of freedom, which are often reported with the statistic and the probability value. Usually abbreviated as *df,* the **degree of freedom** is the freedom of a score's value to vary depending on the other scores and the sum of these scores; thus, $df = N - 1$. For example, imagine you have four numbers represented by letters (*a, b, c,* and *d*) that must add up to a total of *x;* you are free to randomly choose the first three numbers, but the fourth must be chosen to make the total equal to *x,* and thus your degree of freedom is 3.

To make statistical inferences from data, many types of tests can be conducted. Tables 16-5 and 16-6 list the tests most commonly used for inferential statistics. The test used depends on the level of the measurement of the variables in question and the type of hypothesis being studied. These statistics test two types of hypotheses: that difference exists between groups (see Table 16-5) and that a relationship exists between two or more variables (see Table 16-6). In addition, many types of regression analyses are available to predict the dependent variable. Simple regression analyses (one independent variable) and multiple regression analyses (several independent variables) are used when the dependent variable is at the interval level or higher. In **logistic regression (logit analysis),** relationships between multiple independent variables and a dependent variable that is binary, ordinal, or polynomial are analyzed.

Helpful Hint

The use of nonparametric statistics in a study does not mean that the study is useless. The use of nonparametric statistics is appropriate when measurements are not made at the interval level or the variable under study is not normally distributed.

Evidence-Informed Practice Tip ____

Try to discern whether the test for analyzing the data was chosen because it gave a significant *P* value. A statistical test should be chosen on the basis of its appropriateness for the type of data collected, not because it gives the answer that the researcher hoped to obtain.

Tests of Differences

The type of test used for any particular study depends primarily on whether the researcher examines differences in one, two, or three or more groups and whether the data to be analyzed are nominal, ordinal, or interval (see Table 16-5). Suppose that a researcher constructs an experimental study with an after-only design (see Chapter 10). What the researcher hopes to determine is that the two randomly assigned groups are different after the introduction of the experimental treatment. If the measurements taken are at the interval level, the researcher would use the *t* test to analyze the data. If the *t* statistic was found to be high enough to be unlikely to have occurred by chance, the researcher would reject the null hypothesis and conclude that the two groups were indeed more different than would have been expected on the basis of chance alone. In other words, the researcher would conclude that the experimental treatment had the desired effect.

Schneider and colleagues' (2011) study illustrated the use of the *t* statistic (see Table 16-4). In this study, the *t* test was used to determine differences in sample characteristics and psychosocial outcome variables by gender. As noted, the women were slightly younger than the men ($t = -2.61$, $df = 271$, $P = .009$), reported more difficulty in managing the costs associated with caregiving and the child's illness ($t = 2.42$, $df = 252$, $P = .016$), spent significantly more hours per week providing care ($t = 4.29$, $df = 237$, $P = .000$), and ascribed more importance to religion ($t =$ 2.16, $df = 269$, $P = .032$). Check for differences in means and standard deviations in Table 16-4.

Evidence-Informed Practice Tip ____

Tests of difference are most commonly used in experimental and quasi-experimental designs that provide level II and level III evidence.

PARAMETRIC TESTS. The *t* **statistic** is commonly used in nursing research. This statistic reflects whether two group means are different. Thus, the *t* statistic is used when the researcher has two groups, and the question is whether the mean scores on some measure are more different than would be expected by chance. To use this test, the variables must have been measured at the interval or ratio level, and the two groups must be independent, meaning that nothing in one group helps determine what is in the other group. If the groups are related in some way, as when samples are matched (see Chapter 12), and the researcher also wants to determine differences between the two groups, a paired, or correlated, *t* test would be used.

The *t* statistic illustrates one of the major purposes of research in nursing: to demonstrate that differences exist between groups. Groups may be naturally occurring collections, such as age groups, or they may be experimentally created, such as treatment and control groups. Sometimes a study has more than two groups, or measurements are taken more than once. For example, Sobieraj and colleagues (2009) used three groups—mothers, fathers, and both parents—to describe and compare distress scores when one or both parents were present in the procedure room (see Table C-2 in Appendix C). These researchers used **analysis of variance (ANOVA),** a test similar to the *t* test, because there were three groups. Like the *t* statistic, the ANOVA statistic is used to test whether group means differ, but instead of testing each pair of means separately,

ANOVA accounts for the variation between groups and within groups. The ANOVA is usually performed with two or more groups by an F test rather than multiple pairs of t tests (see Practical Application box). If multiple pairs of t tests are done, the type I error rate would increase.

Practical Application ───────────

Wagner and associates (2009) described perceptions of workplace safety culture among nurses in a long-term care setting. One of their analyses consisted of examining whether place of employment (a for-profit corporation, a nonprofit corporation, or a governmental agency) had an effect on perceptions of safety culture. They found that safety culture perceptions were significantly less positive among participants working in nonmanagement positions: $F(2, 545) = 6.943$, $P < .001$. The ANOVA indicated that there were differences among the three groups in perceptions. From the post hoc analyses, Wagner and associates determined that licensed nurses working in nonprofit settings reported more positive safety culture perceptions than did those working in for-profit and governmental settings.

When more than two groups are compared over time, a repeated-measures ANOVA is used because this variation of the ANOVA takes into account the fact that multiple measures at several times affect the potential range of scores.

Leung and colleagues (2007) examined exercise behaviour patterns in patients with cardiac disease and investigated the sociodemographic, clinical, environmental correlates of exercise patterns. Data were collected at baseline and 9 and 18 months after discharge. Leung and colleagues used repeated-measures ANOVA to determine whether changes had occurred between the baseline and 6-month collection times. Another expansion of the notion of ANOVA is **multiple analysis of variance (MANOVA),** which is also used to determine differences in group means, but only with more than one dependent variable.

POST HOC ANALYSIS. When the decision according to the ANOVA is to reject the null hypothesis, this indicates that at least one of the means is not the same as the other means, as in Wagner and associates' (2009) study. To determine where the difference in means lies, a **post hoc analysis** is conducted; in this analysis, pairs of means in the main effects and interaction effects are compared to determine whether they are statistically different. Many post hoc analyses are available; the most common include Tukey's Honestly Significant Difference (HSD), the Scheffé analysis, and the Bonferroni analysis. This type of analysis is also known as *paired comparisons.*

Helpful Hint───────────────────

A research report may not always refer to the test that was done. The reader can find this information by looking at the tables. For example, a table with t statistics contains a column for t values, and an ANOVA table lists F values.

Schneider and colleagues (2011) reported that the women were slightly younger than the men ($t = -2.61$, $df = 271$, $P = .009$), reported more difficulty in managing the costs associated with caregiving and the child's illness ($t = 2.42$, $df = 252$, $P = .016$), spent significantly more hours per week providing care ($t = 4.29$, $df = 237$, $P = .000$), and ascribed more importance to religion ($t = 2.16$, $df = 269$, $P = .032$) In other cases, particularly in experimental work, researchers use t tests or ANOVA to determine whether random assignment to groups was effective in creating groups that are equivalent before the experimental treatment is introduced. In this case, a researcher wants to show that no difference exists among the groups.

In many cases, researchers check whether groups are different at the beginning of a study or baseline by using the technique of **analysis of covariance (ANCOVA).** ANCOVA also entails measuring differences among group means and helps researchers equate the groups under study on an important variable.

Fox and associates (2010) investigated the relationship between bed rest and sitting orthostatic intolerance in adults residing in chronic care facilities. They used the ANCOVA to examine the between-group differences in self-reported orthostatic intolerance, while controlling for drugs with known orthostatic effects.

NONPARAMETRIC TESTS. As mentioned previously, Schneider and colleagues (2011) tested whether differences existed between men and women in marital status, employment, change in employment status, and whether their employer allowed them to take time off work. These variables are not interval-level data but categorical, and so this difference could not be analyzed with any of the tests discussed thus far.

When data are at the nominal or ordinal level and the researcher wants to determine whether groups are different, the chi-square, another commonly used statistic, is helpful. The **chi-square** (χ^2) is a nonparametric statistic used to determine whether the frequency in each category is different from what would be expected by chance. As with the *t* test and ANOVA, if the calculated chi-square is high enough, the researcher would conclude that the frequencies found would not be expected on the basis of chance alone, and the null hypothesis would be rejected. Although this test is robust and can be used in many different situations, it cannot be used to compare frequencies when samples are small and expected frequencies are less than six in each cell. In those instances, **Fisher's exact probability test** is used.

When the data are ranks, or are at the ordinal level, several other nonparametric tests may be used: the Kolmogorov-Smirnov test, the sign test, the Wilcoxon matched-pairs test, the signed-rank test for related groups, the median test, and the Mann-Whitney *U* test for independent groups. Explanation of these tests is beyond the

scope of this chapter; readers who desire further information should consult a general statistics book.

In nursing research studies, several different statistical tests are often used. Schneider and colleagues' (2011) study illustrated the use of several of these statistical tests. They were interested in comparing the psychological outcomes between two groups, and although the patients could not be randomly assigned to the group because of the attribute of gender, the researchers needed to determine whether the convenience sampling procedure succeeded in creating equivalent groups. For data measured at the nominal level, such as marital status, the chi-square statistic was used, as mentioned previously. For data measured at the interval level, such as the age, hours per week spent providing care, self-esteem, and spiritual involvement and beliefs scales, the *t* test was used. Finally, to test the differences between the two groups, the chi-square method was used for nominal variables, such as change in employment status and community (see Table 16-4).

Tests of Relationships

Researchers often are interested in exploring the *relationship* between two or more variables. In such studies, they use statistics that determine the **correlation,** or the degree of association, between two or more variables. Tests of the relationships between variables are sometimes considered to be descriptive statistics when they are used to describe the magnitude and direction of a relationship of two variables in a sample and when the researcher does not wish to make statements about the larger population. Such statistics also can be inferential when they are used to test hypotheses about the correlations that exist in the target population.

In tests of the null hypothesis, no relationship is assumed to exist between the variables. Thus, when a researcher rejects this type of null hypothesis, the conclusion is that the variables are, in fact, related. Suppose that a researcher is interested in the relationship between the age of patients and the length of time it takes them to recover from surgery. As with other statistics discussed, the researcher would design a study to collect the appropriate data and then analyze the data by using measures of association. In this example, age and length of time until recovery can be considered interval measurements. The researcher would use the **Pearson correlation coefficient** (**Pearson** *r;* also called the *Pearson product-moment correlation coefficient*) in which the calculation reflects the degree of relationship between two interval variables. The distribution of the Pearson *r* enables the researcher to determine whether the value obtained is likely to have occurred by chance. Again, the research reports both the value of the correlation and its probability of occurring by chance.

Correlation coefficients can range in value from −1.0 to +1.0 and also can be zero. A zero coefficient means that no relationship exists between the variables. A *perfect positive correlation* is indicated by a coefficient of +1.0, and a *perfect negative correlation* by a coefficient of −1.0. The meaning of these coefficients is illustrated by the example from the previous paragraph. If no relationship exists between the age of the patient and the time required for the patient to recover from surgery, the correlation would be zero. However, a correlation of +1.0 would mean that the older the patient is, the longer the

recovery time is. A negative coefficient would imply that the younger the patient is, the longer the recovery time is. Figure 16-6 illustrates a perfect positive correlation, a perfect negative correlation, and a zero correlation. A correlation value of 0 to .2 is considered extremely weak, a value of .2 to .4 is weak, a value of .4 to .6 is moderate, a value of .6 to .8 is strong, and a value of .8 to 1.0 is very strong (Bluman, 2009).

Of course, relationships are rarely perfect. The magnitude of the relationship is indicated by how close the correlation is to the absolute value of 1 (see the Practical Application box). Thus, a correlation of −.76 is just as strong as a correlation of +.76, but the direction of the relationship is opposite. In addition, a correlation of .76 is stronger than a correlation of .32. In testing hypotheses about the relationships between two variables, the researcher considers whether the magnitude of the correlation is large enough not to have occurred by chance. This is the meaning of the probability value, or the *P* value, reported with correlation coefficients. As with other statistical tests of significance, the larger the sample is, the greater is the likelihood of finding a significant correlation. Therefore, researchers also report the degrees of freedom associated with the test performed.

Nominal- and ordinal-level data also can be tested for relationships by nonparametric statistics. When two variables being tested are only

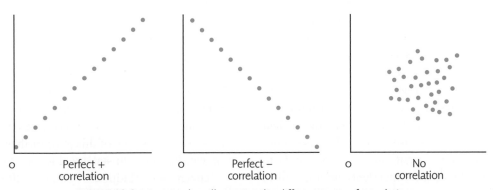

FIGURE 16-6   Scatter plots illustrating the different types of correlations.

Practical Application

An example of a descriptive, correlational study is that of Bailey and colleagues (2010), who described family member perception of informational support, anxiety, satisfaction with care, and their interrelationships in the intensive care setting. Bailey and colleagues found a significant positive correlation between informational support and satisfaction with care ($r = 0.741$, $P < .001$).

Schneider and colleagues (2011) also conducted correlations between two interval variables and found positive correlations for women between meaningfulness in caregiving and self-esteem ($r = .34$, $P = .000$), optimism ($r = .19$, $P = .006$), spirituality ($r = .48$, $P = .000$), and post-trauma growth ($r = .66$, $P = .000$). All of these variables were measured with validated scales.

dichotomous (e.g., male/female; yes/no), the phi coefficient can be used to express relationships. When the researcher is interested in the relationship between a nominal variable and an interval variable, the point-biserial correlation is used. Spearman's rho is used to determine the degree of association between two sets of ranks, as is Kendall's tau. All these correlation coefficients may range in value from -1.0 to $+1.0$. These tests are listed in Table 16-6.

Nursing problems are rarely so simple that they can be explained by only two variables. When researchers are interested in studying complex relationships among more than two variables, they use techniques other than those discussed thus far. When researchers are interested in understanding more about a problem than just the relationship between two variables, they often use **multiple regression,** in which the relationship between one dependent variable at the interval level and several independent variables is measured. Multiple regression is the expansion of correlation to include more than two variables and is used when the researcher wants to determine what variables contribute to the explanation of the dependent variable and to what degree.

For example, a researcher may be interested in determining what factors help women decide to breast-feed their infants. A number of variables—such as the mother's age, previous experience with breast-feeding, number of other children, and knowledge of the advantages of breast-feeding—might be measured and then analyzed to determine whether they, separately and together, are predictive of the length of breast-feeding. Such a study would require the use of multiple regression. The results of such a study might help nurses know that a younger mother with only one other child might be more likely to benefit from a teaching program about breast-feeding than would an older mother with several other children.

In reading research reports, you will often see multiple regression techniques described as *forward solution, backward solution,* or *stepwise solution.* These techniques are used in multiple regression to find the smallest group of variables that will account for the greatest proportion of variance in the dependent variable. In the forward solution, the independent variable that has the highest correlation with the dependent variables is entered first, and the next variable is the one that will increase the explained variance the most. In the backward solution, all variables are entered into the solution, and each variable is deleted to determine whether the explained variance drops significantly. The stepwise solution is a combination of the two approaches. In general, all of the approaches yield similar, although not identical, results.

Suppose that the individual who was researching breast-feeding was interested in not just breast-feeding but also maternal satisfaction. *Canonical correlation* is used with more than one dependent variable. If the data are nominal or ordinal, the contingency coefficient or discriminant function analyses are used. These three tests are beyond the scope of this text; further information can be found in statistical texts.

Janzen and Hadjistavropoulos (2008) were interested in understanding to what extent anxiety sensitivity, health anxiety, depression, and anxiety were predictive of coping, concern for waiting, and anxiety about surgery in individuals waiting for surgery. Three regression analyses were conducted. The results indicated that health anxiety ($\beta = .43$, $P > .05$) and anxiety sensitivity ($\beta = .50$, $P > .05$) were statistically significant predictors of emotional coping. These data allowed them to build on the past research that they had reviewed and to suggest both future descriptive and intervention research, thus moving the data toward evidence-informed practice.

Evidence-Informed Practice Tip ____

Tests of relationship are usually associated with nonexperimental designs that provide level IV evidence. A strong, statistically significant relationship between variables often provides support for replicating the study, in order to increase the consistency of the findings and provide a foundation for developing an intervention study.

The Use of Confidence Intervals

A **confidence interval** is a range of values, based on a random sample, that is often described with measures of central tendency and measures of association and provides the nurse with a measure of precision or uncertainty about the sample findings. In other words, the confidence interval is an estimated range of values, which is likely to include an unknown population parameter calculated from a given set of sample data.

Typically, investigators record their confidence interval results as a 95% degree of certainty; sometimes, the degree of certainty is recorded as 99%. Today, professional journals often require investigators to report confidence intervals as one of the statistical methods used to interpret study findings. Even when confidence intervals are not reported, they can be easily calculated from study data. The method for performing these calculations is widely available in statistical texts.

Ostry and associates (2010) explored whether differences in mental health outcomes were observable between a cohort of sawmill workers living in rural areas and a cohort living in urban places in British Columbia (Table 16-7). The confidence interval helps place the results in context for all patients in the study. The results shown in Table 16-7 demonstrate, for example, that workers who remain at an urban mill have higher odds for neurotic disorder (value greater than 1.0), adjustment reaction, and acute reaction to stress.

TABLE **16-7**

UNIVARIATE ANALYSES: ODDS RATIOS FOR FOUR MENTAL HEALTH DIAGNOSES AMONG SAWMILL WORKERS, 1994 TO 2001

	MENTAL HEALTH DIAGNOSIS*			
LOCATION	NEUROTIC DISORDER: ICD-9 CODE 300 ($N = 6306$)	ACUTE REACTION TO STRESS: ICD-9 CODE 308 ($N = 4104$)	ADJUSTMENT REACTION: ICD-9 CODE 309 ($N = 2133$)	ANXIETY/DEPRESSION: ICD-9 CODE 311 ($N = 7816$)
Urban stay	1.14 (1.02–1.27)	1.04 (0.84–1.29)	1.42 (1.08–1.87)	0.99 (0.85–1.15)
Migrate from urban	0.67 (0.48–0.93)	1.19 (0.82–1.72)	0.82 (0.48–1.38)	0.94 (0.73–1.21)
Rural stay	0.94 (0.79–1.11)	0.68 (0.54–0.86)	0.74 (0.55–0.99)	1.04 (0.89–1.21)
Migrate from rural to urban	1.58 (1.28–1.94)	1.69 (1.30–2.19)	1.54 (1.11–2.13)	1.30 (1.09–1.56)
Migrate from urban to rural	0.95 (0.60–0.94)	0.86 (0.66–1.11)	0.63 (0.44–0.99)	0.77 (0.63–0.92)

Adapted from Ostry, A., Maggi, S., Hershler, R., Chen, L., & Hertzman, C. (2010). Mental health differences among middle-aged sawmill workers in rural compared to urban British Columbia. *Canadian Journal of Nursing Research, 42*(3), 84-100.
ICD-9, *International Classification of Diseases and Related Health Problems,* Ninth Revision (World Health Organization, 1977).
*Numbers in parentheses are 95% confidence intervals.

Helpful Hint

When evaluating whether you should spend time reviewing an article, examine the article's tables. The information you need to answer your clinical question should be contained in one or more of the tables.

Harm Studies

The odds ratio in logistic regression can be used in exploring clinical questions of harm, when investigators want to determine whether an individual has been harmed by being exposed to a particular event. In this type of study, investigators select the outcome of interest (e.g., pressure ulcers) and try to determine whether any one factor explains why a patient has or does not have the outcome of interest. The measure of association that best describes the analyzed data is the **odds ratio,** which communicates that one event is likelier to occur than other events. An odds ratio is calculated by dividing the odds in the treated or exposed group by the odds in the control group. Investigators present an odds ratio of factors in study tables; thus, calculation of the odds ratio is rarely necessary. The interpretation of the odds ratio is straightforward and presented in Table 16-8. Note that the null value for the odds ratio is equal to 1.

The use of the odds ratio to describe the probability of an event is illustrated by a study in which investigators sought to determine risk factors for the postneonatal death of full-term, healthy infants born to young mothers (Phipps, Blume, & DeMonner, 2002). The authors used a large data set ($N = 1,830,350$) of mothers 12 to 29 years of age who had delivered healthy babies. The investigators wanted to determine whether the death within the first year after birth was more likely to occur among infants of young mothers than among infants of older mothers. The main finding of the study, stratified by age, is described in Table 16-9. For both unadjusted and adjusted odds, as the mother's age declined, the probability of death of an infant in the postneonatal period increased (the odds ratio became larger). Healthy, full-term infants born to mothers younger than 15 years of age were three to four times more likely to die within their first year than were infants born to mothers 23 to 29 years of age. The study was not designed to determine which factors are associated with death. However, Phipps and associates (2002) indicated that unmeasured social factors could have a potential association; further studies are needed to test the validity of this association. With this evidence, a nurse could justify the need for increased home care visits to younger mothers

TABLE **16-8**

INTERPRETATION OF ODDS RATIOS

ODDS RATIO	ADVERSE OUTCOME (E.G., MYOCARDIAL INFARCTION)	BENEFICIAL OUTCOME (E.G., ADHERENCE TO MEDICATION REGIMEN)
<1 (e.g., 0.375)	Intervention produced better results	Intervention produced worse results
1	Intervention produced no better/worse results	Intervention produced no better/worse results
>1 (e.g., 4.0)	Intervention produced worse results	Intervention produced better results

TABLE **16-9**

ODDS RATIOS* FOR POSTNEONATAL MORTALITY ASSOCIATED WITH MATERNAL AGE GROUPS

MATERNAL AGE (YEARS)	CRUDE ODDS RATIO	ADJUSTED ODDS RATIO[†]
≤15	4.1 (3.4–4.8)	3.0 (2.5–3.6)
16–17	3.1 (2.8–3.5)	2.4 (2.1–2.7)
18–19	2.5 (2.3–2.8)	2.0 (1.8–2.3)
20–22	1.8 (1.6–2.0)	1.5 (1.4–1.7)
23–29	1.0	1.0

Modified from Phipps, M., Blume, J., & DeMonner, S. (2002). Young maternal age associated with increased risk of postneonatal death. *Obstetrics and Gynecology, 100,* 481–486.
*Numbers in parentheses are 95% confidence intervals.
[†]Adjusted for maternal race/ethnicity, adequacy of prenatal care utilization, and marital status.

in the immediate postpartum period. Another nurse can use this evidence to start a nurse-managed support group for younger mothers.

Harm data, with their measure of probabilities, help nurses identify factors that may or may not contribute to an adverse or beneficial outcome.

Meta-analysis

Meta-analysis is not a type of study design but a research method in which the results of multiple studies (usually randomized controlled trials) are statistically combined to answer focused clinical questions through an objective appraisal of carefully synthesized research evidence (see Chapter 11). People sometimes use the terms *meta-analysis* and *systematic review* interchangeably; however, a meta-analysis is a quantitative analysis used in a systematic review.

Systematic review is the process whereby the investigators evaluate all relevant studies, published and unpublished, on the topic or question (Higgins & Green, 2009). At least two members of the review team independently assess the quality of each study, include or exclude studies on the basis of preestablished criteria, statistically combine the results of individual studies, and present a balanced and impartial summary of the findings that represents a "state-of-the-science" conclusion about the evidence supporting the benefits and risks of a given health care practice.

In the evidence-informed hierarchy, the findings of a systematic review are considered to provide the strongest evidence available to the clinician because they summarize large amounts of information derived from multiple experimental studies of the effect of the same intervention. A methodologically sound systematic review with a rigorous meta-analysis is more likely than an individual study to identify the true effect of an intervention because the meta-analysis limits bias.

In a systematic review, the researcher quantitatively combines the data from the selected experimental studies by using their measures of association (see Table 16-6). An odds ratio is the statistic of choice for use in a meta-analysis. The same interpretation of odds ratio described in Table 16-8 applies to the odds ratios obtained in a meta-analysis.

The usual manner of displaying data from a meta-analysis is by a pictorial representation known as a *blobbogram,* accompanied by a summary measure of effect size in odds ratios. In the meta-analysis depicted in Figure 16-7, the investigators were interested in comparing the efficacy of a beta-agonist given by a metered-dose inhaler with a chamber versus a nebulizer on hospital admission in children younger than 5 years (Castro-Rodriquez & Rodrigo, 2004). The investigators searched the literature for randomized controlled trials with children younger than 5 years with acute asthma who were treated in the emergency department and were randomly assigned to receive treatment either a metered-dose inhaler with a chamber or a nebulizer. The investigators found six trials that met this criterion (see Figure 16-7). The study groups are represented by a fraction; for example, in the first trial listed, of 17 children who received metered-dose inhalers with a chamber, 4 were admitted to the hospital, and of 17 children who received nebulizers, 4 were admitted to the hospital. In the centre of the figure, each trial in the analysis is represented by a horizontal line. The findings from each study are represented as a blob or square (the measured effect) on the vertical line. The size of the blob or square (sometimes just a small vertical line) reflects the amount of information in that study. The width of the horizontal line represents the 95% confidence interval. A vertical line is the line of no effect (odds ratio = 1). When the confidence interval of the result (horizontal line) crosses the line of no effect (vertical line), then the differences in the effect of the treatment are not statistically significant. If the confidence interval does not cross the vertical line, then the study results are statistically significant.

Study	MDI + VHC n/N	Nebulization n/N	OR (95% CI Random)	Weight %	OR (95% CI Random)
Closa	4/17	4/17		12.2	1.00 (0.20–4.88)
Delgado	5/83	20/85		28.7	0.21 (0.07–0.59)
Leversha	10/30	18/30		27.6	0.33 (0.12–0.96)
Mandelberg	6/23	7/19		17.7	0.61 (0.16–2.26)
Ploin	3/32	3/32		10.8	1.00 (0.19–5.37)
Rubilar	0/62	1/61		3.0	0.32 (0.01–8.08)
Total (95% CI)	28/247	53/244		100.0	0.42 (0.24–0.72)

Test for heterogeneity chi-square = 4.46, df = 55, p = .49
Test for overall effect z = –3.10, p = .002

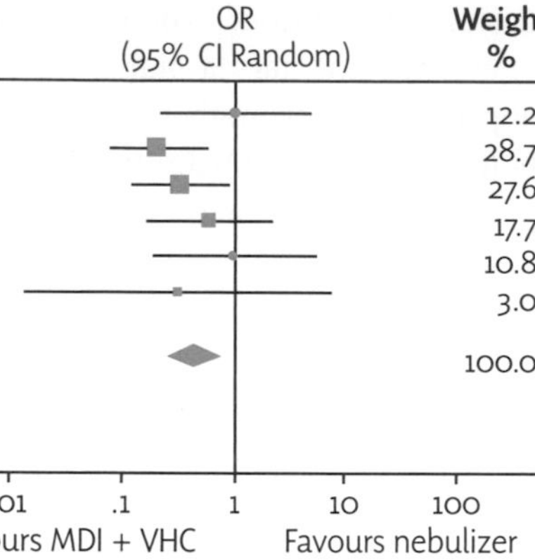

```
        .01      .1       1      10     100
```
Favours MDI + VHC   Favours nebulizer

FIGURE 16-7   Tabular display of systematic review with meta-analysis data. These data reflect the efficacy of administering a β-agonist by metered-dose inhaler (MDI) with a valved holding chamber (VHC) versus a nebulizer in children younger than 5 years who had acute exacerbation of wheezing or asthma in the emergency department on hospitalization.
CI, confidence interval; OR: odds ratio.
From Castro-Rodriquez, J., & Rodrigo, G. (2004). Beta-agonists through metered-dose inhaler with valved holding chamber versus nebulizer for acute exacerbation of wheezing or asthma in children under 5 years of age: A systematic review with meta-analysis. *Journal of Pediatrics, 145*(2), 172–177. doi:10.1016/j.jpeds.2004.04.007, Copyright 2004, with permission from Elsevier.

In the blobbograms in Figure 16-7, only two of the six studies (the second and third listed) yielded analysis lines that did not cross the line of no effect. Because the analysis lines did not cross the line of no effect, these studies have statistically significant findings. In the two right columns of the figure, Castro-Rodriquez and Rodrigo (2004) also provided the numerical equivalent of each blobbogram. Other important information and additional statistical analysis may accompany the blobbogram, such as a test to determine the degree to which the results of each of the individual trials are mathematically compatible (heterogeneity). For more information, refer to a book of advanced research methods.

In Figure 16-7, the summary odds ratio for all of the studies combined is represented by a diamond. In this case, after the results of each of the controlled trials are statistically pooled, these statistically combined results favour the metered-dose inhaler with a chamber for preventing hospitalization of children younger than 5 years of age, and this option is statistically significant. If this meta-analysis were methodologically sound,

it would support the clinical practice of providing metered-dose inhalers with a chamber to children younger than 5 years of age with asthma exacerbation in order to prevent hospitalization.

Advanced Statistics

Sometimes, researchers are interested in even more complex problems. For example, Linton and colleagues (2009) conducted a cross-sectional study to identify predictors of human immunodeficiency virus (HIV) status in homeless youth. Linton and colleagues had a sample size of nearly 140 patients who accessed preventive health and social services. The results of the logistic regression revealed that the variables of age and ethnicity were significant predictors of self-reported HIV status. In comparison with 18- to 25-year-old participants, participants who were 26 to 30 years of age were at increased odds (11 times higher) to self-report their HIV status as being positive (β = 2.413, P < .001, odds ratio = 11.17, 95% confidence interval = 3.344 to 37.303). On the basis of a proposed model, the relationships between the independent and dependent variables were tested through logistic regression analysis. Logistic regression is a form of advanced statistics used when a researcher wishes to confirm the relationship of a set of categorical data (data that have a discrete value).

This notion of testing specific relationships in a specific order can be extended further to test hypothesized variables that are made up of several measures. In structural equation modelling, path models made up of variables that are not actually measured are tested. For example, a researcher might study the concept of self-esteem and use three different measures to determine participants' levels of self-esteem. The researcher would test how carefully these three measures gauge self-esteem by testing a measurement model; for example, Samuels-Dennis and associates (2010) tested the validity of the intersectionality model of trauma and posttraumatic stress disorder.

Another advanced technique often used in nursing research is factor analysis. Factor analysis helps researchers understand concepts more fully and contributes to their ability to measure concepts reliably and validly (see Chapter 14). In **factor analysis,** a large number of variables are grouped into a smaller number of factors to reduce a set of data so that it may be easily described and used; this statistical procedure is used to determine the underlying dimensions or components of a variable. Factor analysis is also used for instrument development and theory development.

In instrument development, factor analysis is used to group individual items on a scale into meaningful factors or subscales. Heaman and Gupton (2009) used factor analysis to refine a new instrument, the Perception of Pregnancy Risk Questionnaire. The original scale contained 11 items, and psychometric analyses were performed on the final 9-item version. Factor analysis was used to determine whether the scale measured the concepts that it was intended to measure. Many other statistical techniques are available to nurse researchers.

The Use of Statistics

Statistics are used in nursing research to describe the samples of research studies and to test for hypothesized differences or associations in the sample. Knowing the characteristics of the sample of a research study allows the researcher to determine the population for whom the results will be generalized. For example, if a study sample was primarily white with a mean age of 42 years ($SD = 2.5$), the findings may not be applicable to elderly Punjabi men and women. The cultural, demographic, or clinical factors of an elderly population of a different ethnic group may contribute to different results. Thus, understanding the descriptive statistics of a study assists in determining the applicability of findings to different practice settings.

Statistics are also used to test hypotheses proposed by the researchers. Inferential statistics used to analyze data (e.g., t test, F test, r coefficient) and the associated significance level (P value) indicate the likelihood that the association or difference found in any study results from chance or because of a true difference between groups. The closer the P value is to zero, the less likely it is for the association or difference of a study to result from chance. Thus, inferential statistics provide an objective way to determine whether the results of the study are likely to be a true representation of reality (Munro, 2004).

Evidence-Informed Practice Tip

A basic understanding of statistics will improve your ability to assess the effect of the independent variable on the dependent variable and related patient outcomes for your patient population and practice setting.

EXAMPLE OF THE USE AND CRITIQUE OF STATISTICS

The purpose of the study by Sobieraj and colleagues' (2009) was to determine the effect of music in distracting parents during laceration repair (see Appendix C). The statement of purpose implies that the investigators were interested in differences between groups; thus, an experimental design that provides level II evidence was appropriate. Therefore, you should expect the analysis to consist of statistical tests in which differences between means were examined, such as *t* tests or ANOVA.

Sobieraj and colleagues (2009; see Appendix C) adequately described sample characteristics. If the participants who did not complete the study differed from those who completed the study, the findings would be difficult to interpret (i.e., those who completed the program had fewer problems). Dependent variables consisted of quality of life, health care utilization, and levels of functioning and were measured over time at discharge and 1 month and 12 months after discharge. Sobieraj and colleagues were interested in looking at differences between the participants who received standard care (control group) and those who received

the transitional discharge intervention. Various statistical tests were used to examine differences, depending on the level of measurement. Dependent variables calculated at the interval level were compared in repeated-measures ANOVA.

These tests are appropriate for the study design and the hypotheses because Sobieraj and colleagues (2009) were interested in differences between the two groups. The results for each of the hypotheses were suggestive of differences in some of the outcomes between the two groups. The tables agreed with the text, and the results were understandable to readers. The discussion pointed out limitations to the study. Clear implications for practice were described, and they supported the practical significance of the study. The statistical level of significance was set at .05 and was consistent throughout the article. Therefore, the researchers' statistics were appropriate to the study's purpose, design, method, sample, and levels of measurement.

APPRAISING THE EVIDENCE

Descriptive and Inferential Statistics

Many students who have not had a course in statistics think they cannot critique the statistics of research. However, students should be able to critically analyze the use of statistics even if they do not understand how the numbers presented were derived. What is most important in critiquing this aspect of a research study is that the procedures for summarizing and analyzing the data make sense in view of the purpose of the study (see the Critiquing Criteria box).

Before you decide whether the statistics used make sense, return to the beginning of the study and determine the purpose. Although descriptive statistics are used in all studies to summarize the data obtained, many investigators use inferential statistics to test specific hypotheses. In a report of an exploratory study, it is possible that only descriptive statistics are presented because the purpose is to describe the characteristics of a population.

Just as the hypotheses or research questions should follow from the purpose of a study, so should the

hypotheses or research questions suggest the type of analysis that follows. The hypotheses or the research questions should indicate the major variables that are expected to be presented in summary form. Each of the variables in the hypotheses or research questions should be presented in the "Results" section along with appropriate descriptive information.

After you study the hypotheses or research questions, proceed to the "Methods" section. Using the operational definition provided, identify the levels of measurement used to measure each of the variables listed in the hypotheses or research questions. From this information, you should be able to determine the measures of central tendency and variability that should be used to summarize the data. For example, you would not expect to see a mean used as a summary statistic for the nominal variable of gender; gender would probably be reported as a frequency distribution. The means and standard deviations should be provided for measurements performed at

APPRAISING THE EVIDENCE

Descriptive and Inferential Statistics—cont'd

the interval level. The sample size is another feature described in the "Methods" section that is helpful for evaluating the researcher's use of descriptive statistics. The larger the sample is, the less chance there is that one outlying score will affect the summary statistics.

If tables or graphs are used, they should agree with the information presented in the text. The tables and charts should be clearly and completely labelled. If the researcher presents grouped frequency data, the groups should be logical and mutually exclusive. The size of the interval in grouped data should not obscure the pattern of the data, nor should it create an artificial pattern. Each table and chart should be referred to in the text, but each should add to the text, not merely repeat it. Each table or graph should have an obvious connection to the study.

In reading a table such as Table 16-4, first look at the table title. The title should give an indication of the information in the table. Next, review the column headings. Do these headings follow from the title? Is each heading clear, and are any nonstandard abbreviations explained? Are the statistics contained in the table appropriate to the level of measurement used? In Table 16-4, the column headings follow from the title. Each study variable is listed, along with its mean and standard deviation. Mean and standard deviation are appropriate statistics because these data were regarded as interval-level data.

After you evaluate the descriptive statistics, evaluate the inferential statistical analysis of a research report, beginning with the hypothesis or research question. If the hypothesis or research question indicates that a relationship will be found, you should expect to find indices of correlation. If the study is experimental or quasiexperimental, the hypothesis should indicate that the author is looking for differences between the groups studied, and you would expect to find statistical tests of differences between means that test the effect of the intervention.

As you read the "Methods" section of the article, again consider the level of measurement used to measure the important variables. If the level of measurement is interval or ratio, the statistics will probably be parametric. If the variables are measured at the nominal or ordinal level, however, the statistics used should be nonparametric. Also, consider the sample size and remember that samples need to be large enough to enable the assumption of normality. If the sample is quite small—for example, 5 to 10 participants—the researcher may have violated the assumptions necessary for inferential statistics to be used (see Chapter 12). Thus, the important question is whether the researcher has provided enough justification to use the statistics presented.

Finally, consider the results as they are presented. Enough data should be presented for each hypothesis or research question for you to determine whether the researcher actually examined each one. The tables should accurately reflect the procedure performed and be in harmony with the text. For example, the text should not say that a test result reached statistical significance, but the tables show that the probability value of the test was higher than .05. If the researcher used analyses that are not discussed in this text, you may want to refer to a statistics text to decide whether the analysis was appropriate for the hypothesis or research question and the level of measurement.

You should critique two other aspects of the data analysis. The study should not read as if it were a statistical textbook. The results should be presented clearly enough that the reader can determine what was done and what the results were. In addition, the author should distinguish between the practical and the statistical significance of the evidence in relation to the findings. Some results may be statistically significant, but their practical importance may be doubtful in terms of applicability to a patient population or clinical setting. In this case, the author should note the deficiency. Alternatively, a research report may be elegantly presented, but the findings do not impress you. Such a feeling may indicate that the practical significance of the study and its findings have not been adequately explained in the report. From an evidence-informed practice perspective, a significant hypothesis or research question should contribute to improving patient care and clinical outcomes.

Note that the critical analysis of a research article's statistical analysis is not conducted in a vacuum. The

Continued

APPRAISING THE EVIDENCE

Descriptive and Inferential Statistics—cont'd

adequacy of the analysis can only be judged in relation to the other important aspects of the article: the problem, the hypotheses, the research question, the design, the data-collection methods, and the sample. If these aspects of the research process are not considered, the statistics themselves have very little meaning. Statistics can be misleading; thus, the researcher must use the appropriate statistic for the problem. For example, a researcher may use a nonparametric statistic when a parametric statistic is appropriate. Because parametric statistics are more powerful than nonparametric statistics, the result of the parametric analysis may not have been what the researcher expected. However, the nonparametric result might be in the expected direction, and so the researcher reports only that result.

CRITIQUING CRITERIA

1. Were appropriate descriptive statistics used?
2. What level of measurement is used for each major variable?
3. Is the sample size large enough to prevent one extreme score from affecting the summary statistics used?
4. What descriptive statistics are reported?
5. Were these descriptive statistics appropriate to the level of measurement for each variable?
6. Are appropriate summary statistics provided for each major variable?
7. Does the hypothesis indicate that the researcher tested for differences between groups or tested for relationships? What is the level of significance?
8. Does the level of measurement enable the use of parametric statistics?
9. Is the sample size large enough to use parametric statistics?
10. Has the researcher provided enough information for you to decide whether the appropriate statistics were used?
11. Are the statistics used appropriate for the problem, the hypothesis, the method, the sample, and the level of measurement?
12. Are the results for each of the hypotheses presented clearly and appropriately?
13. If tables and graphs are used, do they agree with the text and extend it, or do they merely repeat it?
14. Are the results clear?
15. Is a distinction made between practical significance and statistical significance? How is it made?

CRITICAL THINKING CHALLENGES

- Discuss the ways a researcher might use a computer to analyze data and present the descriptive statistical results of a study.
- What is the relationship between the level of measurement used and the choice of a statistical procedure? How is the level of measurement related to the level of evidence in the study design?
- What type of visual depiction can be used to show the use of correlations? Use examples from clinical practice to illustrate the difference between positive and negative correlations.
- A classmate states that it is ridiculous for the instructor to have students critique the descriptive statistics used in a study when none of the students has taken a statistics course. Would you agree or disagree? Defend your position.
- What assumptions are violated when a clinical research study uses a convenience sample and applies inferential statistics?
- What are the advantages and disadvantages of decreasing the alpha level for a study? What is the relationship between setting an alpha level and type I and type II errors?
- Discuss the parameters for using nonparametric statistics in a study and their effect on the usefulness of applying the evidence provided by the findings in practice.
- A research study's findings are not considered significant at the .05 level; are they deemed to provide evidence that is applicable to practice? Justify your answer.

KEY POINTS

- Descriptive statistics are a means of describing and organizing data gathered in research.
- The four levels of measurement are nominal, ordinal, interval, and ratio. Measurement at each level is performed with appropriate descriptive techniques.
- Measures of central tendency describe the average member of a sample. The mode is the score that occurs most frequently, the median is the middle score, and the mean is the arithmetical average of the scores. The mean is the most stable and useful of the measures of central tendency and, with the standard deviation, forms the basis for many inferential statistics.
- The frequency distribution is depicted in tabular or graphic form and allows calculation or observation of characteristics of the data distribution, including skewness, symmetry, modality, and kurtosis.
- In nonsymmetrical distributions, the degree and direction of the pull of the off-centre peak are described in terms of skew.
- The ranges reflect differences between high and low scores.
- The standard deviation is the most stable and most useful measure of variability. It is derived from the concept of the normal curve. In the normal curve, sample scores and the means of large numbers of samples cluster around the midpoint in the distribution, and a fixed percentage of the scores is within given distances of the mean. This tendency of means to approximate the normal curve is called the *sampling distribution of the means*. A Z score is the standard deviation converted to standard units.
- Because the sampling distribution of the means follows a normal curve, researchers are able to estimate the probability that a certain sample will have the same properties as the total population of interest. Sampling distributions provide the basis for all inferential statistics.
- Inferential statistics allow researchers to estimate population parameters and to test hypotheses about populations from sample data. The use of these statistics allows researchers to make objective decisions about the outcome of the study. Such decisions are based on the rejection or acceptance of the null hypothesis, which is that no relationship exists between the variables.
- If the null hypothesis is supported, then the findings are likely to have occurred by chance. If the null hypothesis is rejected, then a relationship does exist between the variables and is unlikely to have occurred by chance.
- Statistical hypothesis testing is subject to two types of errors: type I and type II.
- A type I error is the researchers' incorrect decision to reject the null hypothesis.
- A type II error occurs when the results from the sample data lead to the acceptance of the null hypothesis when it is actually false; this error is also known as beta (β).
- The researcher controls the risk of making a type I error by setting the alpha level, or level of significance. Unfortunately, reducing the risk of a type I error by reducing the level of significance increases the risk of making a type II error.
- The results of statistical tests are reported to be significant or nonsignificant. For a result to be statistically significant, the probability of occurring must be less than .05 or .01, depending on the level of significance set by the researcher.
- Commonly used parametric and nonparametric statistical tests include tests for differences between means, such as the *t* test and ANOVA, and tests for differences in proportions, such as the chi-square test.
- Tests in which data are examined for the presence of relationships include the Pearson *r*, the sign test, the Wilcoxon matched-pairs test, the signed-rank test, and multiple regression.
- Advanced statistical procedures include path analysis and factor analysis.
- The most important aspect of critiquing statistical analyses is the relationship between the statistics used and the problem, design, and method used in the study. Clues to the appropriate statistical test to be used by the researcher should stem from the researcher's hypotheses. You also should determine whether all of the hypotheses have been presented in the article.
- A basic understanding of statistics will improve your ability to think about the level of evidence provided by the study design and findings and their relevance to patient outcomes for your patient population and practice setting.

REFERENCES

Arnold, J. M., Liu, P., Demers, C., Dorian, P., Giannetti, N., Haddad, H., et al.(2006). Canadian Cardiovascular Society consensus conference recommendations on heart failure 2006: Diagnosis and management. *Canadian Journal of Cardiology, 22*(1), 23-45.

Bailey, J. J., Sabbagh, M., Loiselle, C. G., Boileau, J., & McVey, L. (2010). Supporting families in the ICU: A descriptive correlational study of informational support, anxiety, and satisfaction with care. *Intensive and Critical Care Nursing, 26*, 114-122.

Bluman, A. J. (2009). *A brief version elementary statistics: A step by step approach.* New York: McGraw-Hill.

Castro-Rodriquez, J., & Rodrigo, G. (2004). Beta-agonists through metered-dose inhaler with valved holding chamber versus nebulizer for acute exacerbation of wheezing or asthma in children under 5 years of age: A systematic review with meta-analysis. *Journal of Pediatrics, 145*(2), 172-177.

Fox, M. T., Sidani, S., & Brooks, D. (2010). The relationship between bed rest and sitting orthostatic intolerance in adults residing in chronic care facilities. *Journal of Nursing and Healthcare of Chronic Illness, 2,* 187-196. doi:10.1111/j/1752-9824.2010.01058.x

Gigerenzer, G. (1993). The superego, the ego, and the id in statistical reasoning. In G. Keren & C. Lewis (Eds.), *A handbook for data analysis in the behavioural sciences: Vol. 1. Methodological issues* (pp. 311-339). Hillsdale, NJ: Erlbaum.

Heaman, M. I., & Gupton, A. L. (2009). Psychometric testing of the Perception of Pregnancy Risk Questionnaire. *Research in Nursing and Health, 32,* 493-503.

Higgins, J. T., & Green, S. (Eds.), (2009). *Cochrane handbook for systematic reviews of interventions.* New York: The Cochrane Collaboration, John Wiley & Sons.

Janzen, J., & Hadjistavropoulos, H. D. (2008). Examination of negative affective responses to waiting for surgery. *Canadian Journal of Nursing Research, 40*(4), 72-91.

Kline, R. B. (2005). *Beyond significance testing: Reforming data analysis methods in behavioral research.* Washington, DC: American Psychological Association.

Leung, Y. W., Ceccato, N., Stewart, D. E., & Grace, S. (2007). A prospective examination of patterns and correlates of exercise maintenance in coronary artery disease patients. *Journal of Cardiopulmonary Rehabilitation and Prevention, 27*(5), 347-357.

Linton, A., Singh, M., Turbow, D., & Legg, T. J. (2009). Street youth in Toronto: An investigation of demographic predictors of high risk behaviors and HIV status. *Journal of HIV/AIDS & Social Services, 8,* 375-396.

Munro, B. H. (2004). *Statistical methods for health care research* (5th ed.). Philadelphia: Lippincott Williams & Wilkins.

Ostry, A., Maggi, S., Hershler, R., Chen, L., & Hertzman, C. (2010). Mental health differences among middle-aged sawmill workers in rural compared to urban British Columbia. *Canadian Journal of Nursing Research, 42*(3), 84-100.

Phipps, M., Blume, J., & DeMonner, S. (2002). Young maternal age associated with increased risk of post-neonatal death. *Obstetrics and Gynecology, 100,* 481-486.

Profetto-McGrath, J., Negrin, K., Hugo, K., & Bulmer Smith, K. (2010). Clinical nurse specialists' approaches in selecting and using evidence to improve practice. *Worldviews on Evidence-Based Nursing, 7*(1), 36-50.

Samuels-Dennis, J., Ford-Gilboe, M., & Ray, S. (2010). Single mother's adverse and traumatic experiences and post-traumatic stress symptoms. *Journal of Family Violence, 26*(1), 9-20.

Schneider, M., Steele, R., Cadell, S., & Hemsworth, D. (2011). Differences on psychosocial outcomes between male and female caregivers of children with life-limiting illnesses. *Journal of Pediatric Nursing, 26*(3), 186-199. doi: 10.1016/j.pedn.2010.01.007

Slakter, M. J., Wu, Y. W. B., & Suzuki-Slakter, N. S. (1991). Statistical nonsense at the .00000 level. *Nursing Research, 40,* 248-249.

Snowdon, A. W., Polgar, J., Patrick, L., & Stamler, L. (2006). Parents' knowledge about use of child safety systems. *Canadian Journal of Nursing Research, 38*(2), 98-114.

Sobieraj, G., Bhatt, M., LeMay, S., Rennick, J., & Johnston, C. (2009). The effect of music on parental participation during pediatric laceration repair. *Canadian Journal of Nursing Research, 41*(4), 68-82.

Wagner, L. M., Capezuti, E., & Rice, J. C. (2009). Nurses' perceptions of safety culture in long-term care settings. *Journal of Nursing Scholarship, 41*(2), 184-192.

Wong, C. A., Laschinger, H., Cummings, G. G., Vincent, L., & O'Connor, P. (2010). Decisional involvement of senior nurse leaders in Canadian acute care hospitals. *Journal of Nursing Management, 18,* 122-133. doi: 10.1111/j.1365-2834.2010.01053.x

World Health Organization. (1977). *International classification of diseases and related health problems,* ninth revision [ICD-9]. Geneva, Switzerland: Author.

FOR FURTHER STUDY

ⓔvolve Go to Evolve at http://evolve.elsevier.com/Canada/LoBiondo/Research for Audio Glossary, how-to instructions for Writing Proposals for Funding, and additional research articles for practice in reviewing and critiquing.

CHAPTER 17

Presenting the Findings

Geri LoBiondo-Wood | Mina D. Singh

LEARNING OUTCOMES

After reading this chapter, you will be able to do the following:

- Discuss the difference between a study's "Results" section and the "Discussion" section.
- Identify the format of the "Results" section.
- Determine whether both statistically supported and statistically unsupported findings are discussed.
- Determine whether the results are objectively reported.
- Describe how tables and figures are used in a research report.
- List the criteria of a meaningful table.
- Identify the format and components of the "Discussion of the Results" section.
- Determine the purpose of the "Discussion" section.
- Discuss the importance of including the generalizations and limitations of a study in the report.
- Determine the purpose of including recommendations in the study report.
- Discuss how the strength, quality, and consistency of evidence provided by the findings are related to a study's limitations, generalizability, transferability, and applicability to practice.

KEY TERMS

confidence interval
findings

generalizability
limitations

recommendations
transferability

STUDY RESOURCES

Go to Evolve at http://evolve.elsevier.com/Canada/LoBiondo/Research for Audio Glossary, how-to instructions for Writing Proposals for Funding, and additional research articles for practice in reviewing and critiquing.

THE ULTIMATE GOALS OF NURSING RESEARCH are to develop nursing knowledge and to promote evidence-informed nursing practice, thereby supporting the scientific basis of nursing. From the viewpoint of the research consumer, the analysis of the results, interpretations, and the conclusions that a researcher makes from a study becomes a highly important piece of the research report. After the analysis of the data, the researcher constructs an overall view of the findings, like putting the pieces of a jigsaw puzzle together to view the total picture. This process is analogous to evaluation, the last step in the nursing process. In the final sections of the report, after the statistical procedures have been applied, the statistical or numerical findings are described in relation to the theoretical framework, literature, methods, hypotheses, and problem statements. In qualitative research, after the content analyses have been concluded, the themes are discussed in relation to the literature, problem statements, and a theoretical framework, as appropriate.

The final sections of published research reports are generally titled "Results" and "Discussion," but other topics, such as limitations of findings, implications for future research and nursing practice, recommendations, and conclusions, may be addressed separately or subsumed within these sections. The format of the "Results" and "Discussion" is contingent on the stylistic considerations of the author and the journal. The function of these final sections is to depict all aspects of the research process, as well as to discuss, interpret, and identify the limitations, generalizations, and applicability relevant to the investigation, thereby furthering research-based practice.

The process that both the investigator and you as the research consumer use to assess the results of a study is depicted in the Critical Thinking Decision Path. The goal of this chapter is to introduce the purpose and content of the final sections of a research investigation, in which the data are presented, interpreted, discussed, and generalized. An understanding of what an investigator

presents in these sections will help you critically analyze the findings.

FINDINGS

The **findings** of a study are the results, conclusions, interpretations, recommendations, generalizations, and implications for future research and nursing practice, which are separated into two major areas: the results and the discussion of the results. The "Results" section focuses on the thematic results or statistical findings of a study, and the "Discussion" section focuses on the remaining topics. For both sections, as well as all other sections of a report, the same rule applies: The content must be presented clearly, concisely, and logically.

Evidence-Informed Practice Tip

Evidence-informed practice is an active process that requires you to consider how, and whether, research findings are applicable to your patient population and practice setting.

Results

In the "Results" section of a research report, the researcher presents the quantitative data or numbers generated by the descriptive and inferential statistical tests or the themes from narratives generated from a content or coding analysis. The results of the data analysis are the foundation for the interpretations or "Discussion" section that follows the results. The "Results" section should then reflect the question being posed or hypothesis tested. The information from each hypothesis or research question should be presented sequentially. The tests used to analyze the data should be identified. If the author does not explicitly state the exact test that was used, then the values obtained should be noted. The researcher typically provides the numerical values of the statistics and states the specific test value and probability level achieved (see Chapter 16). Examples of statistical tests and the corre-

CRITICAL THINKING DECISION PATH

Assessing Study Results

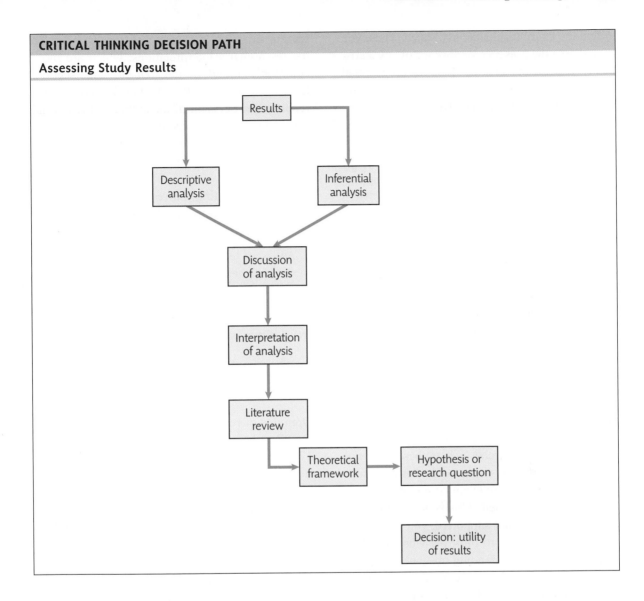

sponding statistical values can be found in Table 17-1. An example of a qualitative analysis with themes and subthemes is given later in this chapter (see Table 17-4).

You should not be intimidated by numbers and symbols. Although these numbers are important, they are only one piece of the whole; the research process is much more important. Whether you superficially understand statistics or have an in-depth knowledge of statistics, you can expect

TABLE **17-1**

EXAMPLES OF REPORTED STATISTICAL RESULTS

STATISTICAL TEST	EXAMPLES OF REPORTED RESULTS
Mean	$M = 118.28$
Standard deviation	$SD = 62.5$
Pearson correlation	$r = .39, P < .01$
Analysis of variance (ANOVA)	$F = 3.59; df = 2, 48; P < .05$
t test	$t = 2.65, P < .01$
Chi-square	$\chi^2 = 2.52, df = 1, P < .05$

df, degrees of freedom.

to find the study results clearly stated. Thus, you should note the presence or absence of any statistically significant results. For the conceptual meanings of the numbers found in studies, refer to the discussion in Chapter 16.

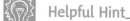

Helpful Hint

In the "Results" section of a research report, the descriptive statistics are generally presented first, followed by the results of each hypothesis or research question tested.

The researcher must present the data for all of the hypotheses posed or research questions asked (e.g., whether the hypotheses were accepted or rejected, supported or not supported). If the data support the hypotheses, you might assume that the hypotheses were proven, but this is not necessarily true. It only means that the hypotheses were supported, and the results suggest that the relationships or differences tested, which were derived from the theoretical framework, were probably logical in that study's sample.

As a novice research consumer, you might also think that if a researcher's hypotheses are not supported statistically or are only partially supported, the study is irrelevant or possibly should not have been published. This is also not true. If the hypotheses are not supported, you should not expect the researcher to bury the work in a file. Reviewing and understanding unsupported hypotheses is as important for a research consumer as it is for the researcher. Information obtained from such studies can often be as useful as data obtained from supported studies.

Unsupported hypotheses can be used to suggest **limitations** (weaknesses) of particular aspects of a study's design and procedures. Data from such studies may suggest that current modes of practice or current theory in an area may not be supported by research and so should be reexamined and researched further. Data help generate new knowledge, as well as prevent knowledge stagnation.

In general, the results are interpreted in a separate section of the report. Sometimes the "Results"

section contains not only the results but also the researcher's interpretations, which are more commonly found in the "Discussion" section. Integrating the results with the discussion in a report is the decision of the author or the journal editor. The two sections may be integrated when a study contains several segments that may be viewed as separate subproblems of a major overall problem.

When presenting the results, the investigator should show objectivity. The following quotation gives the appropriate way to express results:

> Analysis of the effect of time was statistically significant for intensity and unpleasantness related to pain ($F = 160.395$, $P < 0.0001$).

Investigators would be accused of lacking objectivity if they stated the results as follows:

> The results were not surprising as we found a significant relationship between effect of time and intensity and unpleasantness, as we expected.

Opinions or reactionary statements to the data in the "Results" section are therefore avoided. Box 17-1 gives examples of objectively stated results.

You should consider the following points when you read a "Results" section:

- The investigators responded objectively to the results in the discussion of the results.
- In the discussion of the results, the investigators interpreted the results, with careful reflection on all aspects of the study that preceded the results.
- The data presented are summarized. Many data are generated, but only the critical summary numbers for each test are presented. Examples of summarized data are the means and standard deviations of age, education, and income. Including all data is too cumbersome. The "Results" section can be viewed as a summary.
- The data are condensed both in the written text and through the use of tables and figures. Tables and figures facilitate the presentation of large amounts of data.

BOX 17-1

EXAMPLES OF OBJECTIVE STATEMENTS IN THE RESULTS SECTION

"There were statistically significant differences within each group in mean of pain-related unpleasantness, between triage and 24 hours post-discharge from the ED [emergency department] (Exp: $t = 4.541$, $P < 0.0001$; Ctrl: $t = 3.847$, $P < 0.0001$)." (LeMay, Johnston, Choiniére, Fortin, Hubert, Fréchette, ... Murray, 2010, p. 2446)

"Health board chairperson reported that seniors accounted for over half of the residents in rural communities and that mortality, in combination with out-migration, had resulted in an overall decrease in the size of the population." (Martin-Misener, Reilly, & Vollman, 2010, p. 35)

"The participants were moderately satisfied with the current system (mean = 7.0; SD = 2.2) as measured on a scale of 1 (completely dissatisfied) to 10 (completely

satisfied). RNs reported less satisfaction (mean = 6.60; SD = 2.42) than RPNs (mean = 7.37; SD = 1.93), and this difference was statistically significant ($t = 2.38$; $P < 0.02$)." (Kaasalainen, Agarwal, Dolovich, Papaioannou, Brazil, Akhtar-Danesh, 2010, p. 65)

"Learning-centered characteristics emerged as an indicator that the teacher valued students, and empowered them in a partnership that increased self-awareness through shared assessment." (Greer, Pokorny, Clay, Brown, & Steele, 2010, p. 5)

"Some survey respondents indicated that bringing family members to the bedside during resuscitation helped families to better understand and thus accept the resuscitation team's decision to discontinue attempts at reviving the patient." (McClement, Fallis, & Pereira, 2009, p. 236)

TABLE 17-2

DEMOGRAPHICS OF STUDY PARTICIPANTS

	SENIOR NURSE LEADER		CEO	
	M	*SD*	*M*	*SD*
Age	50.4	4.8	51.97	6.01
Years of management experience	20.8	6.7		
Years in role	3.7	3.3	5.32	4.10
	n	*%*	*n*	*%*
Gender				
Male	0	0	37	75.5
Female	63	100	11	22.4
Highest (educational) level				
Diploma	2	3.4	1	2.1
Baccalaureate	19	32.2	5	10.4
Masters	34	57.6	40	8
PhD	4	6.8		3.3
Other			2	4.2

From Wong, C. A., Laschinger, H. A., Cummings, G. G., Vincent, L., & O'Connor, P. (2010). Decisional involvement of senior nurse leaders in Canadian acute care hospitals. *Journal of Nursing Management, 18,* 122–133.
CEO, chief executive officer; *M,* mean; *SD,* standard deviation.

- Results for the descriptive and inferential statistics for each hypothesis or research question are presented. No data should be omitted even if insignificant.

In the study in Appendix B, Wong and colleagues (2010) developed tables to present the results visually. Table 17-2 lists demographic descriptive results about the study's participants; Table 17-3 lists the correlations among the study variables. Tables allow researchers to provide a more visually thorough explanation and discussion of the results. If tables and figures are used, they must be concise. Although the text is the major mode of communicating the results, the tables and figures serve a supplementary but independent role. The role of tables and figures is to report results with details that the investigator does not enter into the text. This does not mean

TABLE 17-3

CORRELATIONS AMONG VARIABLES REGARDING SENIOR NURSE LEADERS

VARIABLE	N	M (SD)	α	1	2	3	4
Timing of involvement	63	1.93 (0.95)	0.84	—			
Breadth of content expertise	63	4.08 (0.98)	0.89	0.133	—		
Number of decision activities	57	3.88 (1.19)	0.90	0.064	−0.022	—	
Decision-making influence	63	4.23 (0.76)	0.83	0.022	0.324*	0.356*	—
Quality of decisions	62	3.80 (0.59)	0.68	0.133	0.219†	0.242†	0.195

From Wong, C. A., Laschinger, H. A., Cummings, G. G., Vincent, L., & O'Connor, P. (2010). Decisional involvement of senior nurse leaders in Canadian acute care hospitals. *Journal of Nursing Management, 18,* 122–133.
M, mean; *SD*, standard deviation.
*$P < 0.01$, one-tailed.
†$P < 0.05$, one-tailed.

TABLE 17-4

THEMES AND SUBTHEMES IN RESULTS FROM A STUDY ON PEER LEARNING

THEMES	SUBTHEMES
Novelty of peer learning	Initial reaction
	Adjustment to peer learning
"You're not alone"	Emotional support
	Physical support
	Need for support vs. independence
Peer-to-peer communication	Positive exchange
	Communication discomforts
Facilitating learning	"Bouncing ideas off each other"
	Sharing tasks

From Chojecki, P., Lamarre, J., Buck, M., St-Sauveur, I., Eldaoud, N., & Purden, M. (2010). Perceptions of peer learning approach to pediatric clinical education. *International Journal of Nursing Education Scholarship, 7*(1), Article 39, 1–12. *International Journal of Nursing Education Scholarship* by Berkeley Electronic Press Copyright 2010 Reproduced with permission of BERKELEY ELECTRONIC PRESS in the format Textbook via Copyright Clearance Center.

that the content of tables and figures should not be mentioned in the text. The amount of detail that the author uses in the text to describe the specific tabular data varies with the needs of the researcher.

A good table meets the following criteria:
- It supplements and economizes the text.
- It has precise titles and headings.
- It does not repeat the text.

Table 17-4 is an example of a table that meets these criteria. This table, which is from the article by Chojecki and associates (2010), lists the study's themes and subthemes. Visualizing the findings of a study is easier if a table clearly summarizes the results, as this table does. Descriptions of each theme in the text of the article would have taken a lot of space, and the results would have been difficult to visualize. The table developed by the researchers allows you not only to visualize the concepts quickly but also to assess the results (see Table 17-4).

Helpful Hint

A well-written "Results" section is systematic, logical, concise, and drawn from all of the analyzed data. All that is written in the "Results" section should be geared to letting the data reflect the testing of the problems and hypotheses. The length of this section depends on the scope and breadth of the analysis.

Evidence-Informed Practice Tip

As you reflect on the results of a study, think about how the results fit with previous research on the topic and the strength and quality of available evidence on which to base clinical practice decisions.

Discussion of the Results

In the final section of the report, the investigator interprets and discusses the results of the study. In the discussion, a skilled researcher makes the data "come alive." The researcher interprets and gives meaning to the numbers in quantitative studies or the concepts in qualitative studies. You may ask how the investigator extracted the meaning that is applied in this section. If the researcher reports properly, the discussion will refer to the beginning of the study, in which a problem statement was identified and independent and dependent variables were related on the basis of a theoretical framework (see Chapter 2) and literature review (see Chapter 5). In this section, the researcher discusses the following:

- The supported and the nonsupported hypotheses
- The limitations, or weaknesses, of a study in view of the design and the sample or data-collection procedures
- How the theoretical framework was supported
- Additional or previously unrealized relationships suggested by the data

Even if the hypotheses are supported, the reviewer should not believe the conclusions to be the final word. Statistical significance is not the endpoint of a researcher's thinking, and low P values may not be indicative of research breakthroughs. Thus, statistical significance in a research study does not always mean that the results of a study are clinically significant. As the body of nursing research grows, so does the profession's ability to critically analyze beyond the test of significance and assess a research study's applicability to practice. Chapter 20 reviews methods for analyzing the usefulness of research findings. Within the nursing literature, discussion of clinical significance and evidence-informed practice has also emerged (Goode, 2000; Ingersoll, 2000; Melnyk & Fineout-Overholt, 2002).

As indicated throughout this text, many important pieces in the research puzzle must fit together for a study to be evaluated as a well-done project. Therefore, researchers and reviewers should accept statistical significance with prudence. Statistically significant findings are not the sole means of establishing the study's merit. Remember that accepting statistical significance only means acceptance that the sample mean is the same as the population mean, which may not be true (see Chapter 16).

Another way to assess whether the findings from one study can be generalized is to calculate a confidence interval. A **confidence interval** is an estimated range of values that quantifies the uncertainty of a statistic; that is, it is the probable value range within which a population parameter—for example, the mean—is expected to lie. The width of the confidence interval gives the researcher some idea about the uncertainty surrounding the unknown parameter. A very wide interval may indicate that more data should be collected before definite assertions can be made about the parameter. Confidence intervals are more informative than the simple results of hypothesis tests (in which a researcher rejects the null hypothesis or fails to reject the null hypothesis) because they provide a range of plausible values for the unknown parameter. For example, Kling and colleagues (2009) used confidence intervals around risk ratios to present risk of violence in health care in British Columbia (Table 17-5).

TABLE **17-5**

RISK FACTORS ASSOCIATED WITH WORK-RELATED VIOLENT INCIDENTS AMONG HEALTH CARE WORKERS IN BRITISH COLUMBIA

VARIABLE: OCCUPATION	NUMBER OF VIOLENT INCIDENTS	RATE (INCIDENTS/100,000 PRODUCTIVE HOURS)	UNADJUSTED RESULTS		ADJUSTED RESULTS (MODEL 2)	
			RISK RATIO	95% CI	RISK RATIO	95% CI
RN	347 (40%)	1.97	6.62	4.63–9.46	6.45	4.37–9.52
LPN	79 (9%)	1.97	10.85	7.23–16.29	8.64	5.56–13.42
Care aide	320 (37%)	3.74	12.55	8.77–17.96	10.05	6.72–15.05

Adapted from Kling, R. N., Yassi, A., Smailes, E., Lovato, C. Y., & Koehoorn, M. (2009). Characterizing violence in health care in British Columbia. *Journal of Advanced Nursing, 65*(8), 1655–1663.
CI, confidence interval; *LPN*, licensed practical nurse; *RN*, registered nurse.

The process used to calculate a confidence interval is beyond the scope of this text, but references are provided for further explanation (Bluman, 2009). Other aspects of the study, such as theory, sample, instrumentation, and methods, should also be considered.

When the results do not statistically support the hypothesis, the researcher refers to the theoretical framework and analyzes the earlier thinking process. The results of nonsupported hypotheses do not require that the investigator find fault with each piece of the project. Such a course can become an overdone process. All research has weaknesses. This analysis is an attempt to identify the weaknesses and to suggest the possible or actual problems in the study. At times, the theoretical thinking is correct, but the researcher finds problems or limitations that could be attributed to the tools (see Chapter 14), the sampling methods (see Chapter 12), the design (see Chapters 10 and 11), or the analysis (see Chapters 15 and 16). Therefore, when the hypotheses are not supported, the investigator attempts to find facts rather than fault. The purpose of the discussion, then, is not to show humility or one's technical competence but rather to enable reviewers to judge the validity of the interpretations drawn from the data and the general worth of the study.

In the "Discussion" section, the researcher summarizes all the aspects of the study and refers to the beginning to assess whether the findings support, extend, or counter the theoretical framework of the study. From this point, you can begin to think about clinical relevance, the need for replication, or the germination of an idea for further research study. Finally, you should find the results discussion either in a separate section or subsumed within the "Discussion" section, and it should include generalizability, applicability, and recommendations for future research, as well as a summary or a conclusion.

Generalizability is the extent to which data can be inferred to be representative of similar phenomena in a population beyond the study's

sample. Reviewers of research are cautioned not to generalize beyond the population on which a study is based. Rarely, if ever, can one study be a recommendation for action. Beware of research studies that may overgeneralize. An example of making a sweeping generalization is concluding that all patients waiting for cardiac bypass can benefit from preoperative teaching and support when the study sample consisted of white men, 50 to 70 years of age. Attention must be paid to the limitations section of an article to note what the researchers have considered to affect the generalizability of their study findings. Generalizations that draw conclusions and make inferences within a particular situation and at a particular time are appropriate.

An example of an appropriate generalization is drawn from the study conducted by Luhanga and colleagues (2010), who explored and described preceptor role support and development within the context of a rural and northern midsized Canadian community. When discussing the sample in light of the results, Luhanga and colleagues appropriately noted the following:

> The main limitation of this study was that the sample was limited to one hospital and one university in northeastern Canada, which limits its generalizability to other settings and geographical locations. Additionally, the specificity of the formal education of the majority of the participants limits transference of findings to other settings. (p. 15)

This type of statement is important for reviewers of research. It helps guide thinking in terms of a study's clinical relevance and suggests areas for further research (see Chapter 20).

In a qualitative study, the limitations may be stated differently, as Chiovitti (2008) wrote:

> One of the purposes of this qualitative study was to specify, not generalize, the conditions and actions of caring. Consequently, as conditions change, it is expected that the theoretical formulation presented will also change to meet new conditions, different settings and samples. Therefore, what cannot be

found in the actual data, at the time of the study, is one of the limitations. (p. 208)

Transferability is the extent to which findings from one qualitative research study have meaning in other studies with similar situations. Authors must note the issues of a qualitative study to prevent a sweeping transferability of findings, which would lead to misinterpretations of the results. In an example of how the limitations in a qualitative study can affect transferability, Cohen and Gregory (2009) conducted a qualitative, descriptive study to explore how baccalaureate nursing programs in Canada address the development of competencies to promote social justice, equity, and the social determinants of health in their community health clinical courses. Cohen and Gregory noted several limitations of the study and that these may affect the transferability of findings. The focus groups were clinical course leaders from programs that submitted course syllabi and supporting documentation. Also, close to 25% of the English language programs did not participate in the study, and no French language programs participated. It is possible that some course leaders may have been using nontraditional placement sites that were not represented in the study. One study does not provide all of the answers, nor should it. The final steps of evaluation are critical links to the refinement of practice and the generation of future research. Evaluation of research, like evaluation of the nursing process, is not the last link in the chain but a connection between findings that may serve to improve nursing theory and nursing practice.

Hall and Irvine (2008) conducted a qualitative study to explain how mothers used a community-based, electronic communication system to build a local community, request and provide emotional support, share information and facilitate learning, and provide validation for mothering experiences. Hall and Irvine noted that an important limitation was the lack of transferability of the study design and findings to mothers who did not have access to electronic communication.

 Helpful Hint_____

It has been said that a good study is one that raises more questions than it answers. Thus, you should not view a study's limitations, generalizations, and implications of the findings for practice as an investigator's lack of research skills but as the beginning of the next step in the research process.

BOX **17-2**

EXAMPLES OF RESEARCH RECOMMENDATIONS AND PRACTICE IMPLICATIONS

RESEARCH RECOMMENDATIONS
- "Future studies are needed to support and verify the findings supporting the relationship between orthostatic intolerance and bed rest." (Fox, Sidani, & Brooks, 2010, p. 194)
- "In the current study, we included some demographic variables to enable description of the sample, but the emphasis was on psychometrics of the scale. Accordingly, we did not perform detailed analysis of the relationships among those variables and scale responses. Future researchers could explore those relationships." (Watson, Oberle, & Deutscher, 2008, p. 592)
- "An important consideration for future research is the use of total number of cues as a self-awareness measure. Many participants lost particular cues for hypo- or hyperglycemia over the study period." (Hernandez, Hume, & Rodger, 2008, p. 51)

PRACTICE IMPLICATIONS
- "Our findings suggest that significant predictors of higher levels of distress during laceration repair are younger age and parental accompaniment." (Sobieraj, Bhatt, LeMay, Rennick, & Johnston, 2009, p. 79; see Appendix C)
- "The higher levels of assaultive and psychological traumas found in this study suggest the need for a gender sensitive approach to violence prevention." (Samuels-Dennis, Ford-Gilboe, & Ray, 2010, p. 18)
- "Learning about the dominant and distinct values, normative practices, and expectations of the critical nursing subculture can help newcomers to understand differences between the critical care nursing subculture and the nursing culture as a whole." (Evans, Bell, Sweeney, Morgan, & Kelly, 2010, p. 339)
- "Further study identifying the relationships between staffing, care-planning practices, and quality improvement initiatives are warranted." (Wagner, Damianakis, Mafrici, & Robinson-Holt, 2010, p. 322)

The final topic that the investigator integrates into the "Discussion" section is that of the recommendations. The **recommendations** are the investigator's suggestions for the study's application to practice, theory, and further research. These suggestions require the investigator to reflect on the question "What contribution to nursing does this study make?" Box 17-2 provides examples of recommendations for future research and implications for nursing practice. This evaluation places the study in the realm of what is known and what needs to be known before being used. Nursing has grown tremendously over the last century through the efforts of many nursing researchers and scholars. This thought is critical and has been reaffirmed by many nurse researchers in the past decade, such as Gortner (2000) and Hinshaw (2000).

APPRAISING THE EVIDENCE

Results and Discussion

The results and the discussion of the results are the researcher's opportunity to examine the logic of the hypothesis or question posed, the theoretical framework, the methods, and the analysis (see the Critiquing Criteria box). This final section requires as much logic, conciseness, and specificity as employed in the preceding steps of the research process.

For quantitative studies, the research consumer should be able to identify statements on the type of analysis that was used and whether the data statistically supported the hypothesis. These statements should be straightforward and not reflect bias (see Tables 17-3 and 17-4 and Box 18-1, p. 402). Auxiliary data or serendipitous findings also may be presented. If such auxiliary findings are presented, they should be stated as dispassionately as were the hypothesis data. The statistical test used also should be noted, as well as the numerical value of the data (see Tables 17-1, 17-3, and 17-5). The presentation of the tests, the numerical values found, and the statements of support or nonsupport should be clear, concise, and systematically reported. For illustrative purposes that facilitate readability, the researchers should present extensive findings in tables rather than in the text.

For qualitative studies, the richness of the data should be described. The consumer must also have sufficient detail about the analysis, the coding, the categories of coding or themes, and the level of coding agreement.

The "Discussion" section should interpret the data, gaps, limitations, and conclusions of the study, as well as provide recommendations for further research. Drawing these aspects into the study should give the research consumer an understanding of the relationship between the findings and the theoretical framework. Statements reflecting the underlying theory are necessary, whether or not the hypotheses were supported.

If the findings were not supported, the consumer should—as the researcher did—attempt to identify, without fault finding, possible methodological problems. Finally, a concise presentation of the study's generalizability and the implications of the findings for practice and research should be evident. The last presentation can help the research consumer begin to rethink clinical practice, provoke discussion in clinical settings (see Chapter 20), and find similar studies that may support or refute the phenomena being studied to more fully understand the problem.

CRITIQUING CRITERIA

1. Are the results of each hypothesis presented?
2. Is the information regarding the results concisely and sequentially presented?
3. Are the tests that were used to analyze the data presented?
4. Are the results presented objectively?
5. If tables or figures are used, do they meet the following standards?
   - They supplement and economize the text.
   - They have precise titles and headings.
   - They do not repeat the text.
6. Are the results interpreted in light of the hypotheses and theoretical framework and all of the other steps that preceded the results?

CRITIQUING CRITERIA

7. If the data are supported, does the investigator provide a discussion of how the theoretical framework was supported?
8. If the data are not supported, does the investigator attempt to identify the study's weaknesses and strengths, as well as suggest possible solutions for the research area?
9. Does the researcher discuss the study's clinical relevance?
10. Are any generalizations made, and, if so, are they within the scope of the findings or beyond the findings?
11. Are any recommendations for future research stated or implied?
12. What is the study's strength of evidence?

CRITICAL THINKING CHALLENGES

- Defend or refute the following statement: "All results should be reported and interpreted whether or not they support the hypothesis (hypotheses)."
- What type of knowledge does the researcher draw on to interpret the results of a study?
- What new knowledge is contributed from the research findings? Are they clinically significant and do they have practice implications?
- Do you agree or disagree with the statement that a good study raises more questions than it answers? Support your view with examples.
- How is it possible for readers of research to critique the findings and recommendations of a reported study? How could you use the Internet for critiquing the findings of a study?
- Now that nursing students and nurses have access to reports of clinical problems (i.e., critiques of multiple studies available on a clinical topic) or critiques of individual studies of a clinical topic published in *Evidence-Based Nursing*, as well as published meta-analyses and meta-syntheses on clinical topics, why is it necessary for them to read and critique research studies on their own? Justify your response.

KEY POINTS

- The analysis of the findings is the final step of a research investigation. In this section, the research consumer will find the results presented in a straightforward manner.
- All results should be reported whether or not they support the hypothesis. Tables and figures may be used to illustrate and condense data for presentation.
- Once the results are reported, the researcher interprets the results. In this presentation, usually titled "Discussion," the consumer should be able to identify the key topics being discussed. The key topics, which include an interpretation of the results, are the limitations, generalizations, implications, and recommendations for future research.
- The researcher draws together the theoretical framework and makes interpretations based on the findings and theory in the section on the interpretation of the results. Both statistically supported and unsupported results should be interpreted. If the results are not supported, the researcher should discuss the results reflecting on the theory, as well as possible problems with the methods, procedures, design, and analysis.
- The researcher should present the limitations or weaknesses of the study. This presentation is important because it affects the study's generalizability. The generalizations or inferences about similar findings in other samples also are presented in light of the findings.
- The research consumer should be alert for sweeping claims or overgeneralizations that a researcher may state. An overextension of the data can alert the consumer to possible researcher bias.
- The recommendations provide the consumer with suggestions regarding the study's application to practice, theory, and future research. These recommendations furnish the reader with a final perspective of the utility of the investigation's findings in practice.

REFERENCES

Bluman, A. J. (2009). *Elementary statistics: A brief version*. New York: McGraw-Hill.

Chiovitti, R. (2008) Nurses' meaning of caring with patients in acute psychiatric hospital settings: A grounded theory study. *International Journal of*

Nursing Studies, *45*(2), 203-223. doi: dx.doi. org/10.1016/j.ijnurstu.2006.08.018

Chojecki, P., Lamarre, J., Buck, M., St-Sauveur, I., Eldaoud, N., & Purden, M. (2010). Perceptions of peer learning approach to pediatric clinical education. *International Journal of Nursing Education Scholarship*, *7*(1), Article 39, 1-12.

Cohen, B. E., & Gregory, D. (2009). Community health clinical education in Canada: Part 2—developing competencies to address social justice, equity, and the social determinants of health. *International Journal of Nursing Education Scholarship*, *6*(1), Article 2.

Evans, J., Bell, J. L., Sweeney, A. E., Morgan, J. I., & Kelly, H. M. (2010). Confidence in critical care nursing. *Nursing Science Quarterly*, *23*, 334-340.

Fox, M. T., Sidani, S., & Brooks, D. (2010). The relationship between bed rest and sitting orthostatic intolerance in adults residing in chronic care facilities. *Journal of Nursing and Healthcare of Chronic Illness*, *2*(3), 187-196. doi: 10.1111/j/1752-9824.2010.01058

Goode, C. J. (2000). What constitutes the "evidence" in evidence-based practice. *Applied Nursing Research*, *13*, 222-225.

Gortner, S. (2000). Knowledge development in nursing: Our historical roots and future opportunities. *Nursing Outlook*, *48*, 60-67.

Greer, A. G., Pokorny, M., Clay, M. C., Brown, S., & Steele, L. L. (2010). Learner-centered characteristics of nurse educators. *International Journal of Nursing Education Scholarship*, *7*(1), Article 6.

Hall, W., & Irvine, V. (2008). E-communication among mothers of infants and toddlers in a community-based cohort: A content analysis. *Journal of Advanced Nursing*, *65*(1), 175-183.

Hernandez, C. A., Hume, M. R., & Rodger, N. W. (2008). Evaluation of a self-awareness intervention for adults with type 1 diabetes and hypoglycemia awareness. *Canadian Journal of Nursing Research*, *40*(3), 38-56.

Hinshaw, A. S. (2000). Nursing knowledge for the 21st century: Opportunities and challenges. *Journal of Nursing Scholarship*, *32*, 117-123.

Ingersoll, G. L. (2000). Evidence-based nursing: What it is and what it isn't. *Nursing Outlook*, *48*, 151.

Kaasalainen, S., Agarwal, G., Dolovich, L., Papaioannou, A., Brazil, K., & Akhtar-Danesh, N. (2010). Nurses' perceptions of and satisfaction with the medication administration system in long-term-care homes. *Canadian Journal of Nursing Research*, *42*(4), 58-79.

Kling, R. N., Yassi, A., Smailes, E., Lovato, C. Y., & Koehoorn, M. (2009). Characterizing violence in

health care in British Columbia. *Journal of Advanced Nursing*, *65*(8), 1655-1663.

LeMay, S., Johnston, C., Choiniére, M., Fortin, C., Hubert, I., Fréchette, G., . . . Murray, L. (2010). Pain management interventions with parents in the emergency department: A randomized trial. *Journal of Advanced Nursing*, *66*, 2442-2449.

Luhanga, F. L., Dickeson P., & Mossey, S. D. (2010). Preceptor preparation: An investment in the future generation of nurses. *International Journal of Nursing Education*, *7*(1), Article 38, 1-15.

Martin-Misener, R., Reilly, S. M., & Vollman, A. R. (2010). Defining the role of primary health care nurse practitioners in rural Nova Scotia. *Canadian Journal of Nursing Research*, *42*(2), 30-47.

McClement, S. E., Fallis, W. M., & Pereira, A. (2009). Family presence during resuscitation: Canadian critical care nurses' perspectives. *Journal of Nursing Scholarship*, *41*, 233-240.

Melnyk, B. M., & Fineout-Overholt, E. (2002). Key steps in evidence based practice: Asking compelling questions and searching for the best evidence. *Pediatric Nursing*, *28*, 262-263, 266.

Samuels-Dennis, J., Ford-Gilboe, M., & Ray, S. (2010). Single mother's adverse and traumatic experiences and post-traumatic stress symptoms. *Journal of Family Violence*, *26*(1), 9-20.

Sobieraj, G., Bhatt, M., LeMay, S., Rennick, J., & Johnston, C. (2009). The effect of music on parental participation during pediatric laceration repair. *Canadian Journal of Nursing Research*, *41*(4), 68-82.

Wagner, L. M., Damianakis, T., Mafrici, N., & Robinson-Holt, K. (2010). Falls communication patterns among nursing staff working in long-term care settings. *Clinical Nursing Research*, *19*(3), 311-326.

Watson, L., Oberle, K., & Deutscher, D. (2008). Development and psychometric testing of the Nurses' Attitudes Toward Obesity and Obese Patients (NATOOPS) scale. *Research in Nursing and Health*, *31*, 586-593.

Wong, C. A., Laschinger, H. A., Cummings, G. G., Vincent, L., & O'Connor, P. (2010). Decisional involvement of senior nurse leaders in Canadian acute care hospitals. *Journal of Nursing Management*, *18*, 122-133.

FOR FURTHER STUDY

ⓔvolve   Go to Evolve at http://evolve.elsevier.com/ Canada/LoBiondo/Research for Audio Glossary, how-to instructions for Writing Proposals for Funding, and additional research articles for practice in reviewing and critiquing.

Critiquing Research

RESEARCH **VIGNETTE**

Evolution in a Program of Research Focusing on Family Violence, Caregiving, and Women's Health

Judith Wuest RN, BScN, MN, PhD
Professor Emerita, Faculty of Nursing
University of New Brunswick
Fredericton, New Brunswick

Programs of research evolve in unpredictable ways, depending on the findings of previous studies, opportunities for collaboration, and successes and failures in applications for funding. My current program of research began with my first research study, the thesis of my master's degree in nursing: a grounded theory study of family caregiving for children with chronic middle ear disease. I had a generous mentor in my supervisor, Phyllis Noerager Stern, who was an expert in grounded theory. This first research experience was exciting and interesting because the research approach enabled me to learn about family issues from the perspective of the families themselves, and developing a beginning theory was useful for both nurses and families.

As a new faculty member who was expected to develop a program of research and to obtain funding locally, I built on my thesis research by conducting a similar study with Aboriginal families. This research was followed by a small study of family caregiving for relatives with Alzheimer's disease. Throughout this research, I became very conscious that family caregivers were largely women who carried the brunt of caring, sometimes at great personal cost, including disruptions of family relationships. I entered the summer doctoral program at Wayne State University with this in mind.

At this same time, my colleague Marilyn Merritt-Gray and I began a grounded theory study of women who left abusive partners. Our goal was to fill the gap in our theoretical knowledge about the process of leaving. As a community mental health nurse, Marilyn felt the need for a framework to guide her practice and to help women understand what stage in life they were in, where they were headed, and how to get there.

Our initial findings, funded by a local grant, allowed us to obtain a larger local grant to develop the *theory of reclaiming self.* We became affiliated with the Muriel McQueen Fergusson Centre for Family Violence Research and began to collaborate with professionals and survivors of abusive relationships, who were concerned that, despite their best efforts, the incidence of intimate partner violence (IPV) in their rural area remained high. Together, we engaged in a participatory action study to determine the sociocultural influences on the meanings of and responses to woman abuse. This participatory study helped enhance the visibility of domestic violence and resulted in community actions to help women and change common understandings or attitudes that allowed abuse to continue.

This work took place over several years, when I was also spending summers in doctoral work at Wayne State University. There I met Jacquelyn Campbell, an international expert in domestic violence, who introduced me to a wide range of feminist thought and emphasized IPV as a nursing and health issue. In my doctoral research, I combined feminist theory and grounded theory and studied women's caring across the life span, developing the theory of *precarious ordering.* An important finding in this study was that women who were caring for family members who in the past had abused them, or with whom they had very strained relationships, had more difficulty gaining control of their health and had poorer health outcomes. My two areas of interest, IPV and women's caring, had begun to intersect!

After graduation, I grappled with the challenge of getting national funding. By combining my and Marilyn Merritt-Gray's interest in IPV and my colleague Marilyn Ford-Gilboe's interest in single motherhood, I began a program of research focusing on single-parent families after they left abusive relationships. This work has been well funded by the Medical Research Council, the National Health Research and Development Program, and, currently, the Canadian Institutes of Health Research (CIHR). Our first study, built on the study of leaving, focused on health promotion in single-parent families after leaving, on the basis of a feminist grounded theory perspective. We developed the theory of *strengthening capacity to limit intrusion* and noted that women in the study had many health issues related to IPV that had persisted for as long as 20 years after they left abusive partners. However, little was known about the long-term health consequences of IPV.

This finding led to the development of a CIHR "New Emerging Team" focusing on the long-term health effects of IPV. With funding from CIHR operating grants, we recruited 309 women who had been out of abusive relationships no longer than 3 years to participate in structured interviews and health assessments annually for 5 years. This study, the Women's Health Effects Study (WHES), demonstrated that physical and mental health problems persist long after leaving an abusive partner, are linked to patterns of cumulative lifetime abuse, and lead to higher use of health service with little symptom relief. Four nurse researchers—Marilyn Ford-Gilbe, Marilyn Merritt-Gray, Colleen Varcoe, and I—have used the findings of the WHES, combined with the intrusion theory we developed, to design a health

intervention for women in the early years after leaving (iHEAL). Currently, feasibility and efficacy studies of the iHEAL are under way in both New Brunswick and Ontario. The New Brunswick study is being conducted in partnership with the provincial domestic violence outreach program, the New Brunswick Women's Issues Branch, and with the New Brunswick Department of Health and Liberty Lane Inc.; it is funded under the Partnerships for Health System Improvement program by CIHR and the New Brunswick Health Research Foundation. Our policy forums, held in New Brunswick and Ontario to share findings from the WHES with policymakers and front-line workers, were key to forming the partnerships necessary to apply for these funds.

Similarly, my research on caregiving has evolved from a qualitative to a quantitative focus. With further CIHR funding, Marilyn Hodgins and I assembled a caregiving team to develop an instrument measuring selected concepts in the grounded theory of precarious ordering, with the goal of testing how past relationships, obligation, health, and health promotion in women caregivers of adult family members are related. We surveyed more than 250 female caregivers and found that past relationships and obligation accounted for significant variance in health outcomes. With funding from the Alzheimer Society of Canada, we completed a second study that replicated the first study but included repeated data

collection to capture changes in health and health promotion over time.

The final portion of my program of research also stems from the study of women who left abusive partners. Although the theory of reclaiming self was useful for these women, it did not help us understand the experiences of some women who remain with their partners and whose relationships become nonviolent. With funding from the Social Sciences and Humanities Research Council (SSHRC), our research team conducted a grounded theory study of how women achieve nonviolence, and we developed a theory: *shifting the pattern of abusive control.* Although violence cessation was important for women staying in relationships, equally important for some women was men reinvesting in the relationship. We realized that to fully understand how relationships shift when they become nonviolent, we needed to understand men's perspective on how their relationships changed when they ceased to be abusive toward their partners. This study was also funded by SSHRC, and the findings will soon be available.

What is most interesting to me is how my program of research has evolved methodologically and substantively in response to each study's findings and the collaborative opportunities that have arisen. I have an affinity for grounded theory research and probably approach most research with the mindset of a grounded theorist. However, each study raises essential questions that cannot always be answered by the method that the researcher likes best. Research partnerships with experts in diverse approaches are essential for building teams with the methodological versatility needed for research to evolve from inductive to deductive to interventional. These partnerships are needed to provide the necessary knowledge for nursing practice to respond to the enormous challenges of the effects of family violence on individuals, families, and communities. ∎

CHAPTER 18

Critiquing Qualitative Research

Helen J. Streubert | Cherylyn Cameron

LEARNING OUTCOMES

After reading this chapter, you will be able to do the following:

- Identify the influence of stylistic considerations on the presentation of a qualitative research report.
- Identify the criteria for critiquing a qualitative research report.
- Evaluate the strengths and weaknesses of a qualitative research report.
- Describe the applicability of the findings of a qualitative research report.
- Construct a critique of a qualitative research report.

KEY TERMS

auditability

credibility

fittingness

phenomena

saturation

theoretical sampling

trustworthiness

STUDY RESOURCES

Go to Evolve at http://evolve.elsevier.com/Canada/LoBiondo/Research for Audio Glossary, how-to instructions for Writing Proposals for Funding, and additional research articles for practice in reviewing and critiquing.

NURSE SCIENTISTS CONTRIBUTE SIGNIFICANTLY TO THE body of health care research. These contributions are evident in nursing, medical, health care, and business journals. Nurse researchers are partnering at an ever-increasing rate with other health care professionals to develop, implement, and evaluate a variety of evidence-informed interventions to improve patient outcomes. The methods used to develop evidence-informed practice include quantitative, qualitative, and mixed research approaches. In addition to the increase in the number of research studies and publications, there is also a significant record of externally funded research by nurses that adds to the **credibility**—accuracy, validity, and soundness—of the work. The willingness of private and publicly funded organizations to invest in nursing research attests to its quality and potential for affecting health care outcomes of individuals, families, groups, and communities.

Because the expansion in nursing research and related interventions affect increasing numbers of patients, the evaluation of this research is crucial. The focus of this chapter is on assessing the quality of qualitative research studies. This chapter demonstrates a set of criteria that can be used to determine the quality of a qualitative research report. Nurses must fully understand how to assess the value of qualitative research, particularly in view of the requirement that nursing practice be evidence based. According to Straus and colleagues (2011), evidence-informed practice requires the integration of critical appraisal with the "clinical expertise and the patient's unique biology, values, and circumstances" (p. 3).

As a framework for understanding the appraisal of qualitative research as a basis for evidence-informed practice, a published research report, as well as critiquing criteria, is presented. The criteria are then used to demonstrate the process of appraising a qualitative research report.

STYLISTIC CONSIDERATIONS

Qualitative research differs from quantitative research in some very fundamental ways. In qualitative research, investigators seek to discover and understand concepts, phenomena, or cultures. Creswell (2009) stated that "qualitative research is exploratory and researchers use it to explore a topic when the variables and theory base are unknown" (p. 98). Jackson and associates (2007) noted that the primary focus of qualitative research is to understand human beings' experiences in a humanistic and interpretive way (p. 21). In a qualitative study, you should not expect to find hypotheses; theoretical frameworks; dependent and independent variables; large, random samples; complex statistical procedures; scaled instruments; or definitive conclusions about how to use the findings. Because the purpose of qualitative research is to describe or explain concepts, phenomena, or cultures, the report is generally written in a way that allows the researcher to convey the full meaning and complexity of the phenomena or cultures being studied. This narrative includes subjective comments that are intended to depict the depth and richness of the phenomena under study. The goal of the qualitative research report is to describe in as much detail as possible the "insider's," or emic, view of the phenomenon being studied. The emic view is the view of the person experiencing the phenomenon that reflects his or her culture, values, beliefs, and experiences. In reports of qualitative research, the investigator hopes to convey an understanding of what it is like to experience a particular phenomenon or to be part of a specific culture.

One of the most effective ways to convey the emic view is to use quotations that reflect the phenomenon as experienced. For this reason, the qualitative research report has a more conversational tone than a quantitative report. In addition, data are frequently articulated in concepts or phrases, which the researcher calls *themes* (see

Chapter 8), as a way of describing large quantities of data in a condensed format.

The richness of the narrative provided in a qualitative research study cannot be shared in its entirety in a journal publication. Page requirements imposed by journals frequently limit research reports to 15 pages. Despite this constraint, investigators in qualitative research need to illustrate the richness of the data and convey to the audience the relationship between the themes identified and the quotes shared. This is essential in order to document the rigour of the research, which is called **trustworthiness,** in a qualitative research study. Of importance is that conveying the depth and richness of the findings of a qualitative study is challenging in a published research report. However, regardless of the page limit, Jackson and associates (2007) suggested that it is the researcher's responsibility to ensure objectivity (use of facts without distortion by personal feeling or bias), ethical diligence (see Chapter 6), and rigour regardless of the method selected to conduct the study. Fully sharing the depth and richness of the data will also help practitioners decide on the appropriateness of applying the findings to their practice.

Some journals, such as *Qualitative Health Research,* are committed to publication of more lengthy reports. Guidelines for publication of research reports are generally listed in each nursing journal or are available from the journal editor. Of importance is that criteria for publication of research reports are not based on a specific type of research method (i.e., quantitative or qualitative). The primary goal of journal editors is to provide their readers with high-quality, informative, timely, and interesting articles. To meet this goal, regardless of the type of research report, editors prefer to publish manuscripts that have scientific merit, present new knowledge, support the current state of the science, and engage their readers. As stated earlier, the challenge in qualitative research is to meet these editorial requirements within the page limit imposed by the journal of interest.

Nursing journals do not generally offer their reviewers specific guidelines for evaluating qualitative and quantitative research reports. The editors try to ensure that reviewers are knowledgeable in the method and subject matter of the study. This determination is often made, however, on the basis of the reviewer's self-identified area of interest. Research reports are often evaluated in accordance with the ideas or philosophical viewpoints held by the reviewer. The reviewer may have strong feelings about particular types of qualitative or quantitative research methods. Therefore, it is important to clearly state the qualitative approach used and, if appropriate, its philosophical base.

The principles for evaluating different qualitative research approaches are very similar fundamentally. Research consumers are concerned with the plausibility and trustworthiness of the researcher's account of the research and its relevance to current or future theory and practice, or both (Horsburgh, 2003). Box 18-1 provides general guidelines for evaluating qualitative research, and Box 18-2 provides guidelines for evaluating grounded theory. For information on specific guidelines for the evaluation of phenomenology, ethnography, grounded theory, and historical and action research, see Streubert and Carpenter (2011). You should review Chapters 7 and 8 in this text before completing this chapter.

APPLICATION OF QUALITATIVE RESEARCH FINDINGS IN PRACTICE

As already stated, one of the purposes of qualitative research is to describe, understand, or explain phenomena. **Phenomena** are events perceived by the senses and may be experienced emotionally, such as pain and losing a loved one. In addition to clarifying phenomena, qualitative research can give voice to people who have been disenfranchised and whose experiences would have otherwise not been documented (Barbour &

BOX 18-1

CRITIQUING GUIDELINES FOR QUALITATIVE RESEARCH

STATEMENT OF THE PHENOMENON OF INTEREST (CHAPTER 4)

1. What is the phenomenon of interest, and is it clearly stated for the reader?
2. What is the justification for using a qualitative method?
3. What are the philosophical underpinnings of the research method?

PURPOSE (CHAPTER 4)

1. What is the purpose of the study?
2. What is the projected significance of the work for nursing?

METHOD (CHAPTER 8)

1. Is the method used to collect the data compatible with the purpose of the research?
2. Is the method adequate for addressing the phenomenon of interest?
3. If a particular approach is used to guide the inquiry, does the researcher complete the study according to the processes described?

SAMPLING (CHAPTER 12)

1. What type of sampling is used? Is it appropriate for the particular method?
2. Are the participants who were chosen appropriate for informing the research?

DATA COLLECTION (CHAPTERS 7, 8, AND 13)

1. Are the data to be collected focused on human experience?
2. Does the researcher describe the data-collection strategies (e.g., interview, observation, field notes)?
3. What are the procedures for collecting the data?
4. Is the protection of human participants addressed?
5. Is saturation of the data described?

DATA ANALYSIS (CHAPTERS 14 AND 15)

1. What strategies are used to analyze the data?
2. Has the researcher reported the data truthfully?
3. Does the researcher describe the steps used for the data analysis?

4. Does the researcher address the credibility, auditability, and fittingness of the data? (See Chapter 14 for a complete discussion.)

Credibility

- Do the participants recognize the experience as their own?
- Has adequate time been allowed to fully understand the phenomenon?

Auditability

- Can the reader follow the researcher's thinking?
- Does the researcher document the research process?

Fittingness

- Are the findings applicable outside of the study situation?
- Are the results meaningful to individuals not involved in the research?
- Is the strategy used for analysis compatible with the purpose of the study?

FINDINGS (CHAPTERS 7 AND 17)

1. Are the findings presented within a context?
2. Is the reader able to apprehend the essence of the experience from the report of the findings?
3. Do the researcher's conceptualizations accurately reflect the data?
4. Does the researcher place the report in the context of what is already known about the phenomenon? Was the existing literature on the topic related to the findings?

CONCLUSION, IMPLICATIONS, AND RECOMMENDATIONS (CHAPTER 17)

1. Do the conclusions, implications, and recommendations give the reader a context in which to use the findings?
2. Do the conclusions reflect the study findings?
3. What are the recommendations for future study? Do they reflect the findings?
4. How has the researcher made explicit the significance of the study for nursing theory, research, or practice?

BOX 18-2

CRITIQUING GUIDELINES FOR RESEARCH CONDUCTED WITH THE GROUNDED THEORY METHOD

FOCUS/TOPIC (CHAPTERS 4 AND 8)

1. What is the focus or the topic of the study? What is it that the researcher is studying? Is the topic researchable? Is it focused enough to be meaningful but not too limited so as to be trivial?
2. Has the researcher identified why the phenomenon requires a qualitative format? What is the rationale for selecting the grounded theory approach as the qualitative approach for the investigation?

PURPOSE (CHAPTER 4)

1. Has the researcher made explicit the purpose for conducting the research?

SIGNIFICANCE (CHAPTER 4)

1. Has the researcher described the projected significance of the work for nursing?
2. What is the relevance of the study to what is already known about the topic?

METHOD (CHAPTER 8)

1. In view of the topic of study and the researcher's stated purpose, how does grounded theory methodology help to achieve the stated purpose?
2. Is the method adequate for addressing the research topic?
3. What approach is used to guide the inquiry? Does the researcher complete the study according to the processes described?

SAMPLING (CHAPTERS 8 AND 12)

1. Does the researcher describe the selection process and protection of human participants?
2. What major categories emerged?
3. What were some of the events, incidents, or actions on which these major categories were based?
4. What categories led to theoretical sampling?

DATA GENERATION (CHAPTERS 8 AND 13)

1. Does the researcher describe the data-collection strategies?
2. Have participants been allowed to guide the direction of the inquiry?

3. How did theoretical formulations guide the data collection?

DATA ANALYSIS (CHAPTERS 8 AND 15)

1. Does the researcher describe the strategies used to analyze the data?
   - Has the theoretical construction been checked against the participants' descriptions of the phenomenon?
   - Are the researcher's views and insights about the phenomenon articulated?
   - Has each category that emerged in the theory been described previously in the literature?
2. How does the researcher address the credibility, auditability, and fittingness of the data?
3. Does the researcher clearly describe how and why the core category was selected?

EMPIRICAL GROUNDING OF THE STUDY FINDINGS (CHAPTERS 8 AND 15)

1. Are the concepts grounded in the data?
2. How are the concepts systematically related?
3. Are conceptual linkages described, and are the categories well developed? Do they have conceptual density (in-depth conceptual discussion)?
4. Are the theoretical findings significant? If so, to what extent?
5. Were the data-collection strategies comprehensive, and were analytical interpretations conceptual and broad?
6. Is variation in the interpretations sufficient to allow for applicability in a variety of contexts related to the phenomenon investigated?

CONCLUSIONS, IMPLICATIONS, AND RECOMMENDATIONS (CHAPTERS 8 AND 17)

1. How do the conclusions, implications, and recommendations provide context in which to use the findings?
2. Are the conclusions drawn from the study appropriate? Explain.
3. What are the recommendations for future research?
4. Are the recommendations, conclusions, and implications clearly related to the findings?

From Streubert, H. J., & Carpenter, D. R. (2011). *Qualitative research in nursing: Advancing the humanistic imperative.* Philadelphia: Wolters Kluwer. Adapted from Chiovitti, R., & Prian, N. (2003). Rigour and grounded theory research. *Journal of Advanced Nursing Practice, 44*(4), 427-435; and from Strauss, A., & Corbin, J. (1990). *Basics of qualitative research: Grounded theory procedures and techniques.* Newbury Park, CA: Sage.

Barbour, 2003; Schepner-Hughes, 1992). In qualitative inquiry, unlike quantitative research, prediction and control of phenomena are not the aim. Therefore, qualitative results are applied differently than more traditional quantitative research findings. As Barbour and Barbour (2003) stated,

> . . . rather than seeking to import and impose templates and methods devised for another purpose, qualitative researchers and reviewers should look . . . for inspiration from their own modes of working and collaborating and seek to incorporate these, forging new and creative solutions to perennial problems, rather than hoping that these will simply disappear in the face of application of pre-existing sets of procedures. (p. 185)

Therefore, findings may be applicable only in certain circumstances. As Lincoln and Guba (1985) stated, "the trouble with generalizations is that they don't apply to particulars" (p. 110). Thus, in qualitative research, if the investigator studies the pain experience of individuals undergoing bone marrow biopsy, for example, the findings will be applicable only to individuals who are similar to those in the study.

In another example, a study of depression in children with chronic disease should not be viewed as having direct application to adults suffering from chronic disease. The findings must be used within a specific context, or additional studies must be conducted to validate the applicability of the findings across contexts. Hence, nurses who wish to use the findings of qualitative research in their practices must first validate them, either through their own observations or through interaction with groups similar to the original study participants, to determine whether the findings accurately reflect wider experiences. In spite of the limitations associated with qualitative research findings, Glesne (2011) stated that qualitative research findings can be used to create solutions to practical problems. Qualitative research also has the ability to contribute to the evidence-informed practice literature (Cesario, Morin, & Santa-Donato, 2002; Gibson & Martin, 2003).

Evidence-Informed Practice Tip

Nurses using qualitative research findings should ask whether the evidence provided in the study enhances their understanding of particular patient care situations.

It is important to view research findings within their context, whether quantitative or qualitative. For instance, a study of survivorship among patients with cancer should not be viewed as applicable to survivors of another illness situation, such as an epidemic. The findings must be used within their given context, or additional studies must be conducted to validate the applicability of the findings across situations and patient populations. This is true in qualitative research as well. Nurses who wish to use the findings of qualitative research in their practice must validate them, through thorough examination and synthesis of the literature on the topic, through their own observations, or through interaction with groups similar to the study participants, to determine whether the findings accurately reflect the experience.

In qualitative outcome analysis (QOA), researchers can use the findings of a qualitative study to develop interventions and then to test them with selected patients. Morse and colleagues (2000) described QOA as a "systematic means to confirm the applicability of clinical strategies developed from a single qualitative project, to extend the repertoire of clinical interventions, and evaluate clinical outcomes" (p. 125). Application of knowledge discovered during QOA adds to clinicians' understanding of clinical phenomena because they can select interventions that are based on the patient's expressed experience of a particular clinical phenomenon. QOA is considered a form of evaluation research and, as such, has the potential to add to the literature on evidence-informed practice at either level V or level VI, depending on how the study was designed.

Another use of qualitative research findings is to initiate examination of important concepts in nursing practice, education, or administration. Caring, for example, is considered a significant concept in nursing; therefore, studying its multiple dimensions is important. Using a qualitative approach, Wilkin and Slevin (2004) explored the meaning of caring for intensive care nurses. Wilkin and Slevin posited that although caring had been studied extensively, little research had been conducted in the highly technological area of critical care. The authors identified caring in an intensive care setting as a "process of competent physical and technical action imbued with affective skills" and confirmed that "to care is human and the capacity to care is affirmed and actualised in caring for the critically ill patient and their relatives" (p. 50). Wilkin and Slevin's study adds to the existing body of knowledge on caring and extends the current state of nursing science because it was an examination of a specific area of nursing practice and the experience of caring by critical care nurses.

Evidence-Informed Practice Tip

Qualitative research studies can be used to guide practice when they are applied within a context. The nurse should ask the following question: "Does this study provide me with a direction for caring for a particular patient group?"

Finally, qualitative research can be used to discover information about phenomena of interest that can lead to instrument development. Usually, qualitative methods are used to direct the development of structured research instruments as part of a larger empirical research project. Instrument development from qualitative research studies is useful to practising nurses because it is grounded in the reality of human experience with a particular phenomenon. For example, after an initial qualitative exploration of the phenomenon, the researcher may develop a survey to collect the data related to specific variables.

CRITIQUING A QUALITATIVE RESEARCH STUDY

CRITIQUE 1

The study "Immunizing Children Who Fear and Resist Needles: Is it a Problem for Nurses?" by Mary Ives and Sherri Melrose (2010) is critiqued here. The article is presented in its entirety and is followed by the critique on pp. 416–418. (From *Nursing Forum*, 45[1], 29–39, reprinted with permission. © 2010 Wiley Periodicals, Inc.)

Immunizing Children Who Fear and Resist Needles: Is It a Problem for Nurses?

Mary Ives, RN, MHS
Chilliwack Health Unit
Chilliwack, British Columbia

Sherri Melrose, RN, PhD
Assistant Professor
Centre for Nursing and Health Studies
Athabasca University
Athabasca, Alberta

BACKGROUND   Despite increasing evidence that immunization procedures can be stressful for children, little is known about what the experience of immunizing frightened and needle-resistant children can be like for nurses.

METHOD   This article presents findings from a qualitative research project designed to explore public health nurses' feelings toward immunizing needle-resistant children. A constructivist theoretical perspective and an action research approach framed the study. Data sources included two survey questions and audio-recorded transcribed data from three focus groups. Participants included 35 public health nurses from five different health units in one Canadian province. The data were analyzed for themes and were confirmed with participants through ongoing member checking.

RESULTS   The following four overarching themes were identified and are used to explain and describe significant features of the immunization experience that were stressful and problematic for nurses: (a) nurses experience stress when immunizing children who fear and resist needle injection; (b) the strength of child resistance and some adult behavior creates an ethical dilemma for nurses; (c) some adult responses make immunizing difficult and unsafe; and (d) resources to help nurses cope with these situations are inconsistent.

INTRODUCTION

This article describes findings from a qualitative research project that investigated the experiences, reflections, and feelings of public health nurses who immunize fearful and needle-resistant children. While the main purpose of the study was to explore nurses' ideas about the experience of immunizing children who are frightened of needles, a secondary purpose was to consider approaches that are helpful in decreasing nurse stress. The research was guided by the question: *What is it about immunizing children who strongly resist needle injection that is a problem for public health nurses?*

LITERATURE REVIEW

A literature review revealed that a significant number of children and adults are frightened of procedures involving needle injections. Considerable research has been undertaken to investigate adult responses that are both non-helpful and helpful in easing children's distress during these procedures (Cohen, Manimala, & Blount, 2000; Duff, 2003; Frank, Blount, Smith, Manimala, & Martin, 1995; French, Painter, & Coury, 1994; Manimala & Blount, 2000; Milgrom, Coldwell, Getz, Weinstein, & Ramsay, 1997; Schecter, Bernstein, Beck, Hart, & Scherzer, 1991; Smalley, 1999). Yet, few resources are available to help nurses understand their own responses or to cope with their feelings of stress. Ives (2007) emphasized how healthcare agencies can begin to address the problem by creating a culture of empathy and respect and by outlining clear policies on the use of force during immunizations. There is a "gap," however, in our understanding of how nurses themselves perceive the experience of immunizing frightened and resistive children.

FEAR OF NEEDLES

Literature from the fields of psychology, nursing, pharmacology, medicine, and dentistry reveals fear of needles as one of children's greatest fears, with claims that up to 93% of some groups of children experience serious immunization-associated stress (Bowen & Dammeyer, 1999; Gaskell, Binns, Heyhoe, & Jackson, 2005; Jacobson et al., 2001; Martin, Ramsay, Whitney, Fiset, & Weinstein, 1994; Peretz & Efrat, 2000; Polillio & Kiley, 1997; Smalley, 1999; Uman, Chambers, McGrath, & Kisely, 2006). Research reflects that as many as 10% of adults experience needle phobia (Bowen & Dammeyer; Hamilton, 1995; Polillio & Kiley; Smalley). Clearly, nurses can expect to encounter both children who are frightened and resistant to needles as well as parents or caregivers who are also fearful.

In his seminal work exploring needle phobia, Hamilton (1995) hypothesized that needle phobia is learned as well as inherited. He noted how negative experiences associated with immunization, laboratory work, dental visits, and other medical procedures can condition children and even those who witness the events toward becoming fearful of needles. Physical restraint and verbal abuse by healthcare personnel during children's medical procedures can lead to life-long fears of situations associated with needles, such as physicians, nurses, examination rooms, and even antiseptic smells (Hamilton). Later, Duff (2003) argued that needle fear centers on anticipatory and procedural stress and advocated for the inclusion of psychological approaches to help children actively gain a sense of control over their reactions.

NON-HELPFUL AND HELPFUL ADULT RESPONSES

Parent and caregiver responses, particularly anxiety-related behaviors, influence how children can reduce stress, gain control, and cope with immunization. Some adult responses have been found to be non-helpful. Parents or caregivers who overly reassured, overly empathized, apologized, criticized, or gave children control of the procedure at the beginning increased children's stress (Cohen et al., 2000; Frank et al., 1995). Further, parents and caregivers who criticized or asked the child to indicate readiness to receive the needle also increased children's stress (Devine et al., 2004). Children coped best when their mothers were present but "watched only" and remained minimally involved. Most children found the presence of their parents during a needle procedure to be helpful (Duff, 2003; O'Laughlin & Ridley-Johnson, 1995).

Distraction strategies were consistently identified as helpful for short-lived pain (Duff, 2003; Gaskell et al., 2005; Lawton & Rose, 2003; Manimala & Blount, 2000; Sparks, 2001). With infants, playing with an object, sucking, belly-to-belly contact, and nonprocedural talk were helpful (Blount, Devine, Cheng, Simons, & Hayutin, 2008). Similarly, with infants, adult verbalizations associated with better pain outcomes reduced crying (Bustos, Jaaniste, Salmon, & Champion, 2008). With children ages 4–6 years, watching cartoons and being coached to attend to the movie helped (Cohen, Blount, & Panopoulos, 1997). With children ages 5–18 years, bubbles, books, music, virtual reality glasses, or handheld video games helped (Windich-Biermeier, Sjoberg, Dale, Eshelman, & Guzzetta, 2007). With most children, preparing ahead (Duff), offering limited choices (Ellis, Sharp, Newhook, & Cohen, 2004), and giving permission to cry (Cohen et al., 2000) reduced stress. Deferring the procedure or referral to an alternate source such as play therapy helped to avoid conflict and coercion (Duff;

French et al., 1994; Milgrom et al., 1997; Smalley, 1999). Distinguishing among adult responses that are helpful and those that are non-helpful offers important guidance to nurses when they work with children who resist needles. However, responses to nurse stress are not as clearly defined.

NURSE STRESS

Stress can be experienced when demands exceed the personal and social resources an individual is able to mobilize (Lazarus & Folkman, 1984). While it is beyond the scope of this article to present a detailed literature review of nurse stress, a snapshot of current work in the area reveals limited attention to nurses immunizing frightened and resistant children. The apparent need to "force" an immunization has been identified as an ethical dilemma for nurses, even constituting "a human rights burden" (Hodges, Svoboda, & Van Howe, 2002, p. 12). Nurses remembered moral dilemmas when they were left to wonder, "Could I have done anything else?" even years later, continuing to justify and absolve themselves from blame (Gunther and Thomas, 2006). Nurses felt powerless, angry, exhausted, and even burned-out following their participation in situations they believed were ethical and moral dilemmas (Thomas, 2009). Coping with the emotional needs of patients and families has consistently been highly stressful for nurses (McVicar, 2003; Sherman, 2004). Avoiding coping rather than identifying that a problem exists and focusing on coping with it was found to be a significant predictor of mood disturbance for nurses (Healy & McKay, 2000). Given our limited understanding of links that may exist between negative immunization experiences and nurse stress, it is essential to explore the problem.

THE RESEARCH APPROACH

This project was framed from a constructivist theoretical perspective (Appleton & King, 2002) and a naturalistic action research design (Kemmis & McTaggart, 1988, 1990; Stringer & Genat, 2004). Action research is a reflective, spiral process where nurses use research techniques to examine their own practice carefully, systematically, and with the intention of applying their findings directly to their own and other nurses' everyday practice. Kemmis and McTaggart offered the seminal explanation that action research is a deliberate, solution-oriented investigation that is group or personally owned and conducted. It is characterized by spiralling cycles of problem identification, systematic data collection, reflection, analysis, data-driven action taken, and, finally, problem redefinition. The linking of the terms "action" and "research" highlights the essential features of this method: trying out ideas in practice as a means of increasing knowledge (Kemmis & McTaggart, 1988). Kemmis and McTaggart (1990) also suggested that the participatory nature of action research, where researchers collaborate with participants in order to understand and improve practice, can reduce the distance between researchers and participants and the ". . . problems they intend to solve, or the lived experience they intend to interpret" (p. 28).

Data sources included two survey questions and audio-recorded transcribed data from three focus groups. The survey was distributed anonymously via employee e-mail to 58 nurses from five different health units in one Canadian province. Survey question one: "Does your practice involve immunizing children?" Survey question two: "Sometimes children who present for immunization strongly resist needle injection. Based on your experience, what is it about this situation that is a problem for you?" This survey generated 35 (60%) responses, all of whom confirmed that their practice did include immunizing children.

The survey was followed by three audio-taped and transcribed focus groups. The focus groups were 2 weeks apart, each with five to six female, English-speaking, Caucasian and Indo-Canadian nurses, from five different health units in one

Canadian province. The participants were those who had responded to the survey, and their experience ranged from novice (less than 1 year experience) to expert (up to 25 years experience) in two groups. The third group had no novice participants. Focus groups are flexible and cost-efficient, generate rich data, and tend to have high face validity (Krueger & Casey, 2009; Morrison-Beedy, Cote-Arsenault, & Feinstein, 2001; Speziale & Carpenter, 2003; Webb & Kevern, 2000). The following questions guided the discussion:

1. When you hear the phrase, "a child who is strongly resistant to needle injection," what comes to mind?
2. What is it about these situations that is challenging for you?
3. What sorts of things have made it easier for you to immunize children who resist the needle injection?
4. What sorts of things have made it harder?
5. Do you have any thoughts on how these situations can be improved?

Content from these data sources was analyzed for themes. The transcripts were thoroughly read and reread, and a systematic process of content analysis was developed (Loiselle, Profetto-McGrath, Polit, & Beck, 2007; Speziale & Carpenter, 2003) to create the categorization and coding scheme that led to the themes. Trustworthiness was established through ongoing interaction and member checking with participants to confirm authenticity. Full ethical approval was granted by a university and a health authority.

The following four themes emerged from analyzing the survey and focus-group data collected from, and confirmed with, nurses who routinely immunized children. The themes represent nurses' perceptions of what it was about immunizing frightened and resistant children that was a problem for them. Verbatim comments are italicized. The themes are as follows: (a) nurses experience stress when immunizing children who fear and resist needle injection; (b) the strength of child resistance and some adult behavior creates

an ethical dilemma for nurses; (c) some adult responses make immunizing difficult and unsafe; (d) resources to help nurses cope with these situations are inconsistent.

THEME ONE: NURSES EXPERIENCE STRESS WHEN IMMUNIZING CHILDREN WHO FEAR AND RESIST NEEDLE INJECTION

Nurses used the word "dread" in all three focus groups to describe their apprehension about immunizing needle-resistant children, especially as a new practitioner. They described the situations as awkward, difficult, and complex, with "too many pieces" or variables. Nurses frequently recounted actual experiences to illustrate specific points. Feeling "flustered" and fearful of making a medication error or harming the child, as well as fear for the nurse's own safety, was reported in the survey and across all groups. Empathy for the child's "incredible panic and fear" was articulated, noting the child's "terror" and "screaming, kicking, and biting" behaviors as very disturbing. "I think of how hard it is to be scared. Like that's so much work on the child's part. It takes so much energy."

Crying was not seen as particularly difficult, but "acting out" behaviors and "struggling to get away, to get out of the room" were problems. "The child's terror, that's what gets to me." "I feel really badly for the child because they're embarrassed . . . and they're kind of ashamed." The nurses felt "torn" about the process. They found it "very disturbing" to witness the child's distress and felt "complicit in an assault." They described feelings of helplessness and uncertainty, wondering how "it might have been done differently." One nurse wrote, "I don't know how to make these situations more comfortable." Nurses felt ". . . pressured to just finish the job, no matter how much the child resists." Novice practitioners were more likely to feel pressured. "Throughout my orientation it was very heavily implied, it does not matter the situation, you always vaccinate children for as many vaccines as they're eligible for. And I just feel a lot of pressure to do that during that clinic visit." Sometimes, the pressure came from parents. "I've had two, three different scenarios where . . . the anger from the parents like, 'Whaddya mean . . .' And they're going to argue with you. 'I (parent) will hold them down and you **will** do it.'"

The nurses reported feeling drained, emotionally exhausted, fatigued, and unsupported. A sense of failure, guilt, "heavy heartedness," and frustration was expressed, as well as a "scary" feeling of being "out of control." One group likened the situation to "a circus," with "moms chasing (children) around to try to get them in and there is a waiting room full of people." Nurses described feeling hurt and annoyed when parents blamed and labeled them "the mean nurse" or "the stabber." Nurses were troubled by the potential for "emotional scarring" and serious erosion of trust in the child's relationship with health professionals. They suspected that past experiences strongly influenced the present and believed children deserve to be better prepared for immunization.

THEME TWO: THE STRENGTH OF CHILD RESISTANCE AS WELL AS SOME ADULT BEHAVIOR CREATES AN ETHICAL DILEMMA FOR NURSES

A major theme that emerged was the conflict around the child's right to refuse versus the right to be protected from preventable diseases. "I think as a nurse, the challenge is combining that gentle persuasion but with letting them make their own decision." "And we're taught in our profession you know, do no harm. So you feel like you're doing harm when you encounter situations where there's such strong resistance." A nurse wanted to find "a balance between helping the child find courage and protecting him from very dangerous diseases." Another stated the problem as

. . . the lack of respect it demonstrates to a child. In deciding on their behalf what is best for them I don't understand what makes that okay and at what age we give the child the control to make that decision. A problem for me is the subjectivity of deciding what's in the child's best interest; subjectivity in assessing potential harm to the child versus benefit of vaccine.

Within each group, two or more nurses recounted stories of especially challenging situations they thought had been handled poorly and felt regret about their involvement in the process. "There's some where you're going—oh that was awful! That didn't feel right. I don't feel good about that." Children kindergarten age and older were viewed as the most challenging, although some nurses also identified "strong toddlers" as difficult.

Nurses wondered, "How much restraint is too much?" A survey responder stated:

The problem becomes one of the child's right to object and refuse . . . some parents like to talk their children into shots; this takes quite a bit of time. Others are quite physical in their restraint methods and I don't know exactly when to step in and say—that's enough!

One nurse remarked:

I don't think the end always justifies the means. Because I had a father who came in with a son and he was really quite brutal with him. And we were really part of that because, you know, it was our end that we wanted to go to and that was the reason why. And I thought, I'm never doing that again. I'm just going to say, "I'm sorry, I can't do this. This is beyond what I can be part of."

Another recalled ". . . a mother actually physically sat on her child and restrained him and slapped his face and told him how much she loved him and told him to just do it. Okay, and that's always going to come to my mind. It was like an assault, us actually harassing him."

A colleague added:

Right, and then being torn between, Do I follow through, give it to him, get it over with for him? Will he have to go through this again? Or do I hold back and say, "Not under these circumstances." . . . It was a very awkward situation. "What do I do?" And I thought, "Let's get it over with for him. He'll have to go through that all over again or be bullied at home." But somehow we were then part of that.

It almost kind of reminds you, you know, of *One Flew Over the Cuckoo's Nest,* where they have to bind them down and they give them the electrical shock treatments and they don't want it.

A survey responder commented: "Immunization of children is recommended, not mandatory, therefore children may have the right to refuse." Another wrote:

The problem I have is with the three to five year olds who clearly verbalize they don't want the shot. We hold them down and do it anyways. From a young age we teach children to use their words. We teach them to say "no" to a stranger who offers candy, rides etc. We teach them to kick, scream, and run when a stranger touches them or they feel threatened by them, yet I am a stranger to this child who is saying "no" to me and I proceed and hurt the child. What message are we sending these children?

Children with developmental delays were particularly challenging. A nurse recalled immunizing a grade six boy with developmental delays, "It was really hard, because he wasn't going to sit still on his own. So we had a lot of hard decisions to make with that and mom held him down. It was awful."

In one group, a few of the more experienced nurses initially seemed somewhat dismissive of the issue as a sort of necessary evil; yet, even these nurses acknowledged with some surprise after the group "how much there was to talk about" on the topic. Challenging variables included "sheer number" of vaccines, complexities of vaccine administration, language barriers, lack of privacy in mass immunization clinics, circulating myths about needles getting stuck or breaking off in people's arms, unpredictability of some resistance, noise levels, too many people involved, and lack of time.

THEME THREE: SOME ADULT RESPONSES MAKE IMMUNIZING MORE DIFFICULT AND UNSAFE

Non-helpful responses by adults, such as parents, school staff, or other caregivers, were defined across all data sources as a burden to nurses. "So often what I find makes it really difficult . . . I'm not quite sure where to go with it when the parenting responses are **so** inappropriate." Most frequently cited non-helpful responses were either inadequate or overly forceful restraint by the parent; shaming, threatening, yelling, slapping, lying; or, alternately, pitying, placating, bribing, wishy-washy, and helpless parental behaviors. Nurses complained of getting kicked and hit by a struggling child and expressed frustration with parents who had not explained the purpose of the visit to the child.

In school situations, nurses felt frustrated when well-meaning adults interfered with the process by attempting to take control.

It isn't suddenly about being poked anymore. There's a bunch of family dynamics there as well and they get the power stuff going, and you put the child in the school situations, sometimes it's with the classroom teacher, you know, that's involved as well, and you think, "Oh boy, how many do we need involved in this really?" We sort of bring in all the skills you have, not just the needle part, but the kind of group skills too.

"It's tough for the nurse because, ultimately . . . we are in charge." Nurses reported that adults sometimes tease students in a way that increases anxiety and that students often "rile up" each other.

Nurses disliked having competitive elements introduced into the situation. For example, parents may complain if the nurse chooses not to proceed with the immunization, with comments such as: "She couldn't do it so I need another nurse." One nurse described her dismay if a parent would tell her, " 'my baby didn't cry at all last time . . . with the other nurse she didn't cry at all.' I don't know why they say that to me because it hurts, it jinxes me." And finally, nurses were frustrated with parents who project their own fears onto the child or communicate to the child expectations of resistant behavior, thus generating a self-fulfilling prophecy.

THEME FOUR: RESOURCES TO HELP NURSES COPE EFFECTIVELY WITH THESE SITUATIONS ARE INCONSISTENT AND INADEQUATE

Nurses voiced how existing strategies and resources to consistently support a positive immunization outcome were inadequate, inconsistently available, and poorly disseminated. Nurses described strategies they used to help in these situations with mixed results. Most of the strategies were learned through trial and error or direct observation. A nurse with more than 10 years of immunization experience stated: "In a school setting, I see it as a learning opportunity of just sitting back and seeing how somebody else handles it. I'm thinking, Thank God, I'm not the one who has to deal with it."

Nurses reported that crude forcible restraint is no longer as common as it once was. "I remember a principal holding a kid against the wall actually, believe that?"

> I think we're better at saying we can't do it than, let's say, fifteen years ago. I think we used to sit on kids more than we do now. I certainly, more now than I used to, just will say, "I can't do this" . . . whereas before . . . we used to get a couple of us in there and really, with the parent's permission of course, but were more forceful.

Several nurses described how they learned, sometimes through bitter experience, where to set boundaries.

> And also, the holding down or the forcing, I think . . . I do not have to give that, force that on that child. So I think that's something I've come to in my practice is that the child does not have to have it. We will not force this child to have it . . . and so that, yes, it is in

your best interest to have this. So let's work together with parents and help them to do this. But as far as the forcing, I will not be a party to this.

"We sort of learn like where **we** draw the line too, and that's hard sometimes." A nurse with less than 2 years experience said: "It's different in different places . . . like its [*sic*] okay for me here, to say we don't do that and I'm comfortable with that. But in another environment there might be more pressure I think, to get the thing done in a time frame."

The nurses described being supported in choosing to defer a vaccine as very important. A novice practitioner stated, "I don't think it's made clear to us that we can say no, that we don't have to do it." One survey response stated:

> Trying to put the child at ease who has become very anxious. This can be very draining and it can be difficult to know when to call it off. If you call it off, then the parent (if a kindergarten immunization) is then quite often angry. Sometimes it seems like there should be a policy or a sign that backs this up. The sign or policy stating we will not use force to immunize.

Collaborating with colleagues and being able to debrief were highly valued. Occasionally, nurses recruited each other to assist with restraint, yet, as one nurse pointed out, "It's the same thing again, like if you're getting another nurse. And then there are two of you holding the kid down." Another agreed, "Yeah, it makes it like a gang mentality. You know, we're all ganging up on him."

The nurses discussed what sorts of things could make it easier for them to effectively manage situations with resistant children. They recommended combination vaccines; labeled trays to hold pre-filled syringes; well-ventilated, soundproof clinic rooms; separate waiting rooms for before and after immunization; and time to debrief after a difficult session. Strategies identified as helpful included giving limited choices, using a calm voice, preparing parents for crying and giving children permission to cry, remaining firm but not threatening, using stickers to celebrate effort, and having distraction and calming tools, such as puppets, bubbles, comfort dolls, and cartoon videos, in waiting areas. Giving children time to express themselves but without engaging in endless negotiation is also important. Anesthesia was not discussed except in one survey response suggesting pre-procedural child sedation.

Nurses desire skills to effectively manage immunization procedures. "I don't have enough skills to know what the best response or techniques are to get the immunization done in a way that is most positive for everyone involved."

> I must admit, I'm better . . . more compassionate with kids that I perceive as being truly afraid (than with) those that I think are . . . just being smart alecks. Sometimes you get a child where you think, "Oh, you're just trying to pull my chain and get things riled up here." Or you see a child that is truly just terrified and I'm better with the kids that are [truly terrified], and maybe I might not even be reading it right.

"[I] . . . would like to learn about more techniques for self-calming." Another wrote, "Parents are often unaware of their child's ability to learn some of these skills and at how young an age it can be taught." Nurses viewed the clinic visit as an opportunity for children to acquire adaptive coping skills and experience mastery in an honest, respectful, supportive environment. Having enough time to prepare and also to debrief with parent and child was seen as important.

> There has been no time to prepare them in anticipation of them being that way [so wound up, not being able to focus and calm down]. We have nothing to offer these families. No opportunity to teach the parents . . . we're rushed and the parents are in a hurry and there's nothing else in place in another time to prepare them. We wind up being a part of it.

They identified a need to provide parents with clear direction about positioning, secure hold, and what not to say to their child, for example, limit bribes and threats, and avoid projecting parent fears onto the child. Referral to parent education sessions was a strategy employed where available. One nurse identified the focus-group session itself as a useful opportunity to "troubleshoot" and "brainstorm ideas." Another talked about "building up your repertoire of tools" and explained how she benefited by learning strategies from other nurses that would have "never occurred to me." The nurses expressed strong interest in educational materials that could be used by parents and children to better prepare for an immunization appointment.

DISCUSSION

These four themes, developed from discussions with nurses who routinely immunize children who fear and resist needles, illustrate how this procedure is problematic and stressful for nurses. The intensity of nurse stress is reflected in the language participants used to describe their experiences and in the vividness of their memories. The words "dread," "awful," "traumatizing," "failure," "assault," "terror," "fear," and "shame" appeared frequently in the data. Casting this response against Lazarus and Folkman's (1984) classic explanation that stress results when "demands exceed the personal and social resources an individual is able to mobilize," study findings lead us to question whether other nurses are also feeling that the demands of immunizing needle-resistant children exceed their ability to cope.

The comments reflect how the experience of forcing compliance from children generates ethical and moral dilemmas for nurses. Bioethicists Hodges et al. (2002) emphasized how heightened scrutiny is essential in situations where children, who are unlikely to be able to provide meaningful consent, are subjected to prophylactic interventions such as immunization. And yet, the issue may not be formally addressed with explicit policies and procedures in the practice arena. With the exception of the present study, the literature has not yet begun to acknowledge that a problem exists.

Nurses' descriptions of their memories of immunizing needle-resistant children were consistent with the moral distress Gunther and Thomas (2006) described in their exploration of patient care events that were unforgettable to nurses. In both studies, nurses wondered whether they could or should have done things differently even years later. Descriptions of their memories in the present study also reflected a sense of powerlessness. Feelings of moral distress, powerlessness, anxiety, and anger all contribute to the stress and burnout Thomas (2009) identified as a persistent issue among nurses. However, nurses' stress related to immunizing needle-resistant children has not been previously included in discussions of moral distress.

CONCLUSION

This article presented findings from a naturalistic action research study that explored nurses' perceptions of immunizing frightened and resistant children. In contrast to other studies that focused mainly on recipients of vaccines, this project extends existing knowledge by describing nurses' reflections on their own experiences with immunizing by identifying four overarching themes. This research found nurses experience stress when immunizing children who fear and resist needle injection, the strength of child resistance and some adult behavior creates an ethical dilemma for nurses, some adult responses make immunizing difficult and unsafe, and resources to help nurses cope with these situations are inconsistent. This article calls for the creation of more opportunities to explore whether or not immunizing needle-resistant children is a problem for other nurses. Articulating that a problem exists, that needle procedures are often stressful, and that the experience can leave nurses feeling morally and ethically conflicted is an important first step. Further study could lead to more consistent support for nurses who are responsible for immunizing children and to more positive outcomes for all.

REFERENCES

Appleton, J. J. V., & King, L. (2002). Journeying from the philosophical contemplation of constructivism to the methodological pragmatics of health services research. *Journal of Advanced Nursing, 40*(6), 641-648.

Blount, R., Devine, K., Cheng, P., Simons, L., & Hayutin, L. (2008). The impact of adult behaviors and vocalizations on infant distress during immunizations. *Journal of Pediatric Psychology, 33*(10), 1163-1174.

Bowen, A., & Dammeyer, M. (1999). Reducing children's immunization distress in a primary care setting. *Journal of Pediatric Nursing, 14*(5), 296-303.

Bustos, T., Jaaniste, T., Salmon, K., & Champion, D. (2008). Evaluation of a brief parent intervention teaching coping-promoting behavior for the infant immunization context. *Behavior Modification, 32*(4), 450-467.

Cohen, L., Blount, R., & Panopoulos, G. (1997). Nurse coaching and cartoon distraction: An effective and practical intervention to reduce child, parent and nurse distress during immunizations. *Journal of Pediatric Psychology, 22*(3), 355-370.

Cohen, L., Manimala, R., & Blount, R. (2000). Easier said than done: What parents say they do and what they do during children's immunizations. *Children's Health Care, 29*(2), 79-87.

Devine, K., Benoit, M., Simons, L., Cheng, P., Seri, L., & Blount, R. (2004). Psychological interventions for acute pediatric pain. *The Suffering Child, 6*, 1-22.

Duff, A. (2003). Incorporating psychological approaches into routine paediatric venipuncture. *Archives of Disease in Childhood, 88*, 931-937.

Ellis, J., Sharp, D., Newhook, K., & Cohen, J. (2004). Selling comfort: A survey of interventions for needle procedures in a pediatric hospital. *Pain Management Nursing, 5*(4), 144-152.

Frank, N., Blount, R., Smith, A., Manimala, R., & Martin, J. (1995). Parent and staff behavior, previous child medical experience, and maternal anxiety as they relate to child procedural distress and coping. *Journal of Pediatric Psychology, 20*(3), 277-289.

French, G., Painter, E., & Coury, D. (1994). Blowing away shot pain: A technique for pain management during immunization. *Pediatrics, 93*(3), 384-388.

Gaskell, S., Binns, F., Heyhoe, M., & Jackson, B. (2005). Taking the sting out of needles: Education for staff in primary care. *Paediatric Nursing, 17*(4), 24-28.

Gunther, M., & Thomas, S. (2006). Nurses' narratives of unforgettable patient care events. *Journal of Nursing Scholarship, 38*(4), 370-376.

Hamilton, J. (1995). Needle phobia: A neglected diagnosis. *Journal of Family Practice, 41*(2), 169-175.

Healy, C., & Mckay, M. (2000). Nursing stress: The effects of coping strategies and job satisfaction in a sample of Australian nurses. *Journal of Advanced Nursing, 31*(3), 681-688.

Hodges, F. M., Svoboda, J. S., & Van Howe, R. S. (2002). Prophylactic interventions on children: Balancing human rights with public health. *Journal of Medical Ethics, 28,* 10-16.

Ives, M. (2007). Model empathy and respect when immunizing children who fear needles. *The Canadian Nurse, 103*(4), 6-7.

Jacobson, R., Swan, A., Adegbenro, A., Ludington, S., Wollan, P., Poland, G., et al. (2001). Making vaccines more acceptable: Methods to prevent and minimize pain. *Vaccine, 19,* 2418-2427.

Kemmis, S., & McTaggart, R. (1988). *The action research planner* (3rd ed.). Geelong, Victoria, Australia: Deakin University Press.

Kemmis, S., & McTaggart, R. (1990). *The action research reader* (3rd ed.). Geelong, Victoria, Australia: Deakin University Press.

Krueger, R. A., & Casey, M. (2009). *Focus groups: A practical guide for applied research* (4th ed.). Thousand Oaks, CA: Sage.

Lawton, L., & Rose, P. (2003). Changing practice in invasive procedures: The experience of the Krishnan Chandran children's centre. *Journal of Child Health Care, 7*(4), 248-257.

Lazarus, R., & Folkman, S. (1984). *Stress, appraisal, and coping.* New York: Springer.

Loiselle, C., Profetto-McGrath, J., Polit, D., & Beck, C. (2007). *Canadian essentials of nursing research* (2nd ed.). Philadelphia: Lippincott, Williams & Wilkins.

Manimala, M., & Blount, R. (2000). The effects of parental reassurance versus distraction on child distress and coping during immunizations. *Children's Health Care, 29*(3), 161-177.

Martin, M., Ramsay, D., Whitney, C., Fiset, L., & Weinstein, P. (1994). Topical anesthesia: Differentiating the pharmacological and psychological contributions to efficacy. *Anesthesia Progress: A Journal for Pain and Anxiety Control in Dentistry, 41*(2), 40-47.

McVicar, A. (2003). Workplace stress in nursing: A literature review. *Journal of Advanced Nursing, 44*(6), 633-642.

Milgrom, P., Coldwell, S., Getz, T., Weinstein, P., & Ramsay, D. (1997). Four dimensions of fear of dental injections. *Journal of the American Dental Association, 128,* 756-762.

Morrison-Beedy, D., Cote-Arsenault, D., & Feinstein, N. (2001). Maximizing results with focus groups: Moderator and analysis issues. *Applied Nursing Research, 14*(1), 48-53.

O'Laughlin, E., & Ridley-Johnson, R. (1995). Maternal presence during children's routine immunizations: The effect of mother as observer in reducing child distress. *Children's Health Care, 24*(3), 175-191.

Peretz, B., & Efrat, J. (2000). Dental anxiety among young adolescent patients in Israel. *International Journal of Paediatric Dentistry, 10,* 126-132.

Polillio, A. M., & Kiley, J. (1997). Does a needless injection system reduce anxiety in children receiving intramuscular injections? *Pediatric Nursing, 23*(1), 46-49.

Schecter, N. L., Bernstein, B. A., Beck, A., Hart, L., & Scherzer, L. (1991). Individual differences in children's response to pain: Role of temperament and parental characteristics. *Pediatrics, 87*(2), 171-177.

Sherman, D. W. (2004). Nurses' stress and burnout. *The American Journal of Nursing, 104*(5), 48-56.

Smalley, A. (1999). Needle phobia. *Paediatric Nursing, 11*(2), 17-20.

Sparks, L. (2001). Taking the "ouch" out of injections for children: Using distraction to decrease pain. *American Journal of Maternal Child Nursing, 26*(2), 72-78.

Speziale, H., & Carpenter, D. (2003). *Qualitative research in nursing: Advancing the humanistic imperative* (3rd ed.). Philadelphia: Lippincott, Williams & Wilkins.

Stringer, E., & Genat, W. (2004). *Action research in health.* Upper Saddle River, NJ: Pearson Prentice Hall.

Thomas, S. (2009). *Transforming nurses' stress and anger: Steps toward healing* (3rd ed.). New York: Springer.

Uman, L. S., Chambers, C. T., McGrath, P. J., & Kisely, S. (2006). Psychological interventions for needle-related procedural pain and distress in children and adolescents. *Cochrane Database of Systematic Reviews, 4.*

Webb, C., & Kevern, J. (2000). Focus groups as a research method: A critique of some aspects of their use in nursing research. *Journal of Advanced Nursing, 33*(6), 798-805.

Windich-Biermeier, A., Sjoberg, I., Dale, J. C., Eshelman, D., & Guzzetta, C. (2007). Effects of distraction on pain, fear, and distress during venous port access and venipuncture in children and adolescents with cancer. *Journal of Pediatric Oncology Nursing, 24*(1), 8-19.

INTRODUCTION TO CRITIQUE 1

The preceding article (Ives & Melrose, 2010) is an example of an action research design. The article is critically examined here for its rigour as an action research study, its contribution to nursing, and its usefulness in practice. The criteria listed in Box 18-1 are used to guide the critique.

Title

The title of the article captured the essence of the study; however, it did not address the secondary purpose of the article to consider approaches that would help reduce nurse stress during immunization.

Abstract

The abstract met the requirements of a good abstract: It contained the background and method (including the purpose and the sample size), and it concluded with the results.

Statement of the Phenomenon of Interest

Ives and Melrose (2010) clearly stated the phenomenon of interest expressed in the research question "What is it about immunizing children who strongly resist needle injection that is a problem for public health nurses?" (p. 29). The authors acknowledged that needle phobia is a common problem and that extensive research has explored nonhelpful and helpful responses of adults to reduce children's distress during a needle injection. Very little research, however, focuses on the nurse's response to immunizing fearful children and how to cope with the subsequent stress. Because nurses' responses are unknown in this field of study, the qualitative research method is appropriate.

Purpose

The purpose of the research project was twofold. First the authors wanted to investigate "the experiences, reflections, and feelings of public health nurses who immunize fearful and needle-resistant children" (p. 29). In addition to exploration of the nurses' perceptions, the authors were interested in approaches that would decrease nurses' stress. The researchers clearly assumed that nurses who immunize children, who in turn fear and resist needles, find the experience stressful. This assumption was supported in the literature review. In many qualitative studies, researchers conduct a cursory literature review so that the findings unfold naturally without a bias. In this case, the literature review probably helped frame the design of the study. The literature review focused on the fear of needles, helpful and nonhelpful adult responses, and nurse stress.

Method

The method was described in a section called "The research approach." The authors used a constructivist theoretical perspective to explore the experiences, reflections, and feelings of the participants. They did not describe the philosophical underpinnings or approach of this method in any detail but were quite explicit in describing the second research method of naturalistic action research design. It is important that the authors identify the theoretical underpinnings of their chosen method and how the two approaches in one study support and inform the other. Appleton and King (2002), referenced in the study, stated that constructivist and participative research (action research) share common methodological steps. It is difficult to assess whether Ives and Melrose's (2010) study adhered to the processes for constructivist and action research, inasmuch as the authors did not clearly explain how they incorporated the methodologies. They did indicate that action research has an action component in which action is taken to improve practice. Although Ives and Melrose did gather the data from the participants on how the situation could be improved, no action was taken in this study to try out new ideas.

Sampling

A survey was sent to a sample of nurses working in five different public health units. Of the 58 nurses who received preliminary survey questions, 35 responded that they immunized children as part of their practice. Although it was not stated explicitly, it appears that of the 35 respondents, 15 to 18 nurses participated in focus groups. In qualitative research, the most common type of sampling is purposive or purposeful sampling. According to Streubert and Carpenter (2011), "individuals are selected to participate in qualitative research based on their first-hand experience with a culture, social process, or phenomenon of interest" (p. 28). This ability to describe an experience from one's own perspective is what makes selection purposive. In this study, all participants had experience with immunizations of children; thus the selection of participants was appropriate.

Data Collection

The primary source of data was a series of three audiorecorded and transcribed focus groups. The researchers described the focus groups as "2 weeks apart, each with five to six female, English-speaking, Caucasian and Indo-Canadian nurses, from five different health units in one Canadian province" (p. 32). The focus groups were selected an early survey that differentiated between nurses who immunized children and those who did not. Five questions were used to guide the discussion:

1. When you hear the phrase, "a child who is strongly resistant to needle injection," what comes to mind?
2. What is it about these situations that is challenging for you?
3. What sorts of things have made it easier for you to immunize children who resist the needle injection?
4. What sorts of things have made it harder?
5. Do you have any thoughts on how these situations can be improved?

The questions were formulated to elicit the participants' descriptions of their experiences and understanding and, in addition, how practice can be improved.

Focus groups are commonly used in qualitative research, and their use was appropriate in this study, although researchers need to be cautious about the development of groupthink. in which one dominant participant can influence other group members (Streubert & Carpenter, 2011). Because the researchers did not identify how they would manage this situation or gather data from other participants through individual interview or observation, this is a potential weakness of the data-collection method.

Ethical approval was sought and received from a university and a health authority who had jurisdiction over the health units.

Data Analysis

The authors indicated that they analyzed the data for themes. Each of the transcripts from the focus groups was "thoroughly read and reread, and a systemic process of content analysis was developed . . . to create the categorization and coding scheme that led to the themes" (p. 32). No further detail was provided.

In general, the measure of rigour in qualitative research is trustworthiness. Trustworthiness includes the concepts of credibility, auditability, and fittingness. It is difficult to determine whether the researchers addressed the **auditability** (to what extent another researcher or a reader can follow method and conclusions drawn by the original researcher[s]) and **fittingness** (how applicable the study findings are to others in similar situations) of the data (see Chapter 14 for complete discussion). Although the researchers did specify that they established trustworthiness by "ongoing interaction and member checking with participants to confirm authenticity" (p. 32), they did not clarify how they accomplished this.

Findings

The authors reported their findings clearly and comprehensively. To provide authenticity of the findings, they provided quotations from the participants, allowing the voices of the nurses to be heard. Each of the four themes that emerged were confirmed with the nurses who participated. The description of each theme was thorough and compelling in the depth of description. The findings seemed to accurately reflect the conceptualization of the emergent themes. The findings were then placed in the context of what is known about nurse stress and immunizations with needle-resistant children, particularly through the literature on stress, ethical and moral dilemmas, and moral distress.

Conclusions, Implications, and Recommendations

The authors resummarized the findings of the nurses' perceptions of immunizing needle-resistant children and called for the creation of more opportunities to explore whether this is a problem for other nurses. Because one of the identified purposes of this study was to consider approaches that are helpful to decrease nurses' stress, the lack of recommendations is a major gap in this study: "Action research is specifically designed as a research method whose outcome is the implementation of an action or change" (Streubert & Carpenter, 2011, p. 308). Because it is clear from the study that administering injections to resistant children is an ethical and moral dilemma for nurses, causing stress and internal conflict, the lack of recommendations is unfortunate. Careful application of action research methods in this study could have resulted in significant changes in practice and contribution to nursing knowledge.

CRITIQUE 2

The study "Women's Decisions to Seek Treatment for the Symptoms of Potential Cardiac Illness" by Sheila A. Turris (2009) is critiqued here. The article is presented in its entirety and is followed by the critique on pp. 430–432. (From *Journal of Nursing Scholarship, 41*[1], 5-12. © 2009 Sigma Theta Tau International.)

Women's Decisions to Seek Treatment for the Symptoms of Potential Cardiac Illness

Sheila A. Turris, RN, PhD
Vancouver Coastal Health
Vancouver, British Columbia

Cardiac disease is the number one killer of Canadian women and therapies are often highly time dependent. Consequently, understanding the forms of knowledge that women draw upon to understand and interpret their symptoms of a potential cardiac event may be important in relation to efforts to reduce treatment-seeking delay. Data for this grounded-theory study were drawn from in-depth interviews with 16 women who went to one of two emergency departments between June 2005 and June 2006 for the treatment of symptoms indicating potential cardiac illness. The basic social process of maintaining integrity explained the women's interpretations of and actions in relation to their symptoms. This paper indicates the findings as they relate to specific forms of knowledge the women used to make decisions about treatment-seeking, including embodied, temporal, rational, and relational ways of knowing.

CLINICAL RELEVANCE: The results of this study contribute to the body of knowledge with regard to women's decisions about seeking treatment for the symptoms of potential cardiac illness.

KEYWORDS: Cardiovascular, grounded theory, women's health, qualitative methodology/qualitative research, research methods

Heart disease is the leading cause of death in Canada (Canadian Institute of Health Information, 2006) and the number one killer of Canadian women (Statistics Canada, 2004). If a cardiac arrest takes place at home, survival rates are dismal (Herlitz, Eek, Holmberg, Engdahl, & Holmberg, 2002). Last year in the United States, an estimated 310,000 people died before reaching an emergency department (ED) for treatment of a cardiac event (American Heart Association, 2008). Attention is being directed to a mandate of treatment within 1 hour of symptom onset, given the number of deaths that occur in the first hour (McKinley et al., 2004). Treatment-seeking delay (TDS), in the context of cardiac illness, is a persistent clinical issue.

When considering the literature with regard to TSD, gender and social support have also garnered a great deal of attention. Specifically, there is considerable debate about gender expectations concerning cardiac symptoms. For example, a persistent belief is held by both men and women that men are more prone than are women to acute myocardial infarction (Hammond, Salamonson, Davidson, Everett, & Andrew, 2007; Harralson, 2007; Lefler & Bondy, 2004). One perception is that women handle stress more effectively and are therefore perceived as being protected from myocardial infarctions (Richards, Reid, & Watt, 2002). Some evidence also exists to show that women are more likely to delay treatment than are men: however, contradictory evidence is reported. Although some researchers have found that being women is associated with greater delay (Bowker et al., 2000; Hannegan et al., 2000; Goldberg, Gurwitz, & Gore, 1999) others have found that gender contributes no unique variance to delay time (Moser, McKinley, Dracut, & Cluing, 2005).

Social support has also been studied with a particular focus on advice seeking after the onset of symptoms indicative of cardiac illness. Researchers have consistently found an association between seeking advice from a physician and prolonged decision time (Bowker el al., 2000; Zerwic, Ryan, DeVon, & Drell, 2003).

Similarly, seeking advice from a relative (Rosenkid, 2004) and living alone (Banks & Dracup, 2006) are typically associated with a delay in seeking treatment. In this grounded theory study, a sample of women explained their decision-making processes in relation to visiting an ED for treatment of symptoms indicating potential cardiac illness. The findings are reported as they relate to the specific forms of knowledge the women used to make decisions about treatment seeking.

METHODS

Grounded theory (GT), the method used for this study, involves a systematic generation of theory from data. These data are constantly compared, at increasing levels of abstraction, searching for evidence of a core category. One goal of GT is to discover the main concern of participants and how they are trying to address that concern. In GT, one does not aim for "the truth;" but rather the goal is to explain what is going on in relation to the phenomenon of concern. The research question was: "In the context of having symptoms suggestive of cardiac illness, what process guides women as they interpret their symptoms, make decisions about their treatment options, and subsequently make sense of their experiences of ED care?"

Setting

This project was undertaken with the approval of the university's behavioural research ethics board, as well as the relevant hospitals' ethics boards. Data were collected from two EDs in a western Canadian province, targeting one tertiary-care and one community hospital, both with more than 50,000 ED visits a year. Hospital A is a tertiary-care referral centre for the province. In contrast,

Hospital B is a community hospital, located in a residential suburb. Hospital B is not designated as a trauma hospital, and staff did not have the infrastructure necessary to carry out rescue angiographic procedures that might be required for the treatment of acute myocardial infarction.

Sampling and Procedures

At the beginning of the study, the sample was a purposive sample drawn from a group of women who sought ED care for the treatment of symptoms of a potential cardiac illness at one of two hospital EDs. To participate in this study, individuals had to be: women, visiting either of the two EDs for treatment of the symptoms of a potential cardiac event, hemodynamically stable, 18 years of age or older, able to speak English, and competent to provide informed consent. If a woman met the inclusion criteria, permission was requested for contact several days following discharge to arrange a convenient time and location for a more formal, audiotaped interview, and she was provided with an information letter about the study. Each participant had more than 24 hours to consider whether she wanted to participate. Following discharge, the women were contacted by telephone and a mutually convenient date, time, and location for an interview was arranged. Before being interviewed, written consent was obtained, and a copy of the consent form was provided. The women were also reminded that they could choose not to respond to particular interview questions, or to request that the tape recorder be turned off at any time. In these ways, ongoing informed consent was addressed. The audiotaped interviews took between 30 and 90 minutes to complete. The transcripts were password protected and identifying data were removed.

Data Analysis

Data collection and analysis were done concurrently. The accounts of 10 participants were obtained as a starting point for this project. Sampling continued to ensure that categories were "dense" and well developed; support for the relationships among the categories and the contributions of categories to the core category were explored. Theoretical sampling was used to collect further information. For example, when analysis of the data suggested age might play a role in women's decisions about treatment seeking, the accounts of younger women were actively sought. Upon the conclusion of the project, a total of 16 women had been interviewed.

Analysis of the data occurred over several months and involved open, selective, and theoretical coding. Each level of coding moved the data analysis toward increasing levels of abstraction. Open coding was the first step. Incidents were compared to other incidents and similarities and differences were sought, compared with other concepts, and subsequently grouped to form categories. This process is termed constant comparative analysis. Initially, labels for the categories were drawn from the interviews directly. As the analysis proceeded, the labels became increasingly explanatory. Gradually, information was grouped according to relationships and interactions; important concepts became apparent in successive accounts.

These concepts contributed to development of increasingly complex categories to explain what was going on in the women's accounts. Categories had two essential features: they were both analytic and sensitizing. The former refers to the quality of being sufficiently abstract and the latter refers to the ability of a code to generate a meaningful picture (Glaser & Strauss, 1999). Initially, the categories were general and broad; they became more specific and better developed as new data were constantly compared with that obtained in earlier interviews. Evidence of the core category was sought throughout the analytic process.

Rigor

The specific criteria for rigor in a GT study includes "fit," "work," "relevance," and "modifiability"

(Bonner & Tolhurst, 2001; Glaser, 1992). In commencing the project, the initial research question was clear and the design of the study was appropriate for the research goals. Each successive interview with a participant allowed confirmation (or obtaining a contrasting account) and further developing themes from earlier accounts. In these ways, the emerging theory was confirmed to fit the data. Fit is described as the extent to which a theory fits or describes the situations in the social area under study. Glaser and Strauss (1999) pointed out that a lack of fit results in the need to force the data to fit the core category emerging. During biweekly meetings of the research team, discussing the early findings allowed identification of gaps in the analysis and contributed to development of an integrated theory.

Relevance, in the context of GT, is the idea that the theory produced should be relevant to action in the area it purports to explain (Lomberg & Kirkevold, 2003). One might ask, to what extent does the theory generated explain actual problems and basic social psychological processes in the research setting? The issue of relevance was addressed in the following specific ways. As data were collected, emerging themes were checked with the participants, as well as with a group of colleagues, asking specifically about the explanatory power of the emerging theory.

Finally, with regard to rigor, the issue of modifiability was considered. Modifiability is a quality of the theory produced (Glaser, 1992). A theory should be able to evolve and encompass new information. For example, a rigorous GT explaining women's decisions in relation to their symptoms might be used as a starting point for researching men's decisions.

In a GT approach, the goal is to formulate hypotheses based on conceptual ideas and to discover participants' main concern and how they continually try to resolve it; this is done through the analysis of empirical data. The findings reported in this manuscript are from a larger study focused on the investigation of women's decisions about the symptoms of potential cardiac events, and their subsequent experiences of care in an ED (Tunis & Johnson, 2008). The following discussion indicates the findings as they relate specifically to the women's decisions about seeking treatment. In the larger study, the basic social process of maintaining integrity was identified encompassing three phases: resisting disruption, suspending agency, and integrating new knowledge and experiences. In the first phase, resisting disruption, participants drew on particular forms of knowledge to make decisions about their symptoms of potential cardiac events. The findings indicated below further our understanding about the decisions women make in relation to the symptoms of potential cardiac events and therefore have potentially important implications for nursing practice.

FINDINGS

Ages of participants ranged from 29 to 89 years. Slightly fewer than half were employed at the time of the interview. Roughly one fourth of the participants were married and half had children. The majority of women experienced the onset of symptoms while at home; 7 participants reported that family members were present when the symptoms began. In relation to the amount of time that elapsed between onset of the symptoms, delay ranged from approximately 30 minutes to more than 48 hours. Twenty percent of the participants were transported to the ED by ambulance; 62% drove in a private vehicle. Roughly one third of the participants received a cardiac-related diagnosis.

According to accounts of the participants, decisions about treatment seeking were influenced primarily by the context of the women's lives as mothers, daughters, and wives and only secondarily by the women's interpretations of, and conclusions about, their symptoms. Resisting disruption of their personal, social, and physical integrity was a dynamic process influenced by particular ways of knowing. Four ways of knowing were evident in the data including: embodied, temporal, rational, and relational knowing. The women used these ways of knowing to understand and interpret their symptoms within a larger personal and social context. The understandings gleaned from particular ways of knowing provided information about specific threats to the women's personal, social, and physical integrity and, most important, shaped decisions about treatment seeking.

Embodied Knowing

Embodied knowing indicated information about the subjective, visceral experience of symptoms in relation to quality, intensity, and effects. The visceral experience of the symptoms was prominent in each account of the participants in this study. For example, one participant reported,

> I didn't feel any stress. I wasn't tense at all . . . I started feeling chest pain . . . chest tightness more than chest pain . . . I remember that I was a little bit short of breath and my head was pounding and I noticed that my hands were shaking.

Important features of embodied knowing included the number of symptoms experienced; the intensity of those symptoms; the development of any new symptoms; and evaluation of symptoms based on past experiences, as well as the degree to which the symptoms interfered with normal daily activities. With rare exceptions, the understanding gained from embodied knowing delayed treatment seeking. In fact, the minimization of symptoms was a recurring theme. The participants made particular assumptions about what constituted an emergency. The criteria for an emergency included visibility. The illness or injury had to be readily apparent to others and not simply an internal experience. For example, when presented with a scenario in which a fall occurred and resulted in an ankle fracture, the women expressed no hesitation about visiting an ED. In contrast, the symptoms of a cardiac event are internal, for the most part, and not always obvious to bystanders or family members. As one women explained,

> If it's not so significant that people are turning around on the street looking as I go past, I could wait . . . until I've got a day off, or I'll find something is open on a Saturday, but it will wait . . . it will definitely wait, it's not that bad. . . . If I had a compound fracture I don't think I'd hesitate to bother somebody, but I think things like whatever was the matter with me that isn't completely debilitating, you can still go to the store, you can still . . . look after your husband, your children, or your dog, you know can certainly wait until tomorrow.

Ideas about gender were used to downgrade the level of threat attached to the experience of the symptoms. For example, participants frequently mentioned the belief that women have "a higher pain tolerance" than men and accordingly the experience of pain was often dismissed or rated as unimportant. One participant said,

> I think if I had been given half a chance, by about 9:30 or l0:00 that morning I might have come home and just lie down and decided I'll just see if it doesn't go away on its own . . . I think women are more stoic than men and I think it would . . . you know, when a man is going [making sound of breathing hard] . . . I think women just think, "Oh, I'll take an aspirin."

Although embodied knowledge primarily delayed treatment seeking, two important exceptions were noted. First, the development of new symptoms usually prompted participants to reconsider their initial evaluation of the significance of their condition, and this reconsideration usually resulted in a prompt visit to the ED. Second, it the symptoms interfered with the women's ability to work, drive, or take care of their families, this constituted appropriate grounds for seeking treatment.

Temporal Knowing

Temporal knowing indicated the contributions of time in relation to the women's interpretation of their symptoms. The women did not measure time in minutes and hours. Instead, time was divided into sections based on social convention (e.g., meal times) and were sometimes pivotal in the women's decisions about treatment seeking. Symptoms could be minimized during the night— that is, a woman might say to herself, "I'll go to the hospital in the morning if I still have the pain." Similarly, symptoms that started before breakfast were judged to be serious only alter additional meals had passed. These time segments were often seen as milestones. Most of the participants in this study expressed a desire to "wait and see" whether the symptoms resolved spontaneously.

Temporal knowing also drew upon the past experiences of the participants. For example, several of the women spoke about interpreting their recent event in light of a past cardiac event, in order to estimate the threat level. One participant had had an acute myocardial infarction 6 months before the interview. She spoke about her need to analyze every ache and pain in light of this event.

> [My] assessment skills before were very on until this whole issue came up and then all of a sudden this . . . it just means that all the ways I looked at discomfort and all the ways I looked at pain and handled them in no nonsense ways and everything and this just makes you sort of second guess it, you know?

The use of a past event to evaluate the current threat was time limited: With the passage of time, the past event became less significant. If a previous cardiac event had occurred relatively recently, the participants were likely to associate the new event with that event and to promptly seek medical attention. However, if the original event was in the distant past, participants were more likely to delay, while considering many other causes for their symptoms.

Rational Knowing

Rational knowing indicated knowledge gleaned from the media, reported statistics, and general information about women and heart disease. Almost without exception, participants in this study noted that women have different symptoms of a heart attack than do men. An assessment of personal risk for heart disease, drawing on their knowledge of their family history and personal health history, was also prominent in their accounts. Yet even when participants expressed concern about their level of risk (i.e., strong family history of premature heart disease), a prompt visit to an ED did not always occur. The only time that rational knowledge was prominent in reducing treatment delay was when such knowledge was taken up by family members. Family members used this knowledge to force action on the part of the participants. Often, the primary reason participants came to the ED for treatment was because a daughter or other family member had insisted on that particular course of action. In this situation, the women were not able to resist disruption and visited an ED, however reluctantly.

Relational Knowing

Relational knowing indicates the knowledge that arises from being part of a social world composed of relationships and interactions that shape behaviour and meaning. Important features of relational knowing included perceptions about the social consequences of seeking or delaying medical treatment. Relational knowing was pivotal in influencing decisions.

In terms of the social costs associated with choosing to seek treatment, four issues of concern were described. First, the participants discussed the dangers associated with not seeking treatment and carrying on with the normal activities of their daily lives. Considerations about the dangers of driving (e.g., colliding with another car in the process of driving oneself to the ED) and the risk to others if one collapsed at work and accidentally injured someone else in the process were examples of the concerns expressed by participants. For example,

> I wasn't doing very much, so it wasn't like it was a big stressful deal, but you know, when you're running out the door to go to work and everything like this and you've got to think about it and you don't want to be . . . you don't want to collapse at work and have somebody say, "You know, you shouldn't have come to work." As it is at work, they're always saying to me. "I always worry about you driving yourself to the hospital," and I'm thinking, "Oh my God!" I said, "I keep to the outside lane."

Second, the effect of treatment-seeking decisions on the social roles held by the women within their families was often a critical influence on their ultimate decisions. In the following example, a participant explained her perspective about the social costs to her if she acted on her experience of symptoms, admitting illness.

> Well . . . my family demographics . . . the whole thing . . . the boys always rule [laughs]. That seems to be sort of how things go . . . just family politics. . . . You sort of feel a bit like the family black sheep and yet I'm the one they all phone. But you just don't want to give them any more . . . anything else that makes you feel like a flake.

Other women emphasized that responsibility at home, particularly in relation to young children, influenced decisions about seeking treatment. One woman explained that she had not told anyone at all about the chest pain, partly because she had children and no child-care. She also refused to call a friend and take that person away from her own children.

Third, relational knowing was to a great extent about understanding treatment-seeking options within a larger social framework. Specifically, the women expressed concern that they would "waste" health-care resources. The women who delayed seeking treatment explained that underlying the decision to "wait and see" was a desire to balance on the one hand, the reality that something might be wrong, and on the other hand, the reality that if nothing was medically wrong, social embarrassment and wasted health-care resources would result.

> I kept thinking, with me, that it . . . will go away on its own and particularly having been into emergency Monday morning, you just looked around and you

thought, "These people have just so much to do, there aren't enough of them, they're overwhelmed, I don't want to bother these people with this little whatever it is I've got because I'm not bleeding, I'm not throwing [up]." And you look around and the place is just jumping. You do feel a bit like, "Oh, wow! What am I doing here? Don't bother them." That probably says it quite well. "Wow! There's sick people here. What am I doing here?"

Finally, relational knowing prompted the women to explore not only the cause of their symptoms, but to interpret those symptoms within the context of their values and the quality of their lives. As one participant stated,

I would prefer to go . . . if I'm going to pop off someday, that I pop off with something that's final: that I don't get rescued to be a "case," you know. But I'm not ready to go yet: I've got things to do.

In contrast, several of the participants in this study shared their experiences of multiple losses such as children, partners, and close friends, as well as being concerned about their growing dependence on their family members. They reported that given their age, and these losses, they were not unhappy at the thought of experiencing a cardiac event that might result in death. Several women provided examples of "perfect days" they had had, and in this context spoke about death and expressed an acceptance that "it may be my time" and "I have lived a good life." One participant stated, "If it is God's will, He will take you home. I have had a good life and I am ready." For these women, the onset of symptoms was, if not welcome, then timely. Not surprisingly, this group of women did not tend to seek treatment in a timely fashion, but rather delayed—often for days—until a family member intervened.

In summary, the women in this study analyzed their symptoms and managed the situation, actively problem solving. Their goal was to resist any disruption to the rhythm of their daily lives or to their images of themselves as healthy and capable of continuing to be good mothers, good wives, and good employees. As discussed above, particular forms of knowledge were employed in the decisions made by the women in relation to their treatment seeking. The findings of this study indicate that attending to role responsibilities as wives and mothers was judged to be vital, whereas attending to symptoms that might indicate cardiac disease was given a lower priority.

DISCUSSION

More than 30 years have passed since Carper (1978) published her paper, "Ways of Knowing." Although this paper does not extend Carper's work, our analysis of these data confirms Carper's theory; specifically, there are many ways to know and understand the world. Women making decisions about treatment seeking draw upon particular forms of knowledge, here characterized as "ways of knowing." In nursing and the social sciences, this terminology is not uncommon. Belenky, Clinchy, Goldberger, and Tarule (1986) used the term to describe received, subjective, procedural, and constructed forms of knowledge. Use of the phrase is in line with Carper's (1978) ways of knowing in nursing practice (e.g., empirical, ethical, esthetic, and personal) or Benner's (1984) case, patient, and person knowledge, which is used by expert nurses.

In terms of the larger body of literature on TSD, several findings of this study are noteworthy. Although the results of this study were in concordance with the findings of other researchers who reported that rational knowledge—that is, knowledge about women's risk of heart disease, or the symptoms of a heart attack—plays little role in reducing TSD (Dempsey, Dracup, & Moser, 1995), the extent to which such information was used by family members to urge action was surprising. In fact, the results of this study are in conflict with reports that consultation with family members increases delay (Hartford, Sjolin, & Herlitz, 1993; Rosenfeld, 2004). For the participants, consulting family members for advice typically resulted in an immediate visit to an ED, a visit that might not have taken place at all without such a consultation. The results of this study indicate that the relationship between TSD and seeking advice should be re-examined. Because women who do not visit an ED are not included in studies, there might be misinterpretation regarding the effect of family intervention.

Although there are consistent reports of women underestimating their risk of heart disease as compared with men (Oliver-McNeil & Artinian, 2002), participants in this study were well aware that women were at equal risk and that women's symptoms might differ from those of men in a similar situation, suggesting that the message is getting out to the public. However, the data from this study do not confirm that this knowledge affected the women's decisions about treatment seeking.

In addition, it was noteworthy that none of the participants in this study had knowledge about medications or medical procedures that might reduce damage to the heart muscle during a myocardial infarction. Therefore, it might be important to consider that particular types of information are more effective than others in relation to reducing TSD. For example, several researchers report that although education about the symptoms of a myocardial infarction did not make a difference, knowledge about thrombolytic therapy and angioplasty did reduce delay (Dracup, McKinley, & Moser, 1997: Moser et al., 2006).

Advancing age is sometimes reported to be associated with longer delays. The results of this study indicate that further exploration of this relationship might be useful. A basic assumption of this study was that reducing TSD is worthwhile because such a reduction addresses the clinical problem of premature death from an acute myocardial infarction. However, the women in this study who were more than 80 years of age reported that when deciding whether to seek treatment, they paused to reflect on their lives and expressed a sense of acceptance that the symptoms they were experiencing might be timely given their situations in relation to age, marital status, and life satisfaction.

Conflicting reports in healthcare literature, regarding the association between past medical history (e.g., previous acute myocardial infarction) and TSD have persisted for the past two decades (Ho, Eisenberg, Litwin, Schaeffer, & Damon, 1989; Leitch, Birbara, Freedman, Wilcox, & Harris, 1989: Wu, Zhang, Li, Hong, & Huang, 2004). The results of the present study show that this might in part be because of the length of time that has passed between the original event and the recurrence, indicating that further exploration of this relationship might be useful. For the participants in this study, if a prior health event occurred within 18 months of the ED visit, the women were likely to attribute their symptoms to a cardiac cause, rather than a more benign gastrointestinal or musculoskeletal cause. If subsequent studies show an association between a reduction in delay and recent past medical history, this might be emphasized in interactions with primary healthcare professionals. For example, a physician or nurse practitioner might say, "As more time passes, you will be tempted to relax and become less vigilant about the symptoms of a heart attack. This would put you at risk."

LIMITATIONS

When interpreting the results of this study, several limitations should be considered, particularly in relation to the design of the study. First, the accounts and experiences of women who did not come to an ED for treatment are missing. It is possible, and indeed probable, that decision making differs for this group in comparison to the sample for this study. Second, women who were critically ill were not recruited for participation in this study because of hemodynamic instability.

Third, one must bear in mind that this is a single study. As such, the results add to our understanding about treatment-seeking delay and experiences of ED care but are an insufficient basis upon which to recommend change. Finally, qualitative findings are not open to generalization but might further add to information about phenomena of interest.

IMPLICATIONS FOR NURSING PRACTICE

The subset of findings reported in this manuscript suggest that TSD is to a great extent a social phenomenon, and not, as currently portrayed in the healthcare literature, primarily a product of individual factors. Participants in this study made decisions about treatment seeking based on particular ways of knowing. They used temporal, embodied, rational, and relational knowledge to understand and interpret their symptoms of a potential cardiac event. Understanding the forms of knowledge used by women in making decisions indicates the process by which decisions about treatment are made and allows us to have conversations with women about those decisions before a crisis arises. For example, understanding that women tend to prioritize family needs above their own health needs might give us an opportunity to open a conversation about decision making in the context of the symptoms of an acute cardiac event during nonurgent healthcare encounters.

Theory about TSD is currently focused primarily on the proximate causes ignoring, for the most part, the larger social context of treatment seeking highlighted by the participants in this study. Understanding TSD as a social phenomenon may widen the focus of research, and this is vital because only 41% of the variance in decision times is explained by a model that includes gender, age, past medical history, comorbidities, educational level, and the presence of family members (Wu et al., 2004). Developing an understanding with regard to the forms of knowledge underpinning women's decisions about their symptoms allows an exploration of decision making from women's perspectives, rather than approaching the discussion exclusively from the perspective of healthcare professionals.

CONCLUSIONS

This project arose from a strong interest in outcomes for women who experience symptoms of potential cardiac illness and seek treatment in an ED. A unique contribution of this study is a broad focus on women's decisions in relation to potential symptoms of cardiac illness rather than an exclusive focus on those who have actually been diagnosed with an acute myocardial infarction. A clear understanding with regard to the decisions undertaken by women experiencing symptoms of potential cardiac illness can "inform" nursing interventions before a cardiac event, preventing death and reducing morbidity. This work advances theory development in relation to TSD, making a contribution to existing theory and research about this clinical issue.

ACKNOWLEDGEMENTS

This research was supported by scholarships and awards from the Canadian Institutes of Health Research (CIHR), the Michael Smith Foundation for Health Research, the Nexus Research Unit at the University of British Columbia, and the *Xi Eta* Chapter of Sigma Theta Tau International. I also acknowledge the helpful comments of Drs. Joy Johnson, Pamela Ratner, and Bonita Long, and thank the study participants.

CLINICAL RESOURCES

- American Diabetes Association: http://www.diabetes.org/diabetes-heart-disease-stroke.jsp
- American Heart and Stroke Foundation: http://www.amhrt.org/presenter.jhtml?identifier=1200000

- British Heart Foundation: http://www.bhf.org.uk/
- Canadian Heart and Stroke Foundation: http://ww2.heartandstroke.ca/splash/
- Framingham Heart Study: http://www.frarningham.com/heart/
- National Heart, Lung, and Blood Institute (2009): http://www.nhlbi.nih.gov//educational/hearttruth/

REFERENCES

American Heart Association. (2008). *Heart disease and stroke statistic, 2008 update* (pp. 1-41). Dallas, TX: Author.

Banks, A. D., & Dracup, K. (2006). Factors associated with prolonged prehospital delay of African Americans with acute myocardial infarction. *American Journal of Critical Care, 15*, 149-157.

Belenky, M. F., Clinchy. B., Goldberger, M., & Tarule, J. (1986). *Women's way of knowing: The development of self, voice, and mind*. New York: Basic.

Benner, P. (1984). *From novice to expert*. New York: Addison Wesley.

Bonner, A., & Tolhurst, G. (2001). Insider-outsider perspectives of participant observation. *Nurse Researcher, 9*(4), 7-19.

Bowker, T. J., Turner, R. M., Wood, T. L., Roberts, T. L., Curzen, M., Gandhi, M., et al. (2000). A national survey of acute myocardial infarction and ischaemia (SAMII) in the UK: Characteristics, management and in-hospital outcome in women compared to men in patients under 70 years. *European Heart Journal, 21*, 1458-1463.

Canadian Institute of Health Information. (2006). *Health care in Canada*. Ottawa: Author.

Carper, B. A. (1978). Fundamental patterns of knowing in nursing. *Advances in Nursing Science, 1*(I), 13-23.

Dempsey, S. J., Dracup, K., & Moser, D. K. (1995). Women's decision to seek care for symptoms of acute myocardial infarction. *Heart and Lung, 24*, 444-456.

Dracup, K., McKinley, S. M., & Moser, D. K. (1997). Australian patients' delay in response to heart attack symptoms. *Medical Journal of Australia, 166*, 233-236.

Finnegan, J. R., Meischke, H., Zapka, J. G., Leviton, L., Meshack, A., Benjamin-Garner, R., et al. (2000). Patient delay in seeking care for heart attack symptoms: Findings from focus groups conducted in five US regions. *Preventive Medicine, 31*, 205-213.

Glaser, B. G. (1992). *Basics of grounded theory*. Mill Valley, CA: Sociology Press.

Glaser, B. G., & Strauss, A. A. (1999). *The discovery of grounded theory: Strategies for qualitative research* (2nd ed.). New York: Aldine de Gruyter.

Goldberg, R. J., Gurwitz, J. H., & Gore, J. M. (1999). Duration of and temporal trends (1994-1997) in prehospital delay in patients with acute myocardial infarction. *Archives of internal Medicine, 159*, 2141-2147.

Hammond, J., Salamonson. Y., Davidson. P., Everett, B., & Andrew, S. (2007). Why do women underestimate the risk of cardiac disease? *Australian Critical Care, 20*(2), 53-59.

Harralson, T. L. (2007). Factors influencing delay in seeking treatment for acute ischemic symptoms among lower income, urban women. *Heart and Lung, 36*(2), 96-104.

Hartford, M., Sjolin, M., & Herlitz, J. (1993). Symptoms, thoughts, and environmental factors in suspected acute myocardial infarction. *Heart and Lung, 22*(1), 64-70.

Herlitz, J., Eek, M., Holmberg, M., Engdahl, J., & Holmberg, S. (2002). Characteristics and outcome among patients having out of hospital cardiac arrest at home compared with elsewhere. *Heart Journal, 88*, 579-582.

Ho, M. T., Eisenberg, M. S., Litwin, P. E., Schaeffer, S. M., & Damon, S. K. (1989). Delay between onset of chest pain and seeking medical care: The effect of public education. *Annals of Emergency Medicine, 18*, 727-711.

Lefler, L. L., & Bondy, K. N. (2004). Women's delay in seeking treatment with myocardial infarction: A meta-synthesis. *Journal of Cardiovascular Nursing, 19*, 251-268.

Leitch, J. W., Birbara, T., Freedman, B., Wilcox, I., & Harris, P. (1989). Factors influencing the time from onset of chest pain to arrival at hospital. *Medical Journal of Australia, 150*, 6-8.

Lomberg, K., & Kirkevold, M. (2003). Truth and validity in grounded theory—a reconsidered realist interpretation of the criteria: Fit, work, relevance and modifiability. *Nursing Philosophy, 4*, 189-200.

McKinley, S. M., Dracup, K., Moser, D. K., Ball, C., Yamasaki, K., Kim, C.-J., et al. (2004). International comparison of factors associated with delay in presentations for AMI treatment. *European Journal of Cardiovascular Nursing, 3*, 225-230.

Moser, D. K., Kimble, L. P., Alberts, M., Alonzo, A. A., Croft, J. B., Dracup, K., et al. (2006). Reducing delay in seeking treatment by patients with acute coronary syndrome and stroke: A scientific statement from the American Heart Association Council on Cardiovascular Nursing and Stroke Council. *Circulation, 114,* 168-182.

Moser, D. K., McKinley, S. M., Dracup, K., & Chung, M. L. (2005). Gender difference in reasons patients delay in seeking treatment for acute myocardial infarction symptoms. *Patient Education and Counselling, 56,* 45-54.

Oliver-McNeil, S., & Artinian, N. T. (2002). Women's perceptions of personal cardiovascular risk and their risk-reducing behaviors. *American Journal of Critical Care, 11,* 221-227.

Richards, H. M., Reid, M. E., & Watt, G. C. M. (2002). Why do men and women respond differently to chest pain? *Journal of the American Medical Women's Association, 57*(2), 79-81.

Rosenfeld, A. G. (2004). Treatment-seeking delay among women with acute myocardial infarction: Decision trajectories and their predictors. *Nursing Research, 53,* 225-236.

Statistics Canada. (2004). Age-standardized mortality rates (female). Retrieved October 26, 2004, from lutp://www.statcan.gc.ca/daily-quotidien/040927/dq040927a-eng.htm

Turris, S. A., & Johnson, J. L. (2008). Maintaining integrity: Women and treatment seeking for the symptoms of potential cardiac illness. *Qualitative Health Research, 18*(11), 1461-1476.

Wu, Y., Zhang, Y., Li, Y., Hong, B., & Huang, C. (2004). Factors associated with the extent of care-seeking delay for patient with acute myocardial infarction in Beijing. *Chinese Medical Journal, 117,* 1772-1777.

Zerwic, J. J., Ryan, C. J., DeVon, H. A., & Drell, M. J. (2003). Treatment seeking for acute myocardial infarction symptoms. *Nursing Research, 52,* 159-167.

INTRODUCTION TO CRITIQUE 2

The preceding article by Turris (2009) is an example of a grounded theory study. The article is critically examined as follows for its rigour as a grounded theory study, its contribution to nursing, and its usefulness in practice. The criteria listed in Box 18-2 are used to guide the critique.

Title

The title of the article concisely captures the essence of the study.

Abstract

The abstract met the requirements of a good abstract: It contained the background, the method (including the purpose and the sample size), and the findings. The abstract also had a statement about the clinical relevance of the study.

Focus/Topic

The phenomenon of interest was stated clearly in the introduction to the study. Turris (2009) was interested in understanding how and why women interpret their symptoms of a potentially deadly cardiac event and in understanding their treatment-seeking behaviour. Many women delay treatment, which is a critical mistake, as life-saving treatment should occur within 1 hour of the onset of symptoms. Although there is a persistent belief that women do not suffer from heart disease, it is the number one killer of women.

Purpose

Turris (2009) was interested in developing a theory to explain women's treatment-seeking delay behaviour in the presence of cardiac symptoms. Her research question concerned what process guided women as they interpreted symptoms suggestive of cardiac illness, chose their treatment options, and subsequently assessed their experiences of care in the emergency department.

Significance

Because of the effects of cardiac disease on the population and the serious repercussion of delay in seeking treatment, this study has the potential to influence nursing practice and the lives of many women. Although treatment-seeking delay has been studied extensively, it continues to be a persistent clinical issue. Some of the explanatory evidence in the literature is conflicting.

Method

The method used in this study was clearly identified as grounded theory. Grounded theory is used to explain basic social processes and to develop theory (Streubert & Carpenter, 2011). In this study, the basic social process under study was the process of maintaining integrity in relation to visiting an emergency department "for treatment of symptoms indicating potential cardiac illness" (Turris, 2009, p. 6). The grounded theory method is appropriate for this study, and the method processes were followed and yielded the expected results.

Sampling

Turris (2009) stated that purposive sampling was used for data collection, which is appropriate for a grounded theory study. Purposive or purposeful sampling provides investigators in qualitative research with the opportunity to recruit participants who are knowledgeable about the phenomenon under study because they can provide rich descriptions of their personal experiences. In this case, Turris recruited women who sought emergency care for the treatment of symptoms of a potential cardiac illness at one of two hospitals. The inclusion criteria included treatment of symptoms that were of a potential cardiac event, hemodynamic stability, age of 18 years or older, English speaking, and ability and willingness to provide informed consent.

Turris (2009) also stated that theoretical sampling was used after the initial purposive sampling. In **theoretical sampling,** which is used primarily in grounded theory, individuals are interviewed in an effort to further develop specific aspects of the emerging theory. In this case, Turris noted that the data suggested that age might play a role in women's decisions about seeking treatment, and therefore the accounts of younger women were actively sought (p. 6). The sample expanded from the original 10 participants to 16 in total. Although this was not explicitly stated, it appears that data collection stopped when no further information was forthcoming or the data **saturation** (repetition of information) was reached.

Turris (2009) carefully described how she recruited the participants and obtained informed consent. She discussed the setting for recruitment, identified as one large urban hospital and one community hospital. The smaller community hospital was not able to offer angiographic procedures often necessary for patients with acute myocardial infarction. Although Turris carefully accounted for these differences between the two settings, she did not describe how the samples of participants differed from each other in each setting.

Data Generation

The primary source of data was a formal audiotaped interview lasting 30 to 90 minutes. Transcripts from the interview were password protected, and any identifying information was removed. Turris (2009) was careful to describe the ethical approval and how informed consent was obtained. She indicated that participants were reminded that they could withdraw from the study at any time, not respond to particular questions, or request to have the tape recorder turned off.

Turris (2009) did not include the interview questions in the study report. This is typical in grounded theory research, in which the use of interview guides are discouraged because they may be based on preconceived notions that may potentially distort the findings. Glaser (1998) recommended that "adjusted conversational interviewing" (p. 173) replace formal questions, whereas Corbin and Strauss (2008) supported interview guides with open-ended questions and opportunities for open dialogue. Because the transcripts in Turris's study were password protected, readers can assume that a series of interview questions were asked. It is not clear whether theoretical notes were used as recommended in grounded theory methodology.

Data Analysis

True to grounded theory methodology, Turris (2009) conducted the data generation and analysis concurrently. Over a period of several months, the data were analyzed through open, selective, and theoretical coding. Beginning with open coding, Turris moved to constant comparative analysis. Important concepts emerged to explain patterns in the women's accounts. She reported that the evidence core category, which occurred over and over in the data, was "sought throughout the analytic process" (p. 6).

Turris (2009) dedicated an entire section of the report to the concept of rigour. She identified how the study met each of the specific criteria of fittingness, work, relevance, and modifiability. For example, fittingness, whereby the theory describes the phenomenon under study, was discussed by the research team on a biweekly basis. In addition, the criterion of relevance was met inasmuch as each of the emerging themes was checked with the participants and colleagues.

Empirical Grounding of the Study Findings

The main finding in this study was that participants make decisions about seeking treatment on the basis of particular ways of knowing. This pattern is part of a large social phenomenon rather than a product of individual factors. Participants were reported to be influenced primarily by the context of their "lives as mothers, daughters, and wives" (Turris, 2009, p. 6) and secondarily by their assessments of their symptoms. The women used ways of knowing (embodied, temporal, rational, and relational) to "understand and interpret their symptoms within a larger personal and social context" (p. 6). Turris then described the findings in sections focusing on each of the ways of knowing, which originated from Carper's seminal work on "Fundamental Patterns of Knowing in Nursing" published in 1978. Participants' quotations supported each of the identified ways of knowing and supported the main finding that their responsibilities in the roles of wives and mothers were more important and vital than attending to their own symptoms of cardiac disease. This thorough discussion of the findings provides credibility that the theory is valid.

In the "Discussion" section, Turris (2009) reported the findings in the literature concerning delay in seeking treatment and claimed that many are noteworthy. For example, Turris found, in contrast to previous studies, that rather than delaying treatment, consultation with a family member resulted in an immediate visit to the emergency department. This and other findings have potentially significant implications for practice. Limitations of Turris's study were appropriately detailed.

Conclusions, Implications, and Recommendations

In the "Implications for Nursing Practice" section, Turris (2009) indicated that the findings on the forms of knowledge that women use to make decisions would allow nurses to have discussions with women about their decisions before a crisis arises. In addition, understanding delay in seeking treatment as a social phenomenon might widen the focus of research. Understanding why women experiencing symptoms of potential cardiac illness make their decisions "can 'inform' nursing interventions before a cardiac event, preventing death and reducing morbidity" (Turris, 2009,

p. 11). The implications for nursing practice are important; however, more specific practical recommendations would have been helpful for the nurse clinician.

The research study by Turris (2009) contributes to the body of nursing knowledge and offers new direction in the area of study on delay in seeking treatment. This area of study can yield information that can potentially reduce death and morbidity from a largely treatable disease process.

Evidence-Informed Practice Tip

Qualitative research may generate basic knowledge, hypotheses, and theories to be used in the design of other types of qualitative or quantitative studies. However, qualitative research is not necessarily a preliminary step to another type of research. It is a complete and valuable end in itself.

CRITICAL THINKING CHALLENGES

- Discuss the similarities and differences between the stylistic considerations of reporting a qualitative study versus a quantitative study in a professional journal.
- Are critiques of qualitative studies by consumers of research, in the role of either a student or a practising nurse, valid? Which type of qualitative study is the most difficult for consumers of research to critique? Discuss what assumptions led you to this determination.
- Discuss how nurses would go about incorporating qualitative research in evidence-informed practice. Give an example.

REFERENCES

Appleton, J. V., & King, L. (2002). Journeying from the philosophical contemplation of constructivism to the methodological pragmatics of health services research. *Journal of Advanced Nursing*, *40*(6), 641-648.

Barbour, R. S., & Barbour, M. (2003). Evaluating and synthesizing qualitative research: The need to develop a distinctive approach. *Journal of Evaluation in Clinical Practice*, *9*, 179-186.

Carper, B. A. (1978). Fundamental patterns of knowing in nursing. *Advanced Nursing Science, 1*, 13-23.

Cesario, S., Morin, K., & Santa-Donato, A. (2002). Evaluating the level of evidence of qualitative research. *Journal of Obstetric, Gynecological and Neonatal Nursing, 31*, 708-714.

Chiovitti, R., & Prian, N. (2003). Rigour and grounded theory research. *Journal of Advanced Nursing Practice, 44*(4), 427-435.

Corbin, J., & Strauss, A. (2008). *Basics of qualitative research* (3rd ed.). Los Angeles: Sage.

Creswell, J. W. (2009). *Research design: Qualitative, quantitative, and mixed methods approaches* (3rd ed.). Thousand Oaks, CA: Sage.

Gibson, B. E., & Martin, D. K. (2003). Qualitative research and evidence-based physiotherapy practice. *Physiotherapy, 89*, 350-358.

Glaser, B. G. (1998). *Doing grounded theory: Issues and discussions* (2nd ed.). Mill Valley, CA: Sociology Press.

Glesne, C. (2011). *Becoming qualitative researchers: An introduction* (4th ed.). Toronto: Allyn & Bacon.

Horsburgh, D. (2003). Evaluation of qualitative research. *Journal of Clinical Nursing, 12*, 307-312.

Ives, M. & Melrose, S. (2010). Immunizing children who fear and resist needles: Is it a problem for nurses? *Nursing Forum, 45*(1), 29-39.

Jackson, R. L., Drummond, D. K., & Camara, S. (2007). What is qualitative research? *Qualitative Research Reports in Communication, 8*(1), 21-28.

Lincoln, Y. S., & Guba, E. (1985). *Naturalistic inquiry.* Beverly Hills, CA: Sage.

Morse, J. M., Penrod, J., & Hupcey, J. E. (2000). Qualitative outcome analysis: Evaluating nursing interventions for complex clinical phenomena. *Journal of Nursing Scholarship, 32*, 125-130.

Schepner-Hughes, N. (1992). *Death without weeping: The violence of everyday life in Brazil.* Berkeley: University of California Press.

Straus, S. E., Glasziou, P., Richardson, W. S., & Haynes, R. B. (2011). *Evidence-based medicine: How to practice and teach it* (4th ed.). Edinburgh: Churchill Livingstone.

Strauss, A., & Corbin, J. (1990). *Basics of qualitative research: Grounded theory procedures and techniques.* Newbury Park, CA: Sage.

Streubert, H. J., & Carpenter, D. R. (2011). *Qualitative research in nursing: Advancing the humanistic imperative* (5th ed.). Philadelphia: Wolters Kluwer.

Turris, S. (2009). Women's decisions to seek treatment for the symptoms of potential cardiac disease. *Journal of Nursing Scholarship, 41*(1), 5-12.

Wilkin, K., & Slevin, E. (2004). The meaning of caring to nurses: An investigation into the nature of caring work in an intensive care unit. *Journal of Clinical Nursing, 13*, 50-59.

FOR FURTHER STUDY

Ǝvolve   Go to Evolve at http://evolve.elsevier.com/Canada/LoBiondo/Research for Audio Glossary, how-to instructions for Writing Proposals for Funding, and additional research articles for practice in reviewing and critiquing.

CHAPTER 19

Critiquing Quantitative Research

Nancy E. Kline | Mina D. Singh

LEARNING OUTCOMES

After reading this chapter, you will be able to do the following:

- Identify the purpose of the critiquing process for a quantitative research report.
- Describe the criteria of each step of the critiquing process for a quantitative research report.
- Evaluate the strengths and weaknesses of a quantitative research report.
- Discuss the implications of the findings of a quantitative research report for nursing practice.
- Construct a critique of a quantitative research report.

KEY TERM

scientific merit

STUDY RESOURCES

Go to Evolve at http://evolve.elsevier.com/Canada/LoBiondo/Research for Audio Glossary, how-to instructions for Writing Proposals for Funding, and additional research articles for practice in reviewing and critiquing.

AS REINFORCED THROUGHOUT EACH CHAPTER of this book, it is important not only to conduct and read research but also to use research for evidence-informed practice. As nurse researchers increase the depth (quality) and breadth (quantity) of research methods from descriptive research designs to randomized clinical trials, the data to support clinical interventions and quality outcomes are becoming more readily available. Each published study, regardless of its design, reflects a *level of evidence,* but the critique of each study covers much more than the level of evidence produced by the design. When you critique a research study, examine each component to determine the merit of the report. Key to the critique is the strength of evidence that each study produces individually and collectively.

This chapter presents critiques of two studies in which research questions were tested with different quantitative designs. The critiquing criteria designed to assist research consumers in judging the relative value of a research report are found at the ends of previous chapters. These critiquing criteria have been summarized to create an abbreviated set of questions that will be used as a framework for the two sample research critiques (Box 19-1). These critiques exemplify the process of evaluating reported research for potential

---

BOX 19-1

MAJOR CONTENT SECTIONS OF A RESEARCH REPORT AND RELATED CRITIQUING GUIDELINES

PROBLEM STATEMENT AND PURPOSE (SEE CHAPTER 4)

1. What is the problem explored in, or the purpose of, the research study?
2. Does the statement about the problem or purpose express a relationship between two or more variables (e.g., between an independent variable and a dependent variable)? If so, what is the relationship? Is it testable?
3. Does the statement about the problem or purpose specify the nature of the population being studied? What is it?
4. What significance of the problem—if any—has the investigator identified?

REVIEW OF THE LITERATURE AND THEORETICAL FRAMEWORK (SEE CHAPTERS 2 AND 5)

1. What concepts are included in the review? Of particular importance, note which concepts are the independent and dependent variables and how they are conceptually defined.
2. Does the literature review make the relationships among the variables explicit or place the variables within a theoretical or conceptual framework? What are the relationships?
3. What gaps or conflicts in knowledge of the problem are identified? How is this study intended to fill those gaps or resolve those conflicts?
4. Are the references cited by the author mostly primary or secondary sources? Give an example of each.
5. What are the operational definitions of the independent and dependent variables? Do they reflect the conceptual definitions?

HYPOTHESES OR RESEARCH QUESTIONS (SEE CHAPTER 4)

1. What hypotheses or research questions are stated in the study? Are they appropriately stated?
2. If research questions are stated, are they used in addition to hypotheses or to guide an exploratory study?
3. What are the independent and dependent variables in the statement of each hypothesis or research question?
4. If hypotheses are stated, is the form of the statement statistical (null) or research?
5. What is the direction of the relationship in each hypothesis, if indicated?
6. Are the hypotheses testable?

SAMPLE (SEE CHAPTER 12)

1. How was the sample selected?
2. What type of sampling method is used in the study? Is it appropriate for the design?
3. Does the sample reflect the population as identified in the problem or purpose statement?
4. Is the sample size appropriate? How is it substantiated?
5. To what population may the findings be generalized? What are the limitations in generalizability?

RESEARCH DESIGN (SEE CHAPTERS 10 TO 11)

1. What type of design is used in the study?
2. What is the rationale for the design classification?
3. Does the choice of design seem logical for the proposed research problem, theoretical framework, literature review, and hypothesis?

Continued

BOX 19-1

MAJOR CONTENT SECTIONS OF A RESEARCH REPORT AND RELATED CRITIQUING GUIDELINES—*cont'd*

INTERNAL VALIDITY (SEE CHAPTER 9)

1. Discuss each threat to the internal validity of the study.
2. Does the design have controls at an acceptable level for the threats to internal validity?

EXTERNAL VALIDITY (SEE CHAPTER 9)

1. What are the limits to generalizability in terms of external validity?

RESEARCH APPROACH (SEE CHAPTERS 7 AND 11)

1. Does the research approach fit with the purpose of the study?
2. Is a mixed-methods approach, if used, appropriate for the study?

METHODS (SEE CHAPTER 13)

1. What data-collection methods are used in the study?
2. Are the data-collection procedures similar for all participants?

LEGAL/ETHICAL ISSUES (SEE CHAPTER 6)

1. Have the rights of participants been protected? How?
2. What indications are given that informed consent of the participants was ensured?

INSTRUMENTS (SEE CHAPTER 13)

1. Physiological measurement
   a. Is a rationale given for why a particular instrument or method was selected? If so, what is it?
   b. What provision is made for maintaining the accuracy of the instrument and its use, if any?
2. Observational methods
   a. Who did the observing?
   b. How were the observers trained to minimize bias?
   c. Did the observers have an observational guide?
   d. Were the observers required to make inferences about what they saw?
   e. Is there any reason to believe that the presence of the observers affected the behaviour of the participants?
3. Interviews
   a. Who were the interviewers? How were they trained to minimize bias?
   b. Is there evidence of any interviewer bias? If so, what is it?
4. Questionnaires
   a. What is the type or format of the questionnaires (e.g., Likert-type, open-ended)? Are they consistent with the conceptual definitions?
5. Available data and records
   a. Are the records that were used appropriate to the problem studied?
   b. Were the data used to describe the sample or for hypothesis testing?

RELIABILITY AND VALIDITY (SEE CHAPTER 14)

1. What type of reliability is reported for each instrument?
2. What level of reliability is reported? Is it acceptable?
3. What type of validity is reported for each instrument?
4. Does the validity of each instrument seem adequate? Why?

ANALYSIS OF DATA (SEE CHAPTERS 15 AND 16)

1. What level of measurement is used to measure each of the major variables?
2. What descriptive or inferential statistics are reported?
3. Were these descriptive or inferential statistics appropriate for the level of measurement for each variable?
4. Are the inferential statistics used appropriate for the intent of the hypotheses?
5. Does the author report the level of significance set for the study? If so, what is it?
6. If tables or figures are used, do they meet the following standards?
   a. They supplement and economize the text.
   b. They have precise titles and headings.
   c. They do not repeat the text.

CONCLUSIONS, IMPLICATIONS, AND RECOMMENDATIONS

1. If hypothesis testing was done, were the hypotheses supported or not supported?
2. Are the results interpreted in the context of the problem or purpose, hypothesis (see this chapter), and theoretical framework or literature reviewed?
3. What does the investigator identify as possible limitations or problems in the study in relation to the design, methods, and sample?
4. What relevance for nursing practice does the investigator identify, if any?
5. What generalizations are made?
6. Are the generalizations within the scope of the findings or beyond the scope of the findings?
7. What recommendations for future research are stated or implied?

APPLICATION AND UTILIZATION (SEE CHAPTER 20)

1. Does the study appear to be valid? In other words, do its strengths for nursing practice outweigh its weaknesses?
2. Do other studies have similar findings?
3. What risks or benefits are involved for patients if the research findings are used in practice?
4. Is direct application of the research findings feasible in terms of time, effort, money, and legal/ethical risks?
5. How and under what circumstances are the findings applicable to nursing practice?
6. Should these results be applied to nursing practice?
7. Would it be possible to replicate this study in another clinical practice setting?

application to practice, thus extending the research base for nursing. For clarification, refer to the earlier chapters for detailed presentations of the critiquing criteria and explanations of the research process. The criteria and examples in this chapter are applicable to quantitative studies in which researchers used experimental, quasiexperimental, and nonexperimental research designs that provided levels II, III, and IV evidence.

STYLISTIC CONSIDERATIONS

As an evaluator, you should be aware of several aspects of publishing before you begin to critique research studies. First, different journals have different publication goals, and they target specific professional nursing specialties. For example, the *Canadian Journal of Nursing Research* publishes articles on the conduct or results of research in nursing. The *Canadian Oncology Nursing Journal* also publishes research articles; however, because its emphasis is broader, this journal also contains clinical and theoretical articles relating to knowledge, experience, trends, and policies in oncological nursing. Consequently, the style and content of a manuscript will vary according to the type of journal to which it is being submitted.

Second, the author of a research article prepares the manuscript by using both personal judgement and specific journal guidelines. *Personal judgement* refers to the researcher's expertise that is developed in the course of designing, executing, and analyzing the study. As a result of this expertise, the researcher is in a position to judge which content is most important to communicate to the profession. The decision is a function of the following:

- The research design: experimental or non-experimental
- The focus of the study: basic or clinical
- The audience to whom the results will be most appropriately communicated

Each journal provides the guidelines for preparing research manuscripts for publication, and usually the following major headings are essential sections of a research manuscript or research report:

- Introduction
- Method
- Results
- Discussion

Depending on the stylistic considerations related to the author's preferences and the journal's requirements, the content included in the research report is specific to each of the sections just mentioned.

Stylistic variations (as factors influencing the presentation of the research study) are very distinct features of a research report and can deter from the focus of evaluating the reported research for **scientific merit:** that is, judging the overall quality or validity of a study. Constructive evaluation is based on objective appraisal of the study's strengths and limitations. This step precedes consideration of the relative worth of the findings for clinical application to nursing practice. Judgements of the scientific merit of a research study are the hallmark of promoting a sound evidence base for quality nursing practice.

CRITIQUING A QUANTITATIVE RESEARCH STUDY

CRITIQUE 1

The study "Older Adults' Awareness of Community Health and Support Services for Dementia Care" by Jenny Ploeg and colleagues (2009), is critiqued here. The article is presented in its entirety and is followed by the critique on pp. 453–455. (From *Canadian Journal of Aging*, 28(4), 359–370. © 2009 by Cambridge University Press. Reprinted by permission.)

Older Adults' Awareness of Community Health and Support Services for Dementia Care

Jenny Ploeg, MScN, PhD
School of Nursing
Department of Health, Aging and Society
McMaster University
Hamilton, Ontario

Margaret Denton, MA, PhD
Department of Health, Aging and Society
Department of Sociology
McMaster Centre for Gerontological Studies
McMaster University
Hamilton, Ontario

Joseph Tindal, PhD
Department of Family Relations and Applied Nutrition
University of Guelph
Guelph, Ontario

Brian Hutchison, MD, MSc, CCFP, FCFP
Department of Epidemiology and Biostatistics
Department of Family Medicine
Centre for Health Economics and Policy Analysis
McMaster University
Hamilton, Ontario

Kevin Brazil, MA, PhD
Department of Epidemiology and Biostatistics
McMaster University
Hamilton, Ontario

Noori Akhtar-Danesh, MSc, PhD
School of Nursing
McMaster University
Hamilton, Ontario

Jean Lillie, PhD
Department of Family Relations and Applied Nutrition
University of Guelph
Guelph, Ontario

Jennifer Millen Plenderleith
McMaster Centre for Gerontological Studies
McMaster University
Hamilton, Ontario

The article examines where older adults seek help in caring for a parent with dementia and the factors associated with their identification of community health and support services as sources of assistance. The authors conducted telephone interviews, using random digit dialing, of 1,152 adults aged 50 and over in the city of Hamilton. Respondents received a vignette that raised issues related to parental dementia. In identifying support sources, over 37 per cent of respondents identified their physician, 33 per cent identified informal support such as family and neighbors, and 31 per cent identified home health services. Only 18 per cent identified community support services. Female participants having higher levels of education were more likely to identify their physician as a source of support. Knowing where to find information about community support services was associated with an increased likelihood of mentioning physicians and home health services as sources of assistance.

KEYWORDS community support services, awareness, dementia, caregivers, vignette methodology

Dementa [*sic*] is an increasingly prevalent and important health concern in Canada (Canadian Study of Health and Aging [CSHA] Working Group, 2000) and globally (Wimo, Winblad, Aguero-Torres, & von Strauss, 2003). Most older adults with dementia continue to live in their homes with the support of informal caregivers (CSHA Working Group, 1994). Informal caregivers of persons with dementia experience a significant burden in their roles. Although many communities have an array of community health and support services to assist older adults with dementia and their caregivers, the literature suggests that these services are underutilized and that one of the barriers to their use is the lack of awareness of such services (Strain & Blandford, 2002). The research literature on service awareness has important methodological limitations: in particular, acquiescence bias, whereby respondents over-report their awareness of services. The purpose of this descriptive study is to describe where older adults would turn to for help in response to vignettes or short stories related to caring for a parent with dementia, and the socio-demographic factors associated with their choice of supports. We used vignette methodology to avoid the acquiescence bias so common in service awareness research.

DEMENTIA

It has been estimated that the global prevalence of dementia in 2001 was more than 24 million people aged 60 years or older, a prevalence rate of approximately 3.9 per cent of that age group (Ferri, Prince, Brayne, Brodaty, Fratiglioni, Ganguli et al., 2005). This prevalence is projected to double every 20 years to more than 81 million people by 2040 (Ferri et al., 2005). In North America, the prevalence of dementia among those aged 60 years and older in 2001 was 6.4 per cent (Ferri et al., 2005). The CSHA Working Group (2000) has estimated that there are 60,150 new cases of dementia per year in Canada. Of those older Canadians with dementia, 64 per cent were diagnosed with Alzheimer's disease (AD), 19 per cent with vascular dementia, and 17 per cent with other forms of dementia (Hill, Forbes, Berthelot, Lindsay, & McDowell, 1996). Dementia has been described as a major burden for health and social care systems (Wimo et al., 2003). The net economic cost of dementia in Canada in 1991 was estimated to be at least CAN $3.9 billion (Østbye & Crosse, 1994), and it is likely to be much higher now, 17 years later.

Dementia also places a significant burden on informal caregivers. About half of all people with dementia in Canada are living in the community, and more than 98 per cent of them have a caregiver, usually an unpaid family member, relative, or friend (CSHA Working Group, 1994). Caregivers of a family member with dementia are more likely to experience chronic health problems, depression, and social isolation, compared to those caring for cognitively intact elderly (CSHA Working Group, 1994). Given the increasing number of people with dementia, the impact on informal caregivers of providing care, and the preference of older adults to "age in place" (Chappell, McDonald, & Stones, 2008), increasing attention is being focused on strategies to support caregivers in their roles. One such strategy involves the use of support provided by community health and support services.

Community Health and Support Services

Many communities have a broad array of community health and support services available to assist persons with dementia and their caregivers. Such services provide an alternative to institutionalization. Service examples include home health services—such as nursing and homemaking—as well as community support services (CSSs). Community support services, as defined here, are delivered in the home or community to assist people with health or social problems to maintain the highest possible level of social functioning and quality of life. Examples of CSSs are (a) adult day programs, (b) volunteer visiting, (c) caregiver support programs, (d) food services, (e) transportation services, and (f) organizations such as the Alzheimer Society. Access to CSSs is particularly challenging because of the multiplicity of small agencies providing these services, the lack of a central access point, and the lack of awareness of such services. Further, the complexity of the health and social support system makes it challenging for older persons, their families, and health care professionals to navigate the system.

There is some evidence that use of community-based services has positive benefits for frail elders (with and without dementia) and their caregivers (Zarit, Gaugler, & Jarrott, 1999). In their review of the literature, Zarit et al. (1999) found that such services resulted in lower levels of care-related stressors, perceived burden, depression, and anger. At the same time, patients with dementia experienced improved life satisfaction and mood, engagement in activities, and fewer behavioural difficulties. In a qualitative study of family caregivers of relatives with AD or a related disorder, community services were found to provide benefits including the experience of community and support, a gain in knowledge, receipt of personal renewal, and benefits to the patient (Winslow, 2003).

LITERATURE REVIEW

Underutilization of community-based services—that is, the gap between expressed need and service use—has been recognized as a general problem in the field of aging (Strain & Blandford, 2002) and a particular problem in dementia care (Brodaty, Thomson, Thompson, & Fine, 2005; Buono, Busato, Mazzetto, Paccagnella, Aleotti, Zanetti et al., 1999; CSHA Working Group, 1994; Collins, Stommel, Given, & King, 1991; Forbes, Morgan, & Janzen, 2006; Vetter, Steiner, Kraus, Moises, Kropp, Moller et al., 1998). Research has suggested that community health and support services are underused, largely due to lack of awareness or knowledge of such services (Strain & Blandford, 2002; Vetter et al., 1998). Krout (1983) distinguished between awareness and knowledge of services. Awareness is a general under-standing that a service exists. Knowledge involves "knowledge of what the program is or does, where it is located, or how one gets involved with it" (Krout, 1983, p. 155). Most of the following research addresses awareness, not knowledge, of services.

Strain and Blandford (2002), in the Manitoba Study of Health and Aging, studied the awareness and use of community-based services among 293 older person-caregiver dyads (44% with cognitive impairment). While they found few people unaware of home-delivered meals (7.9%), in-home nursing (9.5%), personal care (10.6%), and homemaking (11.2%), a much larger proportion was unaware of hospital respite (49.5%), nursing home respite (47.4%), in-home respite (43.8%), day hospitals (43.3%), and day centres (35.7%). For these latter services (i.e., day centres, day hospitals, in-home respite, nursing home respite), the second most common reason given for non-use was that caregivers were not aware of the service. In that study, researchers provided participants with the categories of available community services.

Studies of persons with dementia and their caregivers have also demonstrated limited awareness and utilization of community health and support services (Brodaty et al., 2005; Buono et al., 1999; Caserta, Lund, Wright, & Redburn, 1987; Collins et al., 1991; Maslow, 1990; Vetter et al., 1998). For example, Collins et al. (1991) found that among caregivers of persons with AD not using specific services, the percentage who were not aware of availability of services varied by service as follows: (a) support group (10%), (b) visiting nurse (18%), (c) home-delivered meals (20%), (d) transportation service (30%), (e) counseling (36%), (f) day respite program (39%), and (g) temporary overnight care (58%). Another study found that the main reason reported for non-use of services (e.g., counseling, support groups, Meals on Wheels, and adult day care) was that over 60 per cent of caregivers of persons with AD ($n = 36$) were unaware of the availability of such services (Vetter et al., 1998). A third study found that 36 per cent of caregivers of dementia patients ($n = 597$) did not know whether community services were available or not (Caserta et al., 1987).

Some research has been conducted on the factors associated with utilization of CSSs for dementia care (Brodaty et al., 2005; Caserta et al., 1987; Strain & Blandford, 2002; Vetter et al., 1998), but relatively little on the factors associated with awareness of such services. Collins et al. (1991), in their study of family caregivers of patients with AD, found that older caregivers were more likely to be uncertain about the availability of services, and that caregiver depression was associated with less knowledge of service availability. Our review of the factors associated with, or assessed for their association with, the use of CSSs for dementia care in the research literature guided our selection of the variables in this study. Specifically, researchers have found that socio-economic variables (i.e., employment, income, education) (Collins et al., 1991; Cox, 1999; Ortiz & Fitten, 2000), demographic variables (i.e., age, sex) (Collins et al., 1991; Robinson, Buckwalter, & Reed, 2005), and social variables (i.e., social support, social networks) (Caserta et al., 1987; Cotrell & Engel, 1998) are associated with the use of dementia care services. To date, little evidence exists of associations between the use of dementia care services and other variables such as language and disability (Brodaty et al., 2005; Ortiz & Fitten, 2000).

There is limited Canadian information on older persons' awareness of community health and support services for situations of parental dementia and the factors associated with such awareness. Instead, the literature has focused on use, availability, and acceptability of services, and barriers to their use (Forbes, Markle-Reid, Hawranik, Peacock, Kingston, Morgan et al., 2008; Jansen, Forbes, Markle-Reid, Hawranik, Kingston, Peacock et al., 2009; Strain & Blandford, 2002). For example, a qualitative study exploring the use and satisfaction with home and community-based services for persons with dementia from the perspective of family caregivers found that issues of availability and acceptability captured caregivers' experiences (Forbes et al., 2008). Caregivers talked about the need for a continuum of home and community-based services and concerns such as inconsistency of care provider, inflexible care, and cost of services.

In addition to the limited research on factors associated with awareness of community-based services, there are important methodological limitations of the service awareness literature, including the literature related to dementia care services. In most studies, respondents have been provided with lists of service or agency names and asked to indicate whether or not they were aware of or using each one (Buono et al., 1999; Caserta et al., 1987; Collins et al., 1991; Strain & Blandford, 2002; Vetter et al., 1998). This methodology leads to acquiescence bias, the tendency of respondents to answer the question positively regardless of the content (Calsyn & Winter, 1999). In several studies, Calsyn, Roades, and Calsyn (1992) provided older adults with a fictitious service or agency name and found that 20–30 per cent of respondents reported familiarity with that service. One approach to address acquiescence bias in studies of service awareness is to use open-ended questions to solicit the name or types of agencies, but this approach has seldom been used in studies of service awareness.

The purpose of this study is to measure older persons' awareness of community health and support services when presented with a scenario related to caring for a parent with dementia. We were also interested in the socio-demographic and other factors, including care-giving status, associated with older adults' identification of community health and support services as sources of help in caring for a parent with dementia. We expected that caregivers might have greater awareness of community health and support services than non-caregivers, as research has found that most caregivers have a viable informal network of secondary supports that may help address barriers to the use of formal services (Cotrell & Engel, 1998).

Our study addressed the following research questions:

1. Where would older adults turn for assistance when faced with a scenario related to caring for a parent with dementia?
2. What factors are associated with the identification of community health and support services as a source of assistance in caring for a parent with dementia?
3. Do caregivers have greater awareness of community health and support services than non-caregivers?

METHOD

The study design was a cross-sectional descriptive survey, best used to obtain a description of a phenomenon (de Vaus, 2002). Although this study design can establish association between variables, it cannot determine causation (Streiner & Norman, 1998). The study involved a telephone survey of adults aged 50 years and older residing in the city of Hamilton, Ontario, Canada. Study methods have been described previously (Denton, Ploeg, Tindale, Hutchison, Brazil, Akhtar-Danesh et al., 2008) and are summarized here.

Study Setting

Hamilton, Ontario, is Canada's ninth largest city with a population of nearly 700,000 (Statistics Canada, 2006a). In 2006, Hamilton had a higher percentage (15.1%) of adults aged 65 years and older compared to Canada (13.7%) as a whole (Statistics Canada, 2006b). Hamilton has an array of community health and support service agencies available for persons with dementia and their caregivers.

Vignette Methodology

We used a vignette methodology to address the issue of acquiescence bias in the literature. The use of vignettes or short stories is an established research methodology (Hughes & Huby, 2002; Schoenberg & Ravdal, 2000; Spalding & Phillips, 2007). Vignettes are short descriptions of hypothetical situations that closely approximate real-life decision-making situations. Respondents are read the vignettes and asked to respond to the hypothetical situations. Advantages of vignettes are that they are interesting to the respondents, they provide context, and they can be used to address sensitive topics such as health care (Hughes & Huby, 2002). In the case of research related to awareness of community health and support services, the use of vignettes helps to avoid acquiescence bias, in which lists of services are presented to respondents, and investigator bias, whereby the list of services is bounded by the investigators' awareness of available services.

The vignettes used in this study were developed by front-line service providers to represent realistic and familiar situations faced by older adults for which community health and support services would be appropriate; thus, they have high face and content validity. The vignettes were pretested and some modifications were made.

Data Collection

Awareness of community health and support services was measured through a telephone survey of older adults. A survey firm was contracted to complete the interviews using a Computer Assisted Dialing Information (CADI) system. Interviews were completed within a six-week period beginning mid-February 2006. English-speaking residents aged 50 years of age and older were invited to participate in the study. The sample was obtained by randomly selecting telephone numbers from a list of telephone numbers for all residents of Hamilton.

Each participant was read four short vignettes. Participants were asked, "If you were in this situation, what would you do?" and prompted with "Anything else?" up to four times, in order to establish multiple sources of assistance. We then asked, "Can you name an organization or program in our community that you would turn to in that situation?" and used up to four prompts until a

CSS was named. We also collected demographic, economic, health, and social information about participants. Participants were asked if they had provided any unpaid care or assistance to one or more seniors in the past 12 months. If required, the following probes were provided as examples of caregiving: visiting seniors; helping them with shopping, banking, personal care (bathing, assisting with dressing); and taking medications. If participants indicated they had provided care, they were considered as caregivers for the purpose of this analysis. The study received ethics approval from McMaster University Research Ethics Board.

Sample Size

Sample size calculation was described in an earlier paper (Denton et al., 2008). Of the total 12 vignettes used in the 2008 study, three vignettes addressed issues of caring for a parent with dementia (see Table 19C1-1), and the responses to these vignettes are reported in this paper. A sample size of 384 was needed for each vignette.

TABLE **19C1-1**

VIGNETTES

VIGNETTE NUMBER	PANEL	VIGNETTE
1	A	You are the main caregiver for your parent who has Alzheimer's disease. You have discovered that your mother has been taking more pills than she should.
2	B	You are an only child of a parent with Alzheimer's disease. For years you have been bringing him meals, doing his laundry, and paying his bills. Your spouse is sick, and now you have to help him/her, too. You are feeling overwhelmed and frustrated.
3	C	Your mother, who lives with you, is very confused and can't be left alone. You want to keep her at home, but you have to go to work. The rest of the family are working and cannot help.

The 12 vignettes were divided into three groups (panels) containing four vignettes; a vignette related to caring for a parent with dementia was included in each group of four vignettes. The total sample size was $3 \times 384 = 1,152$. Thus, 384 older adults responded to each vignette, with 1,152 participants responding in total.

Data Analysis

Interviewers entered participants' responses to the vignettes as verbatim responses. These responses were coded and recoded by the survey firm's coders, working collaboratively with the research team, into 150 initial categories and then into 20 meaningful categories for the purpose of analysis (see Table 19C1-2). We had several rounds of peer checking with community partners to ensure that the reduction from 150 to 20 categories was accurate and appropriate. The survey

TABLE **19C1-2**

CATEGORIES OF PARTICIPANT RESPONSES TO VIGNETTES

1. Community support services
2. Spouse
3. Son/daughter
4. Friends and neighbours
5. Relatives
6. Physician
7. Emergency
8. Clinics/hospitals
9. Other health professionals
10. Non-health professionals
11. Pastor/clergy/faith community
12. Social and recreation services
13. Nothing
14. Home health services
15. Long-term care/residential care
16. Self-help/personal strategy
17. Government
18. Information and referral sources
19. Disease-specific agencies
20. Community Care Access Centre

Note: For the purpose of this analysis: Informal supports included spouse, son/daughter, friends, neighbours, relatives, and self-help strategies. Home health services included home health services and Community Care Access Centre. Community support services included 37 agencies such as adult day programs, Alzheimer Society, transportation ser-vices, and Meals on Wheels.

firm provided a Statistical Package for the Social Sciences (SPSS) file of the data to the researchers.

Age was measured as a categorical variable (age 50–60, age 61–70, and 71 and older, with age 50–60 as the reference category). Sex was measured as 1 for females and 0 for males (reference category). Marital status was measured as a categorical variable but was recoded to 1 = married and 0 = not married (reference category) for the purpose of the regression analysis. Four levels of education were measured: (a) less than high school (reference category), (b) some high school or graduated from high school, (c) other post-secondary education including community college and apprenticeship to the trades, and (d) university or higher education. Income was measured in four categories. Being foreign born was measured as 1 = yes and 0 = born in Canada (reference category). Self-rated health was measured as a categorical variable (excellent or very good as the reference category; good, and fair or poor). The respondent's functional health was measured as having a limitation at home or outside the home (1 = yes, 0 = no as the reference category). Membership in clubs or voluntary organizations such as seniors centres, church, or social groups was measured as 1 = member and 0 = non-member (reference category). Caregiving status was measured as 1 = caregiver for a senior in the past year and 0 = non-caregiver (reference category). Participants were asked where they would find information about CSSs with three opportunities to respond. The number of sources of information was summed and ranged from 0 to 3.

To answer the first question, "Where would older adults turn for assistance when faced with a scenario related to caring for a parent with dementia?", we focused on the five most frequent responses given by respondents: (a) informal sources including family, friends, and neighbours as well as self-help strategies; (b) home health services (including the Community Care Access Centre [CCAC] which is a one-stop access centre for home health services covered under the Ontario Health Insurance Plan); (c) CSSs; (d) long-term or institutional care; and (e) their physician. These responses were given by 81.3 per cent of participants as their first response.

To answer the second question, "What factors are associated with the identification of community health and support services as a source of assistance in caring for a parent with dementia?", we used logistic regression, as the identification was measured as a dichotomous variable. We included the following variables in the regression analysis: age, sex, education, country of birth, self-rated health, marital status, membership in clubs or organizations, and functional limitations of the care recipient. The inclusion of caregiver status as a variable in the regression analysis permitted us to address the third question: "Do caregivers have greater awareness of community health and support services than non-caregivers?" Using logistic regression, we regressed the identification of services on the variables just identified.

Odds ratios are presented. An odds ratio greater than 1.0 indicates an increased likelihood of identification of services; a 95 per cent confidence interval of an odds ratio that does not include 1.0 indicates a statistically significant result.

RESULTS

Participants

A total of 22,072 different telephone numbers in Hamilton were called, and 15,857 households were contacted. We were unable to contact 6,215 households because either the number was not in service, the line was busy, an answering machine took the call, or there was no answer. Of the 15,857 households contacted, 10,373 had a resident aged 50 years or older. Following exclusion of 1,034 households due to language barriers and illness, and 8,180 refusals, we conducted 1,159 interviews; seven of these were removed from the database due to incomplete data, leaving 1,152 usable interviews, for a response rate of 12.4 per cent (1,159/9,339) of eligible households.

Participants represented a wide cross-section of older adults living in Hamilton. The demographic profile of the sample is described in Table 19C1-3. Over two thirds of participants were female and most were married (63%), over the age of 60 (57%), and born in Canada (71%). Almost half had high school education or less (47%), and 28 per cent had university education. Household income varied with the most frequent category being CAN $60,000 or more (39%). A high proportion reported excellent, good, or very good self-rated health (54%), and most reported no functional limitations (60%). A high proportion (56%) reported two or more information sources. A comparison of our sample to Hamilton data from the 2006 and 2001 Census of Population was presented earlier (Denton et al., 2008). Our sample included a higher proportion of females, people who were Canadian born, and people with incomes higher than the Hamilton population had (Denton et al., 2008).

Analysis was conducted on the full sample ($n = 1,152$) instead of the three separate groups responding to each vignette. To ensure that the three groups were not significantly different on demographic variables, a chi-square test was conducted to compare each demographic variable between the three groups. No significant differences were found between groups on any of the demographic variables (education, sex, marital status, language, country of birth, health) except age: $\chi^2 (4, n = 1,152) = 11.2, p = 0.03$. Based on these findings, our groups were similar enough to combine into one group for analysis.

Of the total sample of 1,152 respondents, 474 (41%) identified themselves as having provided care to a senior in the previous 12 months. A chi-square test was conducted to compare each variable between caregiver and non-caregiver groups. There were no statistically significant differences between caregivers and non-caregivers on the variables of sex, country of birth, language, and marital status (see Table 19C1-3). However, caregivers were younger, had higher education and income levels, better self-rated health, more information sources, and were less likely to have functional limitations than non-caregivers.

Most caregivers (54%) provided care to one person, while 46 per cent provided care to two or more persons. For the first care recipient mentioned, the care recipient was most likely to be a parent (46%) or friend (31%). Most of the first care recipients (88%) described by the caregivers had a physical or mental condition or a health problem that reduced the amount or kind of activity they could perform. Most caregivers provided care daily (26%) or at least once per week (45%).

Services and Supports Identified by Participants

Across all three vignettes, the percentage of participants who identified each type of community health and support service as a source of assistance in a situation of parental dementia is illustrated in Figure 19C1-1. The bottom part of each bar illustrates the percentage of respondents by first response, and the top part of each bar illustrates the percentage of respondents who mentioned a specific care source after prompting. When faced with a situation of parental dementia, the highest percentage of participants identified a physician and the physician's office staff as sources of support. This source was named by 25 per cent of the respondents as their first choice, and overall (i.e., multiple response) by 37 per cent of respondents. This response was closely followed by those who mentioned informal sources (20% first response, 34% overall) and home health services (19% first response, 31% overall). Only nine per cent of participants mentioned a CSS as their first choice (18% overall), and eight per cent mentioned long-term care as their first choice (13% overall).

TABLE 19C1-3

DEMOGRAPHIC DESCRIPTION OF PARTICIPANTS

DEMOGRAPHIC VARIABLE	TOTAL SAMPLE ($n = 1,152$) %	CAREGIVERS ($n = 474$) %	NON-CAREGIVERS ($n = 678$) %	CHI SQUARE
AGE*				
50–60	42.6	49.2	38.1	χ^2 (2, $n = 1,152$) = 23.1, $p = 0.000$
61–70	29.5	30.2	29.1	
71+	27.9	20.7	32.9	
GENDER				
Male	28.7	26.8	30.1	χ^2 (1, $n = 1,152$) = 1.5, $p = 0.224$
Female	71.3	73.2	69.9	
EDUCATION*				
Less than high school	5.0	2.3	6.9	χ^2 (3, $n = 1,142$) = 18.9, $p = 0.000$
Some or all of high school	41.9	39.1	44.0	
Community college non-university certificate, trade	25.4	26.5	24.6	
University or higher	27.7	32.1	24.6	
COUNTRY OF BIRTH				
Born in Canada	71.4	72.4	70.6	χ^2 (1, $n = 1,142$) = 0.4, $p = 0.529$
Foreign born	27.8	26.8	28.5	
LANGUAGE				
English	94.6	95.4	94.1	χ^2 (2, $n = 1,152$) = 1.0, $p = 0.593$
French	0.6	0.6	0.6	
Other	4.8	4.0	5.3	
MARITAL STATUS				
Married, common law	63.1	67.2	60.2	χ^2 (3, $n = 1,151$) = 7.1, $p = 0.068$
Widowed	19.2	16.5	21.1	
Divorced, separated	11.6	9.9	12.7	
Single, never married	6.5	6.3	6.0	
HOUSEHOLD INCOME ($)*†				
$20, 000 or less	15.0	9.6	18.8	χ^2 (4, $n = 912$) = 24.9, $p = 0.000$
$20, 001–$40, 000	27.6	25.5	29.1	
$40, 001–$60, 000	18.6	18.4	18.8	
$60, 001–$80, 000	16.7	21.3	13.4	
$80,001+	22.0	25.3	19.8	
SELF-REPORTED HEALTH*				
Excellent, very good	54.5	60.7	50.1	χ^2 (2, $n = 1,147$) = 13.5, $p = 0.001$
Good	28.2	25.6	30.1	
Fair, poor	17.3	13.7	19.7	
FUNCTIONAL LIMITATIONS*				
No	60.2	66.7	55.9	χ^2 (1, $n = 1,137$) = 12.6, $p = 0.000$
Yes	39.8	33.6	44.1	
NUMBER OF INFORMATION SOURCES*				
0	13.8	9.5	16.8	χ^2 (3, $n = 1,152$) = 31.6, $p = 0.000$
1	29.8	26.8	31.9	
2	30.6	30.2	30.8	
3	25.9	33.5	20.5	

Number of study respondents varies across independent variables due to missing data.
*Significant difference found between caregiver and non-caregiver groups.
†The number of study responses to the household income was 376 (caregiver), 536 (non-caregiver), 912 (both males and females) respectively.

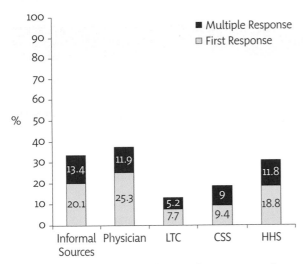

FIGURE 19C1-1 Percentage of respondents stating where they would turn for help by first and multiple responses. [CSS: community support services; HHS: home health service; LTC: long-term care.]

Factors Associated with Identification of Sources of Help

Next, we turn to the socio-demographic and other factors that may be associated with the choice of support service. Here we focus on the overall response, that is, when participants mentioned a home health or CSS at any point in their answer, either as their first response or in response to the prompt "Anything else?". Table 19C1-4 presents the odds ratios and 95 per cent confidence intervals for each variable by type of community health or support service: (a) informal sources, (b) physician, (c) long-term care, (d) CSSs, and (e) home health services.

Findings from the logistic regressions showed the following explanatory variables not to be statistically significantly associated with any type of community health or support service: country of birth, self-rated health, membership in clubs or organizations, being a caregiver, and having any functional limitations in or outside the home. In contrast, holding all other explanatory variables within the model constant when faced with a situation of parental dementia, the odds of turning to

informal sources such as family, friends, and neighbours decreased significantly with age. Looking at the effects of sex, the odds of identifying their physicians as a source of support increased by 40 per cent if caregivers were female rather than male.

The odds of mentioning their physician as a source of support increased by 250 per cent for those participants with higher levels of education (i.e., community college, trade school, or university) compared to those with less than high school education. Knowing where to obtain information about CSSs increased the likelihood of mentioning physicians and home health services as supports for situations of parental dementia. Married participants had lower odds of identifying informal sources of support for situations of parental dementia, compared to those who were unmarried.

DISCUSSION

Our study results provide insight into where older Canadians would turn for help when faced with a situation of parental dementia and the factors associated with their choice of supports. When older adults were presented with vignettes that described situations of parental dementia, they most frequently indicated they would turn to their physician, informal sources of help such as family and friends, home health services, CSSs, and long-term care services. Many CSSs are specifically targeted to assist older adults and their caregivers, yet only 18 per cent of middle-aged or older adults mentioned these services as sources of help in situations of parental dementia.

The most frequently mentioned CSS was the Alzheimer Society, mentioned by an average of 18 per cent of respondents across the three vignettes and the 10 opportunities to respond. These results are much lower than the 50 per cent to 92 per cent of participants who were aware of selected community health and support services in the study by Strain and Blandford (2002). It is

TABLE 19C1-4

LOGISTIC REGRESSION: COMMUNITY HEALTH AND SUPPORT SERVICES AND ASSOCIATIONS WITH DETERMINANTS

VARIABLES	INFORMAL SOURCES OR	(95% CI)	PHYSICIAN OR	(95% CI)	LONG-TERM CARE OR	(95% CI)	COMMUNITY SUPPORT SERVICES OR	(95% CI)	HOME HEALTH SERVICES OR	(95% CI)
AGE (YEARS)										
50–60 (ref)	1.0		1.0		1.0		1.0		1.0	
61–70	0.7	(0.5–1.0)	0.8	(0.6–1.1)	1.3	(0.9–2.0)	1.0	(0.7–1.5)	1.1	(0.8–1.5)
71+	0.6**	(0.4–0.8)	0.8	(0.6–1.2)	1.2	(0.7–2.0)	0.6	(0.4–1.0)	1.2	(0.8–1.7)
GENDER										
Male (ref)	1.0		1.0		1.0		1.0		1.0	
Female	1.0	(0.7–1.3)	1.4*	(1.1–1.9)	1.0	(0.7–1.4)	1.3	(0.9–1.9)	1.4	(1.0–1.8)
EDUCATION										
Less than high school (ref)	1.0		1.0		1.0		1.0		1.0	
Some or all high school	1.0	(0.5–1.9)	3.0**	(1.4–6.5)	1.0	(0.4–2.6)	1.0	(0.4–2.2)	0.9	(0.5–1.8)
Community college; non-university; trade	0.9	(0.5–1.8)	3.6**	(1.6–8.2)	1.5	(0.6–3.7)	1.1	(0.5–2.7)	1.1	(0.5–2.3)
University or higher	0.9	(0.5–1.7)	3.5**	(1.6–7.9)	1.2	(0.5–3.2)	1.6	(0.7–3.9)	1.4	(0.7–2.7)
COUNTRY OF BIRTH										
Canadian (ref)	1.0		1.0		1.0		1.0		1.0	
Foreign born	1.2	(0.9–1.6)	0.9	(0.7–1.2)	1.2	(0.8–1.8)	0.9	(0.7–1.3)	0.9	(0.6–1.2)
SELF-RATED HEALTH										
Excellent, very good (ref)	1.0		1.0		1.0		1.0		1.0	
Good	1.0	(0.7–1.4)	0.9	(0.7–1.2)	1.4	(0.9–2.1)	0.7	(0.5–1.0)	1.0	(0.7–1.4)
Fair, poor	1.0	(0.7–1.6)	0.9	(0.6–1.4)	1.0	(0.5–1.7)	0.7	(0.4–1.2)	0.7	(0.5–1.1)
MEMBERSHIP										
No (ref)	1.0		1.0		1.0		1.0		1.0	
Yes	0.9	(0.7–1.2)	0.9	(0.7–1.2)	0.9	(0.6–1.4)	1.3	(1.0–1.8)	1.3	(1.0–1.7)
CAREGIVER										
No (ref)	1.0		1.0		1.0		1.0		1.0	
Yes	0.9	(0.7–1.1)	1.1	(0.9–1.5)	1.3	(0.9–1.9)	1.1	(0.8–1.6)	1.3	(1.0–1.8)
SUM OF INFORMATION SOURCES†										
Continuous variable (0–3)	1.2	(1.0–1.3)	1.2**	(1.1–1.4)	0.9	(0.8–1.1)	1.1	(1.0–1.3)	1.3***	(1.2–1.5)
MARRIED										
No (ref)	1.0		1.0		1.0		1.0		1.0	
Yes	0.7*	(0.5–0.9)	1.0	(0.7–1.3)	1.5	(1.0–2.2)	1.0	(0.7–1.4)	1.0	(0.8–1.4)
FUNCTIONAL LIMITATION—IN OR OUTSIDE HOME										
No (ref)	1.0		1.0		1.0		1.0		1.0	
Yes	1.0	(0.8–1.4)	1.4	(1.0–1.9)	1.1	(0.7–1.6)	1.2	(0.8–1.7)	0.8	(0.6–1.1)
Chi-Square	22.664		44.000***		13.239		38.083***		61.465***	
−2 Log Likelihood	1,399.157		1,430.218		844.508		1,037.466		1,315.740	
Cox & Snell R Square	0.020		0.039		0.012		0.034		0.054	
Nagelkerke R Square	0.028		0.053		0.022		0.054		0.076	
Overall Percentage Correctly Predicted	66.3		62.5		87.1		81.2		69.1	

* $p < 0.05$, ** $p < 0.01$, *** $p < 0.001$
OR = odds ratio
† The OR represents each unit increase in the variable.

possible that our vignette methodology, by avoiding acquiescence bias, provides a more accurate estimate of older adults' awareness of CSSs.

The highest percentage of participants (37%) indicated they would turn to their physician for help in situations where a parent has dementia. These results are similar to previous research findings that 40 per cent of adults aged 65 and older spontaneously mentioned the facilitating role played by physicians in formal, community-based or home health services (Schoenberg, Campbell, & Johnson, 1999). However, other researchers have found that physicians have insufficient information about available services for dementia (Bruce & Paterson, 2000; Fortinsky, 1998) and that they do not refer patients to support services early enough, despite prolonged and often severe caregiver stress (Bruce & Paterson, 2000; Bruce, Paley, Underwood, Roberts, & Steed, 2002). One of the issues is that CSSs for dementia care are not currently integrated within a privately or publicly funded system. For example, accessing home health services or a family doctor does not necessarily provide a link to CSSs for dementia care. Integrated access to such services would likely benefit older adults and their caregivers.

The analysis revealed that few of the socio-demographic and other determinants we assessed were significantly associated with identification of CSSs, home health services, long-term care, physicians, and informal sources as sources of support. The use of physicians as sources of help for situations of parental dementia may be less likely for some groups than others, including men and those with less education. The use of informal sources of help such as family and neighbours may decrease with age. Knowing where to look for information about CSSs was associated with increased likelihood of mentioning physicians and home health services as potential sources of assistance. Further research is needed on the factors associated with identification of dementia care services. For example, Lillie

(2008), in using data from this project for her PhD studies, found that people who provide care are much more likely to have knowledge of CSSs than those who do not provide care.

Several factors limit the generalizability of study findings. First, we had a low response rate to the telephone survey, consistent with other studies of access to services (Calsyn & Winter, 2000). The barrage of telemarketing and the use of caller ID and telephone answering services make it difficult to achieve high response rates in telephone interviews. Our sample over-represented older adults who were female, Canadian born, and had high levels of education. As a result, the levels of awareness of community health and support services found in this study are likely inflated, since previous research has shown that women and those with higher education levels have higher levels of service awareness (Calsyn & Roades, 1993; Calsyn, Roades, & Klinkenberg, 1998). Further, we have limited information about the caregivers in this study. For example, we do not know if they were caring for a person with dementia. Although we studied older adults from one city only, limiting our ability to generalize our results, we believe that our findings have wider applicability.

The largest proportion of these older adults indicated they would turn to their physicians and informal supports as sources of help in situations of parental dementia. Research has found that both professionals and informal supports play important mediating roles in linking dementia caregivers to formal services (Cotrell & Engel, 1998). Physicians take on a range of important mediation roles such as ordering services, providing linkages or facilitating connections between services/agencies, advising or recommending services, supplying information on services, and providing reassurance about services (Schoenberg et al., 1999). There is a need to develop and evaluate strategies to help physicians and other health care providers to improve the links between older adults and their caregivers with appropriate

CSSs. Such strategies may include educational initiatives, promoting effective interprofessional teamwork and collaboration, and the use of technology such as Internet and email to provide information specific to available community supports for persons with dementia and their caregivers (Cantegreil-Kallen, Turbelin, Angel, Flahault, & Rigaud, 2006; Fortinsky, 2001).

Our study results suggest that efforts should also be made to increase the awareness of older persons and their caregivers related to available services for situations of parental dementia. Harris, Bayer, and Tadd (2002) suggested that older persons may differ in their preferred ways of obtaining information and that multiple approaches should be used including health professionals, organizations providing information and advice, family and friends, leaflets or written documents, television and radio or video, telephone, and the Internet. Some Ontario communities are introducing 211 as a telephone information service, and this may be a promising approach to the lack of awareness (www.211canada.ca). Particular efforts should be made to address the information needs of immigrant and culturally diverse groups.

In our evolving program of research in this area, we are conducting a study on how primary care physicians and allied health care providers working in their offices help to link older adults to CSSs. We are also writing a paper that examines how useful a social-determinants-of-health model is in predicting knowledge of community health services.

CONCLUSION

Lack of awareness of where to turn for help when faced with situations of parental dementia is a serious problem that needs to be addressed so that older adults may continue to live in their own homes using available supports, and so that caregivers avoid unnecessary burden. The lack of awareness of community support services, in particular, is troubling, given that the very purpose of these services is to help people retain social functioning and quality of life in the community. Action must be taken to improve the ability of physicians and other health care providers to help make these linkages possible.

ACKNOWLEDGEMENTS

We thank the following organizations and their employees for the valuable contribution that they have made in the development and analysis of this research: Catholic Family Services of Hamilton—Linda Dayler; Coalition of Community Health and Support Services—Lynne Edwards; Community Information Hamilton—Lesley Russell; Seniors Activation Maintenance Program—Lynne Edwards and Dave Banko; Grocer-Ease—Bev Morgan; Hamilton Community Care Access Centre—Sherry Parsley, Tom Peirce, and Dianne Thompson; Ontario Community Support Association (OCSA)—Susan Thorning and Taru Virkamaki; Regional Geriatric Program (Central)—David Jewell; Social Planning and Research Council of Hamilton (SPRC)—Don Jaffray; and United Way of Burlington and Greater Hamilton—Monica Quinlan. This research was funded by Canadian Institutes of Health Research—Institute on Aging; Ontario Ministry of Health and Long-term Care; United Way of Burlington and Greater Hamilton; and Social Sciences and Humanities Research Council through funding of the MCRI (Social and Economic Dimensions of an Aging Population).

REFERENCES

Brodaty, H., Thomson, C., Thompson, C., et al. (2005). Why caregivers of people with dementia and memory loss don't use services. *International Journal of Geriatric Psychiatry, 20*, 537-546.

Bruce, D. G., Paley, G. A., Underwood, P. J., Roberts, D., & Steed, D. (2002). Communication problems between dementia carers and general practitioners: Effect on access to community support services. *Medical Journal of Australia, 177*, 186-188.

Bruce, D. G., & Paterson, A. (2000). Barriers to community support for the dementia carer: A qualitative study. *International Journal of Geriatric Psychiatry, 15,* 451-457.

Buono, M. D., Busato, R., Mazzetto, M., Paccagnella, B., Aleotti, F., Zanetti, O., et al. (1999). Community care for patients with Alzheimer's disease and non-demented elderly people: Use and satisfaction with services and unmet needs in family caregivers. *International Journal of Geriatric Psychiatry, 14,* 915-924.

Calsyn, R. J., & Roades, L. A. (1993). Predicting perceived service need, service awareness, and service utilization. *Journal of Gerontological Social Work, 21*(1), 59-76.

Calsyn, R. J., Roades, L. A., & Calsyn, D. S. (1992). Acquiescence in needs assessment studies of the elderly. *The Gerontologist, 32,* 246-252.

Calsyn, R., Roades, L. A., & Klinkenberg, W. D. (1998). Using theory to design needs assessment studies of the elderly. *Evaluation and Programming Planning, 21,* 277-286.

Calsyn, R., & Winter, J. (1999). Understanding and control-ling response bias in needs assessment studies. *Evaluation Review, 23,* 399-417.

Calsyn, R. J., & Winter, J. P. (2000). Predicting different types of service use by the elderly: The strength of the behavioral model and the value of interaction terms. *Journal of Applied Gerontology, 19,* 284-303.

Canadian Study of Health and Aging Working Group. (1994). Patterns of caring for people with dementia in Canada. *Canadian Journal on Aging, 13,* 470-487.

Canadian Study of Health and Aging Working Group. (2000). The incidence of dementia in Canada. *Neurology, 55,* 66-73.

Cantegreil-Kallen, I., Turbelin, C., Angel, P., Flahault, A., & Rigaud, A. (2006). Dementia management in France: Health care and support services in the community. *Dementia, 5,* 317-326.

Caserta, M. S., Lund, D. A., Wright, S. D., & Redburn, D. E. (1987). Caregivers to dementia patients: The utilization of community services. *The Gerontologist, 27,* 209-214.

Chappell, N., McDonald, L., & Stones, M. (2008). *Aging in contemporary Canada* (2nd ed.). Toronto, Ontario, Canada: Pearson-Prentice Hall.

Collins, C., Stommel, M., Given, C. W., & King, S. (1991). Knowledge and use of community services among family caregivers of Alzheimer's disease patients. *Archives of Psychiatric Nursing, 5,* 84-90.

Cotrell, V., & Engel, R. J. (1998). The role of secondary supports in mediating formal services to dementia caregivers. *Journal of Gerontological Social Work, 30*(3/4), 117-132.

Cox, C. (1999). Race and caregiving: Pattern of service use by African American and white caregivers of persons with Alzheimer's disease. *Journal of Gerontological Social Work, 32*(2), 5-19.

Denton, M., Ploeg, J., Tindale, J., Hutchison, B., Brazil, K., Akhtar-Danesh, N., et al. (2008). Where would you turn for help? Older adults' awareness of community support services. *Canadian Journal on Aging, 27,* 359-370.

de Vaus, D. (2002). Survey research. In T. Greenfield (Ed.), *Research methods for postgraduates* (2nd ed., pp. 172-182). New York: Oxford.

Ferri, C. P., Prince, M., Brayne, C. H., Fratiglioni, L., Ganguli, M., et al. (2005). Global prevalence of dementia: A Delphi consensus study. *Lancet, 366,* 2112- 2117.

Forbes, D. A., Markle-Reid, M., Hawranik, P., Peacock, S., Kingston, D., Morgan, D., et al. (2008). Availabil-ity and acceptability of Canadian home and community-based services: Perspectives of family caregivers of persons with dementia. *Home Health Care Services Quarterly, 27,* 75-99.

Forbes, D. A., Morgan, D., & Janzen, B. L. (2006). Rural and urban Canadians with dementia: Use of health care services. *Canadian Journal on Aging, 25,* 321-330.

Fortinsky, R. H. (1998). How linked are physicians to community support services for their patients with dementia? *Journal of Applied Gerontology, 17,* 480-498.

Fortinsky, R. H. (2001). Health care triads and dementia care: Integrative framework and future directions. *Aging & Mental Health, 5*(Suppl. 1), S35-S48.

Harris, M., Bayer, A., & Tadd, W. (2002). Addressing the information needs of older patients. *Reviews in Clinical Gerontology, 12,* 5-11.

Hill, G., Forbes, W., Berthelot, J. M., Lindsay, J., & McDowell, I. (1996). Dementia among seniors. *Health Reports, 8*(2), 7-10.

Hughes, R., & Huby, M. (2002). The application of vignettes in social and nursing research. *Journal of Advanced Nursing, 37,* 382-386.

Jansen, L., Forbes, D. A., Markle-Reid, M., Hawranik, P., Kingston, D., Peacock, S., et al. (2009). Formal care providers' perceptions of home and community-based services: Informing dementia care quality. *Home Health Care Services Quarterly, 28,* 1-23.

Krout, J. A. (1983). Knowledge and use of services by the elderly: A critical review of the literature. *International Journal of Aging and Human Development, 17,* 153-167.

Lillie, J. (2008). *Older adults' knowledge of community support services: Does social support make a difference?* Unpublished doctoral dissertation. University of Guelph, Ontario, Canada.

Maslow, K. (1990). Linking persons with dementia to appropriate services: Summary of an OTA study. *Pride Institute Journal of Long Term Home Health Care, 9,* 42-50.

Ortiz, F., & Fitten, L. J. (2000). Barriers to healthcare access for cognitively impaired older Hispanics. *Alzheimer Disease and Associated Disorders, 14,* 141-150.

Østbye, T., & Crosse, E. (1994). Net economic costs of dementia in Canada. *Canadian Medical Association Journal, 151,* 1457-1464.

Robinson, K. M., Buckwalter, K. C., & Reed, D. (2005). Predictors of use of services among dementia caregivers. *Western Journal of Nursing Research, 27,* 126-140.

Schoenberg, N. E., Campbell, K. A., & Johnson, M. M. (1999). Physicians and clergy as facilitators of formal services for older adults. *Journal of Aging & Social Policy, 11,* 9-26.

Schoenberg, N. E., & Ravdal, H. (2000). Using vignettes in awareness and attitudinal research. *International Journal Social Research Methodology, 3,* 63-74.

Spalding, N. J., & Phillips, T. (2007). Exploring the use of vignettes: From validity to trustworthiness. *Qualitative Health Research, 17,* 954-962.

Statistics Canada. (2006a). Age and sex, 2006 counts for both sexes, for Canada and census metropolitan areas and census agglomerations—100% Data. Retrieved September 30, 2008, from http://www12.statcan.ca/english/census06/data/highlights/agesex/pages/Page.cfm?Lang=E&Geo=CMA&Code=01&Table=1&Data=Count&Sex=1&Sta rtRec=1&Sort=7&Display=Page&CSDFilter=5000

Statistics Canada. (2006b). Population and dwelling counts, for Canada and census subdivisions (municipalities), 2006 and 2001 censuses. Retrieved September 30, 2008, from http://www12.statcan.ca/english/census06/data/popdwell/Table.cfm?T=201&S=3&O=D&RPP=150

Strain, L., & Blandford, A. (2002). Community-based services for the taking but few takers: Reasons for nonuse. *Journal of Applied Gerontology, 21,* 220-235.

Streiner, D. L., & Norman, G. R. (1998). *PDQ Epidemiology* (2nd ed.). Hamilton, Ontario, Canada: B.C. Decker.

Vetter, P., Steiner, O., Kraus, S., Moises, H., Kropp, P., Moller, W. D., et al. (1998). Factors affecting the utilization of home-care supports by caregiving relatives of Alzheimer patients. *Dementia and Geriatric Cognitive Disorders, 9,* 111-116.

Wimo, A., Winblad, B., Aguero-Torres, H., & von Strauss, E. (2003). The magnitude of dementia occurrence in the world. *Alzheimer Disease & Associated Disorders, 17,* 63-67.

Winslow, B. W. (2003). Family caregivers' experiences with community services: A qualitative analysis. *Public Health Nursing, 20,* 341-348.

Zarit, S. H., Gaugler, J. E., & Jarrott, S. E. (1999). Useful services for families: Research findings and directions. *International Journal of Geriatric Psychiatry, 14,* 165-181.

INTRODUCTION TO CRITIQUE 1

The article "Older Adults' Awareness of Community Health and Support Services for Dementia Care" (Ploeg et al., 2009) is examined here in terms of its quality and the potential usefulness of the findings for application to nursing practice. The design of this study is level VI, inasmuch as it is a descriptive study.

Title

The title of the article captured the essence of the study succinctly.

Abstract

The abstract met the requirements of a good abstract; it included the purpose, the sample size, the method, the findings, and a short concluding statement.

Problem and Purpose

Ploeg and colleagues (2009) stated that the overall objective of the study was "to measure older persons' awareness of community health and support services when presented with a scenario related to caring for a parent with dementia" (p. 362); this objective was met. The significance of the problem was introduced clearly at the beginning of the article in the following statement: "Although many communities have an array of community health and support services . . . , the literature suggests . . . that one of the barriers to their use is the lack of awareness of such services" (p. 360). This problem statement was very concise, cited an appropriate reference, and presented a persuasive argument. In addition, Ploeg and colleagues specified the prevalence of Alzheimer's disease and stated that "this prevalence is projected to double every 20 years to more than 81 million people by 2040" (p. 360). This adds more credence to the rationale for the research.

Review of Literature and Definitions

Ploeg and colleagues' (2009) article contained a formal section titled "Literature Review," even though literature about dementia and community health and support services is also cited later in the article. The formal section of the literature review guides the reader through three main areas: (1) the concept of underutilization, highlighting the difference between "awareness" and "knowledge"; (2) factors associated with utilization of CSSs; and (3) methodological limitations in previous studies.

Ploeg and colleagues (2009) noted the gaps in each section. Regarding underutilization of community-based services, they suggested that most of the research "addresses awareness, not knowledge, of services" (p. 361). Under factors associated with utilization, they further noted that very little research on the factors associated with awareness of CSSs for dementia care had been conducted. In regard to methodological limitations, they noted that acquiescence bias—in which a respondent answers questions on a survey in a positive manner without paying attention to the content—was a problem. To support this assertion, they stated that in several studies, Calsyn and colleagues (1992) had provided older adults with the name of a fictitious agency and 20% to 30% of respondents reported "familiarity with that service" (p. 362).

Several studies cited were more than 10 years older than the article itself, which may suggest the paucity of research in this area. All of the references were apparently primary sources. The literature review provided a logical argument for Ploeg and colleagues' (2009) study.

Development of a Conceptual Framework

Ploeg and colleagues did not use a conceptual framework for the study. Using a conceptual framework could have provided a structure for the overarching concept of resource utilization.

Hypotheses and Research Question

Ploeg and colleagues (2009) explicitly stated the research questions as follows (p. 362):

1. Where would older adults turn for assistance when faced with a scenario related to caring for a parent with dementia?
2. What factors are associated with the identification of community health and support services as a source of assistance in caring for a parent with dementia?
3. Do caregivers have greater awareness of community health and support services than non-caregivers? (p. 362).

They offered no hypotheses, but an example could have been that greater awareness of support services would lead to increased utilization.

Sample

Ploeg and colleagues (2009) described the random sample, which consisted of 22,072 different telephone numbers, and the final sample included 1,152 individuals (a response rate of 12.4% of eligible particpants). The inclusion criteria were a minimum age of 50 years and ability to speak English. There were no exclusion criteria. Ploeg and colleagues stated that a power analysis was performed and described in another paper. Restating the analysis in this article would have been helpful for readers to assess whether the sample size was adequate and to determine the type of statistical test for which the power analysis was performed. Note that each type of statistical test—such as a *t* test, an analysis of variance (ANOVA), or regression—would have a different sample size.

Research Design

Ploeg and colleagues (2009) stated that their design was a cross-sectional descriptive survey, which was appropriate for this study. The authors used vignettes to address the methodology issue of acquiescence bias. The sample was divided into three groups, and each group received vignettes, one of which was about caring for a parent with dementia. Ploeg and colleagues focused on the responses to that vignette. The variables of this study were socioeconomic, demographic, and social.

Internal Validity

Although threats to internal validity are germane to experimental research, researchers need to pay attention to factors in a nonexperimental design that may potentially compromise a study. Possible threats to internal validity include history which is important to acknowledge in this age of widespread media campaigns around resources directed at Alzheimer's disease. Acquiescence bias was eliminated with the vignette methodology.

External Validity

Generalizability is limited to the sample because the individuals were from a specific geographical area in Canada; thus, generalizing to other populations would be questionable. Ploeg and colleagues (2009) also stated the sample "over-represented older adults who were female, Canadian born, and had high levels of education" (p. 368). To assess selection effects, Ploeg and colleagues compared the demographics of the sample with the Hamilton census data. The sample included higher proportions of women, people who were Canadian born, and people with incomes higher than the the average of the Hamilton population; thus, they did not represent the population.

Legal/Ethical Issues

Ethical approval was received from an ethics review board at the university; this was necessary before the study could proceed.

Instruments

From the literature review, you would anticipate that Ploeg and colleagues would collect information on socioeconomics, demographics, and social supports, which they did. They provided a detailed explanation of the vignette methodology with samples of the vignettes and questions posed.

Reliability and Validity

For the the narrative vignettes, reliability was not necessary. The authors stated that face and content validity of the vignettes was high inasmuch as the "vignettes . . . were developed by front-line service providers to represent realistic and familiar situations faced by older adults for which community health and support services would be appropriate" (p. 362).

Analysis and Findings of the Data

The variables mentioned in the article are on either a nominal or an ordinal scale of measurement. Gender, country of birth, marital status, language, and functional limitations are measured on a nominal scale, whereas age, education, household income, self-reported health, and number of information sources constitute ordinal levels of measurement.

Descriptive statistics were reported as means and standard deviations in both Table 19C1-1 (see p. 443) and the text; a small amount of repetition of the results highlighted the findings. Chi-square analyses at the .05 level of significance were appropriately conducted for obtaining information on the association between the variables and the total sample, caregivers, and noncaregivers before logistic regression analyses were performed. The responses to the first question were outlined clearly in the listing of the top five places from which older adults would seek assistance. Figure 19C1-1 showed that the number one resource for assistance was the physician. This finding was further noted in the text: "When faced with a situation of parental dementia, the highest percentage of participants identified a physician and the physician's office staff as sources of support" (Ploeg et al., 2009, p. 366).

Examples of results for the second question showed that the older the caregivers were, the less likely they were to turn to "informal sources such as family, friends, and neighbours"; this change "decreased significantly with age" (odds ratio = 0.6; Ploeg et al., 2009, p. 366). Furthermore, "identifying their physicians as a source of support" was 40% more likely if caregivers were female (odds ratio = 1.4) and 250% more likely (odds ratio = 3.5) if participants had higher levels of education (Ploeg et al., 2009, p. 366).

The answer to the third question—"Do caregivers have a greater awareness of community health and support services than non-caregivers?"—is unclear, inasmuch as it is not mentioned.

Discussion

The findings were explained within the context of previous research and the CSSs with the comment "There is a need to develop and evaluate strategies to help physicians and other heath care providers to improve the links between older adults and their caregivers with appropriate CSSs" (Ploeg et al., 2009, p. 368).

Also in this section, Ploeg and colleagues noted that they were conducting another study of how primary care physicians and allied health care providers working in their offices help older adults access CSSs. In addition, they were writing another paper in which they used an approach of social determinants of health.

Conclusions, Implications, and Recommendations

Ploeg and colleagues (2009) commented briefly on participants' lack of awareness of CSSs and stated that action must be taken to assist physicians and other allied health care providers in linking individuals to CSSs that are focused on persons with Alzheimer's disease.

CRITIQUING A QUANTITATIVE RESEARCH STUDY

CRITIQUE 2

The study "Self-Harm Intentions: Can They Be Distinguished Based Upon a History of Childhood Physical and Sexual Abuse?" by Elaine E. Santa Mina (2010) is critiqued here. The article is presented in its entirety and is followed by the critique on pp. 470–472. (From *Canadian Journal of Nursing Research, 42*[4], 122–143.)

Self-Harm Intentions: Can They Be Distinguished Based Upon a History of Childhood Physical and Sexual Abuse?

Elaine E. Santa Mina, RN, PhD
Associate Director, Post-Diploma Degree Program
Daphne Cockwell School of Nursing, Ryerson University
Toronto, Ontario

A non-experimental, comparative design is used to measures self-harm intention in clients with and without a history of childhood physical and sexual abuse (CP/SA) presenting to an emergency department with an episode of self-harm behaviour. The traditional suicide literature identifies the key intention concepts of wish-to-die, lethality, hopelessness, and depression. However, the trauma literature understands self-harm behaviour to be an adaptive response to CP/SA and as such possibly helpful for managing intense affect and dissociation. The findings of this study demonstrate that a CP/SA history is not a distinguishing factor in self-harm intention. Almost all participants, regardless of abuse history, gave multiple reasons for their self-harm behaviour, in addition to or other than the wish-to-die. The striking similarity between the non-abused and abused groups with regard to self-harm intention challenges clinicians to assess for the full range of intentions of people who engage in self-harm and suicidal behaviour.

KEYWORDS: child abuse, mental health/pyschosocial, psychiatric nursing, stress and coping, theory

Persistently high rates of self-harm/suicidal behaviours, and their potential outcome of death by suicide, challenge clinicians to develop assessments that direct efficacious treatments and thereby reduce the incidence. Thorough clinical assessments of self-harm/suicidal behaviours include an understanding of the motivations or intentions that drive them. It remains clinically and empirically uncertain whether self-harm and suicidal intentions are distinguishable (Fliege, Lee, Grimm, & Klapp, 2009) and what factors might account for any differences. Conceptualizations of self-harm/suicidal intentions vary from the wish-to-relieve disturbing thoughts and feelings to the wish-to-die (Gratz, 2003; Leenaars, 1988). In addition, there is evidence that a history of childhood physical/sexual abuse (CP/SA) may play a key role in self-harm intentions (Pagura, Cox, Sareen, & Enns, 2008). However, it has not been definitively determined that a history of CP/SA distinguishes between self-harm intentions and suicidal behaviours.

This study investigates the influence of CP/SA in differentiating between self-harm intentions and suicidal behaviour in a clinical sample of adults admitted to an inner-city teaching hospital with self-harm/suicidal behaviour.

BACKGROUND

There are disparities in the reported rates of self-harm/suicidal behaviours, suicides, and CP/SA. These disparities result from differences in conceptual and operational definitions and corresponding measures to report each phenomenon (Santa Mina & Gallop, 1998). Despite reported inconsistencies, the incidences remain high and point to a continuing global health problem. In Western countries, adolescent self-harm rates range from 5% to 9% (Skegg, 2005) and in college students the prevalence may be as high as 14% (Gratz, Dukes Conrad, & Roemer, 2002). Of further concern is evidence that people who engage in self-harm and suicidal behaviours have an increased risk of death by suicide (De Munck, Portzky, & Van Heeringen, 2009). Canadian and American rates of death by suicide are comparable, at approximately 20 males and 5 females per 100,000 population (Langois & Morrison, 2002; U.S. National Center for Health Statistics, 2008). Also, CP/SA is known to be a risk factor for both self-harm and suicide in adults (Pagura et al., 2008; Santa Mina & Gallop, 1998). Investigations to better understand the possible distinguishing role played by CP/SA in self-harm/suicidal intentions could lead to strategies for reducing the incidence of suicide through the use of more precise assessments and interventions.

The theoretical and research literatures describe different suicide and self-harm etiologies and intentions (Walsh & Rosen, 1988). The earliest empirical work describes suicide as an act of self-annihilation (Freud, 1917) and suicidal intention as a phenomenon that fluctuates along a life–death continuum. The research literature supports associations between the wish-to-die, multiple etiologic risk factors, and the severity of depression and hopelessness (Fuse, 1997). However, contemporary trauma theorists suggest that self-harm is a phenomenon separate from but related to suicide and that self-harm intentions may counter the death wish and be a method for coping (Alexander, 1999; Arnold, 1995). Theorists suggest that many adults with a history of childhood CP/SA cope with the overwhelming feelings (affect dysregulation) and disturbances in memories and thoughts (dissociation) by engaging in self-harm. The literature does support an association between CP/SA, the experience of intense emotional and cognitive sequelae, and adult self-harm (Browne & Finkelhor, 1986; Santa Mina & Gallop, 1998). Although an association between CP/SA and adult psychiatric disorders has been widely reported (Brown & Anderson, 1991; Welch, Patterson, Shaw, & Stewart-Brown, 2009), its influence on self-harm and suicidal intentions is not clear. Knowledge about the influence of CP/SA in self-harm

intentions may serve to guide assessments of and interventions for either similar or disparate clinical populations.

LITERATURE REVIEW

Association Between CP/SA and Self-Harm/Suicidal Behaviour

Three major reviews report the impact of CP/SA on adult suicide and self-harm (Beitchman et al., 1992; Browne & Finkelhor, 1986; Santa Mina & Gallop, 1998). These reviews report that adults with a history of CP/SA are more likely to engage in suicide and self-harm. Despite methodological problems related to definitions, small sample sizes, and the lack of control and comparison groups, there is evidence of a link between CP/SA and adult self-harm, suicidal ideation, suicidal behaviours, and suicide. Research also supports an association between self-harm and suicide. Many people who engage in self-harm behaviour eventually attempt suicide or die by suicide (Mann & Currier, 2007).

Childhood Physical and Sexual Abuse

Conceptual and operational definitions of CP/SA differ (Santa Mina & Gallop, 1998). The most common definitions are incorporated into this study and are supported by the literature. Physical abuse is "deliberate striking, hitting, punching, or burning a child less than 18 resulting in physical injury such as: bruises or fractures requiring medical intervention, distinguished from single slaps, or interfamilial fights" (Windle, Windle, Scheidt, & Miller, 1995, p. 1323). Sexual abuse is "sexual contact, ranging from fondling to intercourse, between a child in mid-adolescence or younger and a person at least five years older" (Briere, 1992, p. 4).

Conceptualization of Suicide and Self-Harm Intention

The suicide and self-harm literature and conceptual reviews do not reach consensus on the extent, if any, of overlap of intentions between the two phenomena, or whether they are in fact the same phenomenon (Fliege et al., 2009; Walsh & Rosen, 1988; Whitlock & Knox, 2007). As this study proposes that the intentions may differ based upon a history of CP/SA, the breadth of intentions—as identified across the literature—is included in the study's conceptualization. For this study, self-harm intention is defined, with the key constructs from the self-harm and suicide literature and adapted from Connors' (1996) work, as "the purpose(s) or meaning(s) of the self-harm behaviour, the regulation of affect, the regulation of dissociation, and/or the termination of life associated with direct self-actions that lie outside the realm of social acceptability and that hurt or harm the body" (Santa Mina, 2005, p. 67). Self-harm behaviour is "the class of actions, outside the realm of social responsibility, that hurt or harm the body...including cutting, burning, slapping, punching, scratching, gouging, harmful enemas and douches, interfering with the healing of wounds, inserting dangerous objects into the vagina or rectum, head-banging, . . . choking, hitting oneself with objects, ingesting sharp objects, and biting" (Connors, 1996, p. 199).

The conceptualization of self-harm/suicidal intention and its measurement are informed by the constructs that are known to be risk factors for the behaviours/sociological risk factors; the key suicide-intention constructs; the wish-to-die; lethality, depression, and hopelessness (Leenaars, 1988; Lester, 1991); and the management of emotions (affect) and cognitive disturbance (dissociation) (Gratz, 2003). Previous investigations have minimally integrated these constructs from sociology and psychology to reflect the complexity of the phenomenon. However, the prevalence of trauma history in people who attempt or die by suicide and people who self-harm suggests that intentions may be broader than the intent-to-die that is articulated in the classic suicide literature (Fliege et al., 2006). Therefore, concepts from traditional suicide theories and empirical studies as well as recent trauma theories and investigations direct this study's conceptualization of the phenomenon and the choice of instruments to measure the variables. The conceptualization for the study is that the sociological factor of gender and the cognitive and affective states of wish-to-die, hopelessness, depression, and affective regulation dissociation, as described below, influence self-harm/suicidal intentions in the presence of a history of CP/SA.

Sociological Risk Factors

Sociological suicide theories articulate broad social factors such as geography, culture, socioeconomic status, marital status, age-related factors, and gender that support a macro level of analysis to explain suicide (Fuse, 1997). For example, suicide attempts are more frequent in females (De Munck et al., 2009) yet males are at least three times more likely than females to die by suicide (Statistics Canada, 2010). Also, females are reported to engage in more self-cutting behaviours than males and are motivated by recurring issues of previous trauma (Arnold, 1995). Therefore, this study investigates CP/SA and gender as possible factors influencing self-harm/suicidal intention.

Suicide Intention

The wish-to-die, which is a quintessential suicide concept, emanates from traditional psychological suicide theories (Freud, 1917; Menninger, 1935) and continues to be fundamental today in the assessment of suicide risk (Registered Nurses Association of Ontario, 2007). Suicide intention fluctuates along a wish-to-live/wish-to-die continuum; the extent to which someone wants to end his or her life is an indication of intention to die (suicide intention). The wish-to-die lays the groundwork for investigation of the lethality of the suicidal behaviour. Highly lethal suicidal behaviour is associated with an increased likelihood of dying by suicide and is interpreted as proximal to the wish-to-die (Linehan, Comtois, Brown, Heard, & Wagner, 2006).

Depression

Depression is a medical diagnosis that includes the presence, in a 2-week period, of one of two symptoms—depressed mood; and decreased interest in daily activities almost all day, most days—and four or more of the following symptoms: an increase or decrease in weight in the absence of dieting; a decrease in appetite; an increase or decrease in sleeping; restlessness or a decrease in physical activity; fatigue or a decrease in energy; feelings of worthlessness; decreased ability to concentrate or make decisions; and recurring thoughts of death or suicide (American Psychiatric Association, 1994). Depression is highly associated with suicidal intention and suicidal behaviour (World Health Organization, 2010) and childhood trauma, such as CP/SA (Herman, 1992).

Hopelessness

Hopelessness is characterized by negative, constricted thought content and patterns regarding the past, present, and future such that pessimism and meaninglessness permeate the experience of living (Beck, Weissman, Lester, & Trexler, 1974; Mitchell, Garand, Dean, Panzak, & Taylor, 2005). People who feel hopeless rigidly believe that their perceptions are accurate and exclude other explanations that lead to realistic interpretations (Lester, 1994). Suicide becomes the only way to escape emotional suffering. Beck, Morris, and Beck (1974) demonstrate the ability of the cognitive state of hopelessness to influence the nature of emotions and the subsequent behaviour. In their seminal work, Beck, Schuyler, and Herman (1974) report that depression combined with hopelessness is a key factor in suicide intention and may result in highly lethal suicidal behaviour and death by suicide.

Affect Regulation

The conceptualization of self-harm without the intent-to-die has evolved within the trauma literature. Prior to the 1980s, few authors (Jung, 1974; Rosenthal, Rinzler, Walsh, & Klausner, 1972) alluded to trauma as a precursor of self-harm. More recently, authors (Klonsky & Moyer, 2008; van der Kolk et al., 1996) have described an association between the constellation of emotional, behavioural, and cognitive disturbances and a history of childhood trauma in people who engage in self-harm behaviour. The emotions of rage, frustration, guilt, and shame are common in trauma survivors and are experienced intensely and rapidly (Herman, 1992). Emotional instability, or sudden fluctuations in overwhelming feelings, is known as affective lability. It is theorized that self-harm is a response to these intense negative feelings as it expresses them and thereby restores emotional stability (Alexander, 1999; Arnold, 1995).

Dissociation

A cognitive disturbance known as dissociation is experienced frequently by survivors of CP/SA. Dissociation is a temporary state of cognitive disintegration such that a person's "consciousness, memory, identity and perception of environment" are momentarily disrupted along a continuum of severity, from inattention to inability to integrate affect, behaviour, and cognition (Mulder, Beautrais, Joyce, & Fergusson, 1998, p. 806). Separation of conscious awareness from traumatic events enables a person to withdraw from the psychological, emotional, and cognitive pain. In the dissociated state, the child "observes" him/herself as though the abuse were happening to someone else. Later in life, the person may re-experience dissociative states in the presence of emotional distress and have temporary perceptual experiences that are out of touch with the real world. The behavioural response to a state of dissociation may be self-harm, which can help the person to regain a sense of what is real (Mangall & Yurkovich, 2008; van der Kolk et al., 1996).

RESEARCH HYPOTHESES

It was hypothesized that, compared to those without CP/SA, clients who engaged in a recent episode of self-harm behaviour and reported a CP/SA history would have (1) less suicide intention, (2) more reasons related to affect regulation and dissociation, (3) greater dissociation, (4) greater affective lability, (5) less hopelessness, and (6) no difference in depression.

METHOD

A non-experimental, comparative design was used. A power analysis for the study was conducted in advance of data collection to determine sample-size adequacy. It was decided that a sample size of 64 per non-abused group and abused group was required in order to detect a moderate effect. Ethics approval was obtained from the research ethics boards of the university and the hospital.

A convenience sample of clients who engaged in self-harm behaviour was recruited from the inpatient and emergency units of the mental health service in an inner-city teaching hospital; the clients were recruited while still in hospital. Recruitment took place weekdays only, due to constraints in providing around-the-clock research assistant support. The principal investigator informed all clinical staff about the study and the clinical staff identified clients who met the inclusion criteria: 18 years of age or older; English-speaking; presenting to the inpatient or emergency unit with an episode of self-harm; and medically deemed as a voluntary admission to the hospital, competent to give consent under the *Mental Health Act of Ontario, Canada, 1990*. Potential participants were asked if they were interested in learning more about the study. If the client expressed interest, then the research assistant, who was not associated with either unit, met with the client at his or her convenience in a private office on the unit. Study details were described in depth, with opportunities for the participant to ask questions and withdraw at any time. Written informed consent was obtained. The research assistant was a graduate student in psychology with experience counselling people with psychiatric disorders and a history of trauma. Clinical staff were available should the participant become distressed. A contact number was provided to participants for crisis support should they become distressed at any time after completion of the study.

The participants completed all self-report instruments in hospital within 3 days of the episode of self-harm behaviour. They received $10 plus public transit or parking expenses, if incurred. No participant reported distress requiring clinical or crisis support.

The instruments for measuring CP/SA were the Childhood Physical Abuse Scale (Briere, 1992) and Russell's Sexual Abuse Scale (Russell, 1999). The instruments for each hypothesis were (1) the Beck Suicide Intent Scale (SIS) (Beck, Morris, et al., 1974) and the Self-Inflicted Injury Severity Form (SIISF) (Potter et al., 1998); (2) the Reasons for Self-Injury Inventory (SIQ) (Alexander, 1999); (3) the Dissociative Experiences Scale (DES) (Bernstein Carlson & Putnam, 1993) and the Structured Interview for Disorders of Extreme Stress (SIDES) dissociative subscale (Pelcovitz et al., 1997); (4) the Trauma Symptom Checklist-40 (Briere, 1996) and the SIDES affective subscale (Pelcovitz et al.); (5) the Beck Hopelessness Scale (BHS) (Beck, Weissman, et al., 1974); and (6) the Beck Depression Inventory II (BDI II) (Beck, Steer, & Garbin, 1988).

DATA ANALYSIS

Descriptive statistics were calculated to characterize the sample on the variables of interest.

Inferential analyses were used to address the study purpose. Two-tailed t tests and chi-square tests for independence (5% level of significance) compared the non-abused and abused groups on suicide intention, lethality, reasons for self-harm, dissociation, affect regulation, hopelessness, and depression. Of the 64 participants with abuse, 31 had CP/SA, 17 had physical abuse only, and 16 had sexual abuse only. Therefore, an ANOVA for four groups—non-abused, physically abused only, sexually abused only, and CP/SA—constituted the secondary analysis.

Three analyses of the SIQ items were conducted. First, the total number of reasons for self-harm per participant was calculated from the sum of the items selected. Next, the "reason" items were categorized into two subscales based on trauma theory, in order to test the hypotheses. Finally, a principal component analysis was conducted to extract five SIQ reason factors conceptually grounded in trauma theory. The findings from this work are reported elsewhere (Santa Mina et al., 2006).

RESULTS

The research assistant approached 113 clients for possible participation. Of these, 83 agreed to take part, for a response rate of 73% (non-abused, $n =$ 19; abused, $n = 64$). The reason given for refusal was lack of interest and/or time.

Descriptive statistics indicated a demographically homogeneous sample. Although gender was distributed evenly, females were more likely than males to be abused rather than non-abused (females, 7:1; males, 2:1; $\chi^2 = 4.723$; $df = 1$; $p = 0.03$). The participants ranged in age from 18 to 69 years, with the majority (82%) being between 21 and 50 years ($\bar{x} = 37.28$; $SD = 11.05$). Due to the small sample size per group, analysis of additional sociological factors did not produce meaningful results. Types of self-harm behaviour varied somewhat (overdose, $n = 42$; cutting, $n = 20$; other, $n = 21$), although overdose was the most frequent type ($\chi^2 = 11.122$; $df = 5$; $p = 0.049$). Self-harm types were evenly distributed between genders. The predominance of overdose as a self-harm method is consistent with method distributions found in other clinical studies (Haw, Houston, Townsend, & Hawton, 2002; Lester & Beck, 1980; Schnyder & Valach, 1997). The majority of the abused participants in the sample reported isolated incidents of CP/SA. They rarely reported incidents of abuse at a very young age (pre-pubescence) or of a prolonged or severe nature (over several years with force and penetration). All participants were moderately suicidal yet reflected an overall low level of lethality (SIISF; 48/77 had no actual injury). The participants had received immediate intervention after the self-harm episode, which may have served to lower the level of lethality.

The sample was highly dissociative, with high affective lability. All participants reported a "lifetime presence" of affective instability and 70% reported a "lifetime presence" of dissociation, with no significant between-group differences. On the SIDES "current presence" items, 40% ($n = 80$) reported "current presence" of affective instability and 34% reported "current presence" of dissociation, also with no between-group differences. Overall, the sample reported moderate hopelessness and severe depression.

Self-harm/suicidal intentions did not differ for the non-abused and abused groups (Table 19C2-1), nor did the level of lethality of the behaviour.

However, the sample overwhelmingly (98%) reported multiple reasons for the self-harm episode. Only 2% of the sample ($n = 2$) reported suicide as the sole reason for the behaviour, while 60% ($n = 50$) reported suicide plus other reasons, such as "to achieve a feeling of peace" or "to regain a sense of reality," and 38% ($n = 31$) reported multiple reasons that did not include suicide. The abused group revealed greater dissociation than the non-abused group, as well as greater affective lability. The secondary ANOVA found no significant difference across the four

TABLE 19C2-1

INSTRUMENTS, SCORING METHODS, AND RELIABILITY AND VALIDITY

CONCEPT	INSTRUMENT	NUMBER OF ITEMS	SCORING METHOD	INTERPRETATION OF SCORES	PREVIOUSLY REPORTED RELIABILITY AND VALIDITY	THIS STUDY'S RELIABILITY AND VALIDITY
Childhood Physical Abuse	Childhood Physical Abuse Scale[a]	3 items	Yes/no and frequency if yes	Yes to any of the items = history of CPA	No reports	Not tested
Childhood Sexual Abuse	Russell's Sexual Abuse Scale[b]	8 items	Yes/no and frequency of events by perpetrator	Yes to any of the items = history of CSA	Test-retest reliability $r = .91-.99$	Not tested
Suicide Intent	Beck's Suicide Intent Scale (SIS)[c]	10 items	Each item scored as 0, 1, or 2; possible range of scores 0–30	Higher score indicative of greater intent; SIS scores in suicidal clients $\overline{x} = 7.68-10.2$	Interrater reliability $r = .82-.95$[d]; $\alpha = .85$[e]	$\alpha = .76$; 95% confidence interval; $\alpha = .67-.83$
Lethality	Self-Inflicted Injury Severity Form (SIISF)[f]	4 categories of lethality severity for each of 7 self-harm behaviour methods	Based on chart review, self-harm behaviour is categorized by self-harm method and severity of lethality	1 (no injury) to 4 (highly lethal trauma penetrating body cavity)	High internal consistency; high interrater reliability; high discriminate and construct validity[f]	Interrater reliability on method of self-harm $r = .94$; interrater reliability SIISF $r = .77$
Reasons for Self-Harm	Self-Injury Questionnaire (SIQ)[g]	31 items total: 2 subscales: (i) reasons due to affect, 7 items; (ii) reasons due to dissociation, 4 items	Yes/no per item; total sum of number of reasons; sum of reasons for subscales; factor analysis for reason themes[h], range of scores: total scale total number of reasons 0–31; subscale reasons due to affect 0–7; subscale reasons due to dissociation 0–4	Yes = reason given by participant for self-harm event; no = not a reason for self-harm given by participant for self-harm event	Good face validity[g]	Strong $\alpha = 0.83$; 95% confidence interval; 0.78–0.86; affective subscale: $\alpha = 0.72$; 95% confidence interval, 0.62–0.80; dissociative subscale: $\alpha = 0.77$; 95% confidence interval, 0.68–0.84; factor analysis: factors I–V: weak significant correlations with SIS, BDI II, BHS, SIISF, TSC-40, DESh

Affect Regulation	Structured Interview for Disorders of Extreme Stress: affect dysregulation subscale, 19 items[i]	(i) symptom current presence; (ii) symptom lifetime presence; (iii) symptom severity 19 items	(i) yes/no; (ii) yes/no; (iii) 0–3 per item mean score on subscale	Yes = present; no = not present; 0 (none) to 3 (frequently) score: ≥ 2 is clinically significant	α = .90[i]	α = .83; 95% confidence interval = .76–.87
Affect Regulation	Trauma Symptom Checklist-40 (TSC-40)	40 items	1 (never) to 4 (often) Range of scores 0–120	Higher score indicates greater affective dysregulation	α = .89–.91[i]	α = .90; 95% confidence interval = .86–.93
Dissociation	Structured Interview for Disorders of Extreme Stress (SIDES): alteration in attention subscale 5 items[i]	(i) symptom current presence; (ii) symptom lifetime presence; (iii) symptom severity 5 items	(i) yes/no; (ii) yes/no; (iii) 1–3 per item mean score on subscale	(i) and (ii) yes = present, no = not present; (iii) 0 (none) to 3 (frequently); range of scores 0–3; score ≥ 2 is clinically significant	Alteration inattention = .76[i]	α = .62; 95% confidence interval = .47–.73
Dissociation	Dissociative Experiences Scale (DES)[k]	28 items 0–100; 0 (never) to 100 (always); mean scores	Mean scores range from 0 to 100	Cut-off scores <10 = low dissociation; 10–29.9 = dissociation common with psychiatric disorders, not trauma; >30 = dissociative disorders[k]	Test-retest reliability r = .79–.96 at intervals of 4 to 8 weeks; internal reliability α = .83–.93 (p < .00)[k]	α = .93; 95% confidence interval = .88–.95

Continued

TABLE 19C2-1

INSTRUMENTS, SCORING METHODS, AND RELIABILITY AND VALIDITY—cont'd

CONCEPT	INSTRUMENT	NUMBER OF ITEMS	SCORING METHOD	INTERPRETATION OF SCORES	PREVIOUSLY REPORTED RELIABILITY AND VALIDITY	THIS STUDY'S RELIABILITY AND VALIDITY
Hopelessness	Beck Hopelessness Scale (BHS)[l]	20-item true/false	Sum total score	0–3 = no hopelessness; 4–8 = mild; 9–14 = moderate; 15–20 = severe; 9 = criteria for sensitivity (attempters correctly identified as eventually dying by suicide) and specificity (attempters identified and did not die by suicide)[l]	$\alpha = .92$[m]	$\alpha = .93$; 95% confidence interval = .82–.95
Depression	Beck Depression Scale (BDI II)[n]	21 items	Scores range from 0 to 63	0–9 = no to minimal depression; 10–18 = mild to moderate; 19–29 = moderate to severe; 30–63 = severe[n]	$\alpha = .81–86$[n]	$\alpha = .87$; 95% confidence interval = .82–.91

Note: α = coefficient alpha.
[a]Briere (1992).
[b]Russell (1999).
[c]Beck, Morris, & Beck (1974).
[d]Beck, Morris, et al. (1974).
[e]Beck & Steer (1989).
[f]Potter et al. (1998).
[g]Alexander (1999).
[h]Santa Mina et al. (2006).
[i]Pelcovitz et al. (1997).
[j]Elliot & Briere (1992).
[k]Bernstein Carlson & Putnam (1993).
[l]Beck, Weissman, Lester, & Trexler (1974).
[m]Beck & Steer (1989).
[n]Beck, Steer, & Garbin (1988).

groups for any of the hypotheses, with one exception: On the SIQ "affect" sub-scale, the physical and sexual abuse group reported the largest mean number of reasons, as compared to the other three groups ($F = 2.88, 3, 79; p = .04$). On the factor analysis, the SIQ mean scores for factors I through V did not differ significantly across the groups. The ANOVA, in the secondary analyses, tested for a difference in dissociation (DES) and depression (BDI II) across the four groups. Although there was no statistically significant difference in dissociation or depression across the four groups, a trend of higher scores in the group with both physical and sexual abuse was noted and examined. A linear trend was calculated on the DES and BDI II and demonstrated a statistically significant increase in dissociation ($F = 5.211; df = 1; p = 0.025$) and depression ($F = 7.796; df = 1; p = 0.01$), with an increase in abuse severity.

DISCUSSION

The results of this study refute the hypothesis that self-harm intentions can be distinguished based on a history of CP/SA. Although the findings are not statistically significant, they are clinically significant. The majority of participants, regardless of abuse history, reported multiple intentions, reflective of the key concepts in both suicide and self-harm intention. This finding provides direction for practice and research. The participants endorsed numerous, seemingly contradictory, intentions for self-destructive behaviours: "to bring myself back to reality," "to achieve a feeling of peace," "to distract from feelings or thoughts [of suicide] and a suicide attempt." Participants also reported moderate levels of suicidality (SIS) and high levels of hopelessness (BHS) and depression (BDI II), even if they did not report "suicide attempt" as a reason on the SIQ. This mixed clinical picture is consistent with the findings of other studies (Brown, Comtois, & Linehan, 2002; Holden & McLeod, 2000). One might argue that it supports the notion of ambivalence

between life and death (Shneidman, 1985). Yet that conjecture misses the breadth of other powerful intentions by narrowly focusing on the wish-to-live/wish-to-die continuum that subsequently may shape assessments and interventions.

Recruitment of an adequate sample size for a non-abused group proved to be very challenging in this inner-city population. When adequacy of sample size for the abused group was achieved ($n = 64$), the non-abused sample remained at 19. As data analysis demonstrated highly non-significant findings and risk of a type II error was low, the decision was made to stop data collection. However, this limitation is important in placing the findings in context. Participants with a broad history of childhood trauma, inclusive of emotional and psychological abuse and physical neglect, may endorse responses to suicide intention, reasons for self-harm, affect regulation, dissociation, depression, and hopelessness that are similar to responses of those with a history of CP/SA. It is possible that some of the participants in the non-abused group had experienced these other types of childhood abuse, but it was beyond the scope of this study to measure them. This could account for the absence of differences between the groups, as the non-abused sample may have had other forms of childhood trauma and may have been as responsive in intentionality as those with CP/SA. Challenges in finding adequate sample sizes for the non-abused clinical group remain, as abuse prevalence is high in psychiatric populations. It is possible that these findings and a propensity towards an abused population are representative of an inner-city population. Comparisons between inner-city/urban and rural populations, as well as between emergency and community populations, may also be helpful for obtaining comparator groups. Future studies should aim for large sample sizes, to accommodate the breadth of abuse types as well as the myriad sociological factors that can affect intentions. Alternative sampling strategies, such as highly resourced consecutive sampling, would serve to reduce sampling bias and ensure the inclusion of all patients with self-harm who are treated and released from emergency departments during evening/night shifts and weekends.

Evidence also points to a complex relationship between numerous types of childhood maltreatment and adult psychopathology that are not limited to overt self-harm and suicidal behaviours (Welch et al., 2009). The relationship between childhood maltreatment and adult addictions, as one specific type of indirect self-harm behaviour, is an example. Indirect types of self-harm, such as risky behaviour inclusive of substance misuse as discussed by Connors (1996), should be added as factors in our understanding of the complexity and breadth of childhood maltreatment and adult self-harm and suicide.

In the present study, the prevalence of CP/SA in both men and women is noteworthy. The findings point to a similarity in self-harm intentions and methods regardless of gender, a notable sociological risk factor for self-harm and suicide. Much of the self-harm literature addresses females who cut themselves in order to cope with overwhelming thoughts and feelings in response to their trauma histories. The reports are often focused on female patients who cut themselves and are diagnosed with borderline personality disorder (BPD) (Andover, Pepper, Ryabchenko, Orrico, & Gibb, 2005). In the present study, interestingly, men as well as women engaged in cutting to relieve intense affect and manage dissociation, and men and women overdosed to achieve the same purposes, regardless of abuse histories. This suggests that males as well as females engage in various types of self-harm behaviours for reasons related to affect and dissociation. As gender did not present as a sociological factor influencing either the type of self-harm behaviour or behavioural intentions, clinicians and researchers may need to rethink intentions in self-harm behaviours, as these may not be exclusively the sequelae of CP/SA and

may not be gender-based or associated with specific methods or diagnoses such as BPD.

The associations amongst the spectrum of childhood maltreatment and adult self-harm and suicide are multifaceted and complex. The natures of both childhood maltreatment and self-harm/suicide are highly sensitive and are fraught with issues of stigma and intense emotion. Although quantitative, psychometrically sound instruments for measuring the full range of types of childhood abuse and types of self-harm and intentions may be useful, the nature of the phenomena may be such that numeric measures do not fully capture the essence of the experience. Qualitative methods may serve to enrich our knowledge of these multifaceted problems. Both positivist and naturalist paradigms need to be incorporated into future research, to fully inform us about how gender and the spectrum of abuse types, methods, lethality, and intentions contribute to self-harm intention. It may be that a triangulation of methods will lead to a better understanding of this intricate issue.

The findings from this study indicate that patients who are thinking about or engaging in self-harm/suicidal behaviours need to be assessed for the full spectrum of intentions, regardless of gender, self-harm method, or known abuse history. Research is needed to direct the development and utilization of clinical self-harm/suicide assessments that are more inclusive of the breadth of self-harm intentions. Fully informed assessments may guide clinicians to develop interventions targeted to patient needs. Efficacious, intention-based interventions have the potential to diminish the tragic impact of self-destructive behaviours on individuals, their families, and societies by reducing self-harm and suicidal behaviours.

CONCLUSION

This is the first published clinical study to investigate the influence of CP/SA on self-harm/suicide intentions among men and women admitted to an acute-care unit for these behaviours. Although the literature points to CP/SA as a possible distinguishing factor for intentions, the present findings demonstrate that self-harm and suicidal intentions may be remarkably similar, regardless of a history of CP/SA. In the majority of individuals across both abused and non-abused groups, regardless of gender or self-harm type and self-harm/suicidal intentions, intentions were overwhelmingly varied, were seemingly contradictory, and reflected a need to manage distressing feelings and thoughts within the context of the wish-to-die. These findings challenge clinicians and researchers to re-evaluate the breadth of their assessments and interventions and to incorporate knowledge from both suicide and trauma theories in order to best care for people with this multidimensional problem.

ACKNOWLEDGEMENTS

This study was funded by a St. Michael's Hospital Community Mental Health Fellowship, St. Michael's Mental Health Service, in Conjunction with the Mental Health Systems Research and Development Program, Department of Psychiatry, University of Toronto.

I gratefully acknowledge the contributions of my committee members for this study: Dr. Ruth Gallop, Dr. Paul Links, Dr. Dorothy Pringle, and Dr. Ron Heslegrave.

REFERENCES

Alexander, L. A. (1999). *The functions of self-injury and its link to traumatic events in college students.* Unpublished doctoral dissertation, University of Massachusetts, Amherst.

American Psychiatric Association. (1994). *Diagnostic and statistical manual of mental disorders* (4th ed.). Washington: Author.

Andover, M., Pepper, C., Ryabchenko, K., Orrico, E., & Gibb, B. (2005). Self-mutilation and symptoms of depression, anxiety, and borderline personality. *Suicide and Life Threatening Behavior*, *35*(5), 581-591.

Arnold, L. (1995). *Women and self injury: A survey of 76 women.* Bristol: Mental Health Foundation, Bristol Crisis Service for Women.

Beck, A. T., Schuyler, D., & Herman I. (1974). Development of suicidal intent scales. In A. T. Beck, H. L. P. Resnick, & D. J. Lettieri (Eds.), *The prediction of suicide* (pp. 45-58). Bowdie, MD: Charles Press.

Beck, A. T., & Steer, R. A. (1989). Clinical predictors of eventual suicide: A 5-10 year prospective study of suicide attempters. *Journal of Affective Disorders*, *17*, 203-209.

Beck, A. T., Steer, R. A., & Garbin, M. G. (1988). Psychometric properties of the Beck Depression Inventory: Twenty-five years of evaluation. *Clinical Psychology Review*, *8*, 77-100.

Beck, A. T., Weissman, A., Lester, D., & Trexler, L. (1974). The measurement of pessimism: The Hopelessness Scale. *Journal of Consulting and Clinical Psychology*, *42*(6), 861-865.

Beck, R. W., Morris, J. B., & Beck A. T. (1974). Cross-validation of the Suicidal Intent Scale. *Psychological Reports*, *34*, 445-446.

Beitchman, J. H., Zucker, K. J., Hood, J. E., Da Costa, G. A., Akman, D., & Cassavia, E. (1992). A review of the long-term effects of child sexual abuse. *Child Abuse and Neglect*, *16*, 101-118.

Bernstein Carlson, B. E., & Putnam, F. W. (1993). An update on the Dissociative Experiences Scale. *Dissociation*, *6*(1), 16-29.

Briere, J. (1992). *Child abuse trauma: Theory and treatment of the lasting effects.* Newbury Park, CA: Sage.

Briere, J. (1996). Psychometric review of the Trauma Symptom Checklist-40. In B. H. Stamm (Ed.), *Measurement of stress, trauma, and adaptation* (pp. 373-376). Lutherville, MD: Sidran Press. Retrieved December 1, 2001, from www.johnbriere.com/tsc.htm.

Brown, G. R., & Anderson, B. (1991). Psychiatric morbidity in adult inpatients with childhood histories of sexual and physical abuse. *American Journal of Psychiatry*, *148*(1), 55-61.

Brown, M. Z., Comtois, K. A., & Linehan, M. M. (2002). Reasons for suicide attempts and non-suicidal self injury in women with borderline personality disorder. *Journal of Abnormal Psychology*, *11*(1), 198-202.

Browne, A., & Finkelhor, D. (1986). Impact of child sexual abuse: A review of the research. *Psychological Bulletin*, *99*(1), 66-77.

Connors, R. (1996). Self-injury in trauma survivors: 1. Functions and meanings. *American Ortho-psychiatric Association*, *66*(2), 197-206.

De Munck, S., Portzky, G., & Van Heeringen, K. (2009). Epidemiological trends in attempted suicide in adolescents and young adults between 1996 and 2004. *Crisis, 30*(3), 115-119.

Elliot, D. M., & Briere, J. (1992). Sexual abuse trauma among professional women: Validating the Trauma Symptom Checklist-40 (TSC-40). *Child Abuse and Neglect, 16*, 391-398.

Fliege, H., Kocalevent, R., Walter, M., Beck, S., Gratz, K., Gutierrez, P. M., et al. (2006). Three assessment tools for deliberate self-harm and suicide behavior: Evaluation and psychopathological correlates. *Journal of Psychosomatic Research, 61*, 113-121.

Fliege, H., Lee, J.-R., Grimm, A., & Klapp, B. (2009). Risk factors and correlates of deliberate self-harm behaviour: A systematic review. *Journal of Psychosomatic Research, 66*, 477-493.

Freud, S. (1917). Mourning and melancholia. In J. Strachey (Ed.), Complete psychological works, *Vol. 14*. London: Hogarth.

Fuse, T. (1997). Theories of suicide. In T. Fuse (Ed.), *Suicide: Individual and society* (pp. 75-163). Toronto: Canadian Scholars' Press.

Gratz, K. L. (2003). Risk factors for and functions of deliberate self-harm: An empirical and conceptual review. *Clinical Psychology, 10*, 192-205.

Gratz, K. L., Dukes Conrad, S., & Roemer, L. (2002). Risk factors for deliberate self-harm among college students. *American Journal of Orthopsychiatry, 72*(1), 128-140.

Haw, C., Houston, K., Townsend, E., & Hawton, K. (2002). Deliberate self-harm patients with depressive disorders: Treatment and outcomes. *Journal of Affective Disorders, 70*(1), 57-65.

Herman, J. L. (1992). *Trauma and recovery*. New York: Basic Books.

Holden, R., & McLeod, L. (2000). The structure of the Reasons for Attempting Suicide Questionnaire (RASQ) in a non-clinical adult population. *Personality and Individual Differences, 29*, 621-628.

Jung, C. G. (1974). The relations between the ego and the unconscious (R. Hull, Trans.). In H. Read, M. Fordam, & G. Adler (Eds.), The collected works of C. G. Jung, *Vol. 7*. London: Routledge & Kegan Paul. (Original published in 1928.)

Klonsky, E. D., & Moyer, A. (2008). Childhood sexual abuse and non-suicidal self-injury: Meta-analysis. *British Journal of Psychiatry, 192*, 166-170.

Langois, S., & Morrison, P. (2002). Suicide deaths and suicide attempts. *Health Records, 13*(2), 9-22.

Leenaars, A. A. (1988). *Suicide notes: Predictive clues and patterns*. New York: Human Sciences Press.

Lester, D. (1991). The study of suicidal lives. *Suicide and Life Threatening Behavior, 21*(2), 164-173.

Lester, D. (1994). Research note: A comparison of 15 theories of suicide. *Suicide and Life Threatening Behavior, 24*(1), 80-88.

Lester, D., & Beck, A. T. (1980). What the suicide's choice of method signifies. *OMEGA, 11*(3), 271-277.

Linehan, M. M., Comtois, K. A., Brown, M. Z., Heard, H. L., & Wagner, A. (2006). Suicide Attempt Self-Injury Interview (SASII): Development, reliability, and validity of a scale to assess suicide attempts and intentional self-injury. *Psychological Assessment, 18*(3), 303-312.

Mangall, J., & Yurkovich, E. (2008). A literature review of deliberate self-harm. *Perspectives in Psychiatric Care, 44*(3), 175-184.

Mann, J. J., & Currier, D. (2007). Prevention of suicide. *Psychiatric Annals, 37*(5), 331-339.

Menninger, K. A. (1935). A psychoanalytic study of the significance of self-mutilations. *Psychoanalytic Quarterly, 4*, 408-466.

Mitchell, A., Garand, L., Dean, D., Panzak, G., & Taylor, M. (2005). Suicide assessments in hospital emergency departments: Implications for patient satisfaction and compliance. *Topics in Emergency Medicine, 27*(4), 302-312.

Mulder, R. T., Beautrais, A. L., Joyce, P. R., & Fergusson, D. M. (1998). Relationship between dissociation, childhood sexual abuse, childhood physical abuse, and mental illness in a general population. *American Journal of Psychiatry, 155*(6), 806-811.

Pagura, J., Cox, B., Sareen, J., & Enns, M. (2008). Factors associated with multiple versus single episode suicide attempts in 1990–1992 and 2001–2003 United States National Comorbidity Surveys. *Journal of Nervous and Mental Disease, 196*(11), 806-813.

Pelcovitz, D., van der Kolk, B., Roth, S., Mandel, F., Kaplan, S., & Resick, P. (1997). Development of a criteria set and a Structured Interview for Disorders of Extreme Stress (SIDES). *Journal of Traumatic Stress, 10*(1), 3-12.

Potter, L. B., Kresnow, M., Powell, K. E., O'Carroll, P. W., Lee, R. K., Frankowski, R., et al. (1998). Identification of nearly fatal suicide attempts: Self-Inflicted Injury Severity Form. *Suicide and Life Threatening Behavior, 28*(2), 174-186.

Registered Nurses Association of Ontario. (2007). *The assessment and care of adults at risk for suicidal ideation and behaviour: Best practice guideline*. Toronto: Author. Retrieved January 8, 2010, from http://www.rnao.org/.

Rosenthal, R. J., Rinzler, C., Walsh, R., & Klausner, E. (1972). Wrist-cutting syndrome: The meaning of a gesture. *American Journal of Psychiatry, 128*(11), 1363-1363.

Russell, D. E. H. (1999). *The secret trauma: Incest in the lives of girls and women.* New York: Basic Books.

Santa Mina, E. E. (2005). *Intentions in self-harm behaviour in an emergency population: Can they be distinguished based upon a history of childhood physical and sexual abuse?* Unpublished doctoral dissertation, University of Toronto.

Santa Mina, E. E., & Gallop, R. (1998). Childhood sexual and physical abuse and adult self-harm and suicidal behavior: A literature review. *Canadian Journal of Psychiatry, 43*, 793-800.

Santa Mina, E. E., Gallop, R., Links, P., Heslegrave, R., Pringle, D., Wekerle, C., et al. (2006). The Self-Injury Questionnaire: Evaluation of the psychometric properties in a clinical population. *Journal of Psychiatric and Mental Health Nursing, 13*, 221-227.

Schnyder, U., & Valach, L. (1997). Suicide attempters in a psychiatric emergency room population. *General Hospital Psychiatry, 19*(2), 119-129.

Shneidman, E. (1985). Classifications and approaches. In E. Shneidman (Ed.), *Definition of suicide* (pp. 23-40). New York: John Wiley.

Skegg, K. (2005). Self-harm. *Lancet, 366*, 1471-1483.

Statistics Canada. (2010). Summary tables: Suicides and suicide rate, by sex and by age group. Retrieved August 31, 2010, from http://www40.statcan.ca/101/cst01/hlth66a-eng.htm.

U.S. National Center for Health Statistics. (2008). Health, United States. Retrieved August 31, 2010, from http://www.cdc.gov/nchs/hus.htm.

van der Kolk, B. A., Pelcovitz, D., Roth, S., Mandel, F. S., McFarlane, A., & Herman, J. L. (1996). Dissociation, somatization, and affect dysregulation: The complexity of adaptation to trauma. *American Journal of Psychiatry, 153*(7), 83-93.

Walsh, B. W., & Rosen, P. M (1988). Distinguishing self-mutilation from suicide: A review and commentary. In B. W. Walsh & P. M. Rosen (Eds.), *Self-mutilation theory, research, and treatment* (pp. 39-53). New York: Guilford.

Welch, S., Patterson, J., Shaw, R., & Stewart-Brown, S. (2009). Family relationships in childhood and common psychiatric disorders in later life: Systematic review of prospective studies. *British Journal of Psychiatry, 194*, 392-398.

Whitlock, J., & Knox, K. L. (2007). The relationship between self-injurious behaviour and suicide in a young adult population. *Archives of Pediatric and Adolescent Medicine, 161*(7), 634-640.

Windle, M., Windle, R. C., Scheidt, D. M., & Miller, G. B. (1995). Physical and sexual abuse and associated mental disorders among alcoholic inpatients. *American Journal of Psychiatry, 152*(9), 1322-1328.

World Health Organization. (2010). Suicide prevention. Geneva: Author. Retrieved January 8, 2010, from http://www.who.int/mental_health/prevention/en/2010.

INTRODUCTION TO CRITIQUE 2

The article "Self-Harm Intentions: Can They Be Distinguished Based Upon a History of Childhood Physical and Sexual Abuse?" (Santa Mina, 2010) is examined in terms of its quality and the potential usefulness of the findings for application to nursing practice. The design of this was level IV, inasmuch as it was a nonexperimental study.

Title

The title reflects the major purpose of this study.

Abstract

The abstract meets most of the requirements of thoroughness, except for the sample size. It contains the purpose, the research design, the findings, and the results.

Problem and Purpose

Santa Mina (2010) stated that the purpose of the study was to investigate "the influence of CP/SA in differentiating between self-harm intentions and suicidal behaviour in a clinical sample of adults admitted to an inner-city teaching hospital with self-harm/suicidal behaviour" (p. 123).

The identification of the research problem is very well organized, with an easy flow of the linkages. Santa Mina (2010) outlined the significance of the study by stating the incidence of self-harm behaviour and suicidal behaviours. Next, the author offered information on the causes of and intentions involved in self-harm. The concepts of affect dysregulation and dissociation were introduced. The rationale for the study was explicitly stated as follows:

> Although an association between CP/SA and adult psychiatric disorders has been widely reported . . ., its influence on self-harm and suicidal intentions is not clear. Knowledge about the influence of CP/SA in self-harm intentions may serve to guide assessments of and interventions for either similar or disparate clinical populations. (p. 124)

Review of Literature and Definitions

The literature review was well organized. In a systematic manner, the relationships among the core elements of CP/SA and adult-harm, suicidal ideation, suicidal behaviours, and suicide were clarified. The use of subheadings increased the readability of the literature review. The references were mostly primary sources (e.g., Connors, 1996; Windle, Windle, Scheidt, & Miller, 1995), with the addition of a few secondary sources (e.g., Santa Mina & Gallop, 1998). Most sources had been published within 10 years of the article's publication, and those more than 10 years older are landmark studies. Although the research on the study's topic is considerable, as articulated in the literature review, Santa Mina (2010) identified a gap in the literature by commenting that "The suicide and self-harm literature and conceptual reviews do not reach consensus on the extent, if any, of overlap of intentions between the two phenomena, or whether they are in fact the same phenomenon" (p. 125).

Theoretical Framework

The theoretical framework helped structure the study, inasmuch as it consisted of conceptualizations from sociological suicide theories, with the following main factors: suicide intention, depression, hopelessness, affect regulation, and dissociation. The linkages of these factors to support the study are clearly articulated. In addition, conceptual definitions serve to enhance the clarity.

Hypotheses and Research Question

Santa Mina (2010) explicitly stated the research hypotheses as follows: that patients who engaged in a recent episode of self-harm behaviour and reported a history of CP/SA, in comparison with those with no such history, would have "(1) less suicide intention, (2) more reasons related to affect regulation and dissociation, (3) greater dissociation, (4) greater affective lability, (5) less hopelessness, and (6) no difference in depression" (p. 128).

No research question is stated, but such a statement could be articulated from the hypotheses as follows: What is the difference in suicide intention, affect regulation and dissociation, affect liability, level of hopelessness, and level of depression in individuals who reported a CP/SA history in comparison with those who did not have a CP/SA history?

Sample

A convenience sample was used; this is appropriate as it is a nonexperimental study. A probability method such as randomization (assignment to a CP/SA group or to a non-CP/SA group) would have been unethical. The inclusion criteria were age of 18 years or older; ability to speak English; presenting to a hospital after an episode of self-harm; and being admitted voluntarily to the hospital, with competence to give consent under the *Mental Health Act of Ontario, Canada, 1990* (Santa Mina, 2010, p. 129). The study had no exclusion criteria.

Recruitment took place weekdays only, because of constraints in support, and Santa Mina informed all clinical staff about the study. These staff members identified patients who met the inclusion criteria. A power analysis indicated that 64 patients were needed in each group (the abused group and the nonabused group). However, the nonabused group contained only 19 participants, and so a final power analysis should have been performed.

Research Design

Santa Mina (2010) explicitly stated that she used a nonexperimental, comparative design. There were two groups: one of abused patients and one of nonabused patients. These were naturally occurring groups. This design is consistent with the purpose of the research.

The independent variable was type of group (abused, nonabused). Also, to conduct the ANOVA,

the abused group was further divided: participants who had been physically abused only, those who had been sexually abused only, and those with a history of CP/SA; thus, the study, with the addition of the nonabused group, had a total of four groups. The major dependent variables for this study were suicide intention, reasons for self-harm, affect regulation and dissociation, hopelessness, and depression. Demographic variables, such as age and gender, were used to determine homogeneity in the sample.

Internal Validity

Santa Mina (2010) made no mention of possible threats to internal validity that would inordinately decrease confidence in the results. This study was based on self-report measures, which could have led to social desirability bias or acquiescence bias, which in turn could have affected the results.

External Validity

Generalizability is limited to the sample because of the effect of nonprobability convenience sampling. Santa Mina (2010) decided to discontinue data collection because the sample size for the nonabused group was very small: data analysis yielded nonsignificant findings, and the risk of a type II error was low (p. 137), and so this study exhibited selection effects.

Legal/Ethical Issues

The university's ethics review board gave approval for the study, and the relevant permissions from hospital leaders were obtained. The informed consent form was obtained, and clinical staff members were available to participants if they became upset. A contact phone number was given to participants for crisis support should they become upset at any time after completion of the study.

Instruments

Santa Mina (2010) used several instruments and provided a very detailed table outlining the concept: number of items, scoring method, and interpretation of scores. She collected demographic information about age and gender.

Reliability and Validity

A very thorough description of the reliability and validity of each instrument was provided in Table 19C2-1 for previous studies and Santa Mina's study.

Results

Santa Mina (2010) used descriptive statistics to determine homogeneity between the abused and nonabused groups. Although gender was distributed evenly, women were more likely to have been abused. Overdose was found to be the most frequent type of self-harm behaviour, and its prevalence was distributed evenly between the genders.

A description of the participants' results is detailed in the text (Santa Mina, 2010, p. 130). Evidence to support the hypotheses was detailed in the text as follows: "Self-harm/suicidal intentions did not differ for the non-abused and abused groups" (p. 130), and "the sample overwhelmingly (98%) reported multiple reasons for the self-harm episode. . . . The abused group revealed greater dissociation than the non-abused group, as well as greater affective liability" (p. 136). These results were, however, not statistically significant.

Santa Mina (2010) also examined the SIQ "affect" subscale and found that participants who had been both physically and sexually abused "reported the largest mean number of reasons" (p. 136); these results were statistically significant. Santa Mina also tested for a difference in dissociation and depression across the four groups. Although the results were not statistically significant, a trend of higher scores in the group with both physical and sexual abuse was noted.

Overall, the findings related to each hypothesis are clearly stated.

Discussion

Santa Mina (2010) stated that although the results were not statistically significant, they had clinical significance inasmuch as participants, regardless of abuse history, reported multiple intentions. Participants also reported moderate levels of suicidality and high levels of hopelessness and depression. The findings of this study were appropriately related to results of previous studies on self-harm and suicidal behaviours and the differences between the genders.

Several considerations for future research were mentioned: for example, "Future studies should aim for large sample sizes, to accommodate the breadth of abuse types as well as the myriad sociological factors that can affect intentions" (Santa Mina, 2010, p. 137).

Clinical implications from the results are made: "patients who are thinking about or engaging in self-harm/suicidal behaviours need to be assessed for the full spectrum of intentions, regardless of gender, self-harm method, or known abuse history" (Santa Mina, 2010, p. 138).

Limitations and Conclusion

Santa Mina (2010) discussed the limitation of the sample size and its effect on type II error and placed it within the context of "suicide intention, reasons for self-harm, affect regulation, dissociation, depression, and hopelessness" (p. 137). She described the significance of her study: "This is the first published clinical study to investigate the influence of CP/SA on self-harm/suicide intentions among men and women admitted to an acute-care unit for these behaviours" (p. 139).

CRITICAL THINKING CHALLENGES

- Discuss the ways in which the stylistic considerations of a journal affect the researcher's ability to present the research findings of a quantitative study.
- Are critiques of quantitative studies valid when a student or a practising nurse writes them? What level of quantitative study is best for you as a consumer of research to critique? What assumptions did you use to make this determination?
- What is essential for you as a consumer of research to use when you critique a quantitative research study? Discuss the ways you might use Internet resources now or in the future when you critique studies.

REFERENCES

Calsyn, R. J., Roades, L. A., & Calsyn, D. S. (1992). Acquiescence in needs assessment studies of the elderly. *The Gerontologist, 32*, 246-252.

Connors, R. (1996). Self-injury in trauma survivors: 1. Functions and meanings. *American Journal of Orthopsychiatry, 66*(2), 197-206.

Ploeg, J., Denton, M., Tindale, J., Hutchison, B., Brazil, K., Akhtar-Danesh, N., . . . Millen Plenderleith, J. (2009). Older adults' awareness of community health and support services for dementia care. *Canadian Journal of Aging, 28*(4), 359-370.

Santa Mina, E. (2010). Self-harm intentions: Can they be distinguished based upon a history of childhood physical and sexual abuse? *Canadian Journal of Nursing Research, 42*(4), 122-143.

Santa Mina, E. E., & Gallop, R. (1998). Childhood sexual and physical abuse and adult self-harm and suicidal behavior: A literature review. *Canadian Journal of Psychiatry, 43*, 793-800.

Windle, M., Windle, R. C., Scheidt, D. M., & Miller, G. B. (1995). Physical and sexual abuse and associated mental disorders among alcoholic inpatients. *American Journal of Psychiatry, 152*(9), 1322-1328.

FOR FURTHER STUDY

evolve   Go to Evolve at http://evolve.elsevier.com/Canada/LoBiondo/Research for Audio Glossary, how-to instructions for Writing Proposals for Funding, and additional research articles for practice in reviewing and critiquing.

Application of Research: Evidence-Informed Practice

RESEARCH **VIGNETTE**
Nursing Best Practices

Barbara Davies, RN, PhD
Professor
School of Nursing
Faculty of Health Sciences
University of Ottawa;
Co-Director, Nursing Best Practice Research
    Unit
University of Ottawa and RNAO
Ottawa, Ontario

*Give to the world the best you have
and the best will come back to you.*
—*Author unknown*

As a graduating student in nursing at the University of Toronto in 1974, I had to supply a quotation about my philosophy of life to accompany my yearbook photograph. I still recall being perplexed about what to state. Eventually, I selected the above quotation about doing your "best." Little did I know that more than 30 years later, I would be the codirector of the Nursing Best Practice Research Unit at the University of Ottawa, a dynamic collaboration with the politically active Registered Nurses' Association of Ontario. Our research unit won the Sigma Theta Tau international practice-academe innovative collaboration award in 2009. In 2011, I received the distinguished alumnus award from my alma mater, now named the Lawrence S. Bloomberg Faculty of Nursing. These awards are two examples of the "best" coming back to me in recognition of many hours of hard work. The "best" also includes teaching undergraduate and graduate students to use research to make a difference in the health of Canadians.

It is fascinating to contemplate the forces that influenced my career development and, in particular, the development of my research program on evidence-informed practice. One of the most influential people in my early career was Donna Diers, the Dean of Nursing at Yale University. I was employed as a clinical instructor at Yale and recall Donna's passionately pleading for nursing research to provide the data to demonstrate the "power" of nursing care to improve health. She strongly encouraged teaching staff at Yale to conduct nursing research that "would make a difference in practice."

My PhD supervisor, Ellen Hodnett, who holds the Heather M. Reisman Chair in Perinatal Nursing Research at the University of Toronto, also substantially influenced my knowledge and skills related to best practices. Ellen is one of the early leaders of the Cochrane Collaboration, an international research initiative to answer clinical questions by conducting systematic reviews. In Cochrane Reviews, authors strive to determine the most effective health care interventions. Ellen was the lead author of a review about the provision of labour support to women at childbirth.

My PhD research built upon Dr. Hodnett's systematic review findings that continuous labour support provides the benefits of reduced use of analgesia or anaes-thesia, reduced number of births by caesarean section, and fewer reports by women of negative labour experiences. In addition, my PhD research also built upon another Cochrane systematic review in which intermittent fetal auscultation was found to reduce rates of Caesarean section for women at low risk for complications and thus concluded that auscultation is preferable to electronic fetal monitoring. Although the provision of labour support and the use of intermittent fetal auscultation were recommended by the Society of Obstetricians and Gynaecologists of Canada and by the World Health Organization, several observational studies revealed that the majority of women at low risk who gave birth in Canada were not receiving either of these beneficial interventions. This lack of knowledge translation became the challenge of my doctoral studies. In other words, the knowledge from the Cochrane reviews was needed so that women at childbirth would receive care that was consistent with clinical practice guidelines.

What could I do to help healthy women at low risk receive support at childbirth without the encumbrance of continuously being hooked up to monitoring machines? In collaboration with my PhD thesis committee—which consisted of an obstetrician, an epidemiologist, and nursing research experts—I designed a multifaceted intervention that included an educational workshop for nurses with tools for applying research results to practice. Assessment forms, protocols based on the research results, and case study exercises were included.

The intervention received positive evaluations from the participating nurses, and the majority of staff nurses (>80%) attended the workshop. I am pleased to report that this labour support workshop and a fetal health surveillance workshop, both of which were first offered in 1995 as part of my PhD research, are still being offered regularly in Ottawa (http://www.cmnrp.ca/en/pppeso/Home_p2974.html).

A note of caution for other professionals who are considering the development of similar knowledge translation interventions to improve practice: Many nurses and physicians have extensive experience, and it is important to recognize their knowledge and expertise. Using a respectful, collaborative approach works well. Ask health care professionals what they think is needed to improve practice to be consistent with research results, and you will probably hear some excellent ideas.

Shortly after completing my PhD in 2000, I received a Career Scientist award from the Ministry of Health and Long-Term Care (Ontario) for a 5-year program of research on maternal-infant knowledge translation. Although I was excited to be selected as one of six awardees (the only nurse) in a tough provincial competition, I was also apprehensive about whether I could be successful in major national research competitions, a requirement to continue to receive the ongoing funding.

Fortunately, a very special opportunity arose at this time to co-lead, with Dr. Nancy Edwards, the evaluation of the emerging Nursing Best Practice Guidelines Program of the Registered Nurses' Association of Ontario. The guidelines include a synthesis of the available research evidence developed by expert panels on priority topics, such as fall prevention, pressure ulcers, asthma control, breast-feeding, and support for families.

Over the next 11 years, Nancy and I—along with many others—conducted studies of implementation interventions, surveys of nurses' attitudes, qualitative interviews of barriers and facilitators, observations of teaching tools, and chart audits of nursing practice and patient outcomes. The mandate of the Nursing Best Practice Research Unit (http://www.nbpru.ca/) is to incorporate the best knowledge into nursing and health care, enhance practice, and improve health and system outcomes. The goal is to promote best nursing knowledge. The research unit has 52 individual members and 22 organizational members.

Currently, my research on best practices addresses sustainability factors, interprofessional collaboration, and system changes. I am supervising or a thesis committee member for 12 graduate students (MScN, PhD, postdoctoral) working on such important topics as audit and feedback of patient outcomes, implementation of guidelines in academic programs, and community environmental health. Some of these graduate students are continuing knowledge

translation research in maternal infant health about public health networks to support smoking cessation and breast-feeding counselling by family practice nurses for pregnant women. What topics would you research as a graduate student?

Some academicians criticize the notion of best practices, commenting on the harm done by a hierarchy of evidence that unduly glorifies the randomized controlled trial as the "gold standard" of research methodology. My view is that a randomized controlled trial is the preferred research design to determine whether one treatment is more effective than another treatment. However, health has multiple determinants, and health care is provided in a complex environment by many types of health care professionals. Thus, it is equally important to conduct qualitative research studies to better understand the factors influencing the promotion of health for all people.

Finally, I offer a few words about values, preferences, and best practices. At the core of best practices is the notion that decisions and interventions need to be patient centred. Assessing preferences, clarifying values, and informing patients and their families about the risks and benefits of options are essential. Early in my research career, while doing my MScN thesis on factors influencing the decisions of women of advanced maternal age to have genetic amniocentesis, I discovered that different women perceived the risk of "1 per 100" very differently. Each woman, her spouse, and the genetic counsellor had their own and sometimes conflicting perspectives. Conducting this genetic research heightened my awareness of differences in patient and provider values and the need for thoughtful reflection about my own values regarding what constitutes best practices. Best practices require the integration of research knowledge with patient preferences and clinical judgement.

In retrospect, although best practice is an admirable goal, I now question whether such a state can ever be achieved. Nevertheless, the quest to achieve excellence in nursing practice and health services still drives my research journey. What drives your work in practice, education, or research? What type of evidence counts for you? What does "best practices" mean to you? ■

CHAPTER 20

Developing an Evidence-Informed Practice

Marita Titler | Susan Adams | Cherylyn Cameron

LEARNING OUTCOMES

After reading this chapter, you will be able to do the following:

- Differentiate among conduct of nursing research, research utilization, and evidence-informed practice.
- Describe the steps of evidence-informed practice.
- Identify three barriers to evidence-informed practice and strategies to address each.
- List three sources for finding evidence.
- Describe strategies for implementing evidence-informed practice changes.
- Identify steps for evaluating an evidence-informed change in practice.
- Use research findings and other forms of evidence to improve the quality of care.

KEY TERMS

conduct of research
dissemination
evaluation
evidence-informed practice

evidence-informed practice
  guidelines
knowledge-focused triggers
opinion leaders

problem-focused triggers
research utilization
translation science

STUDY RESOURCES

Go to Evolve at http://evolve.elsevier.com/Canada/LoBiondo/Research for Audio Glossary, how-to instructions for Writing Proposals for Funding, and additional research articles for practice in reviewing and critiquing.

EVIDENCE-INFORMED HEALTH CARE PRACTICES ARE available for a number of conditions, such as asthma, smoking cessation, heart failure, and management of diabetes. However, these practices are not always implemented in care delivery, and variation in practices abound (Ward, Evans, Spies, Roberts, & Wakefield, 2006). Availability of high-quality research does not ensure that the findings will be used to affect patient outcomes. Research findings in the United States and the Netherlands suggest that 30% to 40% of patients are not receiving evidence-informed care, and 20% to 25% of patients are receiving unneeded or potentially harmful care (Graham, Logan, Harrison, Straus, Tetroe, Caswell, Robinson, 2006). The use of evidence-informed practices is now an expected standard in many institutions to prevent nosocomial events such as injury from falls, Foley catheter–associated urinary tract infections, and stages 3 and 4 pressure ulcers. However, implementing such evidence-informed safety practices is a challenge and requires use of strategies that address the complexity and systems of care, individual practitioners, senior leadership, and ultimately changing health care cultures to be evidence-informed practice environments (Leape, 2005).

Conduct of research is only the first step in improving practice through the use of research. Because of the gap between discovery and use of knowledge in practice (Bootsmiller, Yankey, Finch, Ward, Vaughn, Welke, & Doebbeling, 2004; Davey, Brown, Fenelon, Finch, Gould, Hartman, … & Wiffen, 2005; Titler, 2008), efforts must be concentrated on developing methods to speed translation of research findings into practice. Development and dissemination of evidence-informed practice guidelines are essential steps, but each alone does little to promote knowledge uptake by direct care providers (Clancy, Slutsky, & Patton, 2004).

Promoting use of evidence in practice is an active process that is facilitated partly by modelling and imitation of other professionals who have successfully adopted the innovation, by an organizational culture that values and supports use of evidence, and by localization of the evidence for use in a specific health care setting (Greenhalgh, Robert, MacFarlane, Bate, & Kyriakdiou, 2004; Rogers, 2003).

Translation of research into practice is a multifaceted, systemic process of promoting adoption of evidence-informed practices in delivery of health care services that goes beyond dissemination of evidence-informed guidelines (Rogers, 2003). **Dissemination** is the communication of research findings; dissemination activities take many forms, including publications, conferences, consultations, and training programs (Adams & Titler, 2010), but promoting knowledge uptake and changing practitioner behaviour requires active interchange with those in direct care (Scott, Plotnikoff, Karunamuni, Bize, & Rodgers, 2008; Titler, Herr, Brooks, Xian-Jin, Ardery, Schilling, … & Clarke, 2009).

Although the science of translation is young, the effectiveness of interventions for promoting adoption of evidence-informed practices is being studied, and funding is supporting research in this area (Bootsmiller et al., 2004; Smith, Williams, Owen, Rubenstein, & Chaney, 2008; Stetler, McQuenn, Demkis, & Mittman, 2008).

In addition, more evidence is now available to guide selection of strategies for translating research into practice (Brooks, Titler, Ardery, & Herr, 2009; Gravel, Légaré, & Graham, 2006; Titler, 2008). This chapter presents an overview of evidence-informed practice, the process of implementing evidence in practice to improve patient outcomes, and a description of translation science.

OVERVIEW OF EVIDENCE-INFORMED PRACTICE

The relationships among conduct, dissemination, and use of research are illustrated in Figure 20-1. **Conduct of research** is the analysis of data collected from a homogeneous group of participants who meet study inclusion and exclusion criteria for the purpose of answering specific research

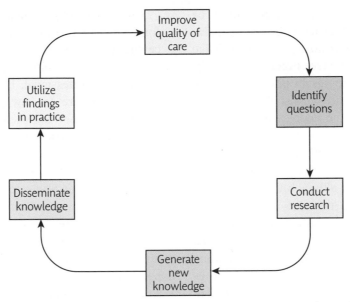

FIGURE 20-1   Model of the relationship among conduct, dissemination, and use of research. Redrawn from Weiler, K., Buckwalter, K., & Titler, M. (1994). Debate: Is nursing research used in practice? In J. McCloskey & H. Grace (Eds.), *Current issues in nursing* (4th ed.). St. Louis: Mosby.

questions or testing specified hypotheses. Research design, methods, and statistical analyses are guided by the state of the science in the area of investigation. Traditionally, conduct of research has included dissemination of findings through research reports in journals and at scientific conferences. In comparison, **research utilization** is the process of using research findings to improve patient care; this process involves implementing sound research-based innovations in clinical practice; dissemination of scientific knowledge; critique of studies; synthesis of research findings; determining applicability of findings for practice; developing an evidence-informed standard or guideline; implementing the standard; and evaluating the practice change with respect to staff, patients, and cost/resource utilization (Titler, Kleiber, Steelman, Rakel, Budreau, Everett, ... & Goode, 2001).

Evidence-informed practice is the conscientious and judicious use of current best evidence in conjunction with clinical expertise and patient values to guide health care decisions (Titler, 2006). As noted in Chapter 1, it is important

to differentiate among the terms *evidence-based practice* and *evidence-informed practice*. Evidence-informed practice extends beyond the early definitions of evidence-based practice. Many of the models explored in this chapter refer to evidence-based practice, inasmuch as they were developed before the use of the term *evidence-informed practice*. The models are still valid and help guide professionals toward actualizing research into best practices. Best evidence includes empirical evidence from systematic reviews, from randomized controlled trials, and from other scientific methods such as descriptive and qualitative research, as well as information from case reports, scientific principles, and expert opinion. When enough research evidence is available, practice should be guided by this evidence, in conjunction with clinical expertise and patients' values. In some cases, however, a sufficient research base may not be available, and health care decision making is derived principally from nonresearch evidence sources such as expert opinion and scientific principles (Titler et al., 2001). When more research is completed in a specific area, the research evidence must be incorporated into evidence-informed practice (Titler, 2006). As illustrated in the knowledge generation and use cycle (see Figure 20-1), application of research findings in practice may not only improve quality care but also create new and exciting questions to be addressed through the conduct of research.

The terms *research utilization* and *evidence-informed practice* are sometimes used interchangeably. However, although these two terms are related, they are not one and the same. *Evidence-informed* is a broader term that encompasses not only research utilization but also the use of case reports and expert opinion in deciding the practices to be used in health care. If evidence-informed practice is defined as the conscious and judicious use of the current "best" evidence in the care of patients and delivery of health care services, then research utilization is a subset of evidence-informed practice that focuses on the application of research findings.

Use of Evidence in Practice

Nursing has a rich history of using research in practice, pioneered by Florence Nightingale, who used data to change practices that contributed to high mortality rates in hospitals and communities (Nightingale, 1858, 1859, 1863a, 1863b). Although during the early and mid-1900s, few nurses built on the solid foundation of research utilization exemplified by Nightingale (Titler, 1993), the nursing profession has provided major leadership for improving care through application of research findings in practice (Kirchhoff, 2004). Today nurses are being prepared as scientists in nursing, leading the way in translation science, and, as a result, the scientific body of nursing knowledge is growing (Estabrooks, Derksen, Winther, Lavis, Scott, Wallin, & Profetto-McGrath, 2008; Titler, 2008; Titler et al., 2009). It is now every nurse's responsibility to facilitate the use of nursing knowledge in practice.

Cronenwett (1995) and others described two forms of using research evidence in practice: conceptual and decision driven (Estabrooks, 2004). Conceptual forms influence the thinking of the health care professional, but not necessarily the action. Exposure to new scientific knowledge occurs, but the new knowledge may not be used to change or guide practice. An integrative review of the literature, formulation of a new theory, or generating new hypotheses may be the result. Use of knowledge in this way is referred to as *knowledge creep* or *cognitive application*. It is often used by individuals who read and incorporate research into their critical thinking (Weiss, 1980). Decision-driven forms of using evidence in practice encompass application of scientific knowledge as part of a new practice, policy, procedure, or intervention. In this type of application of research findings, a critical decision is reached to endorse current practice or to change it on the basis of review and critique of studies applicable to that practice. Examples of decision-driven models of using research in practice are the Iowa Model of Evidence-Based Practice to Promote Quality Care (Titler et al., 2001), the Ottawa Model of Research Use (OMRU; Logan & Graham, 1998), the Promoting Action on Research Implementation in Health Services (PARIHS) model (Rycroft-Malone, Kitson, Harvey, McCormack, Seers, Titchen, & Eastabrooks, 2002), and the Conduct and Utilization of Research in Nursing (CURN) model (Haller, Reynolds, & Horseley, 1979; Horsley, Crane, Crabtree, & Wood, 1983).

Multifaceted active dissemination strategies are needed to promote use of research evidence in clinical and administrative health care decision making, and they must address both the individual practitioner's and the organization's perspectives (Titler, 2008). When nurses decide individually what evidence to use in practice, considerable variability in practice patterns results, which can potentially lead to adverse patient outcomes. For example, a solely "individual" perspective of evidence-informed practice would leave the decision about use of pressure ulcer prevention practices to each nurse. Some nurses may be familiar with the research findings for pressure ulcer prevention, whereas others may not be. As a result, different nurses may use conflicting practices, especially inasmuch as shifts change every 8 to 12 hours. From an organizational perspective, policies and procedures are based on research, and then adoption of these practices by nurses is systematically promoted in the organization (Squires, Moralejo, & LeFort, 2007).

Models of Evidence-Informed Practice

Multiple models of evidence-informed practice and translation science are available. Common elements of these models are syntheses of evidence, implementation, evaluation of the effect on patient care, and consideration of the context/setting in which the evidence is implemented. Grol and associates (2007) provided a summary of models. Included in their summary relevant to quality improvement and implementation of change in health care were cognitive, educational, motivational, social interactive, social learning, social network, and social influence theories, as well as models related to team effectiveness, professional development, and leadership. Additional work by the Improved Clinical Effectiveness through Behavioural Research Group (ICEBeRG) resulted in the development of a database consisting of planned action models, frameworks, and theories that explicitly describe both the concepts and action steps to be considered or taken. This database was developed from a search of social science, education, and health literature that focused on practitioner or organizational change (http://www.iceberg-grebeci.ohri.ca/research/kt_theories_db.html).

Although review of these models is beyond the scope of this chapter, implementing evidence in practice must be guided by a conceptual model to organize the strategies being used and to clarify

extraneous variables (e.g., behaviours and facilitators) that may influence adoption of evidence-informed practices (e.g., organizational size, characteristics of users; ICEBeRG, 2006). Two models are explored in this chapter: the Iowa Model of Evidence-Based Practice to Promote Quality Care and the Ottawa Model of Research Use.

The Iowa Model of Evidence-Based Practice to Promote Quality Care

An overview of the Iowa Model of Evidence-Based Practice to Promote Quality Care, as an example of a practice model, is illustrated in Figure 20-2. This model has been widely disseminated and adopted in academic and clinical settings. Since the original publication of this model in 1994 (Titler, Kleiber, Steelman, Goode, Rakel, Barry-Walker, … & Buckwalter, 1994), Titler and colleagues have received more than 300 written requests to use the model for publications, presentations, graduate and undergraduate research courses, and clinical research programs. It is an organizational, collaborative model that incorporates conduct of research, use of research evidence, and other types of evidence (Titler et al., 2001). Titler and colleagues adopted the definition of *evidence-based practice* as the conscientious and judicious use of current best evidence to guide health care decisions. Levels of evidence range from randomized controlled trials to case reports and expert opinion.

In this model, knowledge- and problem-focused "triggers" lead staff members to question current nursing practice and whether patient care can be improved through the use of research findings. If, through the process of literature review and critique of studies, staff members find that the number of scientifically sound studies is not sufficient for use as a base for practice, they consider conducting a study. Nurses in practice collaborate with scientists in nursing and other disciplines to conduct clinical research that addresses practice problems encountered in the care of patients.

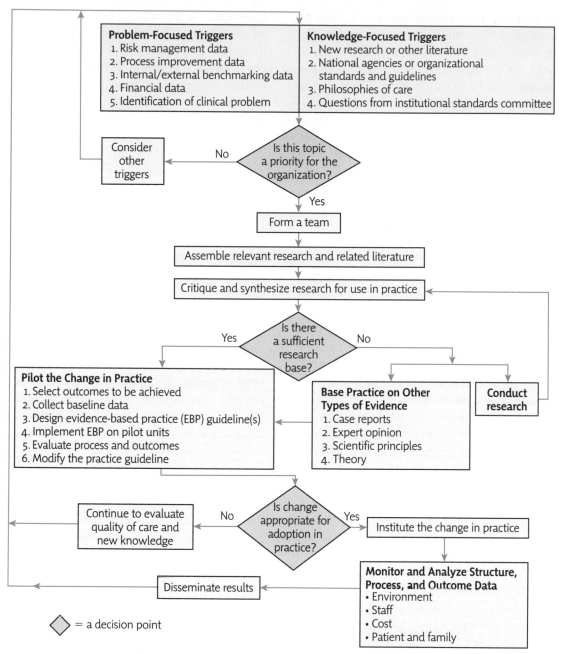

FIGURE 20-2 The Iowa Model of Evidence-Based Practice to Promote Quality Care. Redrawn from Titler, M. G., Kleiber, C., Steelman, V. J., Rakel, B. A., et al. (2001). The Iowa Model of Evidence-Based Practice to Promote Quality Care. *Critical Care Nursing Clinics of North America, 13*(4), 497–509. Copyright Elsevier 2001.

Findings from such studies are then combined with findings from existing scientific knowledge to develop and implement these practices. If research is insufficient for guiding practice, and if conducting a study is not feasible, other types of evidence (e.g., case reports, expert opinion, scientific principles, theory) are used or combined with available research evidence to guide practice. Priority is given to projects in which a high proportion of practice is guided by research evidence. Practice guidelines usually reflect research and nonresearch evidence and therefore are called *evidence-informed practice guidelines.*

An evidence-informed practice guideline is developed from the available evidence. The recommended practices, based on the relevant evidence, are compared with current practice, and a decision is made about the necessity for a practice change. If a practice change is warranted, changes are implemented through a process of planned change. The practice is first implemented with a small group of patients, and it is evaluated. The evidence-informed practice is then refined on the basis of evaluation data, and the change is implemented with additional patient populations for which it is appropriate. Patient/family, staff, and fiscal outcomes are monitored. Organizational support and administrative support are important factors for success in the use of evidence in care delivery.

The Ottawa Model of Research Use

Logan and Graham (1998) developed the OMRU, a model for interdisciplinary health care research use. The framework was created to "be used by policymakers seeking to increase the use of health research by practitioners, as well as by researchers interested in studying the process by which research becomes integrated into practice" (p. 228). They identified the following six components of research utilization: (1) the practice environment, (2) potential adopters, (3) the evidence-informed innovation, (4) transfer strategies, (5) adoption, and (6) health-related and other outcomes (Figure 20-3). Constant assessment, monitoring, and evaluation parallel the

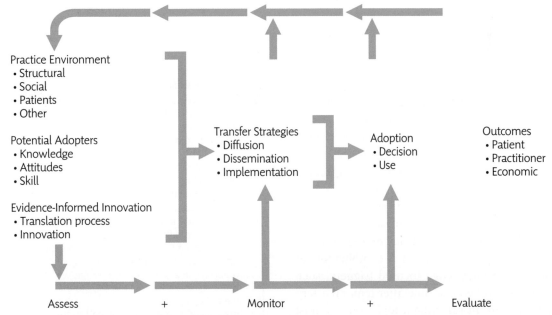

FIGURE 20-3 The Ottawa Model of Health Care Research Use.
Adapted from Logan, J., & Graham, I. (1998). Toward a comprehensive interdisciplinary model of health care research use. *Science Communication, 20*(2), 229. Reprinted by Permission of SAGE Publications.

progression through the components. As barriers are identified, strategies are developed to surmount them and to enhance supports.

STEPS OF EVIDENCE-INFORMED PRACTICE

The Iowa Model of Evidence-Based Practice to Promote Quality Care (Titler et al., 2001; see Figure 20-2), in conjunction with Rogers' (1995, 2003) diffusion of innovations model, provides guiding steps in actualizing evidence-informed practice. A team approach is most helpful in fostering a specific evidence-informed practice, with one person in the group providing leadership for the project.

Selection of a Topic

The first step in carrying out an evidence-informed practice project is to select a topic. Ideas for evidence-informed practice come from several sources categorized as problem- and knowledge-focused triggers. **Problem-focused triggers** are research ideas identified by staff through quality improvement, risk surveillance, benchmarking data, financial data, or recurrent clinical problems. For example, the increased incidence of *Clostridium difficile* on a long-term care unit, resulting in increased morbidity, is a problem-focused trigger because it raises concern among hospital staff.

Knowledge-focused triggers are research ideas generated when staff members read research, listen to scientific papers at research conferences, or encounter evidence-informed practice guidelines published by federal agencies or specialty organizations. Examples of such triggers include ideas about pain management, assessing placement of nasogastric and nasointestinal tubes, and use of saline to maintain patency of arterial lines. Sometimes topics arise from a combination of problem- and knowledge-focused triggers, such as the length of bed rest time after femoral artery catheterization. In selecting a topic, nurses must consider how the topic fits with organization, department, and unit priorities in order to garner support from leaders within the organization and the necessary resources to successfully complete the project.

Individuals should work collectively to achieve consensus in topic selection. Working in groups to review performance improvement data, brainstorm about ideas, and achieve consensus about the final selection is helpful. For example, a unit staff meeting may be used to discuss ideas for evidence-informed practice; quality improvement committees may identify several practice areas in need of attention (e.g., urinary tract infections in older patients, reducing the incidence of pressure ulcers); an evidence-informed practice task force may be appointed to select and address a clinical practice issue (e.g., pain management); or surveying a panel of experts may be used to prioritize areas for evidence-informed practice. Criteria to consider when a topic is selected are outlined in Box 20-1. Table 20-1 is a helpful chart for selecting a topic.

Helpful Hint

Regardless of which method is used to select an evidence-informed practice topic, it is critical that the staff members who will implement the potential practice changes are involved in selecting the topic and view it as contributing significantly to the quality of care.

BOX 20-1

SELECTION CRITERIA FOR AN EVIDENCE-INFORMED PRACTICE PROJECT

1. The priority of this topic for nursing and for the organization
2. The magnitude of the problem (small, medium, large)
3. Applicability to several or few clinical areas
4. Likelihood of the change to improve quality of care, decrease length of stay, contain costs, or improve patient satisfaction
5. Potential problems associated with the topic and capability to diffuse them
6. Availability of baseline quality improvement or risk data that will be helpful during evaluation
7. Multidisciplinary nature of the topic and ability to create collaborative relationships to effect the needed changes
8. Interest and commitment of staff to the potential topic
9. Availability of a sound body of evidence, preferably research evidence

TABLE 20-1

TOOL TO USE IN SELECTING A TOPIC* FOR EVIDENCE-INFORMED PRACTICE

RATING ITEM	TOPIC A	TOPIC B	TOPIC C
Priority for nursing (1 = low; 5 = high)	☐	☐	☐
Priority for organization (1 = low; 5 = high)	☐	☐	☐
Magnitude of the problem (1 = small; 5 = large)	☐	☐	☐
Applicability (1 = narrow; 5 = broad)	☐	☐	☐
Likelihood to improve quality of care (1 = low; 5 = high)	☐	☐	☐
Likelihood to decrease length of stay/contain costs (1 = low; 5 = high)	☐	☐	☐
Likelihood to improve satisfaction (1 = low; 5 = high)	☐	☐	☐
Body of science (1 = little; 5 = multiple studies)	☐	☐	☐
Total	☐	☐	☐

Modified from Titler, M. G. (2002). *Toolkit for promoting evidence-based practice.* Iowa City: University of Iowa Hospitals and Clinics, Department of Nursing Services and Patient Care.
*Each topic should be rated with regard to the scoring criteria and on a 1-to-5 scale. The topic or topics receiving the higher scores should be considered for selection.

Forming a Team

A team is responsible for development, implementation, and evaluation of the evidence-informed practice. The team or group may be an existing committee such as the quality improvement committee, the practice council, or the research committee. A task force approach also may be used, in which a group is appointed to address a specific practice issue and use research findings or other evidence to improve practice. The composition of the team is directed by the topic selected and should include interested stakeholders in the delivery of care. For example, a team working on evidence-informed pain management should be interdisciplinary and include pharmacists, nurses, physicians, and psychologists. In contrast, a team working on the evidence-informed practice of bathing might include a nurse expert in skin care, assistive nursing personnel, and staff nurses.

In addition to forming a team, key stakeholders who can facilitate the evidence-informed practice project or put up barriers against successful implementation should be identified. A stakeholder is a key individual or group of individuals who are directly or indirectly affected by the implementation of the evidence-informed practice. Some stakeholders may already be members of the team. Others may not be team members but are key individuals within the organization or unit who can adversely or positively influence the adoption of the evidence-informed practice. Examples of key stakeholders are nurse managers, nurse educators, researchers, nursing supervisors, chairs of committees or councils that must approve system changes (e.g., policy/procedure revisions; changes in documentation forms), and patients/families. Questions to consider in identification of key stakeholders include the following:

- How are decisions made in the practice areas in which the evidence-informed practice will be implemented?
- What types of system changes will be needed?
- Who is involved in decision making?
- Who is likely to lead and champion implementation of the evidence-informed practice?
- Who can influence the decision to proceed with implementation of an evidence-informed practice?
- What type of cooperation is needed from which stakeholders to be successful?

Failure to involve or keep supportive stakeholders informed may place the success of the evidence-informed practice project at risk because they are unable to anticipate or defend the rationale for changing practice, particularly with resistant (nonsupportive) stakeholders who have a great deal of influence among their peer group. Use Figure 20-4 to think about the status of key stakeholders and to strategize about interventions to engage various types of stakeholders for your evidence-informed practice project.

An important early task for the evidence-informed practice team is to formulate the evidence-informed practice question. This helps set boundaries around the project and assists in retrieval of the evidence. A clearly defined question should specify the types of people/patients, interventions or exposures, outcomes, and relevant study designs (Higgins & Green, 2011). For types of people, the team should specify the

STAKEHOLDER INFLUENCE

	High	Low
High	• Can positively affect dissemination and adoption • Need information to gain their buy-in Strategies: • Collaborate • Involve and/or provide opportunities where they can be supportive • Encourage feedback • Empower	• Can positively affect dissemination and adoption if given attention • Need attention to maintain buy-in and prevent development of ambivalence Strategies: • Collaborate • Encourage feedback • Elicit support via their professional status • Encourage participation, prn • Involve at some level
	High support High influence	High support Low influence
	Low support High influence	Low support Low influence
Low	• Can negatively affect dissemination and adoption • Need great amount of attention and information to obtain and maintain neutrality and work towards buy-in Strategies: • Consensus • Build relationships • Detail benefits for them • Involve some (1 or 2) of these individuals on team • Monitor their support	• Least able to influence dissemination and adoption • May have some negative impact • Some attention to obtain neutrality and to work towards buy-in Strategies: • Consensus • Build relationships • Involve at some level—team member

(Left axis label: STAKEHOLDER SUPPORT — High / Low)

FIGURE 20-4   Characteristics of stakeholders (resistors and facilitators). Redrawn from Titler, M. G. (2002). *Toolkit for promoting evidence-based practice.* Iowa City: University of Iowa Hospitals and Clinics, Department of Nursing Services and Patient Care.

diseases or conditions of interest, the patient population (e.g., age, gender, educational status), and the setting. For example, if the topic for the evidence-informed practice project is pain, the team needs to specify the type of pain (e.g., acute, persistent, cancer), the age of the population (e.g., children, neonates, adults, older adults), and the setting (e.g., inpatient, outpatient, ambulatory care, home care, primary care). For intervention, the types of interventions of interest to the project and the comparison interventions (e.g., standard care, alternative treatments) need to be specified. In the example of pain, the interventions of interest might include pharmacological treatment, analgesic administration methods (e.g., patient-controlled analgesia, epidural, intravenous), pain assessment, nonpharmacological treatment, and patient/family education regarding self-care pain management. For outcomes, the team should select outcomes of primary importance and consider the type of outcome data that will be needed for decision making (e.g., benefits, harm, cost). Outcomes that may be interesting but of little importance to the project should be excluded.

Finally, it is important to consider the types of study designs that are likely to provide reliable data to answer the question, and the team must search for the highest level of evidence available. A similar type of approach to formulating the practice question is PICOT: patient, population, or problem; intervention/treatment; comparison intervention/treatment; outcomes; and time frame (Melnyk & Fineout-Overholt, 2011). This approach is illustrated in Table 20-2.

Evidence Retrieval

Once a topic is selected, relevant research and related literature must be retrieved and should include clinical studies, meta-analyses, integrative literature reviews, and existing evidence-informed practice guidelines. As more evidence is available to guide practice, professional organizations and federal agencies are developing and

---

TABLE **20-2**

PICOT: COMPONENTS OF AN ANSWERABLE, SEARCHABLE QUESTION

Patient population/disease: The patient population or disease of interest; for example:
- Age
- Gender
- Ethnicity
- With certain disorder (e.g., hepatitis)

Intervention or issue of interest: The intervention or range of interventions of interest, for example:
- Therapy
- Exposure to disease
- Prognostic factor A
- Risk behaviour (e.g., smoking)

Comparison intervention or issue of interest: What you want to compare the intervention or issue against, for example:
- Alternative therapy, placebo, or no intervention/ therapy
- No disease
- Prognostic factor B
- Absence of risk factor (e.g., nonsmoking)

Outcome: Outcome of interest, for example:
- Outcome expected from therapy (e.g., pressure ulcers)
- Risk of disease
- Accuracy of diagnosis
- Rate of occurrence of adverse outcome (e.g., death)

Time: The time involved to demonstrate an outcome, for example:
- The time it takes for the intervention to achieve the outcome
- The time over which populations are observed for the outcome (e.g., quality of life) to occur, given a certain condition (e.g., prostate cancer)

From Melnyk, B. M., & Fineout-Overholt, E. (2011). *Evidence-based practice in nursing and healthcare: A guide to best practice* (2nd ed., p. 30, Table 2-1). New York: Wolters Kluwer.

---

making available evidence-informed practice guidelines. It is important that these guidelines are accessed as part of the literature retrieval process.

In October 2007, the Agency for Healthcare Research and Quality (AHRQ) announced the third award of 5-year contracts for evidence-informed practice centres (EPC-III) to 14 evidence-informed practice centres to continue and expand the work performed by the previous group of evidence-informed practice centres. Three Canadian universities are among the 14: McMaster University, University of Alberta, and University of Ottawa. Contacts and additional information about the current participating evidence-informed practice centres are available at http://www.ahrq.gov/clinic/epc/epcenters.htm.

The AHRQ also sponsors a National Guideline Clearinghouse in which abstracts of evidence-informed practice guidelines are set forth on a Web site (http://www.guideline.gov). Other professional organizations that publish evidence-informed practice guidelines are the American Pain Society (http://www.ampainsoc.org); Oncology Nursing Society (http://www.ons.org); American Association of Critical-Care Nurses (http://www.aacn.org); Registered Nurses' Association of Ontario (RNAO; http://www.rnao.org); National Institute for Health and Clinical Excellence (http://www.nice.org.uk); Association of Women's Health, Obstetric and Neonatal Nurses (http://www.awhonn.org); and the American Thoracic Society (http://www.thoracic.org). Current best evidence from specific studies of clinical problems can be found in an increasing number of electronic databases such as the Cochrane Library (http://www.thecochranelibrary.com/view/0/index.html), the Centre for Health Evidence (http://www.cche.net), the Joanna Briggs Institute (http://www.joannabriggs.edu.au), and the American College of Physicians (http://www.acponline.org) (Straus, Richardson, Glasziou, & Haynes, 2005).

In 1999, the RNAO initiated the Nursing Best Practice Guidelines Project to develop practice guidelines for nurses providing patient care. The project had published 32 completed guidelines as of January 2012, with several additional guidelines are under development. Each best practice guideline is developed in phases: planning, development, implementation, evaluation, and dissemination. The topics covered by these guidelines range from smoking cessation to screening for delirium, dementia, and depression in older adults.

The plan for dissemination of the guidelines is threefold. First, the RNAO requested proposals from interested and eligible health care organizations to work in collaboration to plan, implement, and evaluate nursing best practice guideline and disseminate knowledge from demonstrated experiences with guidelines. Second, the Best Practice Champions Network was established to prepare nurses to disseminate the best practice guidelines in their practices throughout Ontario. Third, the RNAO sponsored 10 demonstration projects for colleges and universities to integrate best practice guidelines into nursing curricula.

The guidelines program now also offers Advanced Clinical/Practice Fellowship (ACPF) for nurses or health care organization. It is designed to provide registered nurses with a "focused self-directed learning experience to develop clinical, leadership or best practices guideline implementation knowledge and skills, with support from a mentor(s), the organization where the [registered nurse] is employed, and the RNAO. This initiative is aimed at developing and promoting nursing knowledge and expertise, and improving patient care and outcomes in Ontario" (RNAO, 2011, p. 1). More than 365 ACPF fellowships have been funded in Ontario.

The RNAO best practice guideline is readily available to nurses through an application for personal electronics devices (e.g., BlackBerry, iPhone, and Android). Details are provided at the Web site at: http://www.rnao.org/Page.asp?PageID=924&ContentID=3282.

Another electronic database, Evidence-Based Medicine Reviews (EBMR) from Ovid Technologies (http://www.ovid.com/site/catalog/DataBase/904.jsp), combines several electronic databases, including the Cochrane Database of Systematic Reviews, Cochrane Database of Methodology Reviews (CDMR), and MEDLINE, plus links to more than 200 full-text journals. EBMR links these databases to one another; if a study on a topic of interest is found on MEDLINE and also has been included in a systematic review in the Cochrane Library, the review also can be readily and easily accessed (Straus et al., 2005).

In using these sources, it is important to identify key search terms and to use the expertise of health science librarians in locating publications relevant to the project. Additional information about locating the evidence is in Chapter 5.

Once the literature is located, it is helpful to classify the articles as clinical (nonresearch), integrative research reviews, theory articles, research articles, synthesis reports, meta-analyses, and evidence-informed practice guidelines. Before you read and critique the research, it is useful to read theoretical and clinical articles to have a broad view of the nature of the topic and related concepts and to then review existing evidence-informed practice guidelines. It is helpful to read articles in the following order:

1. Clinical articles, to understand the state of the practice
2. Theory articles, to understand the various theoretical perspectives and concepts that may be encountered when you critique studies
3. Systematic review articles and synthesis reports, to understand the state of the science
4. Evidence-informed practice guidelines and evidence reports
5. Research articles, including meta-analyses

Schemas for Grading the Evidence

There is no consensus among professional organizations or across health care disciplines regarding the best system to use for denoting the type and quality of evidence or for grading schemas to denote the strength of the body of evidence (Atkins, Briss, Eccles, Flottorp, Guyatt, Harbour, … & The GRADE Working Group, 2005; Guyatt, Oxman, Vist, Kunz, Falck-Ytter, Alonso-Coello, & Schunemann, 2008c). For example, the Scottish Intercollegiate Guidelines Network has an extensive method detailed on their Web site for appraising research and setting forth guideline recommendations (http://www.sign.ac.uk/

methodology/index.html). The Grading of Recommendations Assessment, Development, and Evaluation (GRADE) Working Group, initiated in 2000, is an informal collaboration of individuals interested in addressing grading schema in health care (http://www.gradeworkinggroup. org). In setting forth practice recommendations, the GRADE system first rates the quality of the evidence as high, moderate, low, or very low and then grades the strength of the evidence as strong or weak (GRADE Working Group, 2004; Guyatt, Oxman, Kunz, Jaeschke, Helfand, Liberati, & Schunemann, 2008a; Guyatt, Oxman, Kunz, Vist, Falck-Ytter, & Alonso-Cuello, 2008b; Table 20-3). Their methods are available on their Web site with grading software (GRADEpro) available. The National Guidelines Clearinghouse classifies submitted guidelines according to methods used by developers to accomplish two goals: (1) to assess the quality and strength of the evidence through expert consensus (committee or expert panel method), through subjective review, through weighting according to a rating scheme provided by the developers, or through weighting according to a rating scheme not provided by the developers; and (2) to formulate recommendations through various types of expert consensus (e.g., expert manual method; nominal group technique, consensus development conference) and balance sheets.

The RNAO (2011) guidelines for best practices are based on scientific evidence after a thorough review of the literature. Each of the studies is rated to determine whether it should be included in the guideline. The rating system used for the level of evidence and the grades of recommendation are illustrated in Table 20-3.

Before critiquing research articles, reading relevant literature, and reviewing evidence-informed practice guidelines, an organization or group responsible for the review must agree on methods for noting the type of research, rating the quality of individual articles, and grading the strength of the body of evidence. Users must evaluate which systems are most appropriate

TABLE 20-3

EXAMPLES OF EVIDENCE-INFORMED PRACTICE RATING SYSTEMS

GRADE WORKING GROUP (GRADE WORKING GROUP, 2004; GUYATT ET AL., 2008A)	REGISTERED NURSES ASSOCIATION OF ONTARIO (2011)	HARRIS ET AL., 2001 (U.S. PREVENTIVE SERVICES TASK FORCE, 2008)

STRENGTH OF EVIDENCE/QUALITY OF THE EVIDENCE

High: Further research is very unlikely to change our confidence in the estimate of effect. Scientific evidence provided by well-designed, well-conducted, controlled trials (randomized and nonrandomized) with statistically significant results that consistently support the guideline recommendation.

Moderate: Further research is likely to have an important impact on our confidence in the estimate of effect and may change the estimate.

Low: Further research is very likely to have an important impact on our confidence in the estimate of effect and is likely to change the estimate.

Very Low: Any estimate of effect is very uncertain.

Note: The type of evidence is first ranked as follows:
Randomized trial = high.
Observational study = low.
Any other evidence = very low.

Limitations in study quality, important inconsistency of results, uncertainty about the directness of the evidence, imprecise or sparse data, and high probability of reporting bias can lower the grade of evidence. Expert opinion that supports the guideline recommendation because the available scientific evidence did not present consistent results or because controlled trials were lacking. Grade of evidence can be increased if there is (1) strong evidence of association—significant relative risk of >2 (<0.5) based on consistent evidence from two or more observational studies, with no plausible confounders (1); (2) very strong evidence of association—significant relative risk of >5 (<0.2) based on direct evidence with no major threats to validity (2); (3) evidence of a dose response gradient (1); and (4) all plausible confounders would have reduced the effect (1).

LEVELS OF EVIDENCE

Ia: Evidence obtained from meta-analysis or systematic review of randomized controlled trials.

Ib: Evidence obtained from at least one randomized controlled trial.

IIa: Evidence obtained from at least one well-designed controlled study without randomization.

IIb: Evidence obtained from at least one other type of well-designed quasiexperimental study.

III: Evidence obtained from well-designed nonexperimental descriptive studies, such as comparative studies, correlation studies and case studies.

IV: Evidence obtained from expert committee reports or opinions and/or clinical experiences of respected authorities.

LEVELS OF CERTAINTY REGARDING NET BENEFIT

High: The available evidence usually includes consistent results from well-designed, well-conducted studies in representative primary care populations. These studies assess the effects of the preventive service on health outcomes. This conclusion is therefore unlikely to be strongly affected by the results of future studies.

Moderate: The available evidence is sufficient to determine the effects of the preventive service on health outcomes, but confidence in the estimate is constrained by such factors as the following:
• The number, size, or quality of individual studies.
• Inconsistency of findings across individual studies
• Limited generalizability of findings to routine primary care practice.
• Lack of coherence in the chain of evidence.

As more information becomes available, the magnitude or direction of the observed effect could change, and this change may be large enough to alter the conclusion.

Low: The available evidence is insufficient to assess effects on health outcomes. Evidence is insufficient because of one or more of the following:
• The limited number or size of studies.
• Important flaws in study design or methods.
• Inconsistency of findings across individual studies.
• Gaps in the chain of evidence.
• Findings not generalizable to routine primary care practice.
• Lack of information on important health outcomes.

More information may allow estimation of effects on health outcomes.

TABLE 20-3

EXAMPLES OF EVIDENCE-INFORMED PRACTICE RATING SYSTEMS—*cont'd*

GRADE WORKING GROUP (GRADE WORKING GROUP, 2004; GUYATT ET AL., 2008A)	REGISTERED NURSES ASSOCIATION OF ONTARIO (2011)	HARRIS ET AL., 2001 (U.S. PREVENTIVE SERVICES TASK FORCE, 2008)
STRENGTH OF RECOMMENDATIONS Strong: Confident that the desirable effects of adherence to a recommendation outweigh the undesirable effects. Weak: The desirable effects of adherence to a recommendation probably outweigh the undesirable effects, but the developers are less confident. Note: Strength of recommendation is determined by the balance between desirable and undesirable consequences of alternative management strategies, quality of evidence, variability in values and preferences, and resource use.	**GRADES OF RECOMMENDATION** A: There is good evidence to recommend the clinical preventive action. B: There is fair evidence to recommend the clinical preventive action. C: The existing evidence is conflicting and does not allow making a recommendation for or against use of the clinical preventive action; however, other factors may influence decision making. D: There is fair evidence to recommend against the clinical preventive action. E: There is good evidence to recommend against the clinical preventive action. I: There is insufficient evidence (in quantity and/or quality) to make recommendations, however other factors may influence decision-making.	**GRADES OF RECOMMENDATION** A: The USPSTF recommends the service. There is high certainty that the net benefit is substantial. Practice: Offer or provide this service. B: The USPSTF recommends the service. There is high certainty that the net benefit is moderate or there is moderate certainty that the net benefit is moderate to substantial. Practice: Offer or provide this service. C: The USPSTF recommends against routinely providing the service. There may be considerations that support providing the service in an individual patient. There is at least moderate certainty that the net benefit is small. Practice: Offer or provide this service only if other considerations support the offering or providing the service in an individual patient. D: The USPSTF recommends against the service. There is moderate or high certainty that the service has no net benefit or that the harms outweigh the benefits. Practice: Discourage the use of this service. I: The USPSTF concludes that the current evidence is insufficient to assess the balance of benefits and harms of the service. Evidence is lacking, of poor quality, or conflicting, and the balance of benefits and harms cannot be determined. Practice: Read the clinical considerations section of USPSTF Recommendation Statement. If the service is offered, patients should understand the uncertainty about the balance of benefits and harms.

From Registered Nurses Association of Ontario (2011) rating system described by Canadian Task Force on Preventive Health Care. (CTFPHC). (1997). *Quick tables by strength of evidence.* Available at http://www.canadiantaskforce.ca.
USPSTF, U.S. Preventive Services Task Force.

for the task being undertaken, the length of time to complete each instrument, and its ease of use (West, King, Carey, Lohr, McKoy, Sutton, & Lux, 2002). It is also important to decide how the strength of the evidence will be reflected in the guideline.

Critique of Evidence-Informed Practice Guidelines

As the number of evidence-informed practice guidelines proliferate, it becomes increasingly important that nurses critique these guidelines with regard to the methods used for formulating them and consider how they might be used in their practice. Critical areas that should be assessed when evidence-informed practice guidelines are critiqued include (1) date of publication or release; (2) authors of the guideline; (3) endorsement of the guideline; (4) a clear purpose of what the guideline covers and patient groups for which it was designed; (5) types of evidence (research, nonresearch) used in formulating the guideline; (6) types of research included in formulating the guideline (e.g., "We considered only randomized and other prospective controlled trials in determining efficacy of therapeutic interventions"); (7) a description of the methods used in grading the evidence; (8) search terms and retrieval methods used to acquire research and nonresearch evidence used in the guideline; (9) well-referenced statements regarding practice; (10) comprehensive reference list; (11) review of the guideline by experts; and (12) whether the guideline has been used or tested in practice and, if so, with what types of patients and in what types of settings.

Evidence-informed practice guidelines are principles that help the researcher better understand the evidence base of certain practices, Such guidelines, formulated through the use of rigorous methods, provide a useful starting point for nurses to understand the evidence base of certain practices. However, more research may have become available since the publication of the guideline,

and refinements may be needed. Although information in well-developed, national, evidence-informed practice guidelines is a helpful reference, it is usually necessary to localize the guideline through the use of institution-specific, evidence-informed policies, procedures, or standards before the guideline is applied within a specific setting. A useful tool for critiquing clinical practice guidelines is the AGREE II tool (available at http://www.agreetrust.org/).

Critique of Research

Critique of each study should involve the same methodology, and the critique process should be a shared responsibility. It is helpful, however, to have one individual provide leadership for the project and design strategies for completing critiques. A group approach to critiques is recommended because it distributes the workload, helps those responsible for implementing the changes to understand the scientific base for the change in practice, arms nurses with citations and research-based "sound bites" to use in effecting practice changes with peers and other disciplines, and provides novices an environment to learn how to critique and apply research findings. Methods to make the critique process fun and interesting include the following:

- Using a journal club to discuss critiques performed by each member of the group
- Pairing a novice and expert to do critiques
- Eliciting assistance from students who may be interested in the topic and want experience performing critiques
- Making a class project of critique and synthesis of research for a given topic

Several resources are available to assist with the critique process, including the Evidence-Based Medicine and accompanying compact disc (Straus et al., 2005) and Evidence-Based Nursing: A Guide to Clinical Practice (DiCenso, Guyatt, & Ciliska, 2005). If you wish to start your own journal club, refer to Silversides (2011) for practical advice and further references.

Synthesis of the Research

Once studies are critiqued, a decision is made regarding use of each study in the synthesis of the evidence for application in clinical practice. Factors that should be considered for inclusion of studies in the synthesis of findings are overall scientific merit of the study; type (e.g., age, gender, pathological condition) of participants enrolled in the study and their similarity to the patient population to which the findings will be applied; and relevance of the study to the topic of question. For example, if the practice area is prevention of deep venous thrombosis in patients after surgery, a descriptive study with a heterogeneous population of medical patients is not appropriate for inclusion in the synthesis of findings.

To synthesize the findings from research critiques, it is helpful to use a summary table (Table 20-4) in which critical information from studies can be documented. Essential information to include in such summary is the following:

- Study purpose
- Research questions/hypotheses
- The variables studied
- A description of the study sample and setting
- The type of research design
- The methods used to measure each variable
- Detailed description of the independent variable/intervention tested
- The study findings

Setting Forth Evidence-Informed Practice Recommendations

On the basis of the critique of evidence-informed practice guidelines and synthesis of research, recommendations for practice are set forth. The type and strength of evidence used to support the practice need to be clearly delineated. Box 20-2 is a useful tool to assist with this activity.

The following are examples of practice recommendation statements:

- "Small, informal group health education classes, delivered in the antenatal period, have a better impact on breastfeeding initiation rates than breastfeeding literature alone or combined with formal, noninteractive methods of teaching." (Strength of recommendation = B; RNAO, 2003, p. 46)
- Older people who have recurrent falls should be offered long-term exercise and balance training. (Strength of recommendation = B; American Geriatrics Society, British Geriatrics Society, American Academy of Orthopaedic Surgeons, & Panel on Falls Prevention, 2001).
- Every patient should be screened to identify those most likely to be affected by asthma. As part of the basic respiratory assessment, nurses should ask every patient two questions:
  1. "Have you ever been told by a physician that you have asthma?"
  2. "Have you ever used a puffer or inhaler or asthma medication for breathing problems?" (Strength of recommendation = D; RNAO, 2004, p. 30).
- Apply dressings that maintain a moist wound environment. Examples of moist dressings include, but are not limited to, hydrogels, hydrocolloids, saline moistened gauze, and transparent film dressings. The ulcer bed should be kept continuously moist. (Evidence Grade = B; Colwell, Foreman, & Trotter, 1992; Folkedahl, Frantz, & Goode, 2002; Fowler & Goupil, 1984; Gorse & Messner, 1987; Kurzuk-Howard, Simpson, & Palmieri, 1985; Neill, Conforti, & Kedas, 1989; Oleske, Smith, White, Pottage, & Donovan, 1986; Saydak, 1990; Sebern, 1986; Xakellis & Chrischilles, 1992).

TABLE 20-4

EXAMPLE OF A SUMMARY TABLE FOR RESEARCH CRITIQUES

CITATION	PURPOSE AND RESEARCH QUESTION	RESEARCH DESIGN	SAMPLE	INDEPENDENT VARIABLES AND MEASURES	DEPENDENT VARIABLES AND MEASURES	STATISTICAL TESTS	RESULTS	IMPLICATIONS	GENERAL STRENGTHS	GENERAL WEAKNESSES	OVERALL QUALITY OF STUDY*	SUMMARY STATEMENTS FOR PRACTICE

*Use a consistent rating system (e.g., good, fair, poor).

CONSISTENCY OF EVIDENCE FROM CRITIQUED RESEARCH AND APPRAISALS OF EVIDENCE-INFORMED PRACTICE GUIDELINES

1. Are studies replicated with consistent results?
2. Are the studies well designed?
3. Are recommendations consistent among systematic reviews, evidence-informed practice guidelines, and critiqued research?
4. Are risks to the patient identified from evidence-informed practice recommendations?
5. Are benefits to the patient identified?
6. Have cost analysis studies been conducted with regard to the recommended action, intervention, or treatment?
7. Are summary recommendations about assessments, actions, and interventions or treatments available from the research, systematic reviews, and evidence-informed guidelines with an assigned evidence grade?
8. Is one of the following examples of grading the evidence used?
   a. Evidence from well-designed meta-analysis or other systematic reviews
   b. Evidence from well-designed controlled trials, both randomized and nonrandomized, with results that consistently support a specific action (e.g., assessment), intervention, or treatment
   c. Evidence from observational studies (e.g., correlational descriptive studies) or controlled trials with inconsistent results
   d. Evidence from expert opinion or multiple cases

Modified from Titler, M. G. (2002). *Toolkit for promoting evidence-based practice.* Iowa City: University of Iowa Hospitals and Clinics, Department of Nursing Services and Patient Care.

Helpful Hint

Use of a summary form helps identify commonalities across several studies with regard to study findings and the types of patients to which study findings can be applied. It also helps in synthesizing the overall strengths and weakness of the studies as a group.

Decision to Change Practice

After studies are critiqued and synthesized and evidence-informed practices are set forth, the next step is to decide whether findings are appropriate for use in practice. The following criteria should be considered in making these decisions:

- Relevance of evidence for practice
- Consistency in findings across studies, guidelines, or both
- A significant number of studies, evidence-informed practice guidelines, or both in which sample characteristics are similar to those to which the findings will be applied
- Consistency among evidence from research and other nonresearch evidence
- Feasibility for use in practice
- The risk/benefit ratio (risk of harm; potential benefit for the patient)

It is recommended that practice changes be based on knowledge/evidence derived from several sources (e.g., several research studies) that demonstrate consistent findings.

Synthesis of study findings and other evidence may result in supporting current practice, making minor practice modifications, undertaking major practice changes, or developing a new area of practice. For example, a project on gauze versus transparent dressings did not result in a practice change because the results of the studies reviewed supported current practice (Pettit & Kraus, 1995). In comparison, Madsen and colleagues (2005) used a combination of research findings and expert consultation to derive a guideline that resulted in a change in practice for assessing bowel motility after abdominal surgery in an adult inpatient population. Madsen and colleagues' project resulted in (1) omitting bowel sound assessment as a marker of return of gastrointestinal motility and (2) using return of flatus, first bowel movement, and absence of abdominal distention as primary indicators of return of bowel motility after abdominal surgery in adults.

Development of Evidence-Informed Practice

The next step is to put in writing the evidence base of the practice (Haber, Feldman, Penney, Carter, Bidwell-Cerone, & Rose Hott, 1994); the grading schema that has been agreed upon should be used. When results of the critique and synthesis of evidence support current practice or suggest a change in practice, a written evidence-informed practice standard (e.g., policy, procedure, guideline) is warranted. This is necessary so that professionals in the organization (1) know that the practices are based on evidence and (2) know which type of evidence (e.g., randomized controlled trial, expert opinion) was used in developing the evidence-informed standard. Several different formats can be used to document evidence-informed practice changes. The format chosen is influenced by what the document is and how it will be used. Written evidence-informed practices should be part of the organizational policy and procedure manual and should include linkages to the references for the parts of the policy and procedure that are based on research and other types of evidence.

Clinicians (e.g., nurses, physicians, pharmacists) who adopt evidence-informed practices are influenced by the perceived participation they have had in developing and reviewing the protocol (Titler, 2008). It is imperative that once the evidence-informed practice standard is written, key stakeholders have an opportunity to review it and provide feedback to the person or persons responsible for writing it. Focus groups can provide discussion about the evidence-informed standard and identify key areas that may be potentially troublesome during the implementation phase. Key questions that can be used in the focus groups are listed in Box 20-3.

> **Helpful Hint**
> Use a consistent approach to writing evidence-informed practice standards and referencing the research and related literature.

Implementing the Practice Change

If a practice change is warranted, the next steps are to make the evidence-informed changes in practice. This step goes beyond writing a policy or procedure that is evidence informed; it requires interaction among direct care providers to champion and foster evidence adoption, leadership

---

BOX 20-3

KEY QUESTIONS FOR FOCUS GROUPS

1. What is needed by (nurses, physicians) to use the evidence-informed practice with patients in units (specify unit)?
2. In your opinion, how will this standard improve patient care in your unit/practice?
3. What modifications would you suggest in the evidence-informed practice standard before you would use it in your practice?
4. What content in the evidence-informed practice standard is unclear? Needs revision?
5. What would you change about the format of the evidence-informed practice standard?
6. What part of this evidence-informed practice change do you view as most challenging?
7. Any other suggestions?

---

support, and system changes. Rogers's (2003) seminal work on diffusion of innovations is extremely useful for selecting strategies for promoting adoption of evidence-informed practices. Other investigators describing barriers to and strategies for adoption of evidence-informed practices have used Rogers's (2003) model (Gravel et al., 2006; Scott et al., 2008; Thompson, Estabrooks, Scott-Findlay, Moore, & Wallin, 2007).

According to this model, adoption of innovations, such as evidence-informed practices, is influenced by the nature of the innovation (e.g., the type and strength of evidence; the clinical topic) and the manner in which it is communicated (disseminated) to members (nurses) of a social system (organization, nursing profession; Rogers, 2003; Titler & Everett, 2001). Strategies for promoting adoption of evidence-informed practices must address these areas within a context of participative, planned change (Figure 20-5).

Nature of the Innovation/Evidence-Informed Practice

Characteristics of an innovation or evidence-informed practice topic that affect adoption include the relative advantage of the evidence-

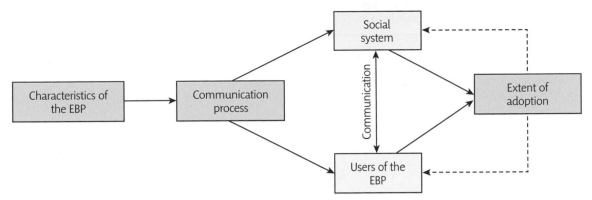

FIGURE 20-5   Implementation model.
Redrawn from Rogers, E. M. (1995). *Diffusion of innovations.* New York: Free Press; and from
Titler, M. G., & Everett, L. Q. (2001). Translating research into practice: Considerations for critical
care investigators. *Critical Care Nursing Clinics of North America, 13*(4), 587–604.

informed practice (e.g., effectiveness, relevance to the task, social prestige); the compatibility with values, norms, work, and perceived needs of users; and complexity of the evidence-informed practice topic (Rogers, 2003). For example, evidence-informed practice topics that are perceived by users as relatively simple (e.g., influenza vaccines for older adults) are more easily adopted in less time than those that are more complex (e.g., acute pain management for hospitalized older adults).

Strategies to promote adoption of evidence-informed practices related to characteristics of the topic include practitioner review and "reinvention" of the evidence-informed practice guideline to fit the local context, use of quick reference guides and decision aids, and use of clinical reminders (Doebbeling, Chou, & Tierney, 2006).

An important principle to remember for planning implementation of an evidence-informed practice is that the attributes of the evidence-informed practice topic as perceived by users and stakeholders (e.g., ease of use, valued part of practice) are neither stable features nor sure determinants of their adoption. Rather, it is the interaction among the characteristics of the evidence-informed practice topic, the intended users, and a particular context of practice that determines the rate and extent of adoption (Greenhalgh et al., 2004; Rogers, 2003).

Studies suggest that clinical systems, computerized decision support, and prompts/quick reference guides that support practice (e.g., decision-making algorithms; paper reminders) have a positive effect on aligning practices with the evidence base (Doebbeling et al., 2006; Shojania & Grimshaw, 2005; Titler, 2006).

Computerized knowledge management has consistently demonstrated significant improvements in provider performance and patient outcomes (Wensing, Wollersheim, & Grol, 2006). Feldman and associates (2005), using a just-in-time e-mail reminder in home health care, demonstrated (1) improvements in evidence-informed care and outcomes for patients with heart failure and (2) reduced pain intensity for cancer patients (McDonald, Pezzin, Feldman, Murtaugh, & Peng, 2005). There is still much to learn about the "best" manner of deploying evidence-informed information through electronic clinical information systems to support evidence-informed care. An example of a quick reference guide is shown in Figure 20-6.

Methods of Communication

Interpersonal communication channels, methods of communication, and influence among social

Use this quick reference guide to help in the assessment of pain:
- Before clients undergo medical procedures or surgeries that can cause pain
- When clients are experiencing pain from recent surgeries, medical procedures, trauma, or other acute illness

General principles for assessing pain in older adults:
- Verify sensory ability (Can the person see you? Hear you?).
- Allow time to respond.
- Repeat questions/instructions as necessary.
- Use printed materials with large type and dark lines.

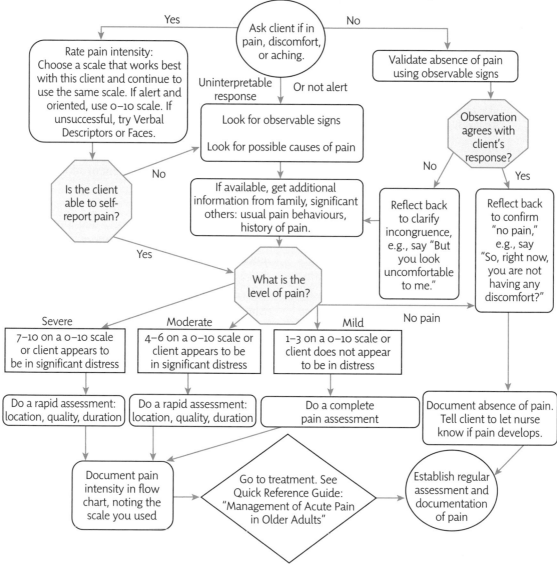

FIGURE 20-6 Quick reference guide: assessment of acute pain in older adults.
Redrawn from Harris, R. P., Helfan, M., Woolf, S. H., Lohr, K. N., Mulrow, C. D., Teutsch, S. M., & Atkins, D. (2001). Current methods of the U.S. Preventive Services Task Force: A review of the process. *American Journal of Preventive Medicine 20*(3S), 21–35; and from Herr, K., Titler, M., Sorofman, B., Ardery, G., Schmitt, M., & Young, D. (2000). Evidence-based guideline: Acute pain management in the elderly. In *From book to bedside: Acute pain Management in the elderly* [Grant No. 1 R01 HS10482-01]. Iowa City: University of Iowa.

networks of users affect adoption of evidence-informed practices (Rogers, 2003). Use of mass media and of consultation with opinion leaders, change champions, and experts, along with education, are among strategies tested to promote use of evidence-informed practices. Interactive education, used in combination with other practice-reinforcing strategies, has more positive effects on improving evidence-informed practice than does education alone (Irwin & Ozer, 2004; Loeb, Brazil, McGeer, Stevenson, Walter, Lohfeld, & Zoutman, 2004).

It is important that staff know the scientific basis for the changes in practice and the improvements in quality of care that are anticipated from the change. This information must be disseminated to staff creatively through various educational strategies. A staff in-service session may not be the most effective method, nor might it reach the majority of the staff. Although it is unrealistic for all staff to have participated in the critique process or to have read all studies used to develop the evidence-informed practice, it is important that they know the myths and realities of the practice. Education of staff also must include ensuring that they are competent in the skills necessary to carry out the new practice. For example, if a pain assessment tool is being implemented to assess pain in cognitively impaired older patients in the long-term care setting, it is essential that caregivers have the knowledge and skill to use the tool in their practice setting.

One method of communicating information to staff is through use of colourful posters that identify myths and realities or describe the essence of the change in practice. Visibly identifying personnel who have learned the information and are using the evidence-informed practice (e.g., buttons, ribbons, pins) stimulates interest in others who may not have internalized the change. As a result, the "new" learner may begin asking questions about the practice and be more open to learning. Other educational strategies such as train-the-trainer programs, Webinars, podcasts,

and competency testing are helpful in education of staff.

Several studies have demonstrated that opinion leaders are effective in changing behaviours of health care practitioners (Cullen, 2005; Greenhalgh et al., 2004; Irwin & Ozer, 2004), especially in combination with educational outreach or performance feedback. **Opinion leaders** are from the local peer group, viewed as a respected source of influence, considered by associates to be technically competent, and trusted to judge the fit between the innovation and the local situation. They have a wide sphere of influence across several microsystems/units and use the innovation, influence peers, and alter group norms (Rogers, 2003). The key characteristic of an opinion leader is that he or she is trusted to evaluate new information in the context of group norms. To do this, an opinion leader must be considered by associates not only to be technically competent but also a full and dedicated member of the local group (Rogers, 2003). Social interactions such as "hallway chats," one-on-one discussions, and addressing questions are important yet often overlooked components of translation (Rogers, 2003). Thus, discussions about the evidence-informed practices between local opinion leaders and members of their peer group is necessary for translating research into practice. If the evidence-informed practice that is being implemented is interdisciplinary in nature, discipline-specific opinion leaders should be used to promote the change in practice (Rogers, 2003). Role expectations of an opinion leader are in Box 20-4.

Change champions are also helpful for implementing innovations (Rogers, 2003; Titler et al., 2006). They are practitioners within the local group setting (e.g., clinic, patient care unit) who are expert clinicians, are passionate about the innovation, are committed to improving quality of care, and have a positive working relationship with other health professionals (Rogers, 2003). They circulate information, encourage peers to

BOX 20-4

ROLE EXPECTATIONS OF AN OPINION LEADER

1. Be or become an expert in the evidence-informed practice.
2. Provide organizational or unit leadership for adopting the evidence-informed practice.
3. Implement various strategies to educate peers about the evidence-informed practice.
4. Work with peers, other disciplines, and leadership staff to incorporate key information about the evidence-informed practice into organizational/unit standards, policies, procedures, and documentation systems.
5. Promote initial and ongoing use of the evidence-informed practice by peers.

Modified from Titler, M. G., Herr, K., Everett, L. Q., Marsh, J. L., Schilling, M., Brooks, J., et al. (2006). *Book to bedside: Promoting and sustaining EBPs in elders* (Final Progress Report to AHRQ, Grant No. 2R01 HS010482-04). Iowa City: University of Iowa College of Nursing.

adopt the innovation, arrange demonstrations, and orient staff to the innovation. The change champion believes in an idea; is undaunted by insults and rebuffs; and, above all, is persistent.

Because nurses prefer interpersonal contact and communication with colleagues rather than Internet or traditional sources of practice knowledge (Estabrooks, Chong, Brigidear, & Profetto-McGrath, 2005), it is imperative that one or two "change champions" be identified for each patient care unit or clinic where the change is being made so that evidence-informed practices can be enacted by direct care providers (Titler et al., 2006). Staff nurses are some of the best change agents for evidence-informed practice. Conferencing with opinion leaders and change champions periodically during implementation is helpful in addressing questions and providing guidance as needed (Titler et al., 2006).

Using a core group in conjunction with change champions is also helpful for implementing the practice change. A *core group* is a select group of practitioners with the mutual goal of disseminating information regarding a practice change and facilitating the change in practice by other staff

in their unit/microsystem (Nelson, Batalden, Huber, Moher, Godfrey, Headrick, & Wasson, 2002). Core group members represent various shifts and days of the week and become knowledgeable about the scientific basis for the practice; the change champion educates and assists them in using practices that are aligned with the evidence. Each member of the core group, in turn, takes the responsibility for imparting evidence-informed information and effecting practice change with several (e.g., two to three) of their peers. They assist the change champion and opinion leader with disseminating the evidence-informed information to other staff, reinforce the practice change on a daily basis, and provide positive feedback to staff members who align their practice with the evidence base (Titler, 2006). Using a core group approach in conjunction with a change champion results in a critical mass of practitioners promoting adoption of the evidence-informed practice (Rogers, 2003).

Clinical nurse specialists can provide one-on-one consultation to staff regarding use of the evidence-informed practice with specific patients, assist staff in troubleshooting issues in application of the practice, and provide feedback on provider performance regarding use of the evidence-informed practices. Studies have demonstrated that when clinical nurse specialists act as facilitators of change, adherence to the evidence-informed practice is promoted (Stetler, Legro, Rycroft-Malone, Bowman, Curran, Guihan, ... & Wallace, 2006; Titler et al., 2009).

Evaluation

Evaluation—the process of determining the value of data—provides an opportunity to collect and analyze data with regard to use of a new evidence-informed practice and then to modify the practice as necessary. It is important that the evidence-informed change be evaluated, both in the area where it is piloted and when the practice is changed in additional patient care areas. The importance of the evaluation cannot be overemphasized; it provides information for performance gap assessment, audit, and feedback, and it provides information necessary to determine whether the evidence-informed practice should be retained, modified, or eliminated.

A desired outcome achieved in a more controlled environment, when a researcher is implementing a study protocol for a homogeneous group of patients (conduct of research), may not be achieved when the practice is implemented in the natural clinical setting, by several caregivers, or to a more heterogeneous patient population. Steps of the evaluation process are summarized in Box 20-5.

Evaluation should include both process and outcome measures. The process component focuses on how the evidence-informed practice change is being implemented. It is important to know whether staff members are using the

practice in care delivery and whether they are implementing the practice as noted in the written evidence-informed practice standard. Evaluation of the process also should include notes about (1) barriers that staff encounter in carrying out the practice (e.g., lack of information, skills, or necessary equipment), (2) differences in opinions among health care professionals, and (3) difficulty in carrying out the steps of the practice as originally designed (e.g., shutting off tube feedings 1 hour before aspirating contents for checking placement of nasointestinal tubes). Process data can be collected from staff reports or patient self-reports, or both; from medical record audits; or from observation of clinical practice. Examples of process and outcome questions are shown in Table 20-5.

Outcome data are an equally important part of evaluation. The purpose of outcome evaluation is to assess whether the patient, staff, or fiscal outcomes expected, or a combination of these, are achieved. Therefore, it is important that baseline data be used for a preintervention/postintervention comparison (Cullen, 2005). Outcome measures should be measured before the change in practice is implemented, after implementation, and every 6 to 12 months thereafter. Findings must be provided to clinicians to reinforce the effects of the change in practice and to ensure that they are incorporated into quality improvement programs.

When process and outcome data are collected for evaluation of evidence-informed practice change, it is important that the data-collection tools are user-friendly, short, concise, and easy to complete and that they have content validity. The evaluation process includes planned feedback to staff members who are making the change. The feedback includes verbal or written (or both) appreciation for the work and visual demonstration of progress in implementation and improvement in patient outcomes. The key to effective evaluation is to ensure that the evidence-informed change in practice is warranted (e.g., will improve quality of care) and that the intervention does not bring harm to patients. For example, when the

---

BOX 20-5

STEPS OF EVALUATION FOR EVIDENCE-INFORMED PRACTICE

1. Identify process and outcome variables of interest.
   Examples:
   Process variable: For patients older than 65 years, a Braden scale will be completed on admission.
   Outcome variable: Presence/absence of nosocomial pressure ulcer; if present, determine stage as I, II, III, or IV.
2. Determine methods and frequency of data collection.
   Example:
   Process variable: Chart audit of all patients older than 65 years, 1 day a month
   Outcome variable: Assessment of all patients older than 65 years, 1 day a month
3. Determine baseline and follow-up sample sizes.
4. Design data-collection forms.
   Example:
   Process variable: chart audit abstraction form
   Outcome variable: pressure ulcer assessment form
5. Establish content validity of data-collection forms.
6. Train data-collectors.
7. Assess interrater reliability of data-collectors.
8. Collect data at specified intervals.
9. Provide "on-site" feedback to staff regarding the progress in achieving the practice change.
10. Provide feedback of analyzed data to staff.
11. Use data to assist staff in modifying or integrating the evidence-informed practice change.

TABLE **20-5**

EXAMPLES OF EVALUATION MEASURES

EXAMPLE OF PROCESS QUESTIONS	STRONGLY DISAGREE	DISAGREE	NEITHER AGREE NOR DISAGREE	AGREE	STRONGLY AGREE
1. I feel well prepared to use the Bracken Scale with older patients.	1	2	3	4	5
2. Malnutrition increases patient risk for pressure ulcer development.	1	2	3	4	5

EXAMPLE OF OUTCOME QUESTION
Patient: On a scale of 0 (no pain) to 10 (worst possible pain), how much pain have you experienced over the past 24 hours?   _____ (Pain intensity)

practice for assessing return of bowel motility after abdominal surgery in adults was changed, it was important to inform staff that using other markers for return of bowel motility, rather than bowel sound assessment, did not result in increased paralytic ileus or bowel obstruction (Madsen et al., 2005).

CREATING A CULTURE OF EVIDENCE-INFORMED PRACTICE

Use of research evidence to guide clinical and operational decisions is a necessity in health care delivery (Cullen & Titler, 2004). Chief nurse executives and their leadership staff set the stage and culture for evidence-informed practice in their settings. How this is done varies, but essential components are necessary for evidence-informed practices (both the process and product) to be an integral part of the organization.

Providing this leadership is a continuous process that involves four major building blocks (Figure 20-7):

- Incorporating evidence-informed practice terminology into the mission, vision, strategic plan, and philosophy of care delivery
- Establishing explicit performance expectations about evidence-informed practice for staff at all levels of the organization
- Integrating the work of evidence-informed practice into the governance structure of

nursing departments and the health care system
- Recognition for and rewarding of evidence-informed practice behaviours

 Helpful Hint_____

Include patient outcome measures (e.g., pressure ulcer prevalence) and cost (e.g., cost savings, cost avoidance) in evaluation.

The first building block involves ensuring that the mission and vision statements of the health care system and nursing services reflect a commitment to the provision of evidence-informed health care; for example: "The vision of the department of nursing services and patient care is to be an international exemplar of using evidence to guide clinical and operational decision-making." For evidence-informed practices to be manifested in everyday work, it is necessary to incorporate into the organization's or department's strategic plan specific action statements that promote and foster evidence-informed practices. Such actions might include offering an annual evidence-informed practice staff nurse internship program; integrating educational content about evidence-informed practice into orientation of new staff; monitoring and acting on the results of key indicators for selected evidence-informed practices (e.g., acute pain management,

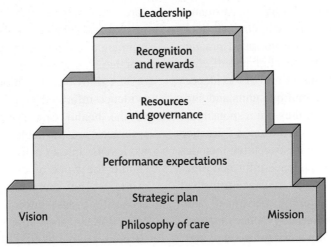

FIGURE 20-7   Four major building blocks in the process of creating a culture of evidence-informed practice.

prevention of pressure ulcers, prevention of falls); and initiating two or three new evidence-informed practices per year that are triggered by operational data, quality improvement data, or both. Equally important to a mission and vision that embrace evidence-informed practice is clarity about (1) the definition and meaning of evidence-informed practice (some departments actually articulate a definition), (2) the organizational process or model of evidence-informed practice, and (3) a philosophy of care that embraces clinical inquiry and questioning of the status quo.

The second building block involves developing and using performance expectations regarding evidence-informed practices. For example, evidence-informed practice performance expectations for staff nurses should include critical thinking, continual questioning of practice, participating in making evidence-informed practice changes, serving as leaders of change in their site of care delivery, and participating in evaluating evidence-informed changes in practice.

The chief nurse executive sets the tone for evidence-informed practice and explicates role expectations of other nurse leaders within the organization regarding the knowledge, skills, and behaviours necessary to promote adoption of evidence-informed practices. Performance expectations for nurse managers include creating a culture that fosters interdisciplinary quality improvement informed by evidence. Clinical nurse specialists' performance expectations include leading a team, finding the evidence, and synthesizing the evidence for practice. Clinical nurse specialists assist staff with focusing their clinical question about improving practice, finding and evaluating the research evidence, and manoeuvring through the committee structures to implement and sustain the changes in practice. The ability of clinical nurse specialists to meet these performance criteria is an essential part of their annual performance appraisals. Similarly, nurse managers set the tone, value, and work culture for the microsystems they lead.

Staff migrate to microsystems that foster professional growth, professional nursing practice, data-informed decision making, and innovative practices; all characteristics of cultures that promote adoption of evidence-informed nursing practices. Nurse managers also foster evidence-informed practices in their units by allocation of resources, which is an important element for staff nurse participation in new evidence-informed practice projects. Consequently, institutions who hire, retain, and value (through performance appraisals) nurse managers and clinical nurse specialists skilled in evidence-informed practice are more likely to observe development of clinical innovations and adoption of evidence-informed practices in the multiple units and sites of care delivery for which they are responsible.

Enactment of evidence-informed practice behaviours by the chief nurse executive includes providing resources for evidence-informed practice such as easy access to evidence-informed practice Web sites, retaining personnel with expertise in evidence-informed practice, supporting programs that develop a critical mass of staff nurses with expertise in evidence-informed practice (e.g., an evidence-informed practice staff nurse internship program; Cullen & Titler, 2004), and providing access to assistance with analysis of data and transforming data into information. Chief nurse executives also enact the value of evidence-informed practice by using information from evaluations of existing and new clinical programs in operational decisions, and by rewarding and recognizing direct care providers who make evidence-informed practice a reality in their daily work. Using evidence in administrative decisions is another behaviour modelled by chief nurse executives who value evidence-informed practice.

One example of an evidence-informed administrative practice involves assessing the work culture of nurses that contribute to job satisfaction and retention and then using this information, along with research evidence, to create administrative interventions that decrease turnover. Because it is difficult to support multiple evidence-informed practice changes simultaneously, chief nurse executives committed to evidence-informed practice lead discussion and decision making regarding priority setting for areas of evidence-informed practice (e.g., skin care, pain). Last, but most important, it is the chief nurse executive's responsibility to ensure that the mission, vision, philosophy of care, strategic plan, and performance criteria incorporate language about the value and commitment of the organization to evidence-informed practice.

The third building block involves integrating evidence-informed practice into the governance of the health care system and ensuring that resources are available to assist staff with this work. One question frequently asked is "Where should the work of evidence-informed practice reside?" The short answer is "Everywhere," because evidence-informed practice saves health care dollars and improves patient outcomes (Brooks et al., 2009; Titler et al., 2009). More explicitly, to sustain a vision of providing evidence-informed health care, the work and accountability for evidence-informed practice must be integrated into the governance structure. This includes interdisciplinary collaboration across departments and services, as well as coordination within discipline-specific areas of practice.

Evidence-informed changes in practice must be coordinated with professional policy and procedure committees in order for the evidence to be reflected in practice standards. Documentation systems, whether electronic or manual, must support the evidence-informed practices through reminder systems, decision-support algorithms, and easy-to-use documentation forms. Too often, personnel providing direct care are expected to change practices without full modification of the documentation systems that capture and reinforce the desired changes. Although the primary responsibility for tracking and promoting evidence-informed practice may reside in a specific department or program (e.g., research, education, quality improvement), evidence-informed practice must be viewed and valued as essential work at all levels of the organization and within the committees/councils that govern the health care system.

The fourth building block involves recognition for and rewarding of evidence-informed practice behaviours. Such recognition can range from (1) submitting staff projects and names to national and international professional organizations that have programs for recognition of excellence in evidence-informed practice to (2) recognizing specific staff members in their unit at the shift change for the care they provide that is informed by evidence. Other recognition activities include an annual recognition day with a display of posters of the evidence-informed practice work occurring in each unit; recognition in a weekly or monthly internal communication; postings on Web sites; and broadcasting the stellar accomplishments in the local, regional, and national media. Some organizations integrate evidence-informed practice expectations into the clinical ladder system, and others provide staff release time from direct patient care to do the work of evidence-informed practice. Recognition by peers, as well as senior administrators, is important.

TRANSLATION SCIENCE

Translation science, mentioned previously in this chapter, is the investigation of strategies to increase the rate and extent of adoption and sustainability of evidence-informed practice by individuals and organizations to improve clinical and operational decision making (Eccles & Mittman, 2006; Titler, Everett, & Adams, 2007). It includes research to (1) understand context variables that influence adoption of evidence-informed practices and (2) test the effectiveness of interventions to promote and sustain use of evidence-informed health care practices. Translation science denotes both the systematic investigation of methods, interventions, and variables that influence adoption of evidence-informed health care practices, as well as the organized body of knowledge gained through such research (Eccles & Mittman, 2006; Rubenstein & Pugh, 2006; Sussman, Valente, Rohrbach, Skara, & Pentz, 2006; Titler et al., 2007).

Because translation research is a young science, there are no standardized definitions of commonly used terms (Graham et al., 2006). This is evidenced by differing definitions and the interchanging of terms that, in fact, may represent different concepts to different people. Adding to the confusion is that terminology may vary depending on the country in which the research was conducted (Adams & Titler, 2010). Graham and colleagues (2006) reported identifying 29 terms in nine countries that refer to some aspect of translating research findings into practice. For example, researchers in Canada may use the terms *research utilization, knowledge-to-action, knowledge transfer,* or *knowledge translation* interchangeably, whereas researchers in the United States, the United Kingdom, and Europe may be more likely to use the term *implementation* or *research translation* to express similar concepts (Graham et al., 2006; Graham & Logan, 2004; Titler & Everett, 2001). The goals of the Canadian Institutes of Health Research (CIHR) are not only to support the development of new knowledge through research but also to ensure that the knowledge is translated into practice. Knowledge translation is defined "as a dynamic and iterative process that includes synthesis, dissemination, exchange and ethically sound application of knowledge to improve the health of Canadians, provide more effective health services and products and strengthen the health care system" (CIHR, 2009).

Building this body of research knowledge mandates development in many areas; theoretical developments are needed to provide frameworks and predictive theories for creating generalizable research such as how to change individual and organizational behaviour. Methodological developments are also required, as well as exploratory studies aimed at understanding the experiential and organizational learning that accompanies implementation. Rigorous evaluations are needed to evaluate the effectiveness and efficiency of implementation interventions (Adams & Titler, 2010). Partnerships are needed to encourage communication among researchers, theorists, and implementers and to understand what types of knowledge are needed and how that knowledge can best be developed (Adams & Titler, 2010; Dawson, 2004; Gold & Taylor, 2007; Tripp-Reimer & Doebbeling, 2004).

FUTURE DIRECTIONS

Use of research across health care systems for improving the quality of care is essential. As professionals continue to understand the science of nursing and synthesize this science for application in practice, it will become increasingly necessary to test and understand how to best promote the use of this science in daily practice.

Ross-Kerr and Wood (2011, p. 136) detailed some of the challenges in the future of the research process:

> Facilitating research utilization in nursing practice is not an easy task, but neither is it an impossible dream. Some activities that might facilitate the research process include the following:
>
> * Funding key research positions
> * Creating institutional infrastructures, including resources needed to access summarized evidence
> * Encouraging and assisting nurses to attend practice-based research workshops and conferences
> * Providing continuing education courses to assist nurses in critiquing research
> * Creating a reward system within the agency for research utilization in practice
> * Promoting collaborative efforts between agency personnel and other health-care agencies or educational institutions
> * Establishing a means for nurses to access research reports relevant to their practice
> * Promoting demonstration projects that illustrate the cost-effectiveness of changing from a traditional, intuitively based practice to one that is research-based
> * Ensuring that research utilization is a role expectation for all nursing positions (management, educational, and clinical) and that it is reinforced in job descriptions, agency policy, and the institution's philosophy of nursing.
>
> Diagnosing barriers, and planning and implementing strategies to overcome them, are challenges. The first challenge is to demonstrate the cost-effectiveness of

nursing research and to justify the allocation of resources and personnel to create the necessary infrastructures. The second challenge is to reduce the time gap between when knowledge is developed and when it is used. The third challenge is to create agency infrastructures that will support the transformation of nursing practice from a ritual base to a research base. Efforts to address these challenges require partnerships among practitioners, researchers, administrators, and disciplines.

Education of nurses must include knowledge and skills in the use of research evidence in practice. Nurses are increasingly being held accountable for practices informed by scientific evidence. Thus, nurses must communicate and integrate into their profession the expectation that all nurses have a professional responsibility to read and use research in their practice and to communicate with nurse scientists the many and varied clinical problems for which a scientific basis for practice does not yet exist.

CRITICAL THINKING CHALLENGES

- Discuss the differences among nursing research, research utilization, and evidence-informed practice. Support your discussion with examples.
- Why would it be important to use an evidence-informed practice model, such as the Iowa Model of Evidence-Based Practice to Promote Quality Care, to guide a practice project focused on justifying and implementing a change in clinical practice?
- You are a staff nurse working on a cardiac step-down unit. Many of your colleagues do not understand evidence-informed practice. How would you help them to understand how evidence-informed practice is relevant to providing optimal care to this patient population?
- What barriers do you see to applying evidence-informed practice in your clinical setting? Discuss strategies to use in overcoming these barriers.

KEY POINTS

- According to the Iowa Model of Evidence-Based Practice to Promote Quality Care, the steps of evidence-informed practice are as follows: selecting a topic, forming a team, retrieving the evidence, grading the evidence, developing an evidence-informed practice standard, implementing the evidence-informed practice, and evaluating the effect on staff, patient, and fiscal outcomes.
- Adoption of evidence-informed practice standards requires education and dissemination to staff and use of change strategies, such as communication with opinion leaders, change champions, a core group, and consultants.
- It is important to evaluate the change. Evaluation provides data for performance gap assessment, audit, and feedback, and provides information necessary to determine whether the practice should be retained.
- Evaluation includes both process and outcome measures.
- It is important for organizations to create a culture of evidence-informed practice. Creating this culture requires an interactive process. To provide this culture, organizations need to provide access to information, access to individuals who have skills necessary for evidence-informed practice, and a written and verbal commitment to evidence-informed practice in the organization's operations.
- The terms *research utilization* and *evidence-informed practice* are sometimes used interchangeably. These terms, although related, are not one and the same. *Research utilization* is the process of using research findings to improve practice. *Evidence-informed practice* is a broad term that not only encompasses use of research findings but also use of other types of evidence such as case reports and expert opinion in deciding the evidence base that informs practice.
- There are two forms of evidence use: conceptual and decision driven.
- There are several models of evidence-informed practice. A key feature of all models is the judicious review and synthesis of research and other types of evidence to develop an evidence-informed practice standard.

REFERENCES

Adams, S. L., & Titler, M. G. (2010). Building a learning collaborative. *Worldviews on Evidence-Based Nursing, 7*(3), 165-173.

American Geriatrics Society, British Geriatrics Society, American Academy of Orthopaedic Surgeons, and Panel on Falls Prevention. (2001). Guideline for the prevention of falls in older persons. *Journal of the American Geriatrics Society, 49*, 664-672.

Atkins, D., Briss, P. A., Eccles, M., Flottorp, S., Guyatt, G. H., Harbour, R. T., . . . & The GRADE Working Group. (2005). Systems for grading the quality of evidence and the strength of recommendations II: Pilot study of a new system. *BMC Health Services Research, 5*(1), 25.

Bootsmiller, B. J., Yankey, J. W., Flach, S. D., Ward, M. M., Vaughn, T. E., Welke, K. F., & Doebbeling, B. N. (2004). Classifying the effectiveness of Veterans Affairs guideline implementation approaches. *American Journal of Medical Quality, 19*(6), 248-254.

Brooks, J. M., Titler, M. G., Ardery, G., & Herr, K. (2009). Effect of evidence-based acute pain management practices on inpatient costs. *Health Services Research, 44*(1), 245-263.

Canadian Institutes of Health Research (2009). About knowledge translation. Retrieved from http://www.canadiantaskforce.ca

Canadian Task Force on Preventative Health Care (CTFPHC). (1997). *Quick tables by strength of evidence*. Retrieved from http://www.ctfphc.org

Clancy, C. M., Slutsky, J. R., & Patton, L. T. (2004). AHRQ moves research to translation and implementation. *Health Services Research, 39*(5), xv-xxiii.

Colwell, J. C., Foreman, M. D., & Trotter, J. P. (1992). A comparison of the efficacy and cost-effectiveness of two methods of managing pressure ulcers. *Decubitus, 6*(4), 28-36.

Cronenwett, L. R. (1995). Effective methods for disseminating research findings to nurses in practice. *Nursing Clinics of North America, 30*, 429-438.

Cullen, L. (2005). Evidence-based practice: Strategies for nursing leaders. In D. Huber (Ed.), *Leadership and nursing care management* (3rd ed., pp. 461-478). Philadelphia: Elsevier.

Cullen, L., & Titler, M. G. (2004). Promoting evidence-based practice: An internship for staff nurses. *Worldviews on Evidence-Based Practice, 1*(4), 215-223.

Davey, P., Brown, E., Fenelon, L., Finch, R., Gould, I., Hartman, G., . . . & Wiffen, P. J. (2005). Interventions to improve antibiotic prescribing practices for hospital inpatients. *Cochrane Database of Systematic Reviews*, (4), CD003543. doi: 003510.001002/14651858.CD14003543.pub14651852

Dawson, J. D. (2004). Quantitative analytical methods in translation research. *Worldviews on Evidence-Based Nursing, 1*(S1), S60-S64.

DiCenso, A., Guyatt, G., & Ciliska, D. (2005). *Evidence-based nursing: A guide to clinical practice.* St. Louis: Elsevier.

Doebbeling, B. N., Chou, A. F., & Tierney, W. M. (2006). Priorities and strategies for the implementation of integrated informatics and communications technology to improve evidence-based practice. *Journal of General Internal Medicine, 21*(S2), S50-S57.

Eccles, M. P., & Mittman, B. S. (2006). Welcome to implementation science. *Implementation Science, 1*, 1.

Estabrooks, C. A. (2004). Thoughts on evidence-based nursing and its science: A Canadian perspective. *Worldviews on Evidence-Based Nursing, 1*(2), 88-91.

Estabrooks, C. A., Chong, H., Brigidear, K., & Profetto-McGrath, J. (2005). Profiling Canadian nurses' preferred knowledge sources for clinical practice. *Canadian Journal of Nursing Research, 37*(2), 119-140.

Estabrooks, C. A., Derksen, L., Winther, C., Lavis, J. L., Scott, S. D., Wallin, L., & Profetto-McGrath, J. (2008). The intellectual structure and substance of the knowledge utilization field: a longitudinal author co-citation analysis, 1945-2004. *Implementation Science, 3*, 49. doi:10.1186/1748-5908-3-49

Feldman, P. H., Murtaugh, C. M., Pezzin, L. E., McDonald, L. E., & Peng, T. R. (2005). Just-in-time evidence-based e-mail "reminders" in home health care: impact on patient outcomes. *Health Services Research, 40*(3), 865-885.

Folkedahl, B., Frantz, R., & Goode, C. (2002). *Evidence-based protocol: Treatment of pressure ulcers* (Series Ed., Titler, M. G.). Iowa City: University of Iowa College of Nursing, Gerontological Nursing Interventions Research Center, Research Dissemination Core (P30 NR03979; PI: T. Tripp-Reimer).

Fowler, E., & Goupil, D. L. (1984). Comparison of the wet-to-dry dressing and a copolymer starch in the management of debrided pressure sores. *Journal of Enterostomal Therapy, 11*(1), 22-25.

Gold, M., & Taylor, E. F. (2007). Moving research into practice: Lessons from the US Agency for Healthcare Research and Quality's IDSRN program. *Implementation Science, 2*, 9.

Gorse, G. J., & Messner, R. L. (1987). Improved pressure sore healing with hydrocolloid dressings. *Archives of Dermatology, 123*(6), 766-771.

GRADE Working Group. (2004). Grading quality of evidence and strength of recommendations. *British Medical Journal, 328*, 1490-1494.

Graham, I. D., Logan, J., Harrison, M. B., Straus, S. E., Tetroe, M. A., Caswell, W., & Robinson, N. (2006). Lost in knowledge translation: Time for a map? *Journal of Continuing Education in the Health Professions, 26*(1), 13-24.

Graham, K., & Logan, J. (2004). Using the Ottawa model of research use to implement a skin care program. *Journal of Nursing Care Quality, 19*(1), 18-24.

Gravel, K., Légaré, F., & Graham, I. D. (2006). Barriers and facilitators to implementing shared decision-making in clinical practice: a systematic review of health professionals' perceptions. *Implementation Science, 1*, 16.

Greenhalgh, T., Robert, G., MacFarlane, F. B., Bate, P., & Kyriakdiou, O. (2004). Diffusion of innovations in health service organisations: A systematic literature review. *The Milbank Quarterly, 82*(4). Retrieved from http://www.milbank.org/quarterly/8204feat.html

Grol, R. P., Bosch, M. C., Hulscher, M. E., Eccles, M. P., & Wensing, M. (2007). Planning and studying improvement in patient care: The use of theoretical perspectives. *The Milbank Quarterly, 85*(1), 93-138.

Guyatt, G. H., Oxman, A. D., Kunz, R., Jaeschke, R., Helfand, M., Liberati, A., . . . & Schunemann, H. J. (2008a). Rating quality of evidence and strength of recommendations: What is "quality of evidence" and why is it important to clinicians? *British Medical Journal, 336*(7651), 995-998. doi:10.1136/bmj.39490.551019.BE

Guyatt, G. H., Oxman, A. D., Kunz, R., Vist, G. E., Falck-Ytter, Y., & Schunemann, H. J. (2008b). Rating quality of evidence and strength of recommendations: Incorporating considerations of resources use into grading recommendations. *British Medical Journal, 336*(7654), 1170-1173. doi:10.1136/bmj.39504.506319.80

Guyatt, G. H., Oxman, A. D., Vist, G., Kunz, R., Falck-Ytter, Y., Alonso-Coello, P., & Schunemann, H. J. (2008c). Rating quality of evidence and strength of recommendations GRADE: An emerging consensus on rating quality of evidence and strength of recommendations. *British Medical Journal, 336*(7650), 924-926. doi: 10.1136/bmj.39489.470347.AD

Haber, J., Feldman, H., Penney, N., Carter, E., Bidwell-Cerone, S., & Rose Hott, J. (1994). Shaping nursing practice through research-based protocols. *Journal of the New York State Nurses Association, 25*(3), 3-8.

Haller, K. B., Reynolds, M. A., & Horsley, J. O. (1979). Developing research-based innovation protocols: Process, criteria, and issues. *Research in Nursing & Health, 2*(2), 45-51.

Harris, R. P., Helfan, M., Woolf, S. H., Lohr, K. N., Mulrow, C. D., Teutsch, S. M., & Atkins, D. (2001). Current methods of the US Preventive Services Task Force: A review of the process. *American Journal of Preventative Medicine, 20*(3S), 21-35.

Higgins, J. P. T., & Green, S. (Eds.). (2011). *Cochrane handbook for systematic reviews of interventions 5.1* [updated March 2011]. Retrieved from http://www.cochrane.org/sites/default/files/uploads/Handbook4.2.6Sep2006.pdf

Horsley, J. A., Crane, J., Crabtree, M. K., & Wood, D. K. (1983). *Using research to improve nursing practice: A guide.* New York: Grune & Stratton.

ICEBeRG. (2006). Designing theoretically informed implementation interventions: The Improved Clinical Effectiveness through Behavioural Research Group. *Implementation Science, 1*, 4.

Irwin, C., & Ozer, E. M. (2004). *Implementing adolescent preventive guidelines. Final progress report to AHRQ* (Grant No. U18HS11095). San Francisco: University of California, San Francisco, Division of Adolescent Medicine.

Kirchhoff, K. T. (2004). State of the science of translational research: From demonstration projects to intervention testing. *Worldviews on Evidence-Based Nursing, 1*(Suppl. 1), S6-S12.

Kurzuk-Howard, G., Simpson, L., & Palmieri, A. (1985). Decubitus ulcer care: A comparative study. *Western Journal of Nursing Research, 7*(1), 58-79.

Leape, L. L. (2005). Where the rubber meets the road. In *Advances in patient safety: From research to implementation, Vol. 3: Implementation issues* (AHRQ pub no 05-0021-3). Rockville, MD: Agency for Healthcare Research and Quality.

Loeb, M., Brazil, K., McGeer, A., Stevenson, K., Walter, S. D., Lohfeld, L., . . . & Zoutman, D. (2004). *Optimizing antibiotic use in long term care. Final progress report to AHRQ* (Project No. 2R18HS011113-03). Hamilton, ON: McMaster University.

Logan, J., & Graham, I. (1998). Toward a comprehensive interdisciplinary model of health care research use. *Science Communication, 20*(2), 229.

Madsen, D., Sebolt, T., Cullen, L., Mueller, T., Richardson, C., et al. (2005). Why listen to bowel sounds? Report of an evidence-based practice project. *American Journal of Nursing, 105*, 40-49.

McDonald, M. V., Pezzin, L. E., Feldman, P. H., Murtaugh, C. M., & Peng, T. R. (2005). Can just-in-time, evidence-based "reminders" improve pain management among home health care nurses and their patients? *Journal of Pain Symptom Management, 29*(5), 474-488.

Melnyk, B. M., & Fineout-Overholt, E. (2011). *Evidence-based practice in nursing and healthcare: A guide to best practice* (2nd ed). New York: Wolters Kluwer.

Neill, K. M., Conforti, C., Kedas, A., et al. (1989). Pressure sore response to a new hydrocolloid dressing. *Wounds, 1*(3), 173-185.

Nelson, E. C., Batalden, P. B., Huber, T. P., Moher, J. J., Godfrey, M. M., Headrick, L. A., & Wasson, J. H. (2002). Microsystems in health care: Earning from high performing front-line clinical units. *Journal of Quality Improvement, 28*(9), 472-493.

Nightingale, F. (1858). *Notes on matters affecting the health, efficiency, and hospital administration of the British Army.* London, England: Harrison and Sons.

Nightingale, F. (1859). *A contribution to the sanitary history of the British Army during the late war with Russia.* London, England: John W. Parker and Sons.

Nightingale, F. (1863a). *Notes on hospitals.* London, England: Longman, Green, Roberts, and Green.

Nightingale, F. (1863b). *Observation on the evidence contained in the statistical reports submitted by her to the Royal Commission on the Sanitary State of the Army in India.* London, England: Edward Stanford.

Oleske, D. M., Smith, X. P., White, P., Pottage, J., & Donovan, M. I. (1986). A randomized clinical trial of two dressing methods for the treatment of low-grade pressure ulcers. *Journal of Enterostomal Therapy, 13*(3), 90-98.

Pettit, D. M., & Kraus, V. (1995). The use of gauze versus transparent dressing for peripheral intravenous catheter sites. *Nursing Clinics of North America, 30*, 495-506.

Registered Nurses Association of Ontario (2003). *Breastfeeding best practice guidelines for nurses.* Retrieved from www.rnao.org/Storage/11/564_BPG_Breastfeeding.pdf

Registered Nurses Association of Ontario (2004). Adult asthma care guidelines for nurses: Promoting control of asthma. Retrieved from http://www.rnao.org/.../2206_Asthma_Guideline_and_Supplement_-_FIN

Registered Nurses Association of Ontario. (2011). *Implementation of clinical practice guidelines.*

Retrieved from http://www.rnao.org/Page.asp?PageID=924&ContentID=823

Rogers, E. (1995). *Diffusion of innovations*. New York: Free Press.

Rogers, E. M. (2003). *Diffusion of innovations* (5th ed.). New York: Free Press.

Ross-Kerr, J. C., & Wood, M. J. (2011). *Canadian nursing: Issues and perspectives* (5th ed). Toronto: Elsevier.

Rubenstein, L. V., & Pugh, J. A. (2006). Strategies for promoting organizational and practice change by advancing implementation research. *Journal of General Internal Medicine, 21*, S58-S64.

Rycroft-Malone, J., Kitson, A., Harvey, G., McCormack, B., Seers, K., Titchen, A., & Eastabrooks, C. (2002). Ingredients for change: Revisiting a conceptual framework. *Quality Safety Health Care, 11*, 174-180.

Saydak, S. J. (1990). A pilot test of two methods for the treatment of pressure ulcers. *Journal of Enterostomal Therapy, 17*(3), 139-142.

Scott, S. D., Plotnikoff, R. C., Karunamuni, N., Bize, R., & Rodgers, W. (2008). Factors influencing the adoption of an innovation: An examination of the uptake of the Canadian Heart Health Kit (HHK). *Implementation Science, 3*, 41. doi:10.1186/1748-5908-3-41

Sebern, M. D. (1986). Pressure ulcer management in home health care: Efficacy and cost effectiveness and moisture vapor permeable dressing. *Archives of Physical Medicine and Rehabilitation, 67*(10), 726-729.

Shojania, K. G., & Grimshaw, J. M. (2005). Evidence-based quality improvement: The state of the science. *Health Affairs, 24*(1), 138-150.

Silversides, A. (2011). Journal clubs: A forum for discussion and professional development. *Canadian Nurse, 107*(2), 18-23.

Smith, J. L., Williams, J. W., Owen, R. R., Rubenstein, L. V., & Chaney, E. (2008). Developing a national dissemination plan for collaborative care for depression: QUERI Series. *Implementation Science, 3*, 59. doi:10.1186/1748-5908-3-59

Squires, J. E., Moralejo, D., & LeFort, S. M. (2007). Exploring the role of organizational policies and procedures in promoting research utilization in registered nurses. *Implementation Science, 2*, 17.

Stetler, C. A., Legro, M. W., Rycroft-Malone, J., Bowman, C., Curran, G., Guihan, M., . . . & Wallace, C. M. (2006). Role of "external facilitation" in implementation of research findings: A qualitative evaluation of facilitation experiences in the Veterans Health Administration. *Implementation Science, 1*, 23.

Stetler, C. B., McQuenn, L., Demkis, J., & Mittman, B. S. (2008). An organizational framework and strategic implementation for system-level change to enhance research-based practice: QUERI Series. *Implementation Science, 3*, 30. doi:10.1186/1748-5908-3-30

Straus, S. E., Richardson, W. S., Glasziou, P., & Haynes, R. B. (2005). *Evidence based medicine: How to practice and teach EBM* (3rd ed.). Philadelphia: Churchill Livingstone.

Sussman, S., Valente, T. W., Rohrbach, L. A., Skara, S., & Pentz, M. A. (2006). Translation in the health professions: Converting science into action. *Evaluation and the Health Professions, 29*(1), 7-32.

Thompson, D. S., Estabrooks, C. A., Scott-Findlay, S., Moore, K., & Wallin, L. (2007). Interventions aimed at increasing research use in nursing: A systematic review. *Implementation Science, 2*, 15. doi: 10.1186/1748-5908-2-15

Titler, M. G. (1993). Critical analysis of research utilization (RU): An historical perspective. *American Journal of Critical Care, 2*(3), 264.

Titler, M. G. (2002). *Toolkit for promoting evidence-based practice*. Iowa City: University of Iowa Hospitals and Clinics, Department of Nursing Services and Patient Care.

Titler, M. G. (2006). Developing an evidence-based practice. In G. LoBiondo-Wood & J. Haber (Eds.), *Nursing research* (6th ed.). St. Louis: Elsevier Mosby.

Titler, M. G. (2008). The evidence for evidence-based practice implementation. In R. Hughes (Ed.), *Patient safety and quality—an evidence-based handbook for nurses*. Rockville, MD: Agency for Healthcare Research and Quality.

Titler, M. G., & Everett, L. Q. (2001). Translating research into practice: Considerations for critical care investigators. *Critical Care Nursing Clinics of North America, 13*(4), 587-604.

Titler, M. G., Everett, L. Q., & Adams, S. (2007). Implications for implementation science. *Nursing Research, 56*(4S), S53-S59.

Titler, M. G., Herr, K., Brooks, J. M., Xian-Jin, X., Ardery, A., Schilling, J., . . . & Clarke, W. R. (2009). A translating research into practice intervention improves management of acute pain in older hip fracture patients, *Health Services Research, 44*(1), 264-287.

Titler, M. G., Herr, K., Everett, L. Q., Marsh, J. L., Schilling, M., Brooks, J., et al. (2006). *Book to bedside: Promoting & sustaining EBPs in elders*

(Final Progress Report to AHRQ, Grant No. 2R01 HS010482-04). Iowa City: University of Iowa College of Nursing.

Titler, M.G., Kleiber, C., Steelman, V., Goode, C., Rakel, B., Barry-Walker, J., . . . & Buckwalter, K. (1994). Infusing research into practice to promote quality care. *Nursing Research*, *43*(5), 307-313.

Titler, M. G., Kleiber, C., Steelman, V. J., Rakel, B. A., Budreau, G., Everett, L. Q., . . . & Goode, C. J. (2001). The Iowa Model of Evidence-Based Practice to Promote Quality Care. *Critical Care Nursing Clinics of North America*, *13*(4), 497-509.

Tripp-Reimer, T., & Doebbeling, B. N. (2004). Qualitative perspectives in translational research. *Worldviews on Evidence-Based Nursing*, *1*(S1), S65-S72.

U.S. Preventive Services Task Force. (2008). *U.S. Preventive Services Task Force grade definitions*. Retrieved from http://www.uspreventiveservicestaskforce.org/uspstf/grades.htm

Ward, M. M., Evans, T. C., Spies, A. J., Roberts, L., & Wakefield, D. (2006). National Quality Forum 30 safe practices: priority and progress in Iowa hospitals. *American Journal of Medical Quality*, *21*(2), 101-108.

Weiss, C. H. (1980). Knowledge creep and decision accretion. *Science Communication*, *1*(3), 381-404.

Wensing, M., Wollersheim, H., & Grol, R. (2006). Organizational interventions to implement improvements in patient care: A structured review of review. *Implementation Science*, *1*(2), doi:10.1186/1748-5908-1-2

West, S., King, V., Carey, T. S., Lohr, K. N., McKoy, N., Sutton, S. F., & Lux, L. (2002). *Systems to rate the strength of scientific evidence*. (Evidence Report/Technology Assessment No. 47, prepared by the Research Triangle Institute-University of North Carolina Evidence-Based Practice Center under Contract No. 290-97-0011, AHRQ Publication No. 02-E016.) Rockville, MD: Agency for Healthcare Research and Quality.

Xakellis, G. C., & Chrischilles, E. A. (1992). Hydrocolloid versus saline gauze dressings in treating pressure ulcers: A cost-effectiveness analysis. *Archives of Physiotherapy and Medical Rehabilitation*, *73*(5), 463-469.

FOR FURTHER STUDY

ℰvolve   Go to Evolve at http://evolve.elsevier.com/Canada/LoBiondo/Research for Audio Glossary, how-to instructions for Writing Proposals for Funding, and additional research articles for practice in reviewing and critiquing.

Understanding Nursing on an Acute Stroke Unit: Perceptions of Space, Time and Interprofessional Practice

Cydnee C. Seneviratne, PhD, RN · Post-Doctoral Fellow and Instructor · Faculty of Nursing · University of Calgary · Calgary, Alberta

Charles M. Mather, PhD · Assistant Professor · Department of Anthropology · University of Calgary · Calgary, Alberta

Karen L. Then, PhD, RN, ACNP · Professor · Faculty of Nursing · University of Calgary · Calgary, Alberta

TITLE. Understanding nursing on an acute stroke unit: perceptions of space, time and interprofessional practice.

AIM. This paper is a report of a study conducted to uncover nurses' perceptions of the contexts of caring for acute stroke survivors.

BACKGROUND. Nurses coordinate and organize care and continue the rehabilitative role of physiotherapists, occupational therapists and social workers during evenings and at weekends. Healthcare professionals view the nursing role as essential, but are uncertain about its nature.

METHOD. Ethnographic fieldwork was carried out in 2006 on a stroke unit in Canada. Interviews with nine healthcare professionals, including nurses, complemented observations of 20 healthcare professionals during patient care, team meetings and daily interactions. Analysis methods included ethnographic coding of field notes and interview transcripts.

FINDINGS. Three local domains frame how nurses understand challenges in organizing stroke care: 1) space, 2) time and 3) interprofessional practice. Structural factors force nurses to work in exceptionally close quarters. Time constraints compel them to find novel ways of providing care. Moreover, sharing of information with other members of the team enhances relationships and improves "interprofessional collaboration". The nurses believed that an interprofessional atmosphere is fundamental for collaborative stroke practice, despite working in a multiprofessional environment.

CONCLUSION. Understanding how care providers conceive of and respond to space, time and interprofessionalism has the potential to improve acute stroke care. Future research focusing on nurses and other professionals as members of interprofessional teams could help inform stroke care to enhance poststroke outcomes.

KEYWORDS: acute stroke unit, ethnography, interprofessional practice, nursing, perceptions, space, time

INTRODUCTION

Stroke can be a devastating and physically debilitating cardio/neurovascular disease (Hickey 2003). It interrupts life, arrests previously cherished activities, and decreases overall quality of life for survivors and their families (Canadian Stroke Network, 2007). According to the World Health Organization (2004), heart attack and stroke are leading causes of death in the world and approximately 15 million people worldwide survive stroke annually.

Dedicated stroke units are part of a widespread effort to ameliorate the impact of stroke. Generally, these units house comprehensive stroke programmes which include interdisciplinary teams of caregivers including nurses, pharmacists,

From the *Journal of Advanced Nursing*, 2009; 65(9):1872-1881. © 2009 Blackwell Publishing Ltd.

physicians, nurse practitioners (NP), social workers, occupational and physical therapists, and speech therapists. The rationale behind the programmes is that the needs of individual patients require caregivers with varied expertise (Teasell *et al.* 2007). Stroke units yield clear benefits to patients (Hill 2002, Stroke Unit Trialists' Collaboration (SUTC) 2007; Indredavik *et al.* 1991, Jorgensen *et al.* 1995a, 1995b, Kalra *et al.* 1993, Kalra 1994). Patients who receive inpatient stroke care vs. care from a conventional or general medical ward stand a better chance of surviving, and living independently at home 1 year post-stroke (SUTC 2007). Patients on stroke units experience greater improvement in functional outcome and quality of life, and a decreased length of stay (Cifu & Stewart 1999).

Researchers have proven the effectiveness of interdisciplinary stroke care (Cifu & Stewart 1999; SUTC 2007). This study looks beyond outcome measures to the daily interactions and beliefs that characterize comprehensive programmes, with a particular focus on the role of nurses. Nurses have long believed that they play an essential role in stroke care, but they remain uncertain about the nature of their contributions (Gibbon 1993, Gibbon & Little 1995, Waters & Luker 1996, Burton 2000). Using an ethnographic approach, we examined nurses' perspectives on the contribution they make to the care of stroke survivors in acute settings. Part of our concern was how nurses see the social connections they have with other members of the interdisciplinary team, and what sort of values they hold toward their practice.

BACKGROUND

Henderson (1980) offered a vision of nurses with a leading role in acute care and rehabilitation, including working with patients to relearn activities, movement, and continence and nutritional care. In contrast to this vision, nurses are moving toward a managerial or understudy role that coordinates rehabilitative tasks under the guidance of other professions (O'Connor 1993, 2000a). This emerging role is "patchy" in that nursing ability in some areas (e.g. feeding and continence care) is advancing while other areas (e.g. mobility and exercise therapies) are lagging behind (Perry *et al.* 2004). Without knowledge and skills in acute stroke care, and accepting rehabilitation as a normal part of nursing, Henderson's vision is unattainable (Myco 1984).

The role of nurses in acute stroke rehabilitation is unclear (O'Connor 1993, 2000a, 2000b, Forster & Young 1996, Kirkevold 1997, Burton 1999, 2000, Elliott 1999, Thorn 2000). Researchers have identified nurses as managers or coordinators (O'Connor 1993, Burton 1999, 2000), clinical specialists (Elliott 1999), community integrators (Forster & Young 1996) and caregivers who perform interpretive, consoling, conserving and integrative tasks (Kirkevold 1997). Kirkevold (1997) describes four unique functions in rehabilitation of stroke survivors that nurses perform but fails to operationalize these functions (O'Connor 2000a).

Nurses vary in their attitudes and perceptions of their role in stroke care. In an early qualitative study, Waters and Luker (1996) found that nurses thought that they were good at basic care, ranging from ensuring that patients were clean and dressed prior to medical assessments to ensuring patients were physically ready prior to therapy sessions, but the [*sic*] considered that they had little time for rehabilitative care. Burton (2000) discovered that nurses provided care, facilitated personal recovery, and managed multidisciplinary care teams, and that these roles suggested that they could provide focused 24-hour coordinated stroke rehabilitation. Perry *et al.* (2004) agreed with Burton (2000) and suggested that nurses must move beyond their traditional role of providing basic care and become active participants in acute and rehabilitative care.

Observational studies of nurses in acute and rehabilitative care settings includes work by Pound and Ebrahim (2000) showing that nurses on a general medical unit and a stroke unit provided impersonal, standardized care, considered rehabilitation secondary to nursing practice and did not regularly consult with therapists. In contrast, nurses on an elder care unit valued and promoted patient independence, and frequently consulted therapists to encourage optimal rehabilitation. The authors concluded that optimal stroke care requires engaging nurses in rehabilitation, increasing training in rehabilitation and compassionate care. Booth *et al.* (2001) compared interventions by nurses with those by occupational therapists (OT) and found that OT used patient prompting and facilitation while nurses favoured supervision. Variation in care practice was because of different intervention and assessment styles and lack of preparation and education in stroke rehabilitation on the par [*sic*] of the nurses.

According to Bukowski *et al.* (1986), neuroscience nurses could implement rehabilitation therapy over the 24 hour period, support treatments recommended by physiotherapists (PT), and ensure that patients and families learn therapy techniques to continue rehabilitation at home. Nurses play an essential role in acute and rehabilitative stroke care (Gibbon 1993, Gibbon & Little 1995, Waters & Luker 1996, Burton 2000) but the broader social construction of stroke rehabilitation and care providers' perceptions toward this construction remains unclear.

THE STUDY

Aim

The aim of the study was to uncover nurses' perceptions of the contexts of caring for acute stroke survivors.

Methodology

Ethnography is a qualitative research approach (Spradley 1979, 1980). In anthropology, ethnography is a tool for describing cultures, and the chief methods ethnographers employ are observation and interviewing. Ethnographers record their observations and interviews in field notes and other media, including audio and visual formats. Post-fieldwork, researchers analyse and interpret the records to uncover dominant themes or understandings among members of the culture (Spradley 1979, 1980, Aamodt 1991). In this study, ethnography provided a means of exploring how stroke unit nurses organized and coordinated care.

Participants and Setting

The study took place on an 18-bed acute stroke unit located in a large tertiary medical centre in Canada. As part of a greater health region, the stroke unit provided specialized interventions, management and investigative care during acute and sub-acute stroke phases. It had 18 beds, two located beside a nursing station and 16 in four-bed rooms with connecting corridors leading to a nursing station. Located on a different floor from the neurosciences department, the stroke unit shared space with another general neurological unit.

Staff on the unit included registered nurses (RN), licensed practical nurses (LPN), patient care attendants (PCA), NP, PT, OT, speech therapists and physicians. The staffing ratio was one RN or LPN to every four patients. We used purposive sampling (Morse & Field 1995, Hammersley & Atkinson 2007) to locate participants, and excluded individuals who could not read, write, or speak English. In total, we followed ten RN, two LPN, one PCA, one NP, two PT, a PT and three physicians ($n = 20$), nine of whom we formally interviewed. Participants ranged in age from 24 to 52 years, 15 were female and five were male. Nurses were the study focus but we also interviewed four other professionals to help contextualize interprofessional perspectives.

Data Collection

Fieldwork took place from February to November of 2006. Observations averaged 2–3 hours on

3 days/week. The fieldworker (CS) made observations during every type of shift. The fieldwork began with 3 months of general observation on the unit with the fieldworker watching at the charting desk, nursing station and walking in the hall. Notes from observations were transcribed via computer. The fieldworker clarified gaps in field notes by returning to the field site and making more focused observations driven by informant comments. To explore work practices, we interviewed participants (Emerson *et al.* 1995) using "grand tour" questions such as "Can you walk me through your typical day?" and asking for examples of nursing practice vs. that of other professions.

Ethical Considerations

The local health research ethics board granted ethical approval for the study. We used several information sessions to introduce the study to members of the stroke unit. During these sessions and interviews we informed stroke unit members about patient confidentiality. We sought written consent only from observation and interview participants and verbal assent from patients when participants were providing direct care.

Data Analysis

Analysis of field notes focused on identifying central domains, specific domain components and related work typologies (Spradley 1979, 1980, Hammersley & Atkinson 2007). We discovered three main themes (domains) and further identified theme components (componential analysis). Finally, we broke work activities into types on the basis of relationships between nurses, and between nurses and other professionals (typological analysis). Through an ongoing process of reading field notes, transcripts and then returning to the field setting for further observations, we crosschecked our findings and were assured that our study domains, components and related subcategories were culturally salient.

Reflexivity

Ethnographers change in the process of conducting research and spending an extensive period learning cultural domains and categories, and from building relationships with study participants (Davies 1999, Hammersley & Atkinson 2007). Indeed, if an ethnographer's ideas, beliefs and values did not change it might indicate that she failed in understanding the culture she was studying. To keep track of the sorts of changes they undergo and the impact of these changes on their fieldwork, ethnographers employ "reflexive" techniques. In this study, the fieldworker used "asides", integrative memos and research journals (Spradley 1979, 1980, Emerson *et al.* 1995) to make explicit her presuppositions and insider relationships, and to maintain awareness of her social position within the culture. Some staff knew the researcher as a nursing instructor or a previous employee. Asides and journaling helped her denote prior relationships, and highlight instances when she might have had "built-in" biases or made priori judgments. Reflexive techniques helped control for potential biases from having an insider perspective, which we did not want to lose because it was essential for gaining access to the study setting, building rapport and building and maintaining trust with staff.

FINDINGS

Space

Participants described "space" as a challenge to patient care. Three themes predominated in the data: "nursing in a submarine", "nursing too close" and "nursing in a state of code burgundy".

Nursing in a Submarine

Staff used the term "submarine" to refer to the unit. Command centres are located near the front of submarines, with missile rooms at the rear. The nursing station was located near the entrance of the unit, while the majority of four-bed rooms were located at the middle and far end. According to one nurse:

> Our submarine . . . it's just a more condensed unit. But the thing that most bothers me is it's not centred. If you have patients in the last room . . . at the other end you are not in close proximity to anything or anybody—you're alone. That drives me crazy because the nursing station is so far away.

Participants connected their feelings of claustrophobia on the unit with being on a submarine. The unit lacked work space and storage space:

> I'm too claustrophobic on this unit. It's like I am closed in . . . if you look down the hall from the nursing station you feel like the walls and curtains are closing in around you. It is so narrow. I feel constricted because I cannot do my work in cramped space. I bump into other people all the time.

Nursing Too Close

Limited space made it difficult to move, to use and relocate equipment, transfer patients, document nursing care and interact with colleagues. Limited space required alternative work strategies to ensure that one did not get in the way of one's colleagues. For example, nurses unlocked the wheels on beds in rooms near the nursing station, wheeled them to an open space, and then transferred patients to stretchers. One nurse said:

> This unit is not set up for us to nurse or do rehab. It is designed so that we are constantly bumping bums, literally *bum to bum* . . . when we transfer patients. We are bashing into one another when we feed patients and when we provide any kind of nursing care.

The layout of the unit caused nurses to bump into each other, and put patients in situations where staff could not ensure appropriate care, privacy or confidentiality.

Nursing Under a State of "Code Burgundy"

A "code burgundy" signals a lack of beds. The unit included an over-capacity bed in a shared

hall. Caring for patients in hallways compounded having to work "too close". Nurses disapproved of nursing under a state of code burgundy:

> [We] feel badly for the lack of privacy for that patient in the hallway. I mean even I had to perform an intimate procedure, a urinary catheter insertion in the hall, and I hated doing it.

Ironically, despite disapproving of these conditions, nurses often faced criticism from patients' families for the conditions:

> I think it really stressed [us] out, because [we] were taking the brunt of family complaints. You try telling the patient that you are just following procedure. This is a region issue and we are obligated to do what the region tells us, but we don't agree.

A state of code burgundy means increased workloads and the ethical challenge of "hallway care".

Time

Participants' talked about time in three major ways: "lack of time", "preserving time" and "time with and without space". Each concept denotes limitations and challenges to providing care.

Lack of Time

Participants complained that care errors, missed therapy or treatment appointments, and awkward patient transfers occurred because of lack of time to plan. Lack of time also compromised nurses' wellbeing. They associated work-related injuries to the pressures of needing to work quickly to complete all the work before the end of a shift:

> We are always injuring ourselves because we rush around. There is just not enough time for us to do things properly with our patients . . . So if things get missed so be it.

Lack of time hindered working on patient rehabilitation. Participants knew that correct positioning and transferring of patients assists in stroke rehabilitation, but they believed that they lacked the time for patients to move and position independently:

It is easier to take over for patients, dressing them or brushing their teeth rather than helping them do the tasks. It is a matter of accomplishing what is required for patients in a specific window of time.

Nurses organized their time according to what they believed they were physically capable of accomplishing during the work day. When patient acuity was high there were time constraints and rehabilitation was not a priority:

The patients need time for us to let them do what they can and . . . for themselves. But, that requires a whole lot of time and effort, which the nurses don't have. So I am sure some of [the patients] are frustrated because they realize that and they aren't able to do as much as they would like to do . . . Some days you just can't wait, you have to get it done and move on.

Preserving Time

To preserve time nurses coordinated their work and cared for patients as a team. They met and identified tasks they could do more efficiently working together. Alternately, individuals who had fewer patients volunteered to "pick-up" patients from colleagues who had a heavier patient load. A more implicit approach to preserving time developed as a consequence of familiarity. As one nurse related:

For me team nursing is knowing who you work with. I don't know whether it's the people I normally work with, but we just know each others [sic] rhythms. It is a matter of not talking about what we should do but just knowing each other.

Participants organized their work to meet timelines and prescribed schedules. They prepoured medications, and arrived early to complete stroke assessments, vital signs and morning care prior to the start of their shift.

Time With and Without Space

Time and space were evolving and interconnected concepts. As result of a lack of space, patients received physiotherapy and occupational therapy in the main therapy department. A PT commented:

I know that it is much easier for [physiotherapists] to do transfers in the main therapy department because the setup is ideal. There is so much of a space conflict on the unit that it's really hard sometimes to set things up optimally, so we would rather work with patients down in the gym without the nurses.

One nurse said it was hard to do rehabilitation on the unit because of limited time and space:

There are limitations on what we can do in the time and space allotted. To be able to come in and have the time to do all of those extra things . . . like assist patients in their room with feeding or mobilization and all of those things . . . that would be great, but it doesn't happen.

Time with and with out adequate space affected nurses' participation in bedside rounds. Unit policy stated that nurses should attend and review patients' neurological status, vital signs and changes in condition. Rounds occurred at 09.00 hours, when nurses were preparing patients for therapy appointments and tests, and/or were providing acute medical care. For nurses attendance at rounds was not a priority:

Then there is the issue of doing rounds on the unit with the docs. I really do not like the idea because your time is so compressed. You have so much going on during the day and to just repeat what the [charge nurse] already knows is . . . well, just repetitive.

One reason to miss bedside rounds was a lack of space in the four-bed rooms. Field observations revealed that the stroke neurologist, stroke residents, one or both NP and the charge nurse attended bedside rounds. Gathered around each bed, the group discussed patient status. According to the nurses there was "never enough room any way", and attendance did not give them new patient information and was thus "a waste of time".

Interprofessional Practice

Participant descriptions of interprofessional practice included two main components: "relationships between stroke professionals" and "communication/collaboration". Each component highlights how participants understood interactions on the stroke unit and interprofessional practice more generally.

Relationships Between Stroke Professionals

Nurses' understanding of stroke care differed from other professionals and this affected how they developed and maintained relationships on the stroke team in three major ways. First, working together and sharing experiences were the cornerstones of relationships between nurses.

Second, relationships between nurses and therapists developed around perceptions of how best to address patient needs. Nurses felt that therapists' failure to recognize and acknowledge the role of nurses in rehabilitation can lead to resentment and half-hearted attempts at rehabilitation. One nurse lamented:

> We are not recognized for the mobility things we do or in any concerns we have about our patients. So, sometimes we don't work hard at it. The physios are only concerned that we get the patients ready for their rehab times in the gym. So we do that for them and then concentrate on our patients' medical needs.

Nurses felt that therapists had a narrow view of nursing practice. In the course of their professional interactions, nurses were responsible for patients' medical needs while therapists were responsible for rehabilitation.

Third, nurses saw their relationships with stroke physicians and NP in terms of interprofessionalism. Participants claimed that in its original state the stroke team was a matter of interprofessional practice. Nurses and physicians candidly discussed patients and collaborated. One of the stroke physicians summarized his view of the situation:

> It should be interprofessional, ideally. In general, stroke units are interdisciplinary. Only a small part of stroke unit care is the physician roles. So during most of stroke care, beyond the acute phase, when you have somebody settled, the physician's role is

relatively minor. It's all about excellent nursing care and rehabilitation. So the team, by accident of history and hierarchy, is led by a physician but we have a NP, all the nurses, the physiotherapist, and social work . . . Everybody is involved in care including home care planning, etc.

Another participant commented:

> We needed something different on our stroke unit. Our unit was not designed to be exclusionary in any way. It was intended to be interprofessional.

The stroke unit was supposed to be an interdisciplinary place where staff felt comfortable sharing information. It would work in a non-hierarchical way, with each professional's opinion being valued and forming part of the plan for medical and rehabilitative care.

Stroke nurses thought that collaboration was important, and that it involved open communication with physicians and NP. They felt that they had positive relationships with the two NP because these professionals were approachable and accessible during acute and non-acute situations. One nurse asserted:

> Having both NP has helped as sort of go between to advocate to the doctors for the things that we need. The NP are more available to come see the patient in an emergent or urgent situation. That helps because you can get the ball rolling for whatever procedures that need to be done.

Communication and Collaboration

Participants claimed that communication and collaboration were critical to the success of the unit. Regular communication ensured everyone understood how other members envisioned patient care. Weekly stroke rounds provided opportunities to discuss patients, collaborate on care and share alternate plans or possibilities. Attendance did not guarantee participation, and inclusion in discussions was predicated on who led rounds. One stroke team member commented:

> When I lead rounds I like to spend more time on the functional and the social end of things than the

medical. I want to make sure the team feels like
they're involved and valued.

This individual thought that it was important to
include all team members, and was concerned
that some did not feel valued or believe that they
were influencing progression and discharge plans
for their patients.

Nurses were the only team members who did
not regularly attend stroke unit rounds because
"[they] did not have enough time to leave [their
required duties] and attend an hour-long stroke
round'. One of the physicians claimed that the
attendance of nurses at the stroke rounds would
have provided more information for both doctors
and nurses:

I think that maybe if we could arrange the time for
once a week in the [stroke unit] rounds for the nurses
to attend. I think that might be beneficial in the long
run for all the staff because we can learn so much
from each other especially about stuff we don't have
time to find out.

The attendance of nurses at stroke rounds would
have reinforced the notion that the unit was
interprofessional.

DISCUSSION

Study Limitations

Ethnography is not a science of generalization.
Ethnographic findings come from certain individuals, situations or single cases from a particular context and a particular time (Hammersley &
Atkinson 2007). Our findings are not necessarily
indicative of what happens on all stroke units and
thus the study is not about how stroke units are,
but rather about how a stroke unit can be. Although
we accept limitations where representativeness is
concerned, we also believe that we have found
common issues in stroke care in particular, and
medical care more broadly.

Space and Time

Space limitations and time constraints are the back-
drop of clinical care throughout North America.

Weinberg (2003) notes that nurses have long
faced a lack of resources to complete daily tasks
safely and effectively, interact with patients, or
attend in-service education sessions. Notwith-
standing the apparent universality of these problems, in our view it is not advisable to dismiss or
devalue the concerns of those who work in caregiving environments. Our investigation presented
an opportunity to re-open dialogue about the
importance of institutional organization and
structure regarding appropriate space and use of
time related to stroke care (Peszczynski *et al.*
1972, Ulrich *et al.* 2004).

A substantial body of literature supports the
view that organized stroke unit care improves
stroke outcomes (Indredavik *et al.* 1991, Kalra
et al. 1993, Kalra 1994, Jorgensen *et al.* 1995a,
1995b, Hill 2002, SUTC 2007). What the literature fails to address is the importance of adequate
work space for providing this care. Our participants perceived lack of space as a constant challenge to providing care. Rather than describe
what they did regarding stroke and rehabilitative
care, nurses talked about what they were forced
to do because of inadequate spaces and insufficient time. They did not take the time to assist
patients to wash, dress and practise mobilization.
They complained about inadequate physical
space for medication delivery, charting and interactions with patients. These comments are concerning because they show that nurses did not
(and probably cannot) make rehabilitation and
patient autonomy (Burton 1999, 2000) priorities
in their acute stroke care.

How conceptions of time affect work practices
in stroke care have not been explored in the literature. In the past, stroke physicians adopted
"watchful waiting" for patient recovery. Thrombolytic therapy changed stroke care in the 1980s,
providing a means of treating a class of acute
cases of ischaemic stroke. The window of opportunity for thrombolysis is three hours after
symptom onset. Members of the stroke team now
use phrases such as "time is brain" as a reminder

that the longer it takes for intervention, the greater the resulting neurological deficit (Barber *et al.* 2005). Team members have a second term, "door to needle time", which refers to the time between a patient's arrival at the hospital and the start of thrombolytic therapy (Hill *et al.* 2000). Temporal metaphors denote boundaries and different dimensions within the work space (Gell 1996, Bluedorn 2002, Hearn & Michelson 2006, Patmore 2006). Thrombolysis made stroke an acute event, and thereby helped radically alter the practice of stroke care. Armed with a novel intervention, stroke teams had to work within the boundaries of a narrow therapeutic window. Both the acknowledgment [*sic*] that organized stroke units improves outcomes and the temporal demands of thrombolysis motivated the adoption of coordinated interprofessional care teams and units such as the stroke unit in this study.

Although the ideal acute stroke care team includes a focus on rehabilitation, the nurses in this study chose not to consistently spend time walking with their patients or taking time to assist with dressing and grooming (all important rehabilitation activities). They believed that if they had the time, they would perform rehabilitative care. A recent study (Vähäkangas *et al.* 2008) showed that nurses who incorporated rehabilitation into their daily care increased the amount of time "working with" patients to maximize patient independence. The question is whether our stroke unit nurses were aware that a re-evaluation of their time from focusing on nursing tasks to facilitating rehabilitation might increase or "preserve" time spent with their patients. Organizing and implementing an education session for the stroke nurses about facilitation of care, as established by Booth *et al.* (2005), could increase their use of facilitative interventions in rehabilitation. They could have advocated for change by documenting their *lack of time* concerns and by requesting more staff through evaluation of patient acuity levels. A recent American study (Neatherlin & Prater 2003) illustrates that nurses are well

positioned to assist in the development and evaluation of appropriate staffing levels on rehabilitation units through documentation of how they spend their time at work.

Interprofessional Practice

The nurses in our study discussed how their role in the interprofessional team developed out of day-to-day working relationships. The stroke team is multidisciplinary because each team member works independently and reports assessments and interventions mainly in team meetings. Nevertheless, participants used the term interprofessional to refer to the stroke team. This suggests a lack of clarity about the type of work relationships and team interactions that exist on the unit. In multidisciplinary teams individuals work separately and come together to share information, while interdisciplinary teams members collaborate to create care plans as they jointly assess and treat patients (Ovretveit 1997, Sorrells-Jones 1997, Payne 2000, Pollard *et al.* 2005). Healthcare professionals commonly use the terms synonymously, although in the case of acute stroke care interprofessional and interdisciplinary teams are the gold standard (Canadian Stroke Network and the Heart and Stroke Foundation of Canada: Canadian Stroke Strategy 2006; SUTC, 2007; Teasell *et al.* 2007).

Despite desiring to work interprofessionally, team members found it difficult to communicate and collaborate consistently. Participants explained that only some nurses wanted to attend rounds and perceived that only some members of the stroke team valued nursing attendance. These findings are consistent with literature exploring team members' perceptions of nurse attendance at unit rounds or team meetings (Cott 1998, Milligan *et al.* 1999). According to Cott (1998), nurses do not regularly attend team meetings except through a representative such as a charge nurse. The exclusion of nurses may be as a result of lack of interest in attending team meetings or to how a culture typically organizes team meetings. In our study, nurses said that whether or not they felt welcome depended on which physicians were present. Ultimately, nurses stopped attending because of time constraints and their perception that the charge nurse could provide requisite information on their behalf.

CONCLUSION

Nurses are an undervalued and underutilized resource in rehabilitation. Our study shows that in some cases nurses hold themselves back from incorporating rehabilitation principles, and that they believe this occurs because of "real world" structural and temporal work issues. An embedded cultural belief exists that nurses only have time for basic care and that rehabilitative care requires expert knowledge usually held by PT and OT. However, nurses do not work in isolation and have the capacity to work with other professionals outside traditional boundaries.

WHAT IS ALREADY KNOWN ABOUT THIS TOPIC
- Stroke is a devastating neurovascular disease that affects over 15 million people worldwide annually.
- Organized stroke units decrease overall mortality and average length of stay, improve quality of life, independence and likelihood of living at home 1 year poststroke.
- Nurses are important and essential members of interprofessional stroke teams as they work with and care for patients 24 hours a day.

WHAT THIS PAPER ADDS
- Limited work space and lack of time to care for patients are important issues for neuroscience nurses.
- Interprofessional practice is a key factor that requires re-evaluation in acute stroke care.
- Nurses should assume a leadership role as rehabilitation practitioners who promote "working with" rather than "doing for" their patients.

IMPLICATIONS FOR PRACTICE AND/OR POLICY
- Providing education sessions for stroke nurses about facilitation of care could increase nursing use of facilitative interventions in rehabilitation.
- Nurses ought to become advocates for change by documenting their space and time concerns and by requesting workspaces and temporal environments appropriate for stroke survivors.

Stroke nurses worldwide must embrace professional development and attend education sessions regarding the use of facilitative interventions in rehabilitation. We see no reason that nurses cannot take on a leadership role as rehabilitation practitioners who promote "working with" rather than "doing for" their stroke survivors. Furthermore, nurses ought to become advocates for work spaces and temporal environments appropriate for patients admitted to acute stroke units.

ACKNOWLEDGEMENT

Many thanks go to Dr Kathryn King for assistance with manuscript preparation and to the late Dr Marlene Reimer, mentor and colleague.

FUNDING

Dr Cydnee Seneviratne received funding for this doctoral research from the Canadian Association of Neuroscience Nurses research fund and from the FUTURE Program for Cardiovascular Nurse Scientists, a CIHR Strategic Training Fellowship.

CONFLICT OF INTEREST

No conflict of interest has been declared by the authors.

AUTHOR CONTRIBUTIONS

CS, SM and KLT were responsible for the study conception and design; CS performed the data collection; CS, CM and KLT performed the data analysis; CS and CM were responsible for the drafting of the manuscript; CS and CM made critical revisions to the paper for important intellectual content; CS and KLT obtained funding; CS provided administrative, technical or material support; KLT supervised the study.

REFERENCES

Aamodt A.M. (1991) Ethnography and epistemology: Generating nursing knowledge. In *Qualitative Nursing Research: A Contemporary Dialogue*, 2nd edn (Morse J.M., ed.), Sage, Newbury Park, pp. 40-53.

Barber P.A., Hill M.D., Eliasziw M., Demchuk A.M., Pexman J.H.W., Hudon M.E., Tomanek A., Frayne R. & Buchan A. (2005) Imaging of the brain in acute ischemic stroke: comparison of computed tomography and magnetic resonance diffusion-weighted imaging. *Journal of Neurology Neurosurgery and Psychiatry 76*, 1528-1533.

Bluedorn A.C. (2002) *The Human Organization of Time: Temporal Realities and Experience*. Stanford University Press, Stanford, CA.

Booth J., Davidson I., Winstanley J. & Waters K. (2001) Observing washing and dressing of stroke patients: nursing intervention compared with occupational therapists. What is the difference? *Journal of Advanced Nursing 33*, 98-105.

Booth J., Hillier V.F., Waters K.R. & Davidson I. (2005) Effects of a stroke rehabilitation education programme for nurses. *Journal of Advanced Nursing 49*, 465-473.

Bukowski L., Bonavolonta M., Keehn M.T. & Morgan K.A. (1986) Interdisciplinary roles in stroke care. *Nursing Clinics of North America 21*, 359-374.

Burton C. (1999) An exploration of the stroke coordinator role. *Journal of Clinical Nursing 8*, 535-541.

Burton C.R. (2000) A description of the nursing role in stroke rehabilitation. *Journal of Advanced Nursing 32*, 174-181.

Canadian Stroke Network (2007) *About Stroke*. Retrieved from http://www.canadianstrokenetwork.ca/eng/about/aboutstroke.php on 29 September 2007.

Canadian Stroke Network and the Heart and Stroke Foundation of Canada: Canadian Stroke Strategy (2006). *Canadian Best Practice Recommendations for Stroke Care*. Canadian Stroke Network and the Heart and Stroke Foundation of Canada, Ottawa.

Cifu D.X. & Stewart D.G. (1999) Factors affecting functional outcome after stroke: A critical review of rehabilitation interventions. *Archives of Physical Medicine and Rehabilitation 80*, S35-S39.

Cott C. (1998) Structure and meaning in multidisciplinary teamwork. *Sociology of Health and Illness 20*, 848-873.

Davies C.A. (1999) *Reflexive Ethnography: A Guide to Researching Selves and Others*. Routledge, London.

Elliott A. (1999) The specialist nurse in rehabilitation. In *Rehabilitation Nursing* (Davis S. & O'Connor S., eds), Edinburgh, Bailliere Tindall, pp. 231-243.

Emerson R.M., Fretz R.I. & Shaw L.L. (1995) *Writing Ethnographic Field Notes*. University of Chicago Press, Chicago and London.

Forster A. & Young J. (1996) Specialist nurse support for patients with stroke in the community: A randomised controlled trial. *British Medical Journal 312*(7047), 1642-1646.

Gell A. (1996) *The Anthropology of Time: Cultural Constructions of Temporal Maps and Images*. Berg, Oxford.

Gibbon B. (1993) Implications for nurses in approaches to the management of stroke rehabilitation: a review of the literature. *International Journal of Nursing Studies 30*, 133-141.

Gibbon B. & Little V. (1995) Improving stroke care through action research. *Journal of Clinical Nursing 4*, 93-100.

Hammersley M. & Atkinson P. (2007) *Ethnography: Principles in Practice*, 3rd edn. Routledge, New York.

Hearn M. & Michelson G. (2006) Time. In *Rethinking Work: Time, Space, and Discourse* (Hearn M. & Michelson G., eds), Cambridge University Press, Cambridge.

Henderson V. (1980) Preserving—the essence of nursing in a technological age. *Journal of Advanced Nursing 5*, 245-260.

Hickey J.V. (2003) *The Clinical Practice of Neurological and Neurosurgical Nursing*, 5th edn. Lippincott Williams & Wilkins, Philadelphia.

Hill M.D. (2002) Stroke units in Canada. *Canadian Medical Association Journal 167*(6), 649-650.

Hill M.D., Barber P.A., Demchuk A.M., Sevick R.J., Newcommon N.J., Green T. & Buchan A. (2000) Building a "brain attack" team to administer thrombolytic therapy for acute ischemic stroke. *Canadian Medical Association Journal 162*(11), 1589-1593.

Indredavik B., Bakke F., Solberg R., Rokseth R., Haheim L.L. & Holme I. (1991) Benefit of a stroke unit: a randomized controlled trial. *Stroke 22*, 1026-1031.

Jorgensen H.S., Nakayama H., Raaschou H.O., Vive-Larson J., Stoier M. & Olsen T.S. (1995a) Outcome and time course of recovery in stroke. Part I: Outcome. The Copenhagen Stroke Study. *Archives of Physical Medicine and Rehabilitation 76*, 399-405.

Jorgensen H.S., Nakayama H., Raaschou H.O., Vive-Larson J., Stoier M. & Olsen T.S. (1995b) Outcome and time course of recovery in stroke. Part II: outcome. The Copenhagen Stroke Study.

Archives of Physical Medicine and Rehabilitation 76, 406-412.

Kalra L. (1994) The influence of stroke unit rehabilitation on functional recovery from stroke. *Stroke 25*, 821-825.

Kalra L., Dale P. & Crome P. (1993) Improving stroke rehabilitation: a controlled study. *Stroke 24*, 1462-1467.

Kirkevold M. (1997) The role of nursing in the rehabilitation of acute stroke patients: toward a unified theoretical perspective. *Advances in Nursing Science 19*, 55-64.

Milligan R.A., Gilroy J., Katz K.S., Rodan M.F. & Subramanian K.N. (1999) Developing a shared language: interdisciplinary communication among diverse health care professionals. *Holistic Nurse Practitioner 13*, 47-53.

Morse J.M. & Field P.A. (1995) *Qualitative Research Methods for Health Professionals*, 2nd edn. Sage Publications, Thousand Oaks.

Myco F. (1984) Stroke and its rehabilitation: The perceived role. *Journal of Advanced Nursing 9*, 429-439.

Neatherlin J.S. & Prater L. (2003) Nursing time and work in an acute rehabilitation setting. *Rehabilitation Nursing 28*, 186-190. 207.

O'Connor S.E. (1993) Nursing and rehabilitation: the interventions of nurses in stroke patient care. *Journal of Clinical Nursing 2*, 29-34.

O'Connor S.E. (2000a) Mode of care delivery in stroke rehabilitation nursing: a development of Kirkevold's unified theoretical perspective of the role of the nurse. *Clinical Effectiveness in Nursing 4*, 180-188.

O'Connor S.E. (2000b) Nursing interventions in stroke rehabilitation: a study of nurses' views of their pattern of care in stroke units. *Rehabilitation Nursing 25*, 224-230.

Ovretveit J. (1997) How to describe interprofessional working. In *Interprofessional Working for Health and Social Care* (Ovretveit J., Mathias P. & Thompson T., eds), Macmillan, Basingstoke, pp. 9-33.

Patmore G. (2006) Time and work. In *Rethinking Work: Time, Space, and Discourse* (Hearn M. & Michelson G., eds), Cambridge University Press, Cambridge, pp. 21-38.

Payne M. (2000) *Teamwork in Multiprofessional Care*. Macmillan Press, Basingstoke.

Perry L., Brooks W. & Hamilton S. (2004) Exploring nurses' perspectives of stroke care. *Nursing Standard 19*, 33-38.

Peszczynski M., Benson F., Collins M.M., Darley F.L., Diller L., Greenhouse A.H., Katzen F.P., Lake L.F.,

Rothberg J.S. & Waggonerm R.W. (1972) Stroke rehabilitation. *Stroke 3*, 375-407.

Pollard K., Sellman D. & Senior B. (2005) The need for interprofessional working. In *Interprofessional Working in Health and Social Care: Professional Perspectives* (Barrett G., Sellman D. & Thomas J., eds), Palgrave MacMillan, New York, NY, pp. 7-17.

Pound P. & Ebrahim S. (2000) Rhetoric and reality in stroke patient care. *Social Science and Medicine 51*, 1437-1446.

Sorrells-Jones J. (1997) The challenge of making it real: interdisciplinary practice in a "seamless" organization. *Nursing Administration Quarterly 21*, 20-30.

Spradley J. (1979) *The Ethnographic Interview*. Holt, Rinehart and Winston, New York.

Spradley J. (1980) *Participant Observation*. Holt, Rinehart and Winston, New York.

Stroke Unit Trialists' Collaboration (2007) Organized inpatient (stroke unit) care for stroke. *Cochrane Database of Systematic Reviews* (4) CD000197.

Teasell R., Foley N., Bhogal S.K. & Speechley M. (2007) *Evidenced based review of stroke rehabilitation: the efficacy of stroke rehabilitation*. Retrieved from http://www.ebrsr.com/modules/module5.pdf on 29 January 2008.

Thorn S. (2000) Neurological rehabilitation nursing: a review of the research. *Journal of Advanced Nursing 31*, 1029-1038.

Ulrich R., Quan X., Zimring C., Joseph A. & Choudhary R. (2004) *The role of the physical environment in the hospital of the 21st century: A once-in-a-lifetime opportunity*. Report to The Center for Health Design for the Designing the 21st Century Project. Retrieved from http://www.rwjf.org/files/publications/other/RoleofthePhysicalEnvironment.pdf on 1 June 2008.

Vähäkangas P., Noro A. & Finne-Soveri H. (2008) Daily rehabilitation nursing increases the nursing time spent on residents. *International Journal of Nursing Practice 14*, 157-164.

Waters K.R. & Luker K.A. (1996) Staff perspectives on the role of the nurse in rehabilitation wards for elderly people. *Journal of Clinical Nursing 5*, 105-114.

Weinberg D.B. (2003) *Code Green: Money-Driven Hospitals and the Dismantling of Nursing*. Cornell University Press, Ithaca, NY.

World Health Organization (2004) *The atlas of heart disease and stroke*. Retrieved from http://www.who.int/cardiovascular_diseases/resources/atlas/en/ on 14 January 2007.

Decisional Involvement of Senior Nurse Leaders in Canadian Acute Care Hospitals

Carol A. Wong, RN, PhD · Associate Professor · Arthur Labatt Family School of Nursing · Faculty of Health Sciences · The University of Western Ontario · London, Ontario

Heather Laschinger, RN, PhD · Professor and Associate Director Nursing Research · Arthur Labatt Family School of Nursing · Faculty of Health Sciences · The University of Western Ontario · London, Ontario

Greta G. Cummings, RN, PhD · Associate Professor · Faculty of Nursing · University of Alberta · CIHR New Investigator and AHFMR Population Health Investigator · Edmonton, Alberta

Leslie Vincent, MSc(A), RN · Senior Vice President Patient Services and Chief Nursing Executive · Mount Sinai Hospital · Toronto, Ontario

Patty O'Connor, MSc(A), CHE · Associate Director of Nursing · Neurosciences · McGill University Health Centre · Montreal, Quebec

AIM   The aim of the present study was to describe the scope and degree of involvement of senior nurse leaders (SNLs) in executive level decisions in acute care organizations across Canada.

BACKGROUND   Significant changes in SNL roles including expansion of decisionmaking responsibilities have occurred but little is known about the patterns of SNL decision-making.

METHODS   Data were collected by mailed survey from 63 SNLs and 49 chief executive officers (CEOs) in 66 healthcare organizations in 10 Canadian provinces. Regression analyses were used to examine whether timing, breadth of content expertise and the number of decision activities predicted SNL decision-making influence and quality of decisions.

RESULTS   Breadth of content expertise and number of decision activities with which the SNL was involved were significant predictors of decision influence explaining 22% of the variance in influence. Overall, CEOs rated SNL involvement in decision-making higher than the SNL.

CONCLUSIONS   Senior nurse leaders contribute to organizational processes in healthcare organizations that are important for nurses and patients, through their participation in decision-making at the senior team level.

IMPLICATIONS FOR NURSING MANAGEMENT   Findings may be useful to current and future SNLs learning to shape the nature and content of information shared with CEOs particularly in the area of professional practice issues.

KEYWORDS   acute care, decision-making, hospitals, influence, leadership, nurse executive

INTRODUCTION

Healthcare restructuring in the 1990s in Canada and the Unites States contributed to significant changes in senior nurse leader (SNL) roles including expansion of their decision-making responsibilities (Murray *et al.* 1998, Mass *et al.* 2006, Smith *et al.* 2006). In some organizations nurse executives were added to senior executive teams and in others, their scope of participation in organizational decisions related to budget, strategic planning, quality of care and a host of challenging

From the *Journal of Nursing Management*, 2010; 18:122-133. © 2010 Blackwell Publishing Ltd.

organizational issues greatly increased. Similarly, healthcare reform in the United Kingdom and other European countries created role changes and new opportunities for nurse leaders in health care organizations (Fedoruk 2000, Filkins 2003, Kirk 2008).

New governance structures and organizational models radically changed disciplinary leadership structures, particularly in nursing (Havens 1998, 2001, Baumann *et al.* 2001, Shannon & French 2005, Sharp *et al.* 2006). Specifically, the programme management structure and regionalized healthcare systems were implemented across Canada (Leatt *et al.* 1994, Smith *et al.* 2006). In regionalization, responsibility for a wide span of health services, frequently spanning community, long-term care and acute care services, were organized under one governing body with consolidation of authority which was previously distributed among many organizations. A goal of this restructuring was greater integration of services with reduced duplication and overlap. Within programme management structures in hospitals, distinct professional departments were eliminated, services were organized around populations of patients and care was provided by multidisciplinary teams. Some claim that these changes provided opportunities for nurse leaders to demonstrate their leadership skills and play a greater role in decision-making within new interdisciplinary and more broad-based programme structures. Others argued that these changes diminished authority and communication links between senior nurse leaders and other nursing personnel and deprived nurses of disciplinary leadership representation at the policy making level (Shamian & Lightstone 1997, Clifford 1998, Canadian Nursing Advisory Committee 2002). Several sources attest to the dissatisfaction that nurses experienced with the reduction in nurse leaders at all levels of organizations with restructuring (Baumann *et al.* 2001, Canadian Nursing Advisory Committee 2002). However, surprisingly little is actually known about the patterns of SNL participation in decision-making (PDM) at the senior executive level of healthcare organizations and in particular, the consequences of organizational changes on nurse executive decision-making. The present study was part of a national survey to describe the profile of nursing leadership structures in Canada and to assess relationships among personal and structural factors, processes and outcomes pertaining to nurse leaders' work post restructuring (Laschinger *et al.* 2008).

Our aim was to describe SNL decision-making processes in terms of the scope and degree of their involvement in strategic and tactical decisions at the executive management level in organizations across Canada. We define the SNL as the nurse who holds the most senior nursing leadership position in the organization with direct responsibility for nursing. While titles such as chief nurse executive, nurse executive or senior nurse leader are often used interchangeably, for clarity we use the SNL term throughout this paper. Specifically, we examined whether timing, breadth of content expertise and the number of decision activities predicted SNL perceptions of their decision-making influence and the quality of management decisions made by the senior team. We also included a description of how chief executive officers (CEOs) perceive SNL decision-making.

LITERATURE REVIEW

SNL Role Changes with Restructuring

Substantial changes in the healthcare system have contributed to new role expectations, higher knowledge requirements and increased responsibility and accountability for nurse leaders including: quality and effective coordination of patient services; managing many clinical areas with a broadened span of control; operating merged facilities and decentralized structures; and decision-making in finance, human resources and quality and safety of patient services across the continuum of care (Duffield *et al.* 2001, Klein-man 2003, Upenieks 2003, Anthony *et al.* 2005, Arnold *et al.* 2006). In many cases restructuring changes provided opportunities for nurse leaders to demonstrate their leadership skills and play a greater role in decision-making within the new multidisciplinary programme structures (Clancy 2003, Thorman 2004, Kirk 2008). As an inte-grated member of the senior leadership team, the SNL has the opportunity to influence team members by ensuring that patient care and nursing practice perspectives are voiced when decisions are being made that affect organizational direc-tions, quality management and resource use. The recent Sharp *et al.* (2006) findings on the effects of service line (similar to programme) manage-ment implementation in U.S. Veterans Health Administration [sic] hospitals supported many of the positive aspects of SNL role changes described previously. However, SNLs in pure service line organizations without a discipline-based nursing service reported decreased direct supervision of nurses and challenges in achieving consistency in quality of nursing care.

SNL Role in Organizational Decision-Making

Decision-making research in nursing has focused primarily on the study of clinical nurses (Orovio-goicoechea 1996, Thompson 1999, Lauri *et al.* 2001). Of the published literature on nurse leader decision-making, there is little coherence in topics such as, risk propensity (Smith & Fried-land 1998), ethical decision-making (Fonville 2002, Berggren & Severinsson 2003), manager role in facilitating staff participation in decision-making (Krairiksh 2000), middle manager involvement in organizational strategic decision-making (Ashmos *et al.* 1998) and personality type and decision-making styles (Freund 1988). Only a small body of research focused on SNLs' organizational decision-making influence (Wangs-ness 1991, Havens 1998, Banaszak-Holl *et al.* 1999, Dwore *et al.* 2000).

The importance of SNLs participation in orga-nizational decision-making is acknowledged in the literature (Fedoruk 2000, Clancy 2003). However, most of the empirical evidence in this area has focused on participation of physicians and registered nurses (RNs) in strategic decision-making (Ashmos & McDaniel 1991, Havens & Laschinger 1997, Ashmos *et al.* 1998, Anderson & McDaniel 1999). Ashmos and McDaniel (1991) determined that the greater the intensity (number and type of decision activities) of par-ticipation in decision-making (PDM) by profes-sionals, the more likely that they will be perceived as having an influence on decisions. Utilizing a survey method that included questions on the timing, breadth and intensity of participation in decision-making to capture overall decision involvement, they examined the effect of clinical, professional and middle manager participation on hospital performance (Ashmos *et al.* 1998). The participation of medical and other clinical profes-sionals (e.g. nurses) in organizational strategic decisions was associated with reduced hospital costs while there was no such effect for middle manager participation. Adding decision influence to the Ashmos *et al.* (1998) measure, Anderson and McDaniel (1998) showed that administrators in nursing homes perceived greater influence of RNs in decisions when RNs were more involved in decision activities. They also showed that increased RN participation in decision-making was associated with improved resident outcomes in nursing homes (Anderson & McDaniel 1999). Thus, these studies suggest that decision-making involvement can be measured and that there is a connection between involvement in decision activities, perceived influence over decisions and organizational outcomes.

A few studies focused on the integration of nurse leaders in executive level organizational decision-making during the healthcare restructur-ing era of the 1990s. In a survey of 115 SNLs in Pennsylvania acute care hospitals, Wangsness (1991) determined that most participants had considerable decision-making authority at the departmental but very little at the organizational level. Havens (1998) studied the involvement of the nurse executive in U.S. hospital governance and policy making in 1990 and again in 1996, reporting little change in SNL involvement at senior executive levels over that time. Another study documenting the integration of SNLs into executive-level administration of 53 acute care hospitals in Utah, found that 80% of the SNLs perceived they were more involved in hospital activities and decisions (Dwore et al. 2000).

There is evidence that the scope and intensity of SNL involvement in strategic decision-making is related to their perceptions of influence in the organization (Banaszak-Holl et al. 1999, Wells et al. 1999). Banaszak-Holl et al. (1999) examined the role of SNLs in organizational decision-making within Veteran's Affairs Medical Centres (VAMCs) in the United States during the mid-1990s. Restructuring led to the inclusion of SNLs on the executive management team as an equal collaborator with the medical chief of staff and other senior directors. All SNLs and their management team colleagues were surveyed in 84 VAMCs using an adapted form of the Ashmos and McDaniel (1991) decision-making instrument. Senior nurse leaders perceived they brought greater breadth of expertise to decisions and participated in more decision activities than non-nurse colleagues' perceptions of the SNL role. There were no significant differences in how SNLs and their colleagues rated SNL influence over decisions or quality of decisions made by management teams, except that SNLs consistently ranked decision quality lower than their non-nurse colleagues. Banaszak-Holl et al. (1999) did not analyse the effect of decision timing, breadth or number of activities on influence or perceived quality of decisions.

Theoretical Framework

Simply stated, a decision is defined as a choice made from two or more alternatives (Robbins &

Langton 2003). More specifically, Mintzberg et al. (1976) emphasized that a decision in organizations is 'a specific commitment to action (usually a commitment of resources)' (p. 246). Decision-making has been described as a complex cognitive process that involves critical thinking, judgement, evaluation and memory (Oetjen et al. 2008). Generally, decision-making occurs as a response to problems or opportunities and thus, decision-makers must address a gap between the current state and some desired future state.

The theoretical framework (Figure B-1) for this study was adapted from the work of Ashmos and McDaniel (1991) and Anderson and McDaniel (1998) who developed an approach to examining health professionals' participation in strategic decision-making in healthcare organizations using information processing and complexity science theories (Anderson & McDaniel 1998, Ashmos et al. 1998). According to information processing theory, increased participation of multiple stakeholders increases both the amount of information and the ability to deal with it (Ashmos et al. 1998). 'Participation is a mechanism for the exchange of information' in decision-making processes (Ashmos & McDaniel 1991, p. 386) and this capacity can be altered by changing the participants but also by changing the '. . . timing, scope, and formalization of the process' (p. 388). Bringing participants into a decision process early expands the capacity of the organization to process information as does widening the scope of participation in various decision activities such as raising issues, clarifying problems and generating alternatives. From the complexity perspective, diversity and expansion of those involved in organizational decision-making increases internal complexity and also enhances an 'organization's ability to create meaning through increased use of connections' among stakeholders (Anderson & McDaniel 1999, p. 8). Such connections also enable interactions among people that may broaden and deepen interpretations of events and actions. Leaders can increase the speed or degree

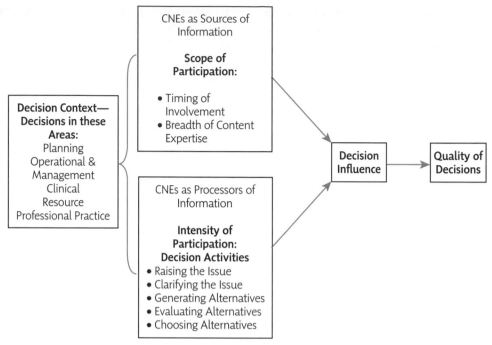

FIGURE B-1   Participation in organizational decision making.

of information flow by increasing the number of people involved and by expanding the number of decision activities in which they are involved using both formal and informal mechanisms for interaction.

In our framework, PDM by SNLs in executive management teams is viewed as creating new organizational connections and mechanisms for exchanging information and enriching interpretation of issues that ultimately influence the quality of management decisions. The scope of decision-making is enhanced by involving SNLs at the beginning of decision-making stages (timing) and the breadth of content expertise is expanded by their clinical and professional knowledge. The intensity of PDM is a function of the number and range of decision-making activities involving SNLs. Any decision-making process entails several different fundamental information processing actions from raising issues, clarifying problems, generating and evaluating solutions to making a final choice (Anderson & McDaniel

1999). The greater the scope and intensity of SNL PDM, the greater the likelihood that they and others perceive them as having an influence on decisions. Last, we propose that decision-making influence is related to the quality of final management decisions reached.

Hypotheses

- The scope (timing and breadth) and intensity (number of decision activities) of SNL participation in executive decision-making processes positively predicts the degree of SNL decision influence.
- SNL decision influence positively predicts perceived quality of operational management decisions.

METHODS

Sample and Data Collection Procedures

To obtain a comprehensive description of nursing management structures in Canada, Academic

Health Centres (AHC) and community hospitals (CH) in 10 provinces were selected as data sources. An AHC is a health care facility that participates in medical research and in teaching undergraduate and graduate medical students. All of the AHCs that focused on acute care in each province were selected to participate in this study. For each of the AHCs, a CH with more than 100 beds was randomly selected from a complete list of CHs in the Health Authority/geographic region of each AHC. Ethics approvals were obtained from a university ethics review board as well as from specific organizations in the study. Data were collected from SNLs and CEOs in 28 academic health centres and 38 community hospitals in 10 Canadian provinces. All SNLs ($n = 66$) and CEOs ($n = 66$) were surveyed by mail. Of the original 132 surveys to SNLS and CEOs, 112 surveys were returned, for an overall response rate of 84.8% (Table B-1).

Instrument

We used the participation in Strategic Decision-Making Scale (Banaszak-Holl *et al.* 1999) to measure SNL decision-making processes. This Likert-type instrument was adapted from a survey developed by Ashmos *et al.* (1998). The SNLs' participation in decision-making processes was evaluated according to five different types of strategic decisions commonly considered by the executive level of the organization:

- planning decisions defined as the formal process of developing organizational goals and strategies;

- operational management decisions that deal with the day-to-day operation of the organization (excluding direct patient care);
- clinical care decisions are policy or administrative issues related to the provision of direct patient care;
- resource decisions address fiscal issues (including budgeting, revenues and spending) and human resources; and
- professional practice decisions relate to standards of nursing practice, discipline, education and research issues (Figure B-2).

The last decisional area, professional practice, was added to the Banaszak-Holl *et al.* (1999) scale because the clinical decision type did not fully represent the range of decisions relevant to nursing as we believe that many organizational decisions made at the top management level affect the professional practice of nurses. For each of these five areas of decision-making, we asked survey participants to rate the SNL's involvement in senior organizational level decision-making over the past 6 months according to the scope of participation (consists of timing and the breadth of content expertise), intensity of participation (the number of decision activities and the mechanisms used), the SNL's influence over decision and the quality of management decisions made.

Timing of decisional involvement was defined as the time point a SNL most often became involved in the decision-making process (1 = beginning of process; 5 = end of the process). No precise timeframes (e.g. days, weeks or months) for decisions are included in the instruments as there is considerable variation in the timeframes for organizational level decisions. For example, strategic planning decisions may take months whereas some clinical decisions may be required within days. Breadth was defined as the scope of expertise the SNL most often offered in the decision-making process (1 = narrow/single area of expertise; 5 = broad/many different areas of expertise). Number of

TABLE B-1

COMPARISON OF RESPONSE RATES

	TOTAL		AHC		CH	
	n	%	n	%	n	%
SNL	63	95.5	30	100.0	33	91.7
CEO	49	74.2	23	82.1	26	68.4

AHC, academic health centre; CEO, chief executive officer; CH, community hospital; SNL, senior nurse leader.

Section 3: Please respond to the questions below in reference to each of the following types of decisions.

PLANNING DECISIONS – The formal process of developing organizational goals and methodologies for achieving those goals. Activities may include addressing critical issues, significant events and major trends, both internal and external, that will impact the overall direction of the hospital. *Examples:* Development of a 5-year plan, addition of a cardiac surgery program, conversion from inpatient to outpatient surgery.

OPERATIONAL MANAGEMENT DECISIONS – Significant decisions dealing with the day-to-day operational management of the hospital; excludes items involving direct patient care. *Examples:* Review/approval of major projects (e.g. interior design renovations), communications deficits/morale issues, review/approval of space for program expansion within the existing facility.

CLINICAL DECISIONS – Policy or administrative issues related to the provision of direct patient care. *Examples:* Plans for addressing a backlog of surgical cases, individual patient care problems not solvable at the unit/service level, clinic waiting time.

RESOURCE DECISIONS – Administrative and policy issues dealing with fiscal (e.g. income, budgeting, expenditure of monies) and human (e.g. employee management) resources. *Examples:* Review/approval of hospital and service-wide budgets, total number and distribution of FTEs, nurse shortage in the ICU.

PROFESSIONAL PRACTICE DECISIONS – Policy or administrative issues relating to decisions about standards of nursing practice, disciplinary issues, quality of patient care, staffing, evidence-based practice, education, and research.

FIGURE B-2   Excerpt from SNL decision-making survey.

decision activities was defined as the total count of decision activities in which the SNL was involved including raising issues, clarifying problems, generating alternatives, evaluating alternatives and choosing options. In addition, SNLs were asked to identify the most frequently used mechanisms through which the SNL is involved in the decision-making process [1 = meeting with top management; 2 = established standing committees; 3 = task forces/ad hoc committees; 4 = meetings with top management team members (excluding CEO); 5 = informal meetings with CEO]. Decision mechanisms were used for descriptive purposes only and not included in the regression analysis. Perceptions of SNL influence over final decisions in the five decision areas were measured according to: 1 = no influence and 5 = great deal of influence. Perceived quality of operational management

decisions was measured by rating their level of agreement (1 = do not agree; 5 = strongly agree) with six items pertaining to: compatibility of decisions with existing constraints and policy, advantageous timing of decisions, appropriate use of information, balance of risks and rewards and whether decisions created conflict of interest (reverse coded item). We evaluated quality of management decisions for all decision areas rather than by each of the five decision areas.

Banaszak-Holl *et al.* (1999) reported Cronbach alphas only for quality of decisions across the original four decisions areas and these ranged from 0.74 to 0.81. In our study, the Cronbach alpha for the six quality scale items was 0.68. The alphas for timing, breadth, number of decision activities, mechanisms and influence subscales ranged from 0.83 to 0.90 (see Table B-5).

Data Analyses

Quantitative survey data were analysed using SPSS 16.0 for Windows (SPSS Inc., Chicago, IL, USA 2005).

Descriptive statistics were analysed by level of management (SNL and CEO) and correlation analyses were used to examine relationships among the decision-making variables in our model. Paired *t*-tests were applied to assess differences in mean scores for SNLs and CEOs. Finally, hierarchical multiple regression was used to test study hypotheses using SNL mean scale scores of the decision-making variables.

RESULTS

Demographics

Demographics of the sample are illustrated in Table B-2. A notable finding was the high average age (50.4 years) of SNLs, suggesting the urgent need for succession planning to ensure the future of nursing leadership. Overall, current SNLs were very experienced individuals as over 80% of senior nurse leaders had at least 15 years of management experience and all had at least 5 years.

All SNLs had a nursing background with university degrees in nursing primarily at master's level (57.6%). In addition, a large percentage of SNLs had earned non-nursing degrees (42%). Twenty-one per cent of SNLs had obtained general or business-related masters degrees whereas others had obtained Masters in Health Administration (MHA) (14%), PhD (8%) and Masters in Education (6%). Thirty-one per cent of SNLs completed the annual 3-week nurse executive development programme sponsored by the Wharton School of Business (University of Pennsylvania) and the Johnson & Johnson Family of companies. Graduates of this programme receive the designation as a Wharton Fellow.

Most CEOs surveyed ($n = 49$) were male (75.5%). The average age of these senior executives was 52 years and on average had been in their present position for 5.3 years. The CEOs most commonly reported their highest education as a masters degree: MHA (36.7%) and Masters in Business Administration (MBA) (20.4%). Other common responses were a combination of an MD and an MBA (18.2%), other Masters degrees (6.1%) and a combination of an MBA and an MHA (4.1%). One respondent reported

TABLE **B-2**

DEMOGRAPHICS

	SENIOR NURSE LEADER		CEO	
	M	*SD*	*M*	*SD*
Age	50.4	4.8	51.97	6.01
Years management experience	20.8	6.7		
Years in role	3.7	3.3	5.32	4.10
	n	*%*	*n*	*%*
GENDER				
Male	0	0	37	75.5
Female	63	100	11	22.4
HIGHEST LEVEL				2.1
Diploma	2	3.4	1	10.4
Baccalaureate	19	32.2	5	8
Masters	34	57.6	40	3.3
PhD	4	6.8		
Other			2	4.2

having a Masters of Science in Nursing (MScN) as the highest earned degree and one reported an MD as their highest earned degree.

Descriptive Results

SNL Perceptions of Decisional Involvement

Means and standard deviations for SNL and CEO ratings of the items and subscales of the decision-making instrument are included in Table B-3. SNLs were involved near the beginning of the decision-making process for all decision areas. The earliest involvement was reported for planning decisions whereas the latest involvement of the SNL was reported for operational and clinical decisions. SNLs reported offering a broad range of expertise in executive decisions with professional practice decisions rated the broadest range of expertise and operational decisions received the lowest mean for range of expertise offered. The highest mean number of decision activities was for professional practice and the lowest was reported for clinical decisions.

Not surprisingly, the types of decision domains (planning, operational, clinical, resources or professional practice issues) require different decision mechanisms (Table B-4). Both CEOs and SNLs rated these forums quite similarly. Planning, operational and resource matters were primarily dealt with in meetings with the top management team (as the decision mechanism), with clinical and professional practice matters included to lesser degrees in these forums. Standing committees were used most frequently for professional practice, operational and clinical decisions and task forces were used most often for clinical decisions. In terms of influence (Table B-3), SNLs reported having a large amount of influence over final decisions across all types of decisions. The highest level of influence was reported for decisions regarding professional ~~ce~~ and the lowest influence was reported ~~rational~~ decisions. Overall quality of

TABLE B-3		
MEANS AND STANDARD DEVIATIONS OF DECISIONAL INVOLVEMENT SUBSCALES		
	SNL ($n = 63$)	CEO ($n = 49$)
DECISIONAL INVOLVEMENT	M(SD)	M(SD)
TIMING*		
Planning	1.49 (1.10)	1.43 (0.89)
Operational	2.25 (1.34)	1.70 (1.13)
Clinical	2.23 (1.33)	1.74 (1.16)
Resource	1.85 (1.17)	1.52 (0.86)
Prof practice	1.83 (1.95)	1.52 (1.17)
Average all decision types	1.93 (0.95)	1.58 (0.85)
BREADTH OF CONTENT EXPERTISE		
Planning	4.16 (1.16)	4.11 (0.89)
Operational	3.89 (1.17)	4.21 (0.88)
Clinical	4.03 (1.15)	4.19 (0.92)
Resource	4.15 (1.08)	4.17 (0.79)
Prof practice	4.46 (1.03)	4.28 (1.06)
Average all decision types	4.08 (0.98)	4.19 (0.76)
NUMBER OF DECISION ACTIVITIES		
Planning	4.25 (1.36)	3.96 (1.56)
Operational	3.62 (1.50)	3.98 (1.55)
Clinical	3.40 (1.56)	3.83 (1.66)
Resource	4.07 (1.37)	3.91 (1.64)
Prof practice	4.15 (1.41)	4.00 (1.62)
Average all decision types	3.88 (1.19)	3.94 (1.54)
DECISION INFLUENCE		
Planning	4.15 (1.08)	4.26 (0.74)
Operational	4.03 (1.14)	4.36 (0.71)
Clinical	4.05 (1.06)	4.66 (0.60)
Resource	4.21 (0.91)	4.28 (0.65)
Prof practice	4.69 (0.83)	4.72 (0.54)
Average all decision types	4.23 (0.76)	4.46 (0.52)
QUALITY OF DECISIONS		
Compatible with constraints	4.11 (0.87)	
Timing for max coverage	3.89 (0.98)	
Optimal information	3.54 (0.85)	
Conflict of interest	3.48 (1.25)	
Balance risk and reward	3.70 (0.76)	
Basis for implementation	3.97 (0.71)	
Average all decision types	3.80 (0.59)	

*Note: Low score = early involvement.

decisions was rated as moderate and the highest agreement was for 'decisions compatible with existing constraints, policies, etc.' and the lowest agreement was for 'implementing decisions caused a conflict of interest'.

TABLE **B-4**

FREQUENCY, MEANS AND STANDARD DEVIATIONS OF DECISION MECHANISMS

DECISION AREAS AND MECHANISMS	SNL		CEO	
	M(SD)	n (%)	M(SD)	n (%)
Planning	1.61 (1.35)		1.37 (1.0)	
Meeting with top management		47 (74.6)		39 (79.6)
Standing committees		3 (4.8)		2 (4.1)
Task forces		1 (1.6)		2 (4.1)
Informal meetings with management		3 (4.8)		1 (2.0)
Informal meetings with CEO		6 (9.5)		2 (4.1)
Operational	1.77 (1.11)		1.74 (1.16)	
Meeting with top management		32 (50.)		27 (55.1)
Standing committees		15 (23.0)		12 (24.5)
Task forces		6 (9.5)		2 (4.1)
Informal meetings with management		4 (6.3)		2 (4.1)
Informal meetings with CEO		2 (3.2)		3 (6.1)
Clinical	2.33 (1.23)		2.07 (1.06)	
Meeting with top management		18 (28.6)		16 (32.7)
Standing committees		16 (25.4)		17 (34.7)
Task forces		16 (25.4)		9 (18.4)
Informal meetings with management		6 (9.5)		2 (4.1)
Informal meetings with CEO		4 (6.3)		2 (4.1)
Resource	1.90 (1/42)		1.57 (1.11)	
Meeting with top management		39 (61.9)		33 (67.3)
Standing committees		7 (11.1)		7 (14.3)
Task forces		4 (6.3)		1 (2.0)
Informal meetings with management		4 (6.3)		3 (6.1)
Informal meetings with CEO		7 (11.1)		2 (4.1)
Professional practice	2.15 (1.67)		1.91 (0.99)	
Meeting with top management		18 (28.6)		16 (32.7)
Standing committees		30 (47.6)		24 (49.0)
Task forces		4 (6.3)		2 (4.1)
Informal meetings with management		4 (6.3)		2 (4.1)
Informal meetings with CEO		5 (7.9)		2 (4.1)
Overall Mean	1.95 (0.98)		1.73 (0.89)	

CEO Perceptions of the SNL Decisional Involvement

CEOs described the SNLs as being involved near the beginning of the decision-making process for all decision areas. The earliest involvement was reported for planning decisions whereas the latest involvement of the SNL was reported for clinical decisions. CEOs reported that SNLs offered a broad range of expertise in top-level decisions. Professional practice decisions rated the broadest range of expertise and planning decisions received the lowest mean for range of expertise offered. The highest mean for number of decision activi-

ties was for professional practice decisions and the lowest was reported for clinical decisions. As for decision mechanisms, CEOs reported the SNLs in their organization were more likely to utilize meetings with top management, especially for planning, operational and resource decisions. SNLs were more likely to use standing committees for professional practice decisions and were least likely to utilize informal meetings with management or CEO and task forces. In terms of influence over final decisions, CEOs reported that SNLs had a large amount of influence over final decisions that were reached across all types of decisions. The highest level of influence was reported for decisions regarding professional practice and the lowest level of influence for planning decisions. Ratings of overall quality of management decisions were not included in the CEO survey. Results of paired t-tests to compare SNL and CEO means of the four decision variables (timing, breadth of involvement, activities and influence) showed no statistically significant differences.

Correlations Among Major Study Variables

Only SNL breadth of content expertise ($r = 0.324$, $P < 0.01$) and of decision-making activities ($r = 0.356$, $P < 0.01$) were significantly correlated with decision-making influence and also with quality of management decisions ($r = 0.219$, $P < 0.05$ for breadth; $r = 0.242$, $P < 0.05$ for number of activities) (Table B-5).

Test of Hypotheses

For hypothesis one, the predictor variables, SNL mean scale scores for timing of involvement, breadth of expertise and number of decision activities, were entered hierarchically with SNL mean scale decision-making influence as the dependent variable. Twenty-two per cent of the variance in SNL decision-making influence was explained by timing of involvement, breadth of content expertise and number of decision activities ($R^2 = 0.223$, $F_{(3, 53)} = 5.06$, $P = 0.004$). However, only breadth of content expertise ($\beta =$

0.312, $t = 2.524$, $P = 0.015$) and number of decision activities ($\beta = 0.364$, $t = 2.997$, $P = 0.004$) were significant predictors of influence and thus, the first hypothesis was partially supported. The second hypothesis was tested by entering mean decision-making influence as the predictor with mean quality of management decisions as the dependent variable. Decision-making influence was not a significant predictor of the quality of management decisions, thus the second hypothesis was not supported.

DISCUSSION

In the present study, we developed a model of SNL participation in organizational decision-making based on the work of Ashmos *et al.* (1998), Anderson and McDaniel (1998) and Banaszak-Holl *et al.* (1999). We found partial support for our hypothesis that SNL timing of involvement, breadth of content expertise and number of decision activities in which they are involved predicted their perception of influence in organizational decisions. Timing was not a significant predictor whereas SNLs reported early involvement in most decision types. Although there is some indication in the healthcare literature that increased involvement in organizational decision-making by physicians and registered nurses was associated with outcomes such as lower costs in hospitals (Ashmos *et al.* 1998) and improved resident outcomes in nursing homes (Anderson & McDaniel 1999), we found that

TABLE **B-5**

MEANS, STANDARD DEVIATIONS AND CORRELATIONS AMONG SNL TIMING, BREADTH OF CONTENT EXPERTISE, NUMBER OF DECISION ACTIVITIES, DECISION INFLUENCE AND QUALITY OF DECISIONS

VARIABLE	n	M(SD)	α	1	2	3	4
Timing of involvement	63	1.93 (0.95)	0.84	—			
Breadth of content expertise	63	4.08 (0.98)	0.89	0.133	—		
Number of decision activities	57	3.88 (1.19)	0.90	0.064	−0.022	—	
Decision-making influence	63	4.23 (0.76)	0.83	0.022	0.324**	0.356**	—
Quality of decisions	62	3.80 (0.59)	0.68	0.133	0.219*	0.242*	0.195

*P < 0.05, one-tailed. **P < 0.01, one-tailed.

SNL decision involvement (timing, breadth and number of activities) and influence in decision-making did not predict their perceived quality of organizational decisions.

There were significant positive, albeit small, correlations between breadth of expertise and number of activities and quality of decisions. Small sample size may have been an issue in why we did not find a significant relationship between influence and quality. Post hoc power analysis showed power was only 0.33. Even although SNLs perceived a significant influence over decisions, there were likely many other factors outside of the control of the SNLs and even the senior leadership team such as government directives, economic constraints or community reactions that ultimately influenced the quality of decisions. The measure of decision quality was a subjective measure and included only SNL ratings. Interestingly, Banaszak-Holl et al. (1999) reported that SNLs rated decision quality significantly lower than did non-nurse members of the senior leadership team in all decision categories but no means were reported so we could not compare them with our decision quality findings. Unfortunately, we could not compare our results to their findings as they did not report quality item or scale means.

In general, CEO ratings of SNL involvement in decision-making were higher than the SNL self ratings. In all decision areas, CEOs rated SNL involvement earlier in the decision process than SNLs reported. CEOs ratings of SNLs breadth of content expertise also were higher than SNL self-ratings in four out of the five decision areas; SNLs rated themselves somewhat higher in professional practice decision-making than did the CEOs. It is possible that the depth of SNL involvement in professional practice decision-making was not readily apparent to the CEO. This could be related to two possible factors:

- professional practice decision-making occurs more frequently within committees, which may not include the CEO, or

- CEOs do not differentiate professional practice decisions from operational ones to the same degree as SNLs.

Some differences in perceptions between CEOs and SNLs were related to number of decision activities: CEOs reported more SNL activities for clinical and operational decisions whereas the SNLs reported a higher number of activities than the CEO for resource, planning and professional practice decisions. CEOs also rated SNL decision influence consistently higher than the SNL did for all decision types. These positive comparative findings may indicate that CEOs have considerable confidence in the decision-making role of their respective SNLs. Wells et al. (1999) reported a similar finding in the Banaszak-Holl et al. (1999) study: directors' (equivalent to the CEO role) perceptions of SNL involvement were similar to SNLs' self-ratings and often were more positive than SNLs were about their participation in decision-making. CEO perceptions of SNL decision-making may provide some insights for current and future SNLs learning to shape the nature and content of information shared with CEOs, particularly in the area of professional practice issues and decision-making.

Concurrence between CEOs and SNLs about the SNL role in executive decision-making is both reassuring and critical to ensuring his/her effectiveness. An essential responsibility of the SNL is to effectively assess, plan, forecast and execute decisions based on the needs within nursing, clinical departments and the patient populations served. But to be successful at this requires that the SNL is able to influence other decision-makers, particularly at the executive and governing board levels. These findings suggest that despite the significant restructuring within Canadian healthcare organizations, CEOs have considerable trust in the leadership competencies of the SNL and view these persons as having a very high degree of influence. This augers [sic] well for members of the nursing workforce, with regard to knowing that frontline clinical issues and concerns will be heard when conveyed by SNLs to the executive team.

Overall, SNLs reported having a large span of influence; the breadth of knowledge and skills the SNL brings to the executive table, allows them to significantly influence not only clinical care, but also organizational policy and strategic directions. In fact, SNLs are in an ideal position to show the linkages between different types of decisions and ensure that there is alignment between the clinical and business decision spheres in organizations. There is likely an overlap among the different decision types. Decisions in organizations are rarely totally independent of other decisions (Mintzberg *et al.* 1976, Oetjen *et al.* 2008). For example, strategic planning decisions determine organizational priorities and ultimately affect most other decision types. Resource decisions are also central to most other decision types and set the boundaries for what is possible within the clinical, human resources and professional practice areas.

When we compared our findings with those of Banaszak-Holl *et al.* (1999), we found substantial similarity in overall decision-making across decision types. Some caution is required with these comparisons given that a new decision-type domain, professional practice, was added in our study. In the earlier study, means for clinical decisions in all the decision variables were generally higher where professional practice decisions were often rated higher than clinical for all decision variables. Some aspects of the clinical domain may be incorporated in SNLs responses to the professional practice domain although we construed these two decision areas to be different. Both the current study and VA results were similar overall for timing of involvement ($M = 1.93$ vs. 1.92, respectively) and breadth of content expertise ($M = 4.08$ vs. 3.90, respectively). Areas of greatest difference were for number of decision activities ($M = 3.88$ vs. 4.31, respectively) where VA mean was higher, and decision influence

($M = 4.23$ vs. 3.83) where our overall mean was higher.

Our findings suggest that concerns about the impact of restructuring (i.e. regionalization of care services, programme management model and elimination of traditional distinct nursing departments) on SNL decision influence may not be warranted. In the present study, the predominant SNL role configuration was operational/line authority for clinical programmes with a direct report to the CEO in 84% of organizations so concern about direct line responsibility for nursing was not an issue. Traditional distinct nursing departments were rare (20%) and were found primarily in Quebec and in community hospitals. Our sample was an experienced group of SNLs suggesting their decision influence skills were well developed. The need for leader succession planning, that is, identifying and developing the next generation of nurse leaders is critical given the average age of SNLs in Canada. Conscious efforts to prepare future nurse leaders in mentored decision-making activities such as learning about organizational decision processes, role shadowing, guided project work and leader development programmes are important to augment their decision-making confidence and expertise.

The demands of 21st century healthcare environments are increasingly characterized as complex, dynamic, unpredictable and somewhat resistant to traditional management solutions to problems (Huston 2008). Strong nursing leadership is required to create cultures of safety and healthier work environments that promote patient safety, excellence in care and recruit and retain staff. To meet these challenges SNLs need expert decision-making skills guided by sound empirical evidence, innovative thinking and effective communication strategies to involve executive team members and other stakeholders in creating new responses to these challenges. SNL decision influence for change is now required on many levels beyond the executive team: at the staff level by creating alignment for organizational decisions, at the board level by providing interpretation of quality concerns, at the community level by raising awareness of health service issues and, at the government level by advocating for policy change.

Study limitations include small sample size for testing the second hypothesis and potential measurement issues with regard to the instrument which may fail to adequately address overlap among decision types and lack of specificity for timing of decisions. Also, the unique aspects of the Canadian healthcare system may limit generalizability to nurse leaders in acute care settings in other countries. While this study shows very positive perceptions of SNLs as executive decision-makers, what is not known are the perceptions of the frontline clinicians and managers about SNL effectiveness in presenting nursing issues. Future studies are needed to examine perceptions at various levels within the organization as a means of validating the overall coherence and confidence in SNL effectiveness.

CONCLUSIONS

Senior nurse leaders play an influential role in the future of healthcare organizations through their participation in decision-making at the senior team level and their ability to influence how nursing is practiced and valued in the organization. Despite variations in how health system restructuring has occurred across Canada, it is clear that SNL involvement is critical and highly valued by CEOs. As a member of the senior leadership team, the SNL has the opportunity to influence team members by ensuring that patient care and nursing practice perspectives are voiced when decisions affect organizational directions, quality management and resource use. In general, we found that SNLs perceived they had early involvement in decision-making processes, contributed breadth of content expertise to most decision types, engaged in a variety of decision activities and had considerable decision-making

influence. Moreover, CEOs validated these findings, rating SNL involvement in decision-making even higher than SNLs. We found support for our contention that involvement in decision-making predicted degree of perceived influence over decisions. In particular, breadth of content expertise and number of decision activities involving SNLs were significant predictors of decision influence, explaining 22% of the variance in influence.

ACKNOWLEDGEMENTS

Funding for this project: Canadian Health Services Research Foundation (CHRSF)/Canadian Institutes of Health Research (CIHR), the Ontario Health Services Research Co-sponsorship Fund from Ontario Ministry of Health and Long-term Care and Nursing Research Fund, Registered Nurses Association of Ontario, Office of Nursing Policy (Health Canada), Centre FERASI, Ministère de la Santé et des Services Sociaux du Québec, CIHR Knowledge Translation Branch, Nursing Leadership Network of Ontario, London Health Sciences Centre, Mount Sinai Hospital and Vancouver Coastal Health Authority.

REFERENCES

Anderson R.A. & McDaniel R.R. (1998) Intensity of registered nurse participation in nursing home decision-making. *The Gerontologist 38* (1), 90-100.

Anderson R.A. & McDaniel R.R. (1999) RN participation in organizational decision-making and improvements in resident outcomes. *Health Care Management Review 24* (10), 7-16.

Anthony M.K., Standing T.S., Glick J. et al. (2005) Leadership and nurse retention: the pivotal role of nurse managers. *Journal of Nursing Administration 35* (3), 146-155.

Arnold L., Drenkard K., Ela S. et al. (2006) Strategic positioning for nursing excellence in health systems—Insights from chief nursing executives. *Nursing Administration Quarterly 30* (1), 11-20.

Ashmos D.P. & McDaniel R.R. (1991) Physician participation in hospital strategic decision-making: the effect of hospital strategy and decision content. *Health Services Research 26* (3), 375-401.

Ashmos D.P., Huonker J.W. & McDaniel R.R. (1998) Participation as a complicating mechanism: the effect of clinical professional and middle manager participation on hospital performance. *Health Care Management Review 23* (4), 7-20.

Banaszak-Holl J., Alexander J., Valentine N.M., Piotrowski M.M., Adams-Watson J.G. & Davis J. (1999) Decision-making activity and influence of nurse executives in top management teams. *Journal of Nursing Administration 29* (4), 18-24.

Baumann A., O'Brien-Pallas L. & Armstrong-Stassen M. et al. (2001) *Commitment and Care: The Benefits of a Healthy Workplace for Nurses, their Patients and the System*. Report submitted to the Canadian Health Services Research Foundation, Ottawa ON.

Berggren I. & Severinsson E. (2003) Nurse supervisors' actions in relation to their decision-making style and ethical approach to clinical supervision. *Journal of Advanced Nursing 41* (6), 615-622.

Canadian Nursing Advisory Committee (2002) *Our Health, Our Future: Creating Quality Workplaces for Canadian Nurses*, Advisory Committee on Health Human Resources, Ottawa, ON.

Clancy T.R. (2003) The art of decision-making. *Journal of Nursing Administration 33* (6), 343-349.

Clifford J.C. (1998) *Restructuring: The Impact of Hospital Organization on Nursing Leadership*, Jossey-Bass Publishing, San Francisco, CA.

Duffield C., Moran P., Beutel J. et al. (2001) Profile of first-line nurse managers in New South Wales, Australia in the 1990s. *Journal of Advanced Nursing 36* (6), 785-793.

Dwore R.B., Murray B.P., Fosbinder D. et al. (2000) Integration of nurse executives into executive level administration in Utah hospitals. *The Health Care Manager 18* (4), 22-36.

Fedoruk M. (2000) The nurse executive: challenges for the 21st century. *Journal of Nursing Management 8* (1), 13-20.

Filkins J. (2003) Nurse directors' jobs—A European perspective. *Journal of Nursing Management 11* (1), 44-47.

Fonville A.G.M. (2002) *How Nurse Executives Acquire and Use Ethics Knowledge in Management Decision-Making*. Unpublished doctoral dissertation, Columbia University Teachers College, New York, NY, USA.

Freund C.M. (1988) Decision-making styles: managerial application of the MBTI and type theory. *Journal of Nursing Administration 18* (12), 5-11.

Havens D.S. (1998) An update on nursing involvement in hospital governance: 1990-1996. *Nursing Economics 16* (1), 6-11.

Havens D.S. (2001) Comparing nursing infrastructure and out-comes: ANCC nonmagnet CNEs report. *Nursing Economics 19* (6), 258-266.

Havens D.S. & Laschinger H.K. (1997) Creating the environment to support shared governance: Kanter's theory of power in organizations. *Journal of Shared Governance 3* (1), 15-23.

Huston C. (2008) Preparing nurse leaders for 2010. *Journal of Nursing Management 16*, 905-911.

Kirk H. (2008) Nurse executive director effectiveness: a systematic review of the literature. *Journal of Nursing Management 16*, 374-381.

Kleinman C.S. (2003) Leadership roles, competencies, and education. *Journal of Nursing Administration 33* (9), 451-455.

Krairiksh M. (2000) *The Relationship among Staff Nurses' Participation in Decision-Making, Nurse Managers' Leadership Competencies, and Nurse-Physician Collaboration*. Unpublished doctoral dissertation, Case Western Reserve University, Cleveland, OH, USA.

Laschinger H.K., Wong C.A., Ritchie J. et al. (2008) A profile of the structure and impact of nursing management in Canadian hospitals. *Healthcare Quarterly 11* (2), 85-94.

Lauri S., Salantera S., Chalmers K. et al. (2001) An exploratory study of clinical decision-making in five countries. *Journal of Nursing Scholarship 33* (1), 83-90.

Leatt P., Lemieux-Charles L. & Aird C. (1994) Program management: introduction and overview. In *Program Management and Beyond: Management Innovations in Ontario Hospitals* (P. Leatt, L. Lemieux-Charles & C. Aird eds), pp. 1-10, Canadian College of Health Services Executives, Ottawa, ON.

Mass H., Brunke L., Thorne S. & Parslow H. (2006) Preparing the next generation of senior nursing leaders in Canada: perceptions of role competencies and barriers from the perspectives of inhabitants and aspirants. *Canadian Journal of Nursing Leadership 19* (2), 75-91.

Mintzberg H., Raisinghani D. & Théorêt A. (1976) The structure of "unstructured" decision processes. *Administrative Science Quarterly 21* (2), 246-275.

Murray B.P., Fosbinder D., Parson R.J. et al. (1998) Nurse executives' leadership roles: perceptions of incumbents and influential colleagues. *Journal of Nursing Administration 28* (6), 17-24.

Oetjen R.M., Oetjen D.M. & Rotarius T. (2008) Administrative decision making: a stepwise method. *The Health Care Manager 27* (1), 4-12.

Oroviogoicoechea C. (1996) The clinical nurse manager: a literature review. *Journal of Advanced Nursing 24*, 1273-1280.

Robbins S.P. & Langton N. (2003) *Organizational Behaviour: Concepts, Controversies, Applications*, Pearson Education Canada, Toronto, ON.

Shamian J. & Lightstone E.Y. (1997) Hospital restructuring initiatives in Canada. *Medical Care 35* (10), OS62-OS69.

Shannon V. & French S. (2005) The impact of the re-engineered world of health-care in Canada on nursing and patient outcomes. *Nursing Inquiry 12* (3), 231-239.

Sharp N.D., Grelner G.T., Li Y. et al. (2006) Nurse executive and staff nurse perceptions of the effects of reorganization in Veterans Health Administration Hospitals. *Journal of Nursing Administration 36* (10), 471-478.

Smith S.L. & Friedland D.S. (1998) The influence of education and personality on risk propensity in nurse managers. *Journal of Nursing Administration 28* (12), 22-27.

Smith D., Klopper H.E., Paras A. & Au A. (2006) Structure in health agencies. In *Nursing Leadership and Management in Canada*, 3rd ed (J.M. Hibberd & D.L. Smith eds), pp. 199-237, Elsevier Canada, Toronto, ON.

Thompson C. (1999) A conceptual treadmill: the need for 'middle ground' in clinical decision making theory in nursing. *Journal of Advanced Nursing 30* (5), 1222-1229.

Thorman K.E. (2004) Nursing leadership in the boardroom. *Journal of Obstetric, Gynecologic, and Neonatal Nursing 33*, 381-387.

Upenieks V.V. (2003) What constitutes effective leadership? Perceptions of magnet and nonmagnet nurse leaders. *Journal of Nursing Administration 33* (9), 456-467.

Wangsness S.I. (1991) *A Study of Decision-Making Activities of Nurse Executives in Acute Care Pennsylvania Hospitals*. Unpublished doctoral dissertation, Pennsylvania State University, Hershey, PA, USA.

Wells R., Alexander J.A., Piotrowski M.M. et al. (1999) How other members of the top management team see the nurse executive. *Nursing Administration Quarterly 23* (3), 38-51.

The Effect of Music on Parental Participation During Pediatric Laceration Repair

Gregory Sobieraj, Maala Bhatt, Sylvie LeMay, Janet Rennick, Celeste Johnston

The purpose of this quasi-experimental study was to test an intervention on the use of music during simple laceration repair to promote parent-led distraction in children aged 1 to 5. Children's songs were broadcast via speakers during laceration repair and parents were encouraged to participate in distracting their child. The proportion of parental participation was determined. Laceration procedures were videotaped and objectively scored using the Procedure Behavior Check List. A total of 57 children participated in the study. There was no difference in parental involvement between the control and intervention groups. When age, sex, and condition were controlled for, distress scores were significantly higher if the father was present in the procedure room than if only the mother was present (43.68 vs. 23.39, $t(54)$ 4.296, $p = < 0.001$). It was concluded that distress varies with the age of the child and the parent who is present during the procedure. Providing music during simple laceration repair did not increase the proportion of parents who were involved in distraction.

KEYWORDS: laccrations, music, intervention studies, pediatrics, pain

INTRODUCTION

In Canada more than 95,000 children visit emergency departments (EDs) annually because of injuries (Public Health Agency of Canada, 2002b) and lacerations and other open wounds account for 25% of injuries among children aged 1 to 4 (Public Health Agency of Canada, 2002a). Although laceration repair is a relatively painless procedure due to the use of topical anesthesia, children experience distress as a result of anti-

cipatory fear. A child's fear, anxiety, and distress must be adequately addressed to ensure successful laceration repair and a positive hospital experience for parents and their children. The focus of this study was the testing of music as an intervention to increase parent-led distraction in the ED.

LITERATURE REVIEW

There is a wealth of research supporting the notion that children who are undertreated for pain suffer long-term deleterious effects. For example, Taddio, Katz, Ilersich, and Koren (1997) found that neonates who were circumcised without analgesia experienced more distress in subsequent routine immunizations than children who were circumcised with topical analgesia. Simple laceration repair, defined in this study as the application of tissue adhesives or sutures to repair torn or damaged tissue without the use of sedatives, is a relatively painless procedure. However, children under 5 years of age are unable to distinguish between the experience and the sensation of fear (Carr, Lemanek, & Armstrong, 1998; Goodenough et al., 1999). Therefore, intense fear experienced by the child during laceration repair may lead to long-term negative outcomes similar to those described by Taddio and colleagues. If we consider distress as "the sum of anxiety and pain" (Walco, Conte, Labay, Engel, & Zeltzer, 2005), any medical procedure resulting in distress in young children may lead to long-term deleterious effects. It should therefore be a priority for all pediatric health-care providers to implement distress reduction in their practice.

From the *Canadian Journal of Nursing Research*, 2009; 41:68–82. © McGill University School of Nursing.

Age has been identified as a significant variable in studies assessing pediatric distress, especially during acute, painful procedures. A study by Goodenough and colleagues (1999) found that ratings of pain and unpleasantness during a painful medical procedure decreased with increasing age. An earlier study, similarly, found a negative correlation between pain (both subjective and objective) and age, indicating that the pain response is attenuated by age (Fradet, McGrath, Kay, Adams, & Luke, 1990).

Psychological interventions have been shown to have a positive effect on procedural distress. Techniques such as distraction have a clear benefit in procedures such as venous cannulation or lumbar puncture (Cohen, 2002; Uman, Chambers, McGrath, & Kisely, 2006). There are, however, very few studies exploring these benefits in painless procedures such as laceration repair using topical anesthesia. Sinha, Christopher, Fenn, and Reeves (2006) attempted to use music as a distraction during laceration repair in children aged 6 to 18. They found that music effectively reduced anxiety in both the children and their parents during the procedure but that it did not have an effect on the sensation of pain. Conversely, a recent Cochrane review concluded that music has a small but measurable effect on the sensation of pain; the authors recommend that although music should not be used as a first-line treatment for pain, it could serve as a useful adjunct to analgesia (Cepeda, Carr, Lau, & Alvarez, 2006). Its positive effect on distress and its unobtrusive nature make music an ideal intervention for testing in a busy environment such as an ED.

Child caregivers are often closely attuned to the child and consequently can have a considerable effect on levels of distress experienced by the child. When a parent is present in the treatment room during a potentially painful event, positive effects include lower distress scores for the parent and the child (Wolfram & Turner, 1996), increased parent satisfaction, and a sense of being helpful (Piira, Sugiura, Champion, Donnelly, & Cole, 2005). Finally, it has been demonstrated that parental engagement in coping behaviours, such as use of humour and non-procedural talk directed at the child, serve to decrease the amount of distress experienced by the child (Blount et al., 1989).

Interestingly, some coping strategies used by parents, such as verbal reassurance (e.g., "it's okay," "don't worry"), empathy, criticism, and apologizing for the child's behaviour, have been shown to heighten the child's distress (Blount et al., 1989; Manimala, Blount, & Cohen, 2000; McMurtry, McGrath, & Chambers, 2006). It is unclear how these parental behaviours directed towards the child serve to increase distress. McMurtry and colleagues (2006) summarize the findings on reassurance and report that this coping strategy may increase distress via three mechanisms. First, reassurance may cue the child to prepare for an unpleasant event and incite fear and anxiety in the child. Second, it may reinforce and encourage distress behaviour: The more the child expresses feelings of distress, the more attention he receives from the parent. Finally, reassurance may provide validation for the child's feelings, effectively telling the child that it is "okay" to be distressed (McMurtry et al., 2006). Showing empathy and apologizing for the child's behaviour likely work via similar mechanisms. Further, it has been demonstrated that parental engagement in these distress-promoting behaviours can result in similar behaviours by those treating the child, such as nurses and physicians (Frank, Blount, Smith, Manimala, & Martin, 1995).

It is therefore important that strategies be developed whereby a parent can actively participate in a procedure and thus be made to feel helpful yet not engage in distress-promoting behaviour. Distress-promoting behaviours may be difficult to prevent, as a parent will intuitively attempt to reassure a child who is experiencing distress. Music, as a recommended adjunct for the treatment of pain, may be a useful tool for distracting the child and involving the parent in an activity that will prevent him or her from engaging in distress-promoting behaviours.

PURPOSE

It has been demonstrated that distraction is an effective means of decreasing distress. The purpose of this study was to test an intervention using children's songs to promote parent-led distraction during simple laceration repair in children aged 1 to 5. Parents were encouraged to participate in their child's treatment by singing along to music being broadcast via speakers. A parent who actively participates by singing will have less opportunity to engage in distress-promoting behaviour and, as reported by Sinha and colleagues (2006), may experience less anxiety during the procedure. Maternal behaviour could account for as much as 53% of the variance in distress experienced by a child (Frank et al., 1995). This finding supports the notion that an intervention targeting both parent and child could have a significant impact on the child's distress. This simple and easily implemented intervention provides parents with a medium through which to distract the child while simultaneously avoiding distress-promoting behaviours. Further, music is an inexpensive, easily implemented, low-burden intervention, requiring only the press of a button. This intervention could lead to a measurable reduction in distress during simple laceration repair by increasing parent-led distraction, thereby improving the hospital experience for both young children and their parents without placing an undue burden on professionals integrating the intervention into their practice.

We hypothesized that parents in the intervention group would demonstrate a greater degree of parent-led distraction than those in the control group. With this objective in mind, we formulated the following research question: *Does music broadcast via speakers have a measurable effect on parent-led distraction during simple laceration repair in children aged 1 to 5?*

METHODS AND MATERIALS

Design

This quasi-experimental study was conducted in a pediatric ED located in a large city. This study design was chosen over randomization because no between-group differences were expected in children presenting at the ED, based on a review of the department's patient-tracking software conducted by one of the investigators. As the study site was experiencing a severe staff shortage at the time of the study, this method also served to minimize any burden associated with randomization (e.g., using randomization software) and to simplify study logistics for participating ED staff.

Recruitment took place in 2-week blocks. Those children presenting during the first 2 weeks of the study had laceration repair as per department protocol, without the music intervention. During the second 2 weeks, consenting patients received the intervention. Recruitment took place over an 8-week period, Monday to Friday from noon to 8 P.M. A review of the patient-tracking software used at the study site, which tracks the presenting complaint, demographic data, and discharge diagnosis, determined that these days and times would allow for the greatest recruitment potential, as they were when lacerations in the 1-to-5 age group were most likely to present at the ED.

Sample

Children aged 12 to 71 months, inclusive, presenting at the ED with a single, simple laceration requiring repair with sutures or tissue adhesives and pretreated topically with lidocaine, epinephrine, and tetracaine (LET) were included in the study. This age range was selected so the intervention could be studied in a narrow developmental range and to facilitate standardization of the intervention and pre-procedural teaching. All children who required suturing received LET followed by injectable lidocaine to ensure that the procedure remained painless. Children were recruited regardless of prior experience with lacerations or laceration repair. Excluded were children who had more than one laceration, required sedation for their laceration repair, presented at the ED without a family member, or were accompanied by a family member who did not speak English or French.

Families were identified as eligible for the study by the triage nurse and flagged for the research assistant. The research assistant then approached the family and requested consent for participation prior to examination by the physician. Recruitment took place over the months of July and August 2008. Of the 69 families screened for the study, 68 agreed to participate (98%). Eleven of the families were excluded from the final analysis because the child did not meet inclusion criteria after being examined by the physician (e.g., required sedation, required complex laceration repair, had multiple injuries). One family did not provide a specific reason for refusal to consent. In total, 57 families were included in the final analysis, 27 of whom received the music intervention.

Intervention

All consenting families were met by a Child Life Specialist (CLS), who provided pre-procedural teaching to the parent and child. The pre-procedural teaching was standardized between the two groups. Children assigned to the intervention group had audiorecorded children's songs played to them during the procedure. The song choices included lullabies, educational songs, and songs performed by popular television characters in both English and French. Three songs were selected by the CLS and the parents prior to the procedure. These were played throughout the procedure on a repeating basis, from the start of the procedure (child placed on bed) to the end of the

procedure (bandage placed over laceration). The parents were encouraged to sing along with the music during the procedure. Participants in the non-intervention group (usual care) had no music played. All laceration-repair procedures were videotaped. The research assistant accompanied the physician, patient, and parents at all the procedures and was responsible for proper positioning of video equipment and for starting the music at the beginning of the procedure.

Approval for the study was obtained from both the Nurse Manager and the Medical Director of the ED. Ethical approval was obtained from the ethical review board prior to implementation. Informed consent was obtained by the research assistant prior to videotaping the procedure. All taped procedures were transferred to a dedicated hard drive in a locked office at the end of each study week. Videotapes were accessed and viewed only by the researchers and objective scorers. Patient confidentiality was ensured through the replacement of patient names with codes on all study materials. Consent forms were kept separate from other study materials at all times.

Instruments

Parental Participation

The video scorers determined the amount of time a parent spent distracting the child during the procedure. They were trained to recognize behaviours that distracted the child. Behaviours such as singing to the child, diverting the child's attention away from the laceration repair, or encouraging the child to sing were considered to be parental participation. The video scorers recorded the number of seconds spent on each distraction event. For example, they timed exactly how long a parent would sing along with the music being broadcast. A parental participation score was then derived by determining the proportion of time spent on distracting the child (time distracting/total procedure time). Interrater reliability for proportion of parental participation was determined (0.767, $p < 0.01$, CI 95% 0.632, 0.923) and judged to be acceptable.

Since the scores given by the two raters were similar, they were averaged to create an objective distress score and a parental participation score (in seconds), which were used in the subsequent analysis.

Procedure Behavior Check List

Videotapes of all laceration repairs were objectively scored using the Procedure Behavior Check List (PBCL) (LeBaron & Zeltzer, 1984). The PBCL is an observational measure of distress that scores the presence and intensity of eight behaviours associated with child pain and anxiety (e.g., muscle tension, verbal stalling, crying). Each behaviour is rated on a Likert-type scale ranging from 0 to 5 (0 = no distress; 1 = very mild distress; 5 = extremely intense distress), for a score ranging from 0 to 40. This tool was originally used to measure observable distress during lumbar punctures in 67 pediatric oncology patients between the ages of 6 and 18 years. Concurrent validity was found to be acceptable, with a correlation of 0.80 ($p < 0.001$) to the children's self-reports of pain and anxiety (Lebaron & Zeltzer, 1984). Subsequent studies have shown the PBCL to be a reliable and valid measure of behavioural distress in children (Cavender, Goff, Hollon, & Guzzetta, 2004; Luhmann, Schootman, Luhmann, & Kennedy, 2006), with observed distress significantly correlated with patient ratings of pain and anxiety (Langer, Chen, & Luhmann, 2005). Finally, a recent review of observational measures of pain rated the PBCL one of the most accurate measures of pain-related distress currently available, with a good balance of evidence, burden, and content validity (von Baeyer & Spagrud, 2007).

Videotapes were scored by two reviewers naive to the study purpose using the PBCL. The reviewers were trained in the use of the PBCL by study investigators prior to the study start date. Interrater reliability was established prior to the study by comparing rater and investigator scores on sample videotapes. Coding of the videotapes was begun by the raters only when reliability was greater than 0.80 on sample videotapes. Following data collection, interrater reliability was strong for the two video scorers on the objective measure of distress (0.884, $p < 0.01$, CI 95% 0.81, 0.93) and the time to complete the procedure (0.995, $p < 0.01$, CI 95% 0.991, 0.997).

RESULTS

The intervention and control groups were similar for age, location of laceration, length of laceration, and family member present, but dissimilar for gender. Children in the intervention group more frequently required sutures to repair the laceration (26% vs. 7%) (Table C-1); however, this difference was not statistically significant.

Linear regression analysis was performed to determine whether parental involvement predicted distress scores and the degree to which age affected distress. In the control group ($n = 30$), 18 parents participated in distracting the child (60%) and the mean proportion of time spent participating in the laceration repair was low (0.0647). Of the 27 parents in the intervention group, 15 distracted their child (56%), with a similar mean proportion of time spent distracting the child (0.0669). There was no significant difference between the two groups in terms of parental participation.

There was no significant difference in distress scores based on parental participation. The greatest predictors of child distress were age ($\beta = -0.434$, $t = -4.017$, $p < 0.01$), with younger children being more distressed, and the presence of the father in the procedure room ($\beta = -0.419$, $t = -3.888$, $p < 0.01$). Children had a significantly higher mean distress score when the father was present (43/100) than when only the mother was present (23/100) ($F (1, 54) = 18.452$, $p < 0.01$). (See Table C-2 for descriptive and comparative data on distress scores.)

TABLE C-1

DEMOGRAPHIC AND PROCEDURAL CHARACTERISTICS OF INTERVENTION AND CONTROL GROUPS

	CONTROL	INTERVENTION	CHI-SQUARED p
Age of child (months)	43.5 ± 14.4	39.9 ± 18.7	ns
Sex (n)			0.047*
Male	24	15	
Female	6	12	
Parent present (n)			ns
Father	4	4	
Mother	19	16	
Both	6	7	
Other	1	0	
Location of laceration (n)			ns
Scalp	9	3	
Face	17	21	
Other	3	3	
Length of laceration (mm)	13.2 ± 7.6	14.5 ± 7.7	ns
Type of repair (n)			ns
Tissue adhesive	28	20	ns
LET[a] + sutures	1	1	
LET + lidocaine + sutures	1	6	
N	30	27	

*Significant at 0.05.
[a]Topical anesthesia.

TABLE C-2

DISTRESS SCORE DATA: TREATMENT GROUP BY PARENTAL PRESENCE (DISTRESS SCORES 0–100)

	CONTROL	INTERVENTION	MEAN	F	P
Mean distress (n)	33.1 (29)	28.6 (26)			ns
Parent present					
Mother (n)	27.1 (19)	19 (16)	23.05	(2, 52) 9.516	<0.01
Father (n)	40.2 (4)	44.7 (4)	42.5		
Both (n)	48.1 (6)	43.4 (6)	45.8		

Note: Two cases were excluded; one child was accompanied by an aunt and one child was missing objective data.

DISCUSSION

There is a paucity of research on distress during laceration repair. Although this is a relatively simple, quick, and painless procedure, it is perceived by observers as extremely distressing (Babl, Mandrawa, O'Sullivan, & Crellin, 2008). As resolution of pain is an important predictor of high patient satisfaction in children (Magaret, Clark, Warden, Magnusson, & Hedges, 2002), it may be inferred that effective resolution of distress during simple laceration repair may also increase patient satisfaction. Further, reducing distress during laceration repair may decrease the need for sedatives such as midazolam, the use of which increases observation time (post-intervention) and the incidence of sequelae (Luhmann, Kennedy, Porter, Miller, & Jaffe, 2001). Our results indicate that the strongest predictors of distress are age and the parent who accompanies the child in the treatment room. The finding that distress is strongly correlated with age is in concordance with the results of several other studies examining pediatric distress (Carr et al., 1998; Goodenough et al., 1999).

Although the intervention did reduce distress in children (see Bhatt, Sobieraj, & Johnston, 2009), in the present study parental participation was not higher in the intervention group. Although parents were encouraged to distract their child during the procedure, the proportion of time spent distracting the child, regardless of condition, was extremely small (6.6% of total procedure time). The intervention may not provide sufficient stimulus to overcome the unpleasantness of seeing one's child in distress. In the future, more time with parents in pre-procedural teaching, to stress the importance of distraction, may serve to increase the proportion of time spent participating. If the proportion of time spent participating is increased, we might observe a lowering of distress scores, as had been expected, since the parents will have less opportunity to engage in distress-promoting behaviours.

Pre-procedural teaching has been demonstrated to reduce anxiety prior to a procedure (Claar, Walker, & Barnard, 2002; Spafford, von Baeyer, & Hicks, 2002). Presumably the older children in our sample had learned more from the pre-procedural teaching and applied the information more effectively. If distress is defined as the "sum of anxiety and pain" (Walco et al., 2005), then older children who are less anxious as a result of pre-procedural teaching will experience less distress. Therefore, we cannot rule out the possibility that the difference in distress levels between age groups is a result of an association between increasing age and pre-procedural teaching and is not in fact an accurate representation of distress scores. In the future it would be imperative to add a third group to the study, one in which no pre-procedural teaching has been provided by a CLS, in order to control for this potential confounding variable.

A novel finding in our study was the difference in distress scores depending upon which family member accompanied the child during the procedure. Children were significantly more distressed if the father was in the treatment room. Although the mean age for the group in which the father was present was slightly lower (38.3 vs. 43.9 months), this is likely not a sufficiently large age difference to explain the stress differences. There are no prior studies reporting a similar finding. As different coping strategies are known to provoke varying degrees of distress (Manimala et al., 2000; McMurtry et al., 2006; Young, 2005), it may be that fathers in our study were using coping strategies known to increase distress, such as reassurance, criticism, or apologizing for the child's behaviour, more frequently than mothers, while mothers may have been using effective coping strategies, such as distraction, humour, or non-procedural talk, with greater frequency. Since families self-selected who would accompany the child in the procedure room, a second possibility for this difference in distress is that fathers chose to accompany "difficult" or expressive children more frequently than mothers alone did. Without collecting more data from parents regarding their relationship with the child, or their preferred method of coping, it is hard to draw conclusions with respect to this difference in distress. A secondary analysis of the videotapes would allow us to determine the frequency and type of coping strategies used by family members, and to validate the hypothesis that different family members use alternative coping strategies.

One study has suggested that distraction loses efficacy in reducing distress if the painful or unpleasant stimulus is prolonged (McCaul & Malott, 1984). Laceration repair in our study took several minutes to complete ($M = 328$ seconds), in stark contrast to immunization, heel sticks, or blood sampling, which may take only seconds. The degree to which a child is distracted may be further influenced by their degree of stimulation. As our intervention was fairly passive, it may not have provided a sufficiently strong stimulus to overcome the unpleasantness of the laceration repair.

The present study had several limitations. A non-randomized design was chosen for the study, because there were no differences expected in children presenting to the ED during the 2-week study blocks. Despite this expectation, groups differed on gender, family member present during the procedure, and type of laceration repair. A single-blind RCT may have prevented the skewing of groups and increased the generalizability of our results. We cannot conclude that the gender composition among groups affected our results, as the literature on gender differences and distress in children is inconclusive (e.g., Carr et al., 1998; Goodenough et al., 1999).

Because audio was recorded and required for proper scoring of the videotapes, the objective scorers were not blind to group assignment. However, the scorers remained blind to study purpose throughout the study, which reduced the risk of bias in video scoring. In any future research it may be useful to apply a measure that does not require audio cues, such as the Child Facial Coding System (CFCS) (Breau et al., 2001), to reduce the risk of bias introduced by scorers who are not blind to group assignment.

The small sample size ($N = 57$) may be a further limitation. A larger sample size would have increased the power of the study and allowed us to detect a smaller clinical effect. Further, no qualitative data were collected from participating families and staff. Data such as satisfaction with the intervention, likelihood of adopting the intervention for future procedures, and parents' and staff members' perceptions of the effectiveness of the treatment might have allowed us to infer the clinical usefulness of the intervention.

Practice Implications

Our findings suggest that significant predictors of higher levels of distress during laceration repair are younger age and paternal accompaniment in the procedure room. This information could influence unit managers/team leaders to more effectively allocate available resources, such as CLSs,

to families where there is greater need. Older children may require less attention by auxiliary staff. This finding suggests that auxiliary staff can spend more time attending to the needs of other patients on the unit. Further, the data suggest that the younger population may require more attention from support staff than they are currently receiving, to lower the increased level of distress experienced by these patients.

CONCLUSION

Although the provision of music and preprocedural teaching did not increase the proportion of parental participation, the study did find that children are more distressed in the presence of fathers—an important finding not described in other studies. This finding will help inform future studies where parent gender may be an important covariate.

ACKNOWLEDGEMENTS

The authors would like to acknowledge the funding support of Groupe de recherche interuniversitaire en interventions en sciences infirmières du Québec (GRIISIQ) and the Montreal Children's Hospital Research Institute; the Emergency Department staff and the Child Life Services Department of the Montreal Children's Hospital; Fonds de la recherche en santé du Québec (FRSQ); and their research assistants, Sushmita Shivkumar and Kamy Apkarian.

Disclosure: There is no conflict of interest.

Gregory Sobieraj, RN, BN, is a PhD student at the School of Nursing, McGill University, Montreal, Quebec, Canada. Maala Bhatt, MD, MSc, is Attending Physician, Division of Pediatric Emergency Medicine, Montreal Children's Hospital. Sylvie LeMay, RN, PhD, is Associate Professor, Faculty of Nursing, Université de Montréal. Janet Rennick, RN, PhD, is Nurse Scientist, Montreal Children's Hospital. Celeste Johnston, RN, DEd, FCAHS, is Professor and Associate Director of Research, School of Nursing, McGill University.

REFERENCES

Babl, F., Mandrawa, C., O'Sullivan, R., & Crellin, D. (2008). Procedural pain and distress in young children as perceived by medical and nursing staff. *Pediatric Anesthesia, 18*(5), 412-419.

Bhatt, M., Sobieraj, G. S., & Johnston, C. C. (2009, May 5). *Improving emergency department treatment of pediatric lacerations with the use of children's songs as a distraction technique.* Poster presentation at meeting of Pediatric Academic Societies, Baltimore, Maryland.

Blount, R. L., Corbin, S. M., Sturges, J. W., Wolfe, V. V., Prater, J. M., & James, L. D. (1989). The relationship between adults' behavior and child coping and distress during BMA/LP procedures: A sequential analysis. *Behavior Therapy, 20*(4), 585-601.

Breau, L., McGrath, P. J., Craig, K. D., Santor, D., Cassidy, K. L., & Reid, G. J. (2001). Facial expression of children receiving immunizations: A principal components analysis of the child facial coding system. *Clinical Journal of Pain, 17*(2), 178-186.

Carr, T. D., Lemanek, K. L., & Armstrong, F. D. (1998). Pain and fear ratings: Clinical implications of age and gender differences. *Journal of Pain and Symptom Management, 15*(5), 305-316.

Cavender, K., Goff, M. D., Hollon, E. C., & Guzzetta, C. E. (2004). Parents' positioning and distracting children during venipuncture: Effects on children's pain, fear, and distress. *Journal of Holistic Nursing, 22*(1), 32-56.

Cepeda, M. S., Carr, D. B., Lau, J., & Alvarez, H. (2006). Music for pain relief. *Cochrane Database of Systematic Reviews, 2,* CD004843.

Claar, L. R., Walker, L. S., & Barnard, J. A. (2002). Children's knowledge, anticipatory anxiety, procedural distress, and recall of esophagogastroduodenoscopy. *Journal of Pediatric Gastroenterology and Nutrition, 34*(1), 68-72.

Cohen, L. L. (2002). Reducing infant immunization distress through distraction. *Health Psychology, 21*(2), 207-211.

Fradet, C., McGrath, P. J., Kay, J., Adams, S., & Luke, B. (1990). A prospective survey of reactions to blood tests by children and adolescents. *Pain, 40*(1), 53-60.

Frank, N. C., Blount, R. L., Smith, A. J., Manimala, M. R., & Martin, J. K. (1995). Parent and staff behavior, previous child medical experience, and maternal anxiety as they relate to child procedural distress and coping. *Journal of Pediatric Psychology, 20*(3), 277-289.

Goodenough, B., Thomas, W., Champion, G. D., Perrott, D., Taplin, J. E., von Baeyer, C. L., et al. (1999). Unravelling age effects and sex differences in needle pain: Ratings of sensory intensity and unpleasantness of venipuncture pain by children and their parents. *Pain, 80,* 179-190.

Langer, D. A., Chen, E., & Luhmann, J. D. (2005). Attributions and coping in children's pain experiences. *Journal of Pediatric Psychology, 30*(7), 615-622.

LeBaron, S., & Zeltzer, L. (1984). Assessment of acute pain and anxiety in children and adolescents by self-reports, observer reports, and a behavior checklist. *Journal of Consulting and Clinical Psychology, 52*(5), 729-738.

Luhmann, J. D., Kennedy, R. M., Porter, F. L., Miller, J. P., & Jaffe, D. M. (2001). A randomized clinical trial of continuous-flow nitrous oxide and midazolam for sedation of young children during laceration repair. *Annals of Emergency Medicine, 37*(1), 20-27.

Luhmann, J. D., Schootman, M., Luhmann, S. J., & Kennedy, R. M. (2006). A randomized comparison of nitrous oxide plus hematoma block versus ketamine plus midazolam for emergency department forearm fracture reduction in children. *Pediatrics, 118*(4), e1078-e1086.

Magaret, N. D., Clark, T. A., Warden, C. R., Magnusson, A. R., & Hedges, J. R. (2002). Patient satisfaction in the emergency department—a survey of pediatric patients and their parents. *Academic Emergency Medicine, 9*(12), 1379-1388.

Manimala, M. R., Blount, R. L., & Cohen, L. L. (2000). The effects of parental reassurance versus distraction on child distress and coping during immunizations. *Children's Health Care, 29*(3), 161-177.

McCaul, K. D., & Malott, J. M. (1984). Distraction and coping with pain. *Psychological Bulletin, 95*(3), 516-533.

McMurtry, C. M., McGrath, P. J., & Chambers, C. T. (2006). Reassurance can hurt: Parental behavior and painful medical procedures. *Journal of Pediatrics, 148*(4), 560-561.

Piira, T., Sugiura, T., Champion, G. D., Donnelly, N., & Cole, A. S. J. (2005). The role of parental presence in the context of children's medical procedures: A systematic review. *Child: Care, Health and Development, 31*(2), 233-243.

Public Health Agency of Canada. (2002a). *Canadian Hospitals Injury Reporting and Prevention Program (CHIRPP) report: Age and sex distribution of injured persons*. Retrieved September 4, 2009, from http://dsol-smed.phac-aspc.gc.ca/dsol-smed/is-sb/c_chrp-eng.phtml.

Public Health Agency of Canada. (2002b). *Canadian Hospitals Injury Reporting and Prevention Program (CHIRPP) report: Indication of the type of injury suffered by the injured person*. Retrieved September 4, 2009, from http://dsol-smed.phac-aspc.gc.ca/dsol-smed/is-sb/c_chrp-eng.phtml.

Sinha, M., Christopher, N. C., Fenn, R., & Reeves, L. (2006). Evaluation of non-pharmacologic methods of pain and anxiety management for laceration repair in the pediatric emergency department. [Comment.] *Pediatrics, 117*(4), 1162-1168.

Spafford, P. A., von Baeyer, C. L., & Hicks, C. L. (2002). Expected and reported pain in children undergoing ear piercing: A randomized trial of preparation by parents. *Behaviour Research and Therapy, 40*(3), 253-266.

Taddio, A., Katz, J., Ilersich, A. L., & Koren, G. (1997). Effect of neonatal circumcision on pain response during subsequent routine vaccination. *Lancet, 349*(9052), 599-603.

Uman, L. S., Chambers, C. T., McGrath, P. J., & Kisely, S. (2006). Psychological interventions for needle-related procedural pain and distress in children and adolescents. *Cochrane Database of Systematic Reviews, 4*, CD005179.

von Baeyer, C. L., & Spagrud, L. J. (2007). Systematic review of observational (behavioral) measures of pain for children and adolescents aged 3 to 18 years. *Pain, 127*(1-2), 140-150.

Walco, G. A., Conte, P. M., Labay, L. E., Engel, R., & Zeltzer, L. K. (2005). Procedural distress in children with cancer: Self-report, behavioral observations, and physiological parameters. *Clinical Journal of Pain, 21*(6), 484-490.

Wolfram, R. W., & Turner, E. D. (1996). Effects of parental presence during children's venipuncture. *Academic Emergency Medicine, 3*(1), 58-64.

Young, K. (2005). Pediatric procedural pain. *Annals of Emergency Medicine, 45*(2), 160-171.

Patient Real-Time and 12-Month Retrospective Perceptions of Difficult Communications in the Cancer Diagnostic Period*

Sally Thorne,[1] Elizabeth-Anne Armstrong,[1] Susan R. Harris,[1] T. Gregory Hislop,[2] Charmaine Kim-Sing,[3] Valerie Oglov,[1] John L. Oliffe,[1] Kelli I. Stajduhar[4]

ABSTRACT

Communication is a notoriously complex challenge in the cancer care context. Our program of research involves exploration of patient–provider communications across the cancer trajectory from the patient perspective. Toward this end, we have been following a cohort of 60 cancer patients, representing a range of tumor sites, from immediately after diagnosis through to recovery, chronic, or advanced disease. Drawing on interpretive description analytic techniques, we documented patterns and themes related to various components of the cancer journey. In this article, we report on findings pertaining to poor communication during the initial diagnostic period, as described by patients at the time of diagnosis and 1 year later. These findings illuminate the dynamics of communication problems during that complex period, and depict the mechanisms by which patients sought to confront these challenges to optimize their cancer care experience. On the basis of these findings, considered in the context of the body of available evidence, suggestions are proposed as to appropriate directions for system-level solutions to the complex communication challenges within cancer care.

[1]University of British Columbia, Vancouver, British Columbia, Canada

[2]British Columbia Cancer Research Centre, Vancouver, British Columbia, Canada

[3]British Columbia Cancer Agency, Vancouver, British Columbia, Canada

[4]University of Victoria, Victoria, British Columbia, Canada

From *Qualitative Health Research*, 2009; 19:1383–1394. © 2009, The Authors and SAGE.

KEYWORDS   cancer, communication, health care, psychosocial issues, quality of life, relationships

A cancer diagnosis marks the experiential beginning of a process that transitions people to patients and takes them on a journey through unfamiliar and frightening territory toward an often uncertain destination. Whether the diagnosis comes as an unanticipated and shattering moment in time, or occurs in the context of a protracted season of anxiety and alarm that culminates in an eventual declaration, it is inherently characterized by meaningful communications with health care providers. Communication during the diagnostic period sets the stage for the relationships cancer patients will have with those who manage and support them on the cancer journey. The diagnostic period is therefore acknowledged as a time when communication between patients and clinicians is particularly important and sensitive.

Until malignant disease is confirmed or strongly suspected, patients with the possibility of a cancer diagnosis tend not to have found their way into a formalized cancer care system; therefore, knowledge about the cancer diagnostic experience is pertinent to a wide range of care contexts, including primary care, ambulatory, and inpatient settings. As recent studies confirm, a minority of patients are first told of their diagnosis by cancer specialists, with a majority officially learning that they have cancer from a family physician or surgeon (Watson, Mooney, & Peterson, 2007). However, some patients also report first "knowing" that they have cancer because of unintentional messages transmitted in the tone or urgency of the clinic-scheduling clerk's voice, nonverbal cues from a radiation technologist, or the subtle shift toward cautious language in a primary care provider. Regardless of its form, the diagnosis experience is retained in vivid memory by patients as a significant and disruptive milestone in their biography and the entry point into a life-altering way of being (Evans, Tulsky, Back, & Arnold, 2006; Walsh & Nelson, 2003). Thus, it is important that we understand the dynamics of communications surrounding diagnosis to ensure that clinicians who encounter patients in and around the diagnostic phase are informed about and sensitive to its impact, and possess the appropriate skills to ensure that patients begin their cancer journey with optimal support and guidance.

BACKGROUND TO THE LITERATURE

Although it is well known that communication will have a strong impact on both the experience and psychosocial outcomes of cancer (Baile & Aaron, 2005; Butow, 2005; Fallowfield & Jenkins, 2004; Fallowfield, 2008; Hack, Degner, Parker, & SCRN Communication Team, 2005; Ong, Visser, Lammes, & de Haes, 2000), poor communication remains a significant problem facing cancer patients across the spectrum of service (Thorne, Bultz, Baile, & SCRN Communication Team, 2005). In part, this is because of the complexity of communication and the variability of the human experience of cancer, both of which create significant challenges for the development of a solid empirical science within this field (Feldman-Stewart, Brundage, Tishelman, & SCRN Communication Team, 2005; Parker, Davison, Tishelman, & Brundage, 2005; Patrick, Intille, & Zabinski, 2005). Recent reviews confirm that the science of cancer communication has been impeded by factors that include the changing

nature of patient needs and goals over the course of disease (Carlson, Feldman-Stewart, Tishelman, Brundage, & SCRN Communication Team, 2005), and the diversity of social and cultural norms and expectations in relation to the communication style preferred by patients (Schofield et al., 2003; Siminoff, Graham, & Gordon, 2006) and by clinicians (Davis, Williams, Marin, Parker, & Glass, 2002; Feldman-Stewart et al., 2005; Ramirez, 2003). This science has also been complicated by the challenge of finding agreement on appropriate measures for cancer communication effectiveness (Carlson et al., 2005; Feldman-Stewart, Brennenstuhl, & Brundage, 2007; Schofield & Butow, 2004).

Studies from the patient perspective have clearly documented that effective communication with health care providers is a high priority concern at diagnosis and throughout the cancer trajectory (Kreps, Arora, & Nelson, 2003). During the diagnostic phase in particular, obtaining and applying information is understood to be a pressing need for patients (Rutten, Arora, Bakos, Aziz, & Rowland, 2005), although there is known to be considerable diversity among patients relative to the type of information that is sought and preference for the manner in which it is delivered (Cox, Jenkins, Catt, Langridge, & Fallowfield, 2006; Eggly et al., 2006).

These conceptual and methodological challenges make it exceedingly difficult to convincingly conclude what is best for all patients in relation to the communications surrounding a cancer diagnosis (Lockhart, Dosser, Cruickshank, & Kennedy, 2007; Schofield & Butow, 2004; Schofield et al., 2003), and the absence of a solid body of evidence-informed communications guidelines further compromises the capacity of concerned clinicians to take the appropriate steps toward skill development (Arora, 2003; Butler, Degner, Baile, Landry, & SCRN Communication Team, 2005). Where clinical guidelines exist, they tend to have been generated on the basis of expert professional opinion, with relatively little interpretation from the patient perspective (Edvardsson, Pahlson, & Ahlstrom, 2006; Hoff, Tidefelt, Thaning, & Hermeren, 2007; Schofield et al., 2001). Although much of the advice available to clinicians is quite general or self-evident, the literature contains considerable depth pertaining to such communication practices as responding to the distress cues of patients (Beach, Easter, Good, & Pigeron, 2005), listening, engaging in compassionate inquiry, and responding empathetically (Back, Arnold, Baile, Tulsky, & Fryer-Edwards, 2005), and ensuring access to psychosocial support services (Ambler et al., 2007; Nelson, 2004; Taylor, Ismail, Hills, & Ainsworth, 2004). Studies from the patient perspective have generally confirmed that these elements during the provision of medical advice are indeed appropriate (Ptacek & Ptacek, 2001). However, because of the significant challenge of tailoring communication practices to the unique and particular needs and contextual circumstances of individual patients, the standardized communication approaches available within the literature have not been widely taken up (Davison & Mills, 2005).

The general problem that this article addresses is the continuing prevalence of poor communication during the diagnostic window of time within the cancer experience. Specifically, we report findings associated with those communication encounters that patients experience as problematic during the diagnostic period within the context of a longitudinal cohort study of patient perspectives of cancer communication across the illness trajectory. By better understanding the dynamics and nature of what patients consider to be difficult communication, we increase our capacity to search for appropriate mechanisms with which to prevent and ameliorate these difficulties for future patients.

STUDY METHOD

The data upon which the current analysis draws is part of an ongoing longitudinal study of cancer care communication from the patient's perspective. In this study, we recruited a cohort of 60 newly diagnosed cancer patients and followed them over time (ideally, at least 2 years) to determine how their communication needs and preferences changed across their cancer trajectory.

Our research uses interpretive description methodology (Thorne, Reimer Kirkham, & MacDonald-Emes, 1997; Thorne, 2008), an established qualitative inquiry approach that extracts elements from the social science tradition (Glaser & Strauss, 1967; Lincoln & Guba, 1985; Miles & Huberman, 1994), integrating their application in a manner that makes them ideally suited to the study of practice-based questions deriving from applied clinical fields (Sandelowski, 2000).

With ethics approval from our university-based review board, we recruited over a 12-month period a cohort of 60 patients representing a range of disease and demographic variables. The study participants who voluntarily responded to our recruitment ads in various parts of the cancer system in a large western Canadian city included 43 women (72%) and 17 men (28%), a majority residing in urban (92%) rather than rural settings and of Euro-Canadian (95%) ethnicity, and the remainder of Chinese or South Asian heritage. Their ages ranged from mid-30s to late 80s, with 22 (37%) in the 50 to 59 bracket and 15 (25%) in each of the 40 to 49 and 60 to 69 groupings. A range of tumor sites was reflected within the cohort, with the primary groupings constituting 23 (38%) breast, 8 (13%) hematological (lymphoma/leukemia), 7 (12%) prostate, 6 (10%) gastrointestinal, and 6 (10%) gynecological (cervix/uterus/ovary), as well as 10 (17%) across other sites.

Each member of the cohort was interviewed initially according to a semi-structured initial interview guide by one of two interviewers, each of whom held a graduate degree in a health professional discipline and had specialized training in qualitative research interview techniques.

Following the initial face-to-face individual interview, interviewers conducted bimonthly follow-up interviews either in person or by telephone, according to the preference and convenience of the study participant. In most instances, the set of follow-up interviews for each cohort member reflected a mixture of the two formats. These follow-up interviews were guided by themes and questions derived from ongoing constant comparative analysis to develop emerging analytic themes and clarify individual variations across accounts (Miles & Huberman, 1994). In this manner, we followed the evolving trajectory of each individual, as well as engaged them in revisiting and reflecting on discrete events.

As might be predicted, the cohort members varied in their trajectory, with some achieving a level of confidence about survivorship, others continuing active treatment, and still others approaching the terminal phase of the disease. At the time of writing, 6 members of the cohort have died of their disease. Thus, we have subsets within the ongoing cohort representing a range of events post-diagnosis. However, as the diagnosis experience was an event common to all, each member was explicitly interviewed at length about that aspect, both in the initial phases of study participation and also in a targeted interview reflecting back on that period of time 12 months later. It is these components of the overall continuing data set on which this article is based.

In the interpretive description method, the collection and analysis of data are considered concurrent processes, with each informing the other iteratively over time. All interviews were transcribed verbatim into electronic format, and we used a qualitative computer software management system to assist with data sorting and management. The analytic process we used involved rigorous engagement in interpretive cross-comparison among and between cases in the context of our emerging thematic synthesis (Sandelowski, Trimble, Woodard, & Barroso, 2006). Findings drawn from interpretive descrip-

tion are not meant to reflect representativeness of the population; rather, when articulated in a manner that is authentic and credible to the reader, they can reflect valid descriptions of sufficient richness and depth that their products warrant a degree of generalizability in relation to a field of understanding.

FINDINGS

Although patient descriptions of communication experiences both at the onset of the study and ongoing were often complex, typically involving multiple health care professionals and circumstances, our trigger questions were specifically designed to prompt elaboration on those elements within communication they found particularly helpful and unhelpful. Within the extensive accounts arising from these prompts, most of the study participants reported a range of helpfulness among and across encounters, with a majority recalling at least one instance of what they considered to be good and poor communication. In a significant number of instances, the overall communications these patients reported in this context were depicted as sufficiently helpful or unhelpful to permit legitimate characterization of their communication experience as generally negative or positive during this time period. Within the cohort of 60 patients in this study, 25 (42%) reported decidedly negative communication experiences pertaining to their diagnostic period, a proportion perhaps not surprising given the evidence in the literature as to the prevalence of poor cancer care communication.

For the purposes of this analysis into dynamics of poor communication, we drew on the reported instances patients characterized as unhelpful; an analysis of helpful communication is reported elsewhere (Thorne et al., in press). Specifically, the current analysis derives from the multiple transcripts from all 60 cohort members for illustrative material relevant to understanding what constitutes difficult communication encounters during the diagnostic time period from the patient perspective, with a particular emphasis on those 25 for whom the experience was predominantly negative. In doing so, we use the language of *difficult* to signal our recognition that this kind of study can pass no judgment on what actually occurred, but rather reflects what the patient perceived to have occurred. Thus, the term *difficult* captures what patients perceived as negative, unhelpful, or poor, without conveying the implication that this situation was associated with poor practice by a clinician. For additional depth, we drew purposively from the 7 of those 25 (representing 28% of the original negative group, and 11% of the cohort) whose characterization of their ongoing cancer communication experiences remained negative 1 year later. Although a majority of the participants in our study ran into occasional problems in communication or encountered individual professionals with whom communication seemed unusually difficult, all members of the cohort considered good communication with their providers as a fundamental requirement of effective cancer care. We found no instances in which an individual whose initial diagnostic cancer communication experience was positive arriving at the 1-year mark with a generally negative view of the current communication context. Thus, careful attention to what we might characterize as *communication casualties* seems of particular significance to understanding the potential negative impact of communication that misses the mark in the early stages of the cancer journey. The findings presented here therefore summarize patterns and themes within descriptions of the diagnostic encounters patients found difficult, and interpret what explains the resolution or continuation of difficult communications 1 year into the cancer journey.

The Dynamics of Difficult Communications

When study participants characterized their diagnostic communication experience as poor, they provided detailed illustrations and examples to explain what it was about that experience that affected them so strongly. Although each patient's story revealed unique features and nuances, we noted clear patterns within the dimensions that constituted what they considered to be poor communication. These patterns pertained to problematic indirect messages, a disrespectful manner, a failure to individualize, or mismatches between the nature and quantity of the information that was received in contrast to what they felt was required.

Indirect Messages

A significant subset of the study participants suspected or "knew" they had cancer because of signals that were inadvertently communicated to them prior to the actual delivery of the formal diagnosis. For example, during her screening colonoscopy, one woman overheard a nurse saying, "It will be okay, because there is enough to resect." Another woman overheard a technician in the diagnostic clinic muttering, "Oh no" when reviewing her scans and then walking away. A third patient reported being phoned by a receptionist to book a radiotherapy work-up prior to being told of his diagnosis or the recommendation for radiation treatment. Yet another patient reported that a relative had been advised to "take very good care of her because it isn't good news" while she was in recovery following surgery.

For some patients, the memory of the diagnostic consultation was strongly shaped by the message implied in the visible discomfort, awkwardness, or anxiety of the health care professional delivering the news. For example, one patient recalled his doctor pacing nervously throughout the session. "He didn't know what to say, you know, he really didn't. He just said, 'Well,' he says, 'that's it.' I didn't know what to do and he didn't really guide me." The sense that a health care professional charged with delivering news as important as a cancer diagnosis ought to be in possession of a particular communication skill set was shared by most of these patients.

However, as one recalled, "I felt like he was in training, that I was a guinea pig to this guy." In another example, a patient remembered the delivery of the diagnostic news as a speech or monologue that was delivered by a specialist who refused to take questions until the end, by which point the patient had forgotten all of the questions he might have incrementally raised. One patient recalled a physician who delivered the news standing rather than sitting in the manner of his usual consultation. A third recalled an encounter in which the clinician demanded that she sit, despite her instinct, in the context of a growing sense of alarm, that an insistence on standing might actually be the only "bit of control" she might legitimately hold onto in that particular moment.

In several instances, patients recalled the indirect use of language as a complicating factor in their understanding of their diagnosis. One described the physician as "pussyfooting around the diagnosis," whereas another remembered being informed that she had a tumor without being told whether or not it was malignant. A third patient described coming out of the diagnostic encounter uncertain as to whether he had lymphoma or stomach cancer because the lesions were referred to simply as "lumps in your stomach."

Another kind of indirect message that compromised the diagnostic communication pertained to system dynamics and processes. For example, one patient was able to interpret from the speed with which a referral to a specialist was enacted that he most likely had cancer. Another, whose cancer diagnosis occurred over the summer when a number of regular members of the health care team were on vacation, experienced the information as fragmented clues to her impending diagnosis from pieces shared by different health care professionals because no one person was prepared or equipped to tell her "the whole story." Thus, for these study participants, the overall climate of communication served as a powerful context within which individual diagnostic messages were received, digested, and interpreted, sometimes with compromising results.

Disrespectful or Unprofessional Manner

The most prevalent context in which diagnostic communication was perceived as negative by participants in this study was associated with the feeling that they were being treated as a "case" or a "number," rather than a unique individual worthy of respect. As one patient angrily expressed it, "I don't think the system gives a damn about the patients. I really think I am a number—'Blah, blah, blah'—in the cancer charts. I'm totally irrelevant, and not an individual at all." Another described the experience of feeling treated as a "piece of meat" rather than a person.

One particularly negative example of a communication encounter that characterized such behavior was an instance in which a patient described the physician as being late for the diagnostic consultation, and then proceeding to accept a personal phone call during which the content of the conversation was sufficiently humorous to occasion audible laughter. The patient perceived this as a violation of sufficient concern that he subsequently reported it to the physician's regulatory body. Other instances in which the affect or language of clinicians was less overtly unprofessional or dismissive could be perceived as equally hurtful to patients. One patient described being informed of her diagnosis by a surgeon who stood at hospital room door and said, "It's cancer," and walked away. Feeling rushed during a diagnostic consultation was also associated with a perception that one was being dismissed or not fully dealt with. One patient recalled a diagnostic encounter in which the clinician said, "I just want you to know it's not that I'm choosing not to spend time with you but you need to realize we have very sick patients here." Another reported a diagnostic exchange in which he felt the clinician's manner was highly abrupt. From his perspective, "I was just somebody that was expendable. That's the way I took it anyway."

Patients described this feeling of being treated as a number or case as an absence of what they considered normal human connection between them and the health care provider with whom they were interacting. For example, one patient described a particularly negative experience when she was unexpectedly given a diagnosis and various details about her cancer although she was both mentally unprepared and physically exposed during a diagnostic procedure. As one participant theorized, health care professionals who deal with cancer might believe they need to keep a "seal" on their emotions because, if they do not, their doctor–patient relationships might get too "messy." For these patients, however, failure to show compassion or attempting to block the inherent emotionality associated with receiving a cancer diagnosis denied them a human connection with their health care provider and added significantly to the distress they were experiencing.

Failure to Individualize

Even when communications were considered generally respectful and professional, a number of the negative experiences reported by the study participants related to what they perceived as a failure to recognize them as unique individuals, different from any other patient, and to tailor approaches accordingly. For example, for some patients, not being called by their preferred name was a symbolic way of communicating that they were in no way memorable or special despite their situation. For others, lack of recognition of their full-time employment status and the challenge it posed for scheduling consultations reflected disinterest in their personal circumstances. Several patients felt that standardized approaches disregarded their particular background and expertise, and believed their special circumstances warranted communications that differed from those that might be appropriate for

the typical patient. For example, a patient who was a professional statistician resented the assumption that he would be satisfied with general statistical information without specific reference to his own demographic or disease features. Others reported what they perceived as standardized approaches to how cancer was discussed as dismissive of their personal communication style and preferences. As one patient cleverly expressed this disjuncture, "I want the abrupt information but I don't want it in an abrupt tone!"

A particular instance of the failure to individualize approaches during the diagnostic phase was evident in the various reports we heard from study participants relative to the use of the telephone to deliver the news that they had cancer. For some patients, the willingness of a physician to call them at home with the news was a powerful signal that they should not have to prolong the anxiety of waiting and that they deserved the information as soon as it was available. In such instances, patients understood that the alternative might have been an urgent request that they make an office appointment, which would have significantly heightened their anxiety. However, for other participants in this study, a telephone diagnosis exemplified a distancing mechanism and a failure to individualize communications. One patient recalled being horrified by a phone message that was left late on a Friday afternoon while she was at work, breaking the news that she had cancer and suggesting she make an appointment for the following week when she had had time to "digest" the information. Another, who was given her cancer diagnosis directly over the phone during a work day, while she was in the midst of running a home-operated business, felt the physician had demonstrated no consideration for her particular professional circumstances. Thus, the issue for these patients seemed not the telephone diagnosis in and of itself, but what that communication approach revealed about the clinician's awareness of and sensitivity to their distinctive needs and circumstances.

Inappropriate Nature or Quantity of Information

A final major problematic communication theme within these accounts of the diagnostic period pertained to what patients perceived as mismatches between the quality and quantity of information they needed and what they received. Although most patients begin the cancer journey with relatively little technical information, many quickly develop considerable sophistication with regard to the complexity associated with a cancer diagnosis and related issues including treatment decision making and prognostication. In a number of instances, study participants ultimately concluded that they had not been given "the complete story" about their cancer based on subsequent understandings of important information that was available to their health professionals at the time of diagnosis. From the perspective of these patients, in some instances this occurred because the communication competencies of the clinician were inadequate to deliver such news, and in others it was because the clinician delivering the diagnosis had knowledge deficits. For example, one patient believed that the physician had withheld information about the cancer stage, even though it was available at the time of diagnosis. Another recalled that his family physician explained that he "did not actually know much about this type of cancer" and therefore simply provided him the name of it on a piece of paper.

Though incomplete information was a distinct worry for some patients, others experienced problematic communication related to "too much" information or information that was badly timed or inappropriate. One patient recalled that, immediately on being told that the diagnosis was cancer, her physician went on to explain that she should not feel guilty and that there were medications to treat depression. Another reported being told that he ought to be pleased about his particular kind of cancer, as it was easier to treat than some of the other cancers. A third felt that she was given far too much information when considerable detail about possible treatments was offered before all her diagnostic test results were fully analyzed and interpreted. In her case, information-induced anxiety emerged as a byproduct of trying to understand and then reinterpret what would happen over time.

In some instances, patients could point to specific information they had been provided that turned out to have been factually or interpretively incorrect. One man reported being initially told that he most likely had bladder wall cancer, only to be later informed that it was actually a stone and that he was "home free." However, he was subsequently notified that both guesses were wrong and that the correct diagnosis was actually prostate cancer. While he was capable of sympathizing with the difficulties posed by differential diagnosis, he found the degree of certainty with which the earlier incorrect conclusions had been put forward made it difficult for him to trust the subsequent recommendations of health care professionals.

A final element associated with the information provided during the diagnostic encounter was associated with the degree of hopefulness that was communicated by the clinician to the patient. Although patients acknowledged that a cancer diagnosis in which there is a bleak outlook is exceedingly difficult to discuss, they were particularly affronted by communications that seemed designed to deprive them of any hope. One woman, diagnosed with a particularly aggressive cancer, vividly recalled asking her physician, "Can you give me any hope?" As she remembered the encounter, his hasty reply was, "That's not my area." Even as patients recognized that they needed accurate information, many found that they also relied on their clinicians to find the "positive spin" they needed to face it. Thus, they were particularly distressed by health care professionals whose perpetual approach seemed to be "knocking my spirits down" rather than helping them find a way forward.

Reflections a Year Later

At the 12-month post-diagnosis mark, the patients in this study were asked to reflect on their experience with communications during the diagnostic period, retelling it from the perspective of time and experience. We were particularly interested in comparing these retrospective accounts with those acquired in the more immediate diagnostic timeframe to determine whether they surfaced any substantive reinterpretation of what effective and problematic communication entailed, or whether elements viewed with a particular valence in the initial experience might have been reframed based on knowledge gained with experience over time. In these accounts, we detected various shifts in the precision of details and the intensity of emotion associated with recall. As one patient described it,

> There's a sort of haziness of memory about the actual sequence of events but the feelings that I felt at the time are still pretty clear, you know. I felt concerned and worried. And you're so thirsty for as much information as I possibly could get, but also cognizant of the fact that I had limited ability to take it in.

In most instances, however, the initial and 12-month accounts were remarkably similar in their content, tone, and quality, even to the point of identical wording in key passages, as if they had been the source of considerable rumination, rendered repeatedly in accounts to others, and committed to memory. This strong emotional tone, even 1 year later, reveals the importance of these early communication experiences in the trajectory of the patient's cancer journey.

Following diagnosis, cancer patients enter a trajectory that might involve various health care professionals, treatments, and care contexts, depending on such factors as their disease type and stage, and the geographical location in which they lived. In some instances, their cancer was managed by clinicians other than those who provided the diagnosis, and in others, the primary management remained fairly constant. Thus some

patients were able to "move on" from the specific clinician with whom the initial problematic communication occurred and others were not. Some patients encountered numerous professionals, in which case the effective communication of one might have buffered the effects of problematic communication with another. Other patients might have had options with regard to switching services to obtain a better communication match. Thus, a progression with regard to the cancer communication experience 1 year later might not reflect a change in the dynamic of any one patient–professional dyad, but rather changing circumstances and opportunities within a comprehensive system of care. Furthermore, regardless of the generally positive or negative communication experience of any individual study participant, a majority reported both positive and negative individual encounters along the way. Nevertheless, it is informative to consider how patients whose communication experiences did and did not improve accounted for their evolving circumstances.

For 7 study participants, the early diagnostic experiences characterized as predominantly difficult were recalled as similarly problematic 12 months later. This group included 2 men and 5 women, aged 49 to 66 years (mean = 55.7), with a range of tumor sites (two lung, two colorectal, and one each of breast, prostate, and leukemia). Among them, 3 had undergone surgery, 3 chemotherapy, and 2 radiation therapy, with 1 having had no treatment. The initial diagnosis was delivered to them by their own family physician (in 4 cases), a locum covering for the usual general practitioner (1), a specialist (2), or a radiologist (1). Over the course of the initial year, 4 had discontinued the relationship with the initial clinician they described as problematic. All of these patients had encountered multiple health care professionals over this period, and 5 described themselves as very happy with the communication of at least one of their specialist practitioners. However, although only 1 patient characterized communication with all of her health care professionals as problematic, all 7 were continuing to receive at least some of their care within a communication context that they characterized as poor. When asked to explain why they thought this to be the case, most cited the continuing sense that they were not being treated as individuals by the clinicians overseeing their care. Though this group was reasonably certain that their clinical care was technically competent, some described feeling highly frustrated that they had never received the compassion they felt they deserved, and reported a litany of continuing communication difficulties, including misinformation, intimidation, and distrust that tainted aspects of their life quality with cancer. Others seemed more resigned to their situation, indicating that they felt they had learned to tolerate problematic communication and accept that the particular clinician overseeing their care was incapable of anything better.

The remaining 18 of the original 25 whose communications were initially characterized as predominantly difficult had resolved that situation and reported their communications to be generally positive at the 1-year point. This group included 14 women and 4 men, aged 35 to 81 years (mean = 54.4), whose tumor sites represented breast (8), lymphoma (4), prostate (3), gynecological (2), and colorectal (1) cancer. All but 1 had undergone cancer treatment, including 13 who had surgery, 9 chemotherapy, and 4 radiation therapy. The initial diagnosis had been delivered to them by an oncologist (5), a radiologist (4), a surgeon (3), another specialist (3), or a general practitioner (2). When asked to account for this change over the course of the year, they described factors relating to their own learning and agency as well as taking advantage of the opportunity to engage with clinicians who were more skilled communicators. For a number of these patients, communication improved immediately on shifting the locus of care to the oncology clinical specialty service. Many noted considerably more attention paid to the value of effective communication as well as skill with enacting it among cancer care specialists compared to the generalist health care professionals who might have been involved during the diagnostic period. Thus, the switch to clinicians with whom communication was more effective occurred as a matter of course within the care trajectory for some patients. In other cases, patients felt that it simply took time to develop rapport, and found that they were able to respond differently to particular clinicians once they better understood how to engage with them and interpret their particular communication approaches.

Among this group of patients whose communications had progressed from difficult to generally positive, a majority attributed this change to their own capacity to take "active control" of the communication circumstances. For example, in some cases, they sought alternative opinions or changed health care professionals. Some study participants reported actively avoiding certain clinicians, through such mechanisms as refusing to be seen by trainees or by clinicians of a certain gender. Others described themselves as actively petitioning to be referred to particular clinicians who came well recommended by fellow patients.

A number of these participants also took control in advocating for themselves in terms of their own communication needs. For example, one patient, who had found her oncologist's serious demeanor highly intimidating, took the initiative of some innocuous joking with him as a strategic way to set the course for the kind of ongoing relationship she felt she needed. From her perspective, her success with this maneuver made their subsequent communications more lighthearted and hopeful. Other patients claimed they had developed an approach of advocating on their own behalf by repeatedly reminding their health care professionals of their particular communication needs. A significant number of these study participants referenced having taught their clinicians how to engage with them in a manner that was supportive of their need for hope. As one patient explained, "I mean let's be truthful, it's pretty grim. But I'll say to them, 'I need hope because I'm such a believer that hope will increase my chances.'" As another reiterated, "I read a lot of body language. And they can tell me something that might be taken as bad news, but if they have a bit of a smile or a twinkle in their eye when they're talking to me, that gives me hope."

Thus, for the participants in this study, communication was a powerfully influential element of their initial cancer care experience and remained important 1 year later. For those whose initial communication experiences were difficult, the impact of those experiences was lasting. Fortunately, many were able, by circumstance or design, to resolve the negative communication for the most part and to find at least one point of effective communication within the system. Their insights into the necessity of ensuring that their communication was as effective as possible reinforce the power of the communication encounter to shape the tone and structure of the cancer experience.

DISCUSSION

Although many of the communication difficulties articulated by these patients as compromising their experience during the cancer diagnosis period are not dissimilar to the kinds of difficult communication patterns that have been reported elsewhere in relation to cancer care in general (Arora, 2003; Hack et al., 2005), these findings orient us to the particularities of these early, initial encounters and reveal the need to thoughtfully consider their potential impact on the journey on which the patient is embarking. The initial diagnosis period stands out for patients as the moment, frozen in time, during which their worst fears are realized (Walsh & Nelson, 2003). In many instances, the clinician delivering that initial news is not a cancer specialist, and is incapable of answering the urgent questions that patients inevitably have. Following the moment of first being informed one has cancer, there is typically a wait

to be seen by the cancer specialist who will determine the course of action. The first consultation with that specialist becomes a time in which treatment plans must be formulated on the basis of the cancer, any comorbidities, and distinctive circumstances. At the same time, the specialist is charged with attempting to establish a rapport with the patient, learning about their concerns and needs, understanding their expectations, and ascertaining how they would prefer to receive and titrate information. From the patient perspective, these encounters become part of the momentum that is starting to build, sweeping them up in a biological, psychosocial, emotional, and experiential turmoil. In this context, complex concepts are to be understood and decisions made that might well have a profound influence on the remainder of their lives.

This situational context helps us appreciate why the diagnostic period plays a particularly meaningful role in creating the foundation for a cancer journey that is characterized by either supportive or compromised communication (Epstein & Street, 2007). As cancer care evolves, the "agenda" for many subsequent clinical consultations often becomes more problem- or treatment-focused. By the time there might be subsequent bad news, such as regarding metastastic [*sic*] disease, many specialists will have formed good working relationships with their patients. Thus, although these subsequent "bad news" occasions remain times of particular vulnerability to poor communication, many patients experience them within a relational context that is more solidly established than was the case during their initial diagnostic experience.

Vivid recall and emotionality associated with poor communication in the initial diagnostic period remained remarkably fresh 12 months later for these patients. This was especially the case for the subset whose communication experiences could be characterized overall as negative. For those unfortunate individuals unable to negotiate a more positive communication environment, whether through circumstance or capacity for self-efficacy, the burden of continuing communication problems added to their distress and deprived them of an important source of comfort. However, except for a small minority of the participants in our study who were unable to fully resolve their communication challenges, most did find their way forward into a cancer care environment within which they had at least some access to helpful and effective communication. This suggests that, although the initial problematic communication might have set the stage for future difficulties, there were also multiple ways in which a "communication rescue" could occur. For many patients, this came about naturally in the course of encountering multiple professionals, especially oncology specialists and allied health professionals with a specialty in cancer care. For other patients, it required active intervention on their part to strategize and develop ways of motivating the specific professionals involved in their care toward more constructive communications. And in a significant number of cases, communication became increasingly effective because of a combination of both professional and patient strategic engagement.

Although the value of communication in cancer care might not have been self-evident prior to their diagnosis, it was strongly recognized thereafter by all of the patients in this study. Their accounts revealed accessing an impressive array of suggestions and techniques for improving their communication experiences from such resources as patient support services, Internet chat sites, mass media consumer advice, and their own social networks. Clearly, the presence of a powerful network of community-based advice and support was instrumental to the development of ideas and options, especially toward preventing future problems in their communications with cancer care providers. Additionally, many attributed important experiential learning associated with effective communication to exposure to

certain cancer care clinicians whose ways of engaging helped them envision what was possible. Thus, though preventing communication problems remains a high priority, it would seem that intervening after they have occurred could be another powerful tool for building a base toward future sensitive communication occasions that might unfortunately become necessary in the course of the cancer illness. Furthermore, the accounts confirmed that although some initially problematic patient–provider relationships can indeed be "rescued," there might be others for which it is feasible and perhaps preferable to change clinicians and "start over."

Among the many features of difficult communication that the participants in this study articulated and that have been reported in the literature, negotiations around hope perpetually stand out as the single most challenging and troublesome battleground (Evans et al., 2006; Hack et al., 2005). Although information, decisional guidance, compassion, and support feature strongly in the substance of cancer care communication across the spectrum, the spectre of hope reflects a pervasive complicating dimension (Thorne, Oglov, Armstrong, & Hislop, 2007). Patients typically report the denial of hope as the most serious violation inherent in poor cancer communication (Clayton, Butow, Arnold, & Tattersall, 2005). Clinicians note the profound complexity inherent in their obligation to provide patients with the level and detail of information to which they have a legal and ethical right, while at the same time supporting their emotional well-being (Salander, Bergenheim, Bergstrom, & Henriksson, 1998; Sardell & Trierweiler, 1993). Fostering unrealistic hope is commonly understood as incompetent practice. The clinician is inevitably caught between the dual requirements of providing accurate information about the seriousness of the bodily condition and concurrent hopefulness for the patient's personal well-being, without inadvertently misleading the patient or causing additional harm (Hagerty et al., 2005; Leydon, 2008).

In the context of newly formed patient–provider relationships, when the emotional shock is profound and the information to be processed complex, the diagnostic period becomes a phase within the cancer trajectory when supportive approaches to ensure optimal communication seem most acutely needed. In this context, diagnostic and prognostic information are most easily conflated in the consideration of what to expect and what can be hoped for. The initial diagnostic phase therefore seems a situation for which adequate time and support ought to be paramount planning concerns. It is well recognized that most cancer care systems are under severe stress (Canadian Strategy for Cancer Control, 2006), and equitable apportioning of scarce expert resources precludes the kind of time and access to medical specialists that most patients would optimally prefer (Epstein & Street, 2007; Thorne, Hislop, Stajduhar, & Oglov, 2008). Although many efforts are under way to minimize undue waiting times in the initial consultation context, delays are likely inevitable. It is therefore unrealistic to expect that medical specialists within existing cancer system structures can accommodate the full range of communication and supportive needs of newly diagnosed patients. Thus, it seems time to consider better ways to capitalize on the communication resources that reside within the allied health professions, especially advanced practice nurses (Ambler et al., 2007; Gentry & Sein, 2007; Jarrett & Payne, 2000; Skrutkowski et al., 2008), as well as the expanding array of available patient/consumer advocacy networks (Decter & Grosso, 2006) and Internet information/support platforms (Decter & Grosso, 2006; Intille & Zabinski, 2005; Weiss & Lorenzi, 2005). Ensuring that patients have a range of options to communicate their needs and concerns, with the proviso that there are effective mechanisms for aligning the insights and issues that arise from these communications into the care management process, seems a logical priority for preventing and ameliorating what we know to be a significant "iatrogenic" problem within cancer care (Parker et al., 2005).

CONCLUSIONS

Although considerable knowledge transfer effort has been directed toward preventing poor communication in cancer care, the problematic practice patterns among a subset of clinicians have proven astonishingly difficult to eradicate (Epstein & Street, 2007; Thorne et al., 2005); analyses of both basic and continuing education communications training outcomes suggest modest results at best (Butler et al., 2005; Fallowfield & Jenkins, 2006; Fellowes, Wilkinson, & Moore, 2004). Thus, studies such as this from the cancer patient perspective provide a valid basis for considering alternative approaches to both strengthening general awareness of the inherent value of communication across the cancer care system and addressing the sequelae of problematic communication when it occurs. In the current context, effective and engaged interprofessional cancer care teams, capitalizing on the distinct competencies of a range of professionals, working collaboratively with patient networks and consumer advocacy systems, seems a highly promising direction for advancement. Aligning the communication challenge with the larger policy mandate of a fully coordinated cancer care system, we can advance services at a population level while continuing to be mindful of the very real needs of the individuals we are privileged to serve.

DECLARATION OF CONFLICTING INTERESTS

The authors declared no conflicts of interest with respect to the authorship and/or publication of this article.

FUNDING

The authors disclosed receipt of the following financial support for the research and/or authorship of this article: Funding was provided by research grant # 74545 from the Canadian Institutes of Health.

REFERENCES

Ambler, N., Rumsey, N., Harcourt, D., Khan, F., Cawthorn, S., & Barker, J. (2007). Specialist nurse counsellor interventions at the time of diagnosis of breast cancer: Comparing "advocacy" with a conventional approach. *Journal of Advanced Nursing*, *29*(3), 445-453.

Arora, N. K. (2003). Interacting with cancer patients: The significance of physicians' communication behavior. *Social Science and Medicine*, *57*, 791-806.

Back, A. L., Arnold, R. M., Baile, W. F., Tulsky, J. A., & Fryer-Edwards, K. (2005). Approaching difficult communication tasks in oncology. *CA: A Cancer Journal for Clinicians*, *55*(3), 164-177.

Baile, W. F., & Aaron, J. (2005). Patient–physician communication in oncology: Past, present, and future. *Current Opinion in Oncology*, *17*(4), 331-335.

Beach, W. A., Easter, D. W., Good, J. S., & Pigeron, E. (2005). Disclosing and responding to cancer "fears" during oncology interviews. *Social Science and Medicine*, *60*, 893-910.

Butler, L., Degner, L., Baile, W., Landry, M., & SCRN Communication Team. (2005). Developing communication competency in the context of cancer: A critical interpretive analysis of provider training programs. *Psycho-Oncology*, *14*(10), 861-872.

Butow, P. (2005). The communication goals and needs of cancer patients: A review. *Psycho-Oncology*, *14*, 846-847.

Canadian Strategy for Cancer Control. (2006). *The Canadian strategy for cancer control: A cancer plan for Canada*. Retrieved January 2, 2008, from http://www.cancer.ca/vgn/images/portal/cit_86751114/10/2/1404842209cw_CSCC_Discussion_Paper_July_2006_v2.pdf

Carlson, L. E., Feldman-Stewart, D., Tishelman, C., Brundage, M. D., & SCRN Communication Team. (2005). Patient–professional communication research in cancer: An integrative review of research methods in the context of a conceptual framework. *Psycho-Oncology*, *14*, 812-828.

Clayton, J. M., Butow, P. N., Arnold, R. M., & Tattersall, M. H. (2005). Fostering coping and nurturing hope when discussing the future with terminally ill cancer patients and their caregivers. *Cancer*, *103*(9), 1965-1975.

Cox, A., Jenkins, V., Catt, S., Langridge, C., & Fallowfield, L. (2006). Information needs and experiences: An audit of UK cancer patients. *European Journal of Oncology Nursing*, *10*(4), 263-272.

Davis, T. C., Williams, M. V., Marin, E., Parker, R. M., & Glass, J. (2002). Health literacy and cancer communication. *CA: A Cancer Journal for Clinicians*, *52*(3), 134-149.

Davison, R., & Mills, M. E. (2005). Cancer patients' satisfaction with communication, information and quality of care in the UK region. *European Journal of Cancer Care*, *14*, 83-90.

Decter, M., & Grosso, F. (2006). *Navigating Canada's health care: A user guide to getting the care you need*. Toronto, ON, Canada: Penguin.

Edvardsson, T. M., Pahlson, A., & Ahlstrom, G. P. (2006). Experiences of onset and diagnosis of low-grade glioma from the patient's perspective. *Cancer Nursing*, *29*(5), 415-422.

Eggly, S., Penner, L. A., Greene, M., Harper, F. W. K., Ruckdeschel, J. C., & Albrecht, T. L. (2006). Information seeking during "bad news" oncology interactions: Questions asked by patients and their companions. *Social Science and Medicine*, *63*(11), 2974-2985.

Epstein, R. M., & Street, R. L. (2007). *Patient-centered communication in cancer care: Promoting healing and reducing suffering*. NIH publication No. 07-6225. Bethesda, MD: National Institutes of Health.

Evans, W. G., Tulsky, J. A., Back, A. L., & Arnold, R. M. (2006). Communication at times of transitions: How to help patients cope with loss and redefine hope. *Cancer Journal*, *12*(5), 417-424.

Fallowfield, L., & Jenkins, V. (2004). Communicating sad, bad, and difficult news in medicine. *Lancet*, *363*, 312-319.

Fallowfield, L., & Jenkins, V. (2006). Current concepts of communication skills training in oncology. *Recent Results in Cancer Research*, *168*, 105-112.

Fallowfield, L. J. (2008). Treatment decision-making in breast cancer: The patient–doctor relationship. *Breast Cancer Research & Treatment*, *112*(Suppl 1), 5-13.

Feldman-Stewart, D., Brennenstuhl, S., & Brundage, M. D. (2007). A purpose-based evaluation of information for patients: An approach to measuring effectiveness. *Patient Education and Counseling*, *65*(3), 311-319.

Feldman-Stewart, D., Brundage, M. D., Tishelman, C., & SCRN Communication Team. (2005). A conceptual framework for patient–professional communication: An application to the cancer context. *Psycho-Oncology*, *14*(10), 801-809.

Fellowes, D., Wilkinson, S., & Moore, P. (2004). Communication skills training for health care professionals working with cancer patients, their families and/or carers. *Cochrane Database of Systematic Reviews, Issue 2, Art No: CD003751. DOI: 10.1002/14651858.CD003751.pub2.*

Gentry, S., & Sein, E. (2007). Taking the wheel. Oncology nurses help patients navigate the cancer journey. *ONS Connect, 22*(3), 8-11.

Glaser, B. G., & Strauss, A. L. (1967). *The discovery of grounded theory: Strategies for qualitative research.* Chicago: Aldine.

Hack, T. F., Degner, L. F., Parker, P. S., & SCRN Communication Team. (2005). The communication goals and needs of cancer patients: A review. *Psycho-Oncology, 14*(10), 831-845.

Hagerty, R. G., Butow, P. N., Ellis, P. M., Lobb, E. A., Pendlebury, S. C., Leighl, N., et al. (2005). Communicating with realism and hope: Incurable cancer patients' views on the disclosure of prognosis. *Journal of Clinical Oncology, 23*(6), 1278-1288.

Hoff, L., Tidefelt, U., Thaning, L., & Hermeren, G. (2007). In the shadow of bad news—Views of patients with acute leukaemia, myeloma or lung cancer about information, from diagnosis to cure or death. *BMC Palliative Care, 6*(1), doi:10.1186/1472-684X-6-1.

Intille, P., & Zabinski, M. F. (2005). An ecological framework for cancer communication: Implications for research. *Journal of Medical Internet Research, 7*(3), e23. Retrieved January 9, 2009, from http://www.jmir.org/2005/3/e23/

Jarrett, N., & Payne, S. (2000). Creating and maintaining "optimism" in cancer care communication. *International Journal of Nursing Studies, 37*, 81-90.

Kreps, G. L., Arora, N. K., & Nelson, D. E. (2003). Consumer/ provider communication research: Directions for development. *Patient Education and Counseling, 50*(1), 3-4.

Leydon, G. (2008). "Yours is potentially serious but most of these are cured": Optimistic communication in UK outpatient oncology consultations. *Psycho-Oncology, 17*, 1081-1088.

Lincoln, Y. S., & Guba, E. G. (1985). *Naturalistic inquiry.* Beverly Hills, CA: Sage.

Lockhart, K., Dosser, I., Cruickshank, S., & Kennedy, C. (2007). Methods of communicating a primary diagnosis of breast cancer to patients [systematic review]. *Cochrane Database of Systematic Reviews 2007;(3), CD006011.*

Miles, M. B., & Huberman, A. M. (1994). *Qualitative data analysis* (2nd ed.). Thousand Oaks, CA: Sage.

Nelson, C. M. (2004). The needs of recently diagnosed cancer patients. *Nursing Standard, 19*(13), 42-44.

Ong, L. M., Visser, M. R., Lammes, F., & de Haes, J. C. (2000). Doctor–patient communication and cancer patients' quality of life and satisfaction. *Patient Education and Counseling, 41*(2), 145-156.

Parker, P. A., Davison, B. J., Tishelman, C., & Brundage, M. D. (2005). What do we know about facilitating patient communication in the cancer care setting? *Psycho-Oncology, 14*, 848-858.

Patrick, K., Intille, S. S., & Zabinski, M. F. (2005). An ecological framework for cancer communication: Implications for research. *Journal of Medical Internet Research, 7*(3), e23.

Ptacek, J. T., & Ptacek, J. J. (2001). Patients' perceptions of receiving bad news about cancer. *Journal of Clinical Oncology, 19*(21), 4160-4164.

Ramirez, A. G. (2003). Consumer–provider communication research with special populations. *Patient Education and Counseling, 50*(1), 51-54.

Rutten, L. J. F., Arora, N. K., Bakos, A. D., Aziz, N., & Rowland, J. (2005). Information needs and sources of information among cancer patients: A systematic review of research (1980-2003). *Patient Education and Counseling, 57*(3), 250-261.

Salander, P., Bergenheim, A. T., Bergstrom, P., & Henriksson, R. (1998). How to tell cancer patients: A contribution to a theory of communicating the diagnosis. *Journal of Psychosocial Oncology, 16*(2), 79-93.

Sandelowski, M. (2000). Whatever happened to qualitative description? *Research in Nursing & Health, 23*, 334-340.

Sandelowski, M., Trimble, F., Woodard, E. K., & Barroso, J. (2006). From synthesis to script: Transforming qualitative research findings for use in practice. *Qualitative Health Research, 16*, 1350-1370.

Sardell, A. N., & Trierweiler, S. J. (1993). Disclosing the cancer diagnosis: Procedures that influence patient hopefulness. *Cancer, 72*(11), 3355-3365.

Schofield, P. E., Beeney, L. J., Thompson, J. F., Butow, P. N., Tattersall, M. H. N., & Dunn, S. M. (2001). Hearing the bad news of a cancer diagnosis: The Australian melanoma patient's perspective. *Annals of Oncology, 12*(3), 365-371.

Schofield, P. E., & Butow, P. N. (2004). Towards better communication in cancer care: A framework for developing evidence-based interventions. *Patient Education and Counseling, 55*(1), 32-39.

Schofield, P. E., Butow, P. N., Thompson, J. F., Tattersall, M. H. N., Beeney, L. J., & Dunn, S. M.

(2003). Psychological responses of patients receiving a diagnosis of cancer. *Annals of Oncology*, *14*(1), 48-56.

Siminoff, L. A., Graham, G. C., & Gordon, N. H. (2006). Cancer communication patterns and the influence of patient characteristics: Disparities in information-giving and affective behaviors. *Patient Education and Counseling*, *62*(3), 355-360.

Skrutkowski, M., Saucier, A., Eades, M., Swidzinski, M., Ritchie, J., Marchionni, C., et al. (2008). Impact of a pivot nurse in oncology on patients with lung or breast cancer: Symptom distress, fatigue, quality of life, and use of health-care resources. *Oncology Nursing Forum*, *35*(6), 948-954.

Taylor, E., Ismail, S., Hills, H., & Ainsworth, S. (2004). Multi-component Psychosocial support for newly diagnosed cancer patients: participants' views. *International Journal of Palliative Nursing*, *10*(6), 287-295.

Thorne, S., Hislop, T., Stajduhar, K., & Oglov, V. (2008). Time-related communication skills from the cancer patient perspective. *Psycho-Oncology*, *Pre-press: DOI: 10.1002/pon.1418*.

Thorne, S., Oglov, V., Armstrong, E.-A., & Hislop, T. G. (2007). Prognosticating futures and the human experience of hope. *Palliative and Supportive Care*, *5*(3), 227-239.

Thorne, S., Oliffe, J., Kim-Sing, C., Hislop, T. G., Stajduhar, K., Harris, S. R., et al. (in press). Helpful communications during the diagnostic period: An interpretive description of patient preferences. *European Journal of Cancer Care*.

Thorne, S., Reimer Kirkham, S., & MacDonald-Emes, J. (1997). Interpretive description: A non-categorical qualitative alternative for developing nursing knowledge. *Research in Nursing & Health*, *20*(2), 169-177.

Thorne, S. E. (2008). *Interpretive description*. Walnut Creek, CA: Left Coast Press.

Thorne, S. E., Bultz, B. D., Baile, W. F., & SCRN Communication Team. (2005). Is there a cost to poor communication in cancer care?: A critical review of the literature. *Psycho-Oncology*, *14*, 875-884.

Walsh, D., & Nelson, K. A. (2003). Communication of a cancer diagnosis: Patients' perceptions of when they were first told they had cancer. *American Journal of Hospice & Palliative Care*, *20*(1), 52-56.

Watson, D. E., Mooney, D., & Peterson, S. (2007). *Patient experiences with ambulatory cancer care in British Columbia, 2005/06*. Retrieved July 20, 2008, from http://www.chspr.ubc.ca/files/publications/2007/chspr_07_4R.pdf

Weiss, J., & Lorenzi, N. (2005). *Online communication and support for cancer patients: A relationship-centric design framework*. Paper presented at the Proceedings of American Medical Informatics Association Annual Symposium, pp. 799-803. Retrieved January 9, 2009, from: http://www.pubmedcentral.nih.gov/articlerender.fcgi?artid=1560480

Glossary

A

a priori From Latin, meaning "the former"; that is, before the study or analysis.

abstract A brief, comprehensive summary of a study at the beginning of an article.

accessible population A population that meets the population criteria and is available.

accuracy The characteristic of all aspects of a study systematically and logically following from the research problem.

after-only design An experimental design with two randomly assigned groups: a treatment group and a control group. This design differs from the true experiment in that both groups are measured only after the experimental treatment. Also known as *posttest-only control group design.*

after-only nonequivalent control group design A quasiexperimental design similar to the after-only experimental design except that participants are not randomly assigned to the treatment group or the control group.

aim of inquiry The goals or specific objectives of the research, which vary with the *paradigm.*

alpha Considered an a priori probability because it is set before the data are collected. Also considered a conditional probability because the null hypothesis is assumed to be true.

alpha coefficient See *reliability coefficient.*

alternate-form reliability A reliability measure in which two or more alternate forms of a measure are administered to the same participants at different times. The scores of the two tests determine the degree of relationship between the measures. Also called *parallel-form reliability.*

analysis The division of the content into parts to understand each aspect of the study.

analysis of covariance (ANCOVA) A statistic that measures differences among group means and uses a statistical technique to equate the groups under study in relation to an important variable.

analysis of variance (ANOVA) A statistic that tests whether group means differ from each other; instead of testing each pair of means separately, ANOVA considers the variation among all groups.

animal rights Guidelines used to protect the rights of animals in the conduct of research.

anonymity A research participant's protection in a study so that no one, not even the researcher, can link the subject with the information given.

antecedent variable A variable that affects the dependent variable but occurs before the introduction of the independent variable.

assent An aspect of informed consent that pertains to protecting the rights of children as research participants.

assumptions Accepted truths, key concepts and ideas, reasons and justifications, supporting examples, parallel experiences, implications and consequences, and any other structural features of the written text used to interpret and assess it accurately and fairly.

attrition The loss of a subject from a study between time 1 data collection and time 2 data collection. Also called *mortality.*

auditability The characteristic of a qualitative study, developed by the investigator's research process, that allows another researcher or a reader to follow the thinking or conclusions of the investigator.

B

behavioural/materialist perspective In ethnographical studies, the observation of culture through a group's patterns of behaviour and customs, its way of life, and what it produces.

beneficence An obligation to do no harm and to maximize possible benefits.

benefits Potential positive outcomes of participation in a research study.

bias A distortion in the interpretation of the results of the data analysis.

biological measurement Use of specialized equipment to determine the biological status of participants in a study.

Boolean operator In a literature search, the word that defines the relationships between words or groups of words; for example, "AND," "OR," "NOT," or "NEAR."

bracketing A process by which the researcher identifies personal biases about the phenomenon of interest to clarify how personal experience and beliefs may colour what is heard and reported. The term comes from the mathematical metaphor of putting "brackets" around our beliefs so they can be put aside.

C

case study The study of a selected phenomenon that provides an in-depth description of its dimensions and processes.

case study method The study of a selected contemporary phenomenon over time to provide an in-depth description of the essential dimensions and processes of the phenomenon.

chance error An error attributable to fluctuations in subject characteristics that occur at a specific point in time and are often beyond the awareness and control of the examiner; an error that is difficult to control, unsystematic, and unpredictable and thus cannot be corrected. Also called *random error.*

chi-square (χ^2) A nonparametric statistic used to determine whether the frequency found in each category is different from the frequency that would be expected by chance.

citation management software A software program that formats and stores the researcher's citations so that they are available for electronic retrieval.

clinical question An inquiry that is the basis of evidence-informed practice. A clinical question concerns five components: population, intervention, comparison, outcome, and time (PICOT).

closed-ended item A question that the respondent may answer with only one of a fixed number of choices.

cluster sampling A probability sampling strategy that involves successive random sampling of units. The units sampled progress from large to small. Also known as *multistage sampling.*

codes Tags or labels that are assigned to themes in a qualitative study.

coding The progressive marking, sorting, resorting, and defining and redefining of the collected data.

cognitive perspective In ethnographical studies, the view that culture consists of beliefs, knowledge, and ideas people use as they live.

cohort The participants of a specific group that are being studied.

community-based participatory research A method by which the voice of a community is systematically accessed in order to plan context-appropriate action.

concealment An observational method that refers to whether or not the participants know that they are being observed.

concept An image or symbolic representation of an abstract idea.

conceptual definition The general meaning of a concept.

conceptual framework A structure of concepts, theories, or both that is used to construct a map for the study.

concurrent validity The degree of correlation between two measures of the same concept that are administered at the same time.

conduct of research The analysis of data collected from a homogeneous group of participants who meet study inclusion and exclusion criteria for the purpose of answering specific research questions or testing specified hypotheses.

confidence interval An estimated range of values, which are likely to include an unknown population parameter calculated from a given set of sample data. Abbreviated *CI.*

confidentiality Assurance that a research participant's identity cannot be linked to the information that was provided to the researcher.

consent Agreement to participate in a study. See *informed consent.*

consistency An aspect of the data collection process that requires that data be collected from each subject in the study in exactly the same way or as close to the same way as possible.

constancy An aspect of control in data collection that ensures that methods and procedures of data collection are the same for all participants; that is, each participant is exposed to the same environmental conditions, timing of data collection, data collection instruments, and data collection procedures.

constant comparative method In the grounded theory method, a process of continuously comparing data as they are acquired during research.

constant error See *systematic error.*

construct validity The extent to which a test measures a theoretical construct or trait.

constructivism The basis for *naturalistic* (qualitative) research, which developed from writers such as Immanuel Kant, who sought alternative ways of thinking about the world; a belief that reality is not fixed but rather is a construction of the people perceiving it.

constructivist paradigm The basis of most qualitative research, which is concerned with the ways in which people construct their worlds.

consumer A person whose activity uses and applies research.

content analysis A technique for the objective, systematic, and quantitative description of communications and documentary evidence.

content validity The degree to which the content of the measure represents the universe of content or the domain of a given behaviour.

context The personal, social, and political environment in which a phenomenon of interest (time, place, cultural beliefs, values, and practices) occurs.

context dependent Condition in which the meaning of an observation is defined by its circumstance or the environment.

contrasted-groups approach A method used to assess construct validity. A researcher identifies two groups of individuals who are suspected of having either an extremely high or an extremely low score on a characteristic; scores from the groups are obtained and examined for sensitivity to the differences. Also called *known-groups approach.*

control The measures used to hold uniform or constant the conditions in a research study.

control group The group in an experimental investigation that does not receive the experimental intervention or treatment; the comparison group.

controlled vocabulary A selected list of words and phrases that are applied to similar pieces of information units (e.g., life skills).

convenience sampling A nonprobability sampling strategy in which the most readily accessible persons or objects serve as participants or participants of a study.

convergent validity A type of construct validity in which two or more tools that theoretically measure the same construct are positively correlated.

correlation The degree of association between two variables.

correlational study A type of nonexperimental research that examines the relationship between two or more variables.

credibility A characteristic of qualitative research that refers to the accuracy, validity, and soundness of data.

criterion-related validity The degree of relationship between performance on the measure and the actual behaviour, either in the present (concurrent) or in the future (predictive).

critical reading An active interpretation and objective assessment of an article, during which the reader is looking for key concepts, ideas, and justifications.

critical social theory The use of both qualitative and quantitative research to highlight historical and current experiences of suffering, conflict, and collective struggles.

critical social thought A philosophical orientation that suggests that reality and a person's understanding of reality are constructed by people with the most power at a particular point in history.

critical thinking The rational examination of ideas, inferences, assumptions, principles, arguments conclusions, issues, statements, beliefs, and actions.

critique The process of objectively and critically evaluating the content of a research report for scientific merit and application to practice, theory, or education.

critiquing criteria The standards, appraisal guides, or questions used for objectively and critically evaluating a research article.

Cronbach's alpha A test of internal consistency in which each item in a scale is simultaneously compared with all others.

cross-sectional study Nonexperimental research in which data at one point in time—that is, in the immediate present—are examined.

culture The system of knowledge and linguistic expressions used by social groups that allows the researcher to interpret or make sense of the world; the structures of meaning through which people shape experiences.

***Cumulative Index to Nursing and Allied Health Literature* (CINAHL)** A print and computerized database; computerized CINAHL is available on CD-ROM and online.

D

data Information systematically collected in the course of a study; the plural of *datum.*

data display Compression and organization of data that promotes understanding and visualization and enables conclusions to be drawn.

data reduction The process of selecting and transforming the data from field notes or transcriptions.

data saturation A point when the information collected by the researcher becomes repetitive; ideas conveyed by the participant have been shared previously by other participants, and inclusion of additional participants does not result in new ideas.

debriefing The opportunity for researchers to discuss the study with the participants and for participants to refuse to have their data included in the study.

deductive Concluded from data.

deductive reasoning A logical thought process in which hypotheses are derived from theory; reasoning moves from the general to the particular.

degree of freedom The number of quantities that are unknown minus the number of independent equations linking these unknowns; a function of the number in the sample. Abbreviated *df.*

delimitations Characteristics that restrict the population to a homogeneous group of participants.

dependent variable In experimental studies, the presumed effect of the independent or experimental variable on the outcome. Variation in the independent variable changes this effect. The dependent variable is observed but not manipulated.

descriptive/exploratory survey A type of nonexperimental research in which descriptions of existing phenomena are collected for the purpose of using the data to justify or assess current conditions or to make plans for improvement of conditions.

descriptive statistics Statistical details used to describe and summarize sample data.

design The plan or blueprint for conduct of a study.

developmental study A type of nonexperimental research that is concerned not only with the existing status and interrelationships of phenomena but also with changes that occur as a function of time.

directional hypothesis A hypothesis that specifies the expected direction of the relationship between independent and dependent variables.

dissemination The communication of research findings.

divergent validity A type of construct validity in which two or more tools that theoretically measure the opposite of the construct are negatively correlated.

domains In an ethnographic study, symbolic categories that include smaller categories.

E

effect size Measurement of the magnitude of a treatment effect; how large of a difference is observed between the groups.

element The most basic unit about which information is collected.

eligibility criteria Characteristics of a population that meet requirements for inclusion in a study.

emic perspective The native's or insider's view of the world.

empirical-analytical A general label for quantitative research approaches that test hypotheses.

empirical factors Those things that can be observed through the senses; the obtaining of evidence or objective data.

empirical literature A synonym for data-based literature.

epidemiological study Examination of factors affecting the health and illness of populations in relation to the environment.

epistemology The theory of knowledge; the branch of philosophy concerned with how people know what they know, or what is known to be "truth."

equivalence Consistency or agreement among observers using the same measurement tool, or agreement among alternative forms of a tool.

error variance The extent to which the variance in test scores is attributable to error rather than to a true measure of behaviours.

ethics The theory or discipline dealing with principles of moral values and moral conduct.

ethnographic method A method that scientifically describes cultural groups. The goal of the ethnographer is to understand the natives' view of their world.

ethnography A qualitative research approach designed to produce cultural theory. Also called *ethnographic research.*

etic perspective An outsider's view of another's world.

evaluation The process of determining the value of data.

evaluation research The use of scientific research methods and procedures to evaluate a program, treatment, practice, or policy outcomes; the analytical means used to document the worth of an activity.

evidence-based practice The conscious, explicit, and judicious use of the current best evidence in the care of patients and the delivery of health care services.

evidence-informed practice Acknowledging and considering the myriad factors beyond such evidence as local indigenous knowledge, cultural and religious norms, and clinical judgement.

evidence-informed practice guidelines Principles that help the researcher better understand the evidence base of certain practices.

ex post facto study A type of nonexperimental research that examines the relationships among variables after variations have occurred. Also known as a *causal-comparative study,* a *comparative study,* and (by epidemiologists) a *retrospective study.*

exclusion criteria Criteria used to exclude individuals from participating in a study.

experiment A scientific investigation in which observations are made and data are collected by means of the characteristics of control, randomization, and manipulation.

experimental design A research design that has the following properties: randomization, control, and manipulation.

experimental group The group in an experimental investigation that receives the experimental intervention or treatment.

external criticism A process used to judge the authenticity of historical data.

external validity The degree to which the findings of a study can be generalized to other populations or environments.

extraneous variable A variable that interferes with the operations of the phenomena being studied. Also called *mediating variable*.

F

face validity A type of content validity in which an expert's opinion is used to judge the accuracy of an instrument.

factor analysis A strategy for assessing construct validity in which a statistical procedure is used to determine the underlying dimensions or components of a variable and to assess the degree to which the individual items on a scale truly cluster around one or more dimensions.

feasibility The capability of the study to be successfully carried out.

findings The statistical results of a study and the conclusions, interpretations, recommendations, generalizations, and implications for future research and nursing practice.

Fisher's exact probability test An analysis used to compare frequencies when samples are small and expected frequencies are less than six in each cell.

fittingness The degree to which study findings are applicable outside the study situation and how meaningful the results are to individuals not involved in the research.

formative evaluation Assessment of a program as it is being implemented, usually focusing on evaluation of the process of a program rather than the outcomes.

frequency distribution A descriptive statistical method for summarizing the occurrences of events under study.

G

generalizability (generalize) The extent to which data can be inferred to be representative of similar phenomena in a population beyond the studied sample.

"grand tour" question A question in a qualitative study that reflects a broad overview of the issue to be studied.

grounded theory A research approach that is constructed inductively from a base of observations of the world as it is lived by a selected group of people.

grounded theory method An inductive approach in which a systematic set of procedures is used to develop theory about basic social processes.

H

Hawthorne effect See *reactivity*.

hermeneutics A theoretical framework in which to understand or interpret human phenomena from the study of those phenomena.

heterogeneity Dissimilarities of a sample group, which inhibit the researchers' ability to interpret the findings meaningfully and make generalizations.

hierarchical linear modelling (HLM) A type of regression analysis that allows for analysis of hierarchically structured data simultaneously at all levels.

historical research method The systematic approach for understanding the past through collection, organization, and critical appraisal of facts.

history threat The threat to internal validity that events outside of the experimental setting may affect the dependent variable.

homogeneity A similarity of conditions. Also called *internal consistency*.

homogeneous Having limited variation in attributes or characteristics.

hypothesis A best guess or prediction about what a researcher expects to find with regard to the relationship between two or more variables.

hypothesis-testing approach A strategy for assessing construct validity in which the theory or concept underlying a measurement instrument's design is used to develop hypotheses that are tested. Inferences are made based on the findings about whether the rationale underlying the instrument's construction is adequate to explain the findings.

I

incidence The number of cases occurring in a particular period.

inclusion criteria Criteria that an individual must satisfy to participate in a study.

independent variable The antecedent or variable that has the presumed effect on the dependent variable. The independent variable is manipulated in experimental research studies.

inductive Generalizing from specific data.

inductive reasoning A logical thought process in which generalizations are developed from specific observations; reasoning moves from the particular to the general.

inferential statistics Statistical details that combine mathematical processes and logic to test hypotheses about a population with the help of sample data.

informed consent An ethical principle that requires a researcher to inform individuals about the potential benefits and risks of a study before the individuals can participate voluntarily.

instrumental case study Research undertaken to pursue insight into an issue or to challenge a generalization.

instrumentation threats Changes in the measurement of the variables that may account for changes in the obtained measurement.

internal consistency The extent to which items within a scale reflect or measure the same concept. Also called *homogeneity.*

internal criticism The process of judging the reliability or consistency of information within a historical document.

internal validity The degree to which the experimental treatment, not an uncontrolled condition, resulted in the observed effects.

interrater reliability The consistency of observations between two or more observers; often expressed as a percentage of agreement between raters or observers or a coefficient of agreement that takes into account the element of chance; generally used with the direct observation method.

intersubjectivity A person's belief that other people share a common world with him or her; an important tenet in phenomenology.

interval measurement A type of measurement in which events or objects are ranked on a scale, with equal intervals between numbers but with a ranking set arbitrarily at zero (e.g., Celsius temperature).

intervening variable A condition that occurs during an experimental or quasiexperimental study that affects the dependent variable.

intervention An observational method that deals with whether or not the observer provokes actions from those who are being observed.

intervention fidelity Consistency in data collection.

interview A method of data collection in which a data collector questions a subject verbally. Such an interview may occur face to face, over the telephone, or by Skype or other electronic media, and may consist of open-ended or close-ended questions.

intrinsic case study Research undertaken to gain a better understanding of the essential nature of the case.

item-to-total correlation The relationship between each item on a scale and the total scale.

J

justice The principle that human participants should be treated fairly.

K

kappa The level of agreement observed beyond the level that would be expected by chance alone.

key informants Individuals who have special knowledge, status, or communication skills and who are willing to share their expertise with the ethnographer.

knowledge-focused triggers Research ideas that are generated when staff read research, listen to scientific papers at research conferences, or encounter evidence-based practice guidelines published by federal agencies or specialty organizations.

known-groups approach See *contrasted-groups approach.*

Kuder-Richardson (KR-20) coefficient The estimate of homogeneity used for instruments in which a dichotomous response pattern is used.

kurtosis The relative peakness or flatness of a distribution.

L

level of significance (alpha level) The risk of making a type I error, set by the researcher before the study begins.

levels of measurement Categorization of the precision with which an event can be measured (nominal, ordinal, interval, and ratio).

Likert-type scale A list of statements for which responses are varying degrees of agreement or opinion; for example, "strongly agree," "agree," "no opinion," "disagree," or "strongly disagree."

limitations The weaknesses of a study.

Linear Structural Relationships (LISREL) A computer program developed to analyze covariance and the testing of complex causal models.

literature review An extensive, systematic, and critical review of the most important published scholarly literature on a particular topic. In most cases, the literature review is not considered exhaustive.

lived experience In phenomenological research, the focus on undergoing events and circumstances (prelingual), as opposed to thinking about these events and circumstances (conceptualized experience).

logistic regression (logit analysis) The analysis of relationships between multiple independent variables and a dependent variable that is binary, ordinal, or polynomial.

longitudinal study A nonexperimental research design in which a researcher collects data from the same group at different points in time. Also called *prospective study* and *repeated-measures study.*

M

manipulation The provision of some experimental treatment, in varying degrees, to some of the participants in the study.

matching A special sampling strategy used to construct an equivalent comparison sample group by filling it with participants who are similar to each subject in another sample group in terms of pre-established variables, such as age and gender.

maturation Developmental, biological, or psychological processes that operate within an individual as a function of time and are external to the events of the investigation.

mean (*M*) A measure of central tendency; the arithmetic average of all scores.

measurement The assignment of numbers to objects or events according to rules.

measurement effects Changes in the generalizability of study findings to other populations, as a result of administration of a pretest.

measures of central tendency Descriptive statistical techniques that describe the average member of a sample (e.g., mean, median, and mode).

measures of variability Descriptive statistical procedures that describe the level of dispersion in sample data.

median A measure of central tendency; in a range of scores, the middle score (50% of the scores are above it and 50% of the scores are below it).

MEDLINE The print or computerized database of standard medical literature analysis and retrieval system online; it is also available on CD-ROM.

member checking In participatory action research, sharing the findings with the participants to know whether the interpretation of their responses is accurate.

meta-analysis A research method in which the results of multiple studies in a specific area are examined and the findings are synthesized to make conclusions regarding the area of focus.

metasynthesis A technique for drawing inferences or synthesizing findings from similar or related studies; a type of systematic review applied to qualitative research.

methodological research The controlled investigation and measurement of the means of gathering and analyzing data; the development and evaluation of data collection instruments, scales, and techniques.

methodology Discipline-specific principles, rules, and procedures that guide the process through which knowledge is acquired.

midrange theory A focused conceptual structure that synthesizes the link between practice and research into ideas central to the discipline of nursing.

mixed-methods research Research in which the investigator collects and analyzes data, integrates the findings, and draws inferences using both qualitative and quantitative approaches or methods in a single study or a program of inquiry; one form of triangulation.

modal percentage A measure of variability; percentage of cases in the mode.

modality The number of modes, or peaks, in a frequency distribution.

mode A measure of central tendency; the most frequent score or result.

model A symbolic representation of a set of concepts that is created to depict relationships.

mortality The loss of a subject from time 1 data collection to time 2 data collection. Also called *attrition.*

multiple analysis of variance (MANOVA) A test used to determine differences in group means when a study has more than one dependent variable.

multiple regression The measure of the relationship between one interval-level dependent variable and several independent variables. Canonical correlation is used when a study has more than one dependent variable.

multistage sampling A sampling method that involves successive random sampling of units (clusters) that progresses from large to small and meets sample eligibility criteria. Also known as *cluster sampling.*

multitrait-multimethod approach A type of validation in which more than one method is used to assess the accuracy of an instrument (e.g., observation and interview of anxiety).

N

narrative inquiry A field of hermeneutics that focuses on the lived experience and perceptions of experience, in which materials such as in-depth interview transcripts, memoirs, stories, and creative nonfiction are used as sources of data.

naturalistic research A general label for qualitative studies that involve the researcher going to a natural setting where the phenomenon being studied is taking place.

naturalistic setting The environment in which people live in every day, such as homes, schools, and communities.

network sampling A strategy used for finding samples that are difficult to locate. It entails the use of social networks and the fact that friends tend to have characteristics in common; participants who meet the eligibility criteria are asked for assistance in getting in touch with others who meet the same criteria. Also known as *snowball effect sampling.*

nominal measurement The level used to classify objects or events into categories without any relative ranking (e.g., gender, hair colour).

nondirectional hypothesis A hypothesis that indicates the existence of a relationship between the variables but does not specify the anticipated direction of the relationship.

nonequivalent control group design A quasi-experimental design that is similar to the true experiment, but participants are not randomly assigned to the treatment or the control group.

nonexperimental research design A research design in which an investigator observes a phenomenon without manipulating the independent variable or variables.

nonparametric statistics Statistics that are usually used when variables are measured at the nominal or ordinal level because they do not estimate population parameters and involve less restrictive assumptions about the underlying distribution. Also called *distribution-free tests.*

nonparametric tests of significance Inferential statistics that make no assumptions about the population distribution.

nonprobability sampling A selection technique in which elements are chosen by nonrandom methods.

normal curve A statistical curve that is unimodal and symmetrical about the mean.

null hypothesis A statement that no relationship exists between the variables and that any relationship observed is a result of chance or fluctuations in sampling. Also known as a *statistical hypothesis* or H_0.

null value When an experimental value indicates no difference between the treatment and control groups; known as *the value of no effect.*

O

objective An adjective describing data that are not influenced by anyone who collects the information.

objectivity The use of facts without distortion by personal feelings or bias.

observed test score The actual score obtained in a measure; the true score plus error.

odds ratio The probability of an event, which is calculated by dividing the odds in the treated or exposed group by the odds in the control group.

one-group pretest–posttest design A study approach used by researchers when only one group is available for study; participants act as their own controls, and no randomization occurs, thus enhancing the internal validity of the study.

online database An Internet collection of journal sources (periodicals) of research and conceptual articles on a variety of topics (e.g., doctoral dissertations), as well as the publications of professional organizations and various governmental agencies.

ontology The science or study of being or existence and its relationship to nonexistence.

open-ended item A question that respondents may answer in their own words.

operational definition The description of how a concept is measured and what instruments are used to capture the essence of the variable.

operationalization The process of translating concepts into observable, measurable phenomena.

opinion leaders Individuals from the local peer group who are viewed as respected sources of influence, considered by associates to be technically competent, and trusted to judge the fit between the evidence-based practice and the local situation.

ordinal measurement A calculation to show rankings of events or objects; numbers are not equidistant, and zero is arbitrary (class ranking).

orientational qualitative inquiry A qualitative approach in which researchers begin with an ideology or orientation (e.g., feminism, Marxism, critical theory) to direct the investigation, including the research question, methodology, fieldwork, and analysis of the findings.

P

P value The conditional probability of obtaining, from the study data, the value of the test statistic that is at least as extreme as that calculated from the data, given that the null hypothesis is true.

paradigm From the Greek word meaning "pattern": a set of beliefs and practices, shared by communities of researchers, that guide the knowledge development process. It is a synonym of *worldview*. See also *philosophical beliefs*.

parallel-form reliability See *alternate-form reliability*.

parameter A characteristic of a population.

parametric statistics Inferential statistics that involve the estimation of at least one parameter, require measurement at the interval level or higher, and involve assumptions about the variables being studied. These assumptions usually include the fact that the variable is normally distributed.

participatory action research A form of orientation research that seeks to change society; the researcher studies a particular setting to identify problem areas to improve practice, identify possible solutions, and take action to implement changes.

path analysis A statistical technique in which the researcher hypothesizes how variables are related and in what order and then tests the strength of those relationships or paths.

Pearson correlation coefficient (Pearson *r*) A statistic that is calculated to reflect the degree of relationship between two interval level variables. Also called *Pearson product-moment correlation coefficient*.

percentile A measure of rank; the percentage of scores that a given score exceeds.

phenomena Occurrences, circumstances, or facts that are perceptible by the senses.

phenomenological method A process of learning and constructing the meaning of human experience through intensive dialogue with persons who are living the experience.

phenomenology A qualitative research approach that aims to describe experience as it is lived through, before it is conceptualized.

philosophical beliefs The system of motivating values, concepts, principles, and the nature of human knowledge of an individual, group, or culture; see also *paradigm* and *worldview*.

physiological measurement The use of specialized equipment to determine the physical status of participants in a study.

pilot study A small, simple study conducted as a prelude to a larger-scale study (which is often called the "parent study").

population A well-defined set that has certain specified properties.

post hoc analysis Comparison of all possible pairs of means after an omnibus ANOVA to determine where the difference lies.

post-positivism The view that a "reality" exists that can be observed, measured, and understood; however, this view is tempered by the belief that science offers an imperfect understanding of the world.

post-positivist paradigm The basis of most quantitative research and, to a smaller extent, qualitative research.

posttest-only control group design See *after-only design*.

power The conditional prior probability that the researcher will make a correct decision to reject the null hypothesis when it is actually false, denoted as $1 - b$.

prediction study A type of nonexperimental research design in which the investigator attempts to make a forecast or prediction on the basis of particular phenomena.

predictive validity The degree of correlation between the measure of a concept and some future measure of the same concept.

prevalence The number of people affected by a disease or health problem.

primary sources Scholarly literature that is written by a person or persons who developed the theory or conducted the research; articles and books by the original author or authors. Primary sources include eyewitness accounts of historical events provided by original documents, films, letters, diaries, records, artefacts, periodicals, and tapes.

print indexes Paper based listings of published material, generally used to find journal sources (periodicals) of data-based and conceptual articles on a variety of topics, as well as publications of professional organizations and various governmental agencies. Most information is now entered onto electronics (online) databases.

probability The long-run relative frequency of an event in repeated trials under similar conditions.

probability sampling A selection technique in which some form of random selection is used when the sample units are chosen.

problem-focused triggers Research ideas that are identified by staff through quality improvement, risk surveillance, benchmarking data, financial data, or recurrent clinical problems.

problem statement A statement in a research article in which the research question is articulated.

process consent A request for the respondent's continued participation in a study.

product testing The testing of medical devices.

proposition A linkage of concepts that lays a foundation for the development of methods that test relationships.

prospective study A nonexperimental study that begins with an exploration of assumed causes and then moves forward in time to the presumed effect. Also called *longitudinal study* and *repeated-measures study*.

psychometrics The theory and development of measurement instruments.

purpose The aims or objectives the investigator hopes to achieve with the research.

purposive sample A group consisting of particular people who can illuminate the phenomenon they want to study.

purposive sampling A sampling strategy in which the researcher's knowledge of the population and its elements is used to select the participants.

Q

qualitative research The systematic, interactive, and subjective research method used to describe and give meaning to human experiences. Qualitative research is often conducted in natural settings and uses data that are words or text, as opposed to numerical data, to describe the experiences being studied.

quantitative research The process of testing relationships, differences, and cause-and-effect interactions among and between variables. These processes are tested with hypotheses and research questions through the use of objective, precise, and highly controlled measurement techniques to gather information that can be analyzed and summarized statistically.

quasiexperiment Research in which the researcher initiates an experimental treatment, but some characteristic of a true experiment is lacking.

quasiexperimental design A research approach in which random assignment is not used, but the independent variable is manipulated and certain mechanisms of control are used.

questionnaire An instrument designed to gather data from individuals.

quota sampling A nonprobability sampling strategy that identifies a specific strata of the population and represents the strata proportionately in the sample.

R

random error See *chance error*.

random selection A selection process in which each element of the population has an equal and independent chance of being included in the sample.

randomization A sampling selection procedure in which each person or element in a population has an equal chance of being assigned to either the experimental group or the control group.

range A measure of variability; the difference between the highest and the lowest scores in a set of sample data.

ratio measurement The ranking of the order of events or objects that has equal intervals and an absolute zero (e.g., height, weight).

reactivity The distortion created when those who are being observed change their behaviour because they know that they are being observed. Also known as the *Hawthorne effect*.

recommendations An investigator's suggestions for the application of a study's results to practice, theory, and future research.

records or available data Information that is collected from existing materials, such as hospital records, historical documents, and audio or video recordings.

refereed (peer-reviewed) journal A scholarly journal that has a panel of external and internal reviewers or editors; the panel reviews manuscripts submitted for possible publication. The review panel uses the same set of scholarly criteria to judge whether the manuscripts are worthy of publication.

reflexivity The situation wherein researchers must monitor whether their own perspectives are affecting their research methods, analyses, or interpretations.

relationship/difference study A study that traces the relationships or differences between variables that can provide a deeper insight into a phenomenon.

reliability The consistency or constancy of a measuring instrument; the extent to which the instrument yields the same results on repeated measures.

reliability coefficient A number between 0 and 1 that expresses the relationship between the error variance, true variance, and the observed score. A correlation of 0 indicates no relationship; the closer to 1 the coefficient is, the more reliable is the tool. Also called the *alpha coefficient*.

representative sample A sample whose key characteristics closely approximate those of the population.

research The systematic, rigorous, logical investigation that aims to answer questions about nursing phenomena.

research-based protocols Practice standards that are formulated from the findings of several studies.

research ethics board (REB) A board established in agencies to review biomedical and behavioural research involving human participants within the agency or in programs sponsored by the agency to assess whether ethical standards are met in relation to the protection of the rights of human participants.

research hypothesis A statement about the expected relationship between variables. Also known as a *scientific hypothesis.*

research question A presentation of an idea that forms the foundation for a study; it is developed from the research problem and results in the research hypothesis.

research utilization A systematic method of implementing sound research-based innovations in clinical practice, evaluating the outcome, and sharing the knowledge through the process of research dissemination.

respect for persons The idea that people have the right to self-determination and to being treated as autonomous agents; that is, they have the freedom to participate or not participate in research.

retrospective data Data that have already been recorded, such as scores on a standard examination.

retrospective study A nonexperimental research design that begins with the phenomenon of interest (the dependent variable) in the present and examines its relationship to another variable (the independent variable) in the past. Also known as a *causal-comparative study,* a *comparative study,* and (by social scientists) an *ex post facto study.*

rigour The strictness with which a study is conducted to enhance the quality, believability, or trustworthiness of study findings.

risk-benefit ratio The extent to which the benefits of the study are maximized and the risks are minimized in such a way that the participants are protected from harm during the study.

risks The potential negative outcomes of participation in a research study.

S

sample A subset of sampling units, or elements, from a population.

sampling A process in which representative units of a population are selected for study in a research investigation.

sampling error The tendency for statistics to fluctuate from one sample to another.

sampling frame A list of all units of the population.

sampling interval The standard distance between the elements chosen for the sample.

sampling unit The element or set of elements used for selecting the sample.

saturation The repetition of information until no further useful data are forthcoming.

scale A self-report measurement tool in which items of indirect interest are combined to obtain an overall score, A set of symbols is used to respond to each item. A rating or score is assigned to each response.

scatter plot A visual representation of the strength and magnitude of the relationship between two variables.

scientific hypothesis The researcher's expectation about the outcome of a study. Also known as the *research hypothesis* or H_1.

scientific literature A synonym for data-based literature.

scientific merit The degree of validity of a study or group of studies.

scientific observation The collecting of data about the environment and participants. The observations undertaken are consistent with the specific objectives of the study; the collection of data is systematically planned and recorded; all observations are checked and controlled; and the observations are related to scientific concepts and theories.

secondary analysis A form of research in which the researcher takes previously collected and analyzed data from one study and reanalyzes the data for a secondary purpose.

secondary source Scholarly material written by a person or persons other than the individual who developed the theory or conducted the research. Secondary sources are usually published. Often a secondary source represents a response to or a summary and critique of a theorist's or researcher's work. Examples are documents, films, letters, diaries, records, artefacts, periodicals, and tapes that provide a view of the phenomenon from another's perspective.

selection The generalizability of the results to other populations.

selection bias The threat to internal validity that arises when pretreatment differences exist between the experimental group and the control group.

selection effects The threat to external validity that occurs when the ideal sample population participants are either too few or unavailable to the researcher.

semiquartile range (semi-interquartile range) A measure of variability; the range of the middle 50% of the scores.

simple random sampling A probability sampling strategy in which the population is defined, a sampling frame is listed, and a subset from which the sample will be chosen is selected; members are randomly selected.

skew The measure of the asymmetry of a set of scores.

snowball effect sampling A strategy used for finding samples that are difficult to locate. This strategy entails the use of social networks and the fact that friends tend to have characteristics in common; participants who meet the eligibility criteria are asked for assistance in getting in touch with others who meet the same criteria. Also known as *network sampling.*

social desirability The tendency of a subject to respond in a manner that he or she believes will please the researcher rather than in an honest manner.

Solomon four-group design An experimental design with four randomly assigned groups: the pretest-posttest intervention group, the pretest-posttest control group, a treatment or intervention group with only posttest measurement, and a control group with only posttest measurement.

split-half reliability An index of the comparison between the scores on one half of a test with those on the other half to determine the consistency in response to items that reflect specific content.

stability An instrument's ability to produce the same results with repeated testing.

standard deviation A measure of variability; measure of average deviation of scores from the mean. In equations, abbreviated *SD.*

standard error of the mean The standard deviation of a theoretical distribution of sample means. It indicates the average error in the estimation of the population mean.

statistic A characteristic of a sample, described in mathematical terms (e.g., percentage).

statistical hypothesis A statement that no relationship exists between the independent and dependent variables. Also known as a *null hypothesis.*

stratified random sampling A probability sampling strategy in which the population is divided into strata or subgroups; members of each strata are homogeneous with regard to certain characteristics. An appropriate number of elements from each subgroup are randomly selected based on their proportion in the population.

summative evaluation Assessment of the outcomes of a program, conducted after the program's completion.

survey study A descriptive, exploratory, or comparative study in which researchers collect detailed descriptions of existing variables and use the data to justify and assess current conditions and practices or to make more plans for improving health care practices.

symmetry When the two halves of a distribution are mirror images of one another (i.e., when folded over, they can be superimposed on each other).

systematic A term used when data collection is carried out in the same manner with all participants and by all persons collecting the data.

systematic error An error attributable to the lasting characteristics of the subject that do not tend to fluctuate from one time to another. Also called *constant error.*

systematic review A summary of research evidence from several studies.

systematic sampling A probability sampling strategy that involves the selection of participants randomly drawn from a population list at fixed intervals.

T

t **statistic** The test of whether two groups' means are more different than would be expected by chance. The groups may be related or independent.

target population A population or group of individuals who meet the sampling criteria and about whom the researcher hopes to make generalizations.

test–retest reliability The stability of the scores of an instrument when it is administered twice to the same participants under the same conditions within a prescribed time interval. The scores from the different times are paired and then compared to determine the stability of the measure.

testability The ability of the variables in a proposed study to be observed, measured, and analyzed by quantitative methods.

testable Measurable by quantitative methods.

testing effect The effect on the scores of a posttest as the result of having taken a pretest.

text Data in a contextual form; that is, narrative or words that were written from recorded interviews and then transcribed.

thematic analysis The process of recognizing and recovering the emergent themes in data.

themes Clusters of data with structured meaning that occur frequently.

theoretical framework A structure for concepts, theories or both used to construct a map for the study based on a philosophical or theorized belief or understanding or why the phenomenon under study exists.

theoretical sampling In the grounded theory method, the sampling method used to select experiences that will help the researcher test ideas and gather complete information about developing concepts.

theory A set of interrelated concepts, definitions, and propositions that present a systematic view of phenomena for the purpose of explaining and making predictions about those phenomena.

time series design A quasiexperimental design used to determine trends before and after an experimental treatment. Measurements are taken several times before the introduction of the experimental treatment, the treatment is introduced, and measurements are taken again at specified times afterward.

transferability The extent to which findings from one qualitative research study have meaning to other studies in similar situations.

translation science The investigation of methods, interventions, and variables that influence the adoption of evidence-based practices.

triangulation The expansion of research methods in a single study or multiple studies to enhance diversity, enrich understanding, and accomplish specific goals.

true experiment A study design in which participants are randomly assigned to an experimental group or a control group, pretest measurements are performed, an intervention or treatment occurs in the experimental group, and posttest measurements are performed. Also known as the *pretest-posttest control group design* or *classic experiment*.

trustworthiness An accurate portrayal of the experience of the study's participants; a measure of rigour in qualitative research that includes the concepts of credibility, audibility, and fittingness.

type I error The researchers' incorrect decision to reject the null hypothesis.

type II error As a result of the sample data, the failure to reject the null hypothesis when it is actually false. Also known as *beta* (β).

V

validation sample The sample that provides the initial data for determining the reliability and validity of a measurement tool.

validity The determination of whether a measurement instrument actually measures what it is purported to measure.

values Personal beliefs of the researcher.

variable A defined concept; a property that takes on different values and is studied by quantitative researchers.

W

Web browser A software program used to connect to or search the World Wide Web (e.g., Internet Explorer).

worldview The way people in society think about the world; a synonym for *paradigm*. See also *philosophical beliefs*.

Z

Z score A rating used to compare measurements in standard units; an examination of the relative distance of the scores from the mean.

Index

Page numbers followed by *f* indicate figures; *t,* tables;
b, boxes.

P

Q